Diagnostic Strategies for Common Medical Problems

For a catalogue of publications available from ACP–ASIM, contact:

Customer Service Center
American College of Physicians–American Society of Internal Medicine
190 N. Independence Mall West
Philadelphia, PA 19106-1572
215-351-2600
800-523-1546, ext. 2600

Visit our web site at www.acponline.org

Diagnostic Strategies for Common Medical Problems

Second Edition

Edgar R. Black, MD, FACP
Clinical Associate Professor of Medicine
University of Rochester School of Medicine and Dentistry
Associate Medical Director
Blue Cross Blue Shield of the Rochester Area
Rochester, New York

Donald R. Bordley, MD, FACP
Associate Professor of Medicine
University of Rochester School of Medicine and Dentistry
Director, Internal Medicine Residency Program
Strong Memorial Hospital
Rochester, New York

Thomas G. Tape, MD, FACP
Associate Professor
Internal Medicine
University of Nebraska College of Medicine
Omaha, Nebraska

Robert J. Panzer, MD, FACP
Associate Professor of Medicine and Medical Informatics
University of Rochester School of Medicine and Dentistry
Chief Quality Officer
Strong Health
Rochester, New York

American College of Physicians
Philadelphia, Pennsylvania

Clinical Consultant: **David R. Goldmann, MD, FACP**
Acquisitions Editor: **Mary K. Ruff**
Manager, Book Publishing: **David Myers**
Administrator, Book Publishing: **Diane McCabe**
Production Supervisor: **Allan S. Kleinberg**
Production Editor: **Victoria Hoenigke**
Cover Design: **Colleen Woods-Esposito**
Interior Design: **Patrick Ward**

Printed in the United States of America
Composition by Fulcrum Data Services, Inc.
Printing/binding by Versa Press

American College of Physicians–American Society of Internal Medicine
190 N. Independence Mall West
Philadelphia, PA 19106-1572

Library of Congress Cataloging-in-Publication Data
Diagnostic strategies for common medical problems /
    edited by Edgar R. Black ... [et al.]. – 2nd ed.
        p.   cm.
    Includes bibliographical references and index.
    ISBN 0-943126-74-6 (alk. paper)
    1. Diagnosis, Laboratory. I. Black, Edgar R.
    [DNLM: 1. Laboratory Techniques and Procedures.
    2. Diagnosis, Differential. QY 4D5355 1999]
    RB37.C57 1999
    616.07′5–dc21
    DNLM/DLC
    for Library of Congress   98-34279
                                                                      CIP

99 00 01 02 03 04/9 8 7 6 5 4 3 2 1

Editors

Edgar R. Black, MD, FACP
Clinical Associate Professor of Medicine
University of Rochester School of Medicine and Dentistry
Associate Medical Director
Blue Cross Blue Shield of the Rochester Area
Rochester, New York

Donald R. Bordley, MD, FACP
Associate Professor of Medicine
University of Rochester School of Medicine and Dentistry
Director, Internal Medicine Residency Program
Strong Memorial Hospital
Rochester, New York

Thomas G. Tape, MD, FACP
Associate Professor
Internal Medicine
University of Nebraska College of Medicine
Omaha, Nebraska

Robert J. Panzer, MD, FACP
Associate Professor of Medicine and Medical Informatics
University of Rochester School of Medicine and Dentistry
Chief Quality Officer
Strong Health
Rochester, New York

Contributors

Joseph A. Aloi, MD
Assistant Professor of Medicine
University of Virginia School of
  Medicine
Charlottesville, Virginia

Eric J. Anish, MD
Primary Care Sports Medicine
  Fellow
University of Pittsburgh Medical
  Center
Pittsburgh, Pennsylvania

Dean A. Arvan, MD
Professor of Pathology and
  Laboratory Medicine
University of Rochester School of
  Medicine and Dentistry
Strong Memorial Hospital
Rochester, New York

Erica Friedman Asch, MD
Associate Professor of Medicine
Mount Sinai School of Medicine
New York, New York

Karai P. Balaji, MD
Internist
Avon Family Medicine
Avon, New York

Michael J. Barry, MD, FACP
Associate Professor of Medicine
Harvard Medical School
Massachusetts General Hospital
Boston, Massachusetts

Nancy M. Bennett, MD, MS
Associate Professor of Medicine
  and Community and Preventive
  Medicine
University of Rochester School of
  Medicine and Dentistry
Monroe County Health Department
Rochester, New York

Lynn S. Bickley, MD
Associate Professor of Medicine
University of Rochester School of
  Medicine and Dentistry
Strong Memorial Hospital
Rochester, New York

Edgar R. Black, MD, FACP
Clinical Associate Professor of
  Medicine
University of Rochester School of
  Medicine and Dentistry
Associate Medical Director
Blue Cross Blue Shield of the
  Rochester Area
Rochester, New York

Donald R. Bordley, MD, FACP
Associate Professor of Medicine
University of Rochester School of
  Medicine and Dentistry
Director, Internal Medicine
  Residency Program
Strong Memorial Hospital
Rochester, New York

James Budd, MD
Clinical Assistant Professor of
 Medicine
University of Rochester School of
 Medicine and Dentistry
Rochester, New York

Diego G. Cahn-Hildalgo, MD
Clinical Instructor of Medicine
University of Rochester School of
 Medicine and Dentistry
Rochester, New York

Joseph D. Cappuccio, MD
Clinical Associate Professor of
 Medicine
University of Rochester School of
 Medicine and Dentistry
Rochester General Hospital
Rochester, New York

Joshua Chodosh, MD
Assistant Professor of Medicine
 and Pediatrics
University of Rochester School of
 Medicine and Dentistry
Strong Memorial Hospital
Rochester, New York

Jules Cohen, MD
Professor of Medicine
University of Rochester School of
 Medicine and Dentistry
Strong Memorial Hospital
Rochester, New York

Julia E. Connelly, MD, FACP
Professor of Medicine
University of Virginia School of
 Medicine
Charlottesville, Virginia

James P. Corsetti, MD, PhD
Associate Professor of Pathology
 and Laboratory Medicine
University of Rochester School of
 Medicine and Dentistry
Strong Memorial Hospital
Rochester, New York

Susan C. Day, MD, MPH, FACP
Adjunct Associate Professor
University of Pennsylvania
Chestnut Hill Healthcare
Philadelphia, Pennsylvania

James G. Dolan, MD, FACP
Associate Professor of Medicine
University of Rochester School of
 Medicine and Dentistry
Highland Hospital
Rochester, New York

John M. Eisenberg, MD, MACP
Administrator
Agency for Health Care Policy and
 Research
Department of Health and Human
 Services
Rockville, Maryland

Robert A. Greene, MD
Clinical Assistant Professor
University of Rochester School of
 Medicine and Dentistry
Rochester, New York

Philip Greenland, MD, FACP
Harry Dinghman Professor of
 Cardiology
Northwestern University School of
 Medicine
Chicago, Illinois

Paul F. Griner, MD, MACP
Vice President and Director,
CAMCAM
Association of American Medical
Colleges
Washington, D.C.

Eric B. Grossman, MD, FACP
Associate Professor of Medicine
University of Rochester School of
Medicine and Dentistry
Strong Memorial Hospital
Rochester, New York

Carmen E. Guerra, MD
Assistant Professor of Medicine
University of Pennsylvania School
of Medicine
University of Pennsylvania Medical
Center
Philadelphia, Pennsylvania

William J. Hall, MD, FACP
Professor of Medicine and
Pediatrics
University of Rochester School of
Medicine and Dentistry
Strong Memorial Hospital
Rochester, New York

R. Brian Haynes, MD, PhD, FACP
Professor of Clinical Epidemiology
and Medicine
McMaster University Faculty of
Health Sciences
Hamilton, Ontario, Canada

N. Paul Hudson, MD
Associate Professor of Clinical
Medicine
Ohio State University College of
Medicine
Columbus, Ohio

Seth M. Kantor, MD
Professor of Clinical Medicine
Ohio State University College of
Medicine
Columbus, Ohio

Anthony L. Komaroff, MD, FACP
Professor of Medicine
Harvard Medical School
Harvard Medical Publications
Boston, Massachusetts

Ruth W. Kouides, MD, MPH
Assistant Professor of Medicine and
Community and Preventive Medicine
University of Rochester School of
Medicine and Dentistry
Rochester, New York

David R. Lambert, MD
Assistant Professor of Medicine
University of Rochester School of
Medicine and Dentistry
Strong Memorial Hospital
Rochester, New York

Jeffrey E. Lancet, MD
Instructor and Fellow in
Hematology/Oncology
University of Rochester School of
Medicine and Dentistry
Rochester, New York

Eric B. Larson, MD, MPH, FACP
Professor of Medicine
University of Washington School of
Medicine
Seattle, Washington

Benson T. Massey, MD, FACP
Assistant Professor of Medicine
Medical College of Wisconsin
Madison, Wisconsin

Raymond J. Mayewski, MD
Dean's Professor of Medicine
University of Rochester School of
  Medicine and Dentistry
Strong Memorial Hospital
Rochester, New York

Daniel J. Mazanec, MD
Department of Rheumatic and
  Immunologic Disease
The Cleveland Clinic Foundation
Cleveland, Ohio

**Wayne C. McCormick, MD, MPH,
FACP**
Associate Professor
University of Washington School of
  Medicine
Seattle, Washington

Alvin I. Mushlin, MD, ScM, FACP
Professor of Community and
  Preventive Medicine and Medicine
University of Rochester School of
  Medicine and Dentistry
Rochester, New York

Rudolph J. Napodano, MD, FACP
Professor of Medicine, Emeritus
University of Rochester School of
  Medicine and Dentistry
Rochester, New York

**Ann Butler Nattinger, MD, MPH,
FACP**
Associate Professor of Medicine
Medical College of Wisconsin
Milwaukee, Wisconsin

Fitzhugh C. Pannill III, MD, FACP
Assistant Clinical Professor of
  Medicine
Yale University School of Medicine
Southbury Medical Associates
Southbury, Connecticut

Robert J. Panzer, MD, FACP
Associate Professor of Medicine
  and Medical Informatics
University of Rochester School of
  Medicine and Dentistry
Chief Quality Officer
Strong Health
Rochester, New York

Mary C. Paris, MPH
Researcher
University of Rochester School of
  Medicine and Dentistry
Rochester, New York

John T. Philbrick, MD, FACP
Professor of Medicine
University of Virginia School of
  Medicine
Charlottesville, Virginia

Robert H. Poe, MD, FACP
Professor of Medicine
University of Rochester School
  of Medicine and Dentistry
Highland Hospital
Rochester, New York

Aaron P. Rapoport, MD
Assistant Professor of Medicine
University of Maryland Greenbaum
  Cancer Center
Baltimore, Maryland

Richard C. Reichman, MD
Professor of Medicine,
  Microbiology, and Immunology
University of Rochester School of
  Medicine and Dentistry
Strong Memorial Hospital
Rochester, New York

Steven A. Rich, MD
Geriatrician
Lifetime Health
Rochester, New York

Eric A. Richard, MD
Assistant Professor of Medicine
St. Mary's Hospital
University of Rochester School of
  Medicine and Dentistry
Rochester, New York

A. Andrew Rudmann, MD
Senior Instructor in Medicine
University of Rochester School of
  Medicine and Dentistry
Strong Memorial Hospital
Rochester, New York

Mark A. Shelly, MD
Assistant Professor of Medicine
University of Rochester School of
  Medicine and Dentistry
Highland Hospital
Rochester, New York

Lawrence G. Smith, MD, FACP
Professor of Medicine
Mount Sinai School of Medicine
New York, New York

Anthony L. Suchman, MD, FACP
Associate Professor of Medicine and
  Psychiatry
University of Rochester School of
  Medicine and Dentistry
Strong Health
Rochester, New York

**J. Thompson Sullebarger, MD,
  FACP**
Associate Professor of Medicine
University of South Florida
Tampa, Florida

Catherine Chiu Tan, MD
Clinical Instructor of Medicine
University of Rochester School of
  Medicine and Dentistry
Rochester, New York

Thomas G. Tape, MD, FACP
Associate Professor
Internal Medicine
University of Nebraska College of
  Medicine
Omaha, Nebraska

Marguerite A. Urban, MD
Assistant Professor of Medicine
University of Rochester School of
  Medicine and Dentistry
Strong Memorial Hospital
Rochester, New York

Gary W. Wahl, MD
Associate Professor of Medicine
University of Rochester School of
  Medicine and Dentistry
Rochester General Hospital
Rochester, New York

Barbara E. Weber, MD, MPH, FACP
Assistant Professor of Medicine
University of Rochester School of
  Medicine and Dentistry
St. Mary's Hospital
Rochester, New York

Steven D. Wittlin, MD
Assistant Professor of Medicine
University of Rochester School of
  Medicine and Dentistry
Strong Memorial Hospital
Rochester, New York

Contents

Respiratory Problems

Musculoskeletal and Immunologic Problems

Endocrinologic Problems

Genitourinary Problems

Hematologic Problems

Neurologic Problems

PREFACE

This book represents a substantial revision of the first edition of *Diagnostic Strategies for Common Medical Problems*. The initial effort that ultimately led to this book was a meeting of an ad hoc committee of the American College of Physicians in 1980 to explore initiatives for stimulating cost containment in health care. The committee decided to sponsor an article on the use of diagnostic tests and procedures, with the premise being that cost containment should be a logical by-product of sound clinical reasoning. The General Medicine Unit of the Department of Medicine at the University of Rochester School of Medicine and Dentistry received a contract to develop the article. Assisted by grants to the College from the National Fund for Medical Education, the Henry J. Kaiser Family Foundation, and the Commonwealth Fund, members of the General Medicine Unit prepared a manuscript titled "Selection and Interpretation of Diagnostic Tests and Procedures: Principles and Applications," which was published as a supplement to the *Annals of Internal Medicine* (1981;94:553–600).

The next phase in the development of this book resulted from the comments of readers of the supplement, who indicated that application of the principles of test selection and interpretation was limited by a lack of readily available information about the operating characteristics of tests and procedures commonly used in clinical practice. In response, *Manual of Test Characteristics* was developed with support from a grant by the Rochester Area Hospitals Corporation. The grant also supported a survey of practicing physicians in Rochester of which clinical problems posed the greatest diagnostic dilemmas. It also made possible the piloting and evaluation of the manual's use by medical students, residents, and attending physicians practicing in several Rochester area hospitals and clinics.

The expansion of the manual into a book occurred through the efforts of many faculty and fellows of the General Medicine Unit and the Department of Medicine at the University of Rochester, as well as through the efforts of several contributors from other institutions. The encouragement and support of Year Book Medical Publishers helped lead to the publication of *Clinical Diagnosis and the Laboratory* in 1986. Prompted by the needs that led to the initial works, we collaborated with the American College of Physicians to publish the first edition of

Diagnostic Strategies for Common Medical Problems in 1991. For that edition, the number of clinical problems addressed was increased to nearly fifty and a new chapter was added on reading the literature to learn about diagnostic tests.

Our efforts have continued for many of the same reasons. Information about the diagnostic value and operating characteristics of most tests and procedures is still not complete and is not always readily available. For this edition, topics covered in the previous edition have been updated with new information from the literature. Much of the updated information related to imaging is in the area of magnetic resonance, which had not been studied widely at the time of the previous edition. The role of genetic testing is also becoming more important and has been included in several chapters. Clinical problems have been expanded to several new areas, including peptic ulcer disease, osteoporosis, and sinusitis.

In this edition, we continue to use the terminology of the previous work: *Pretest probability* and *post-test probability* are used throughout, rather than the older terms *prevalence, positive predictive value,* and *negative predictive value.* We have found our preferred terms to be easier to use, especially in considering multiple tests in sequence and in applying the concept of thresholds. Likelihood ratios, which are most helpful in dealing with tests that have multiple levels of abnormality, are listed, along with the sensitivities and specificities of tests and procedures. This should allow the use of odds and likelihood ratios as an alternative approach to test selection and interpretation.

We cannot emphasize enough the importance of a well-performed history and physical examination in guiding the intelligent use of diagnostic tests. The section "Estimating Pretest Probability" in each chapter is intended to provide the reader with information on the diagnostic value of symptoms and signs, which can often modify disease probability as much as or more than do formal tests.

Readers should not place undue reliance on the precise numbers that can be derived using the quantitative methods presented here. Much of the information presented is based on primary data that are less certain than the tables in this book appear to indicate. However, as discussed in Chapter 2, modest errors in estimates of pretest probability or in test operating characteristics do not substantially impair the ability of the quantitative approach to assist clinical decision making.

With the increasing emphasis on evidence-based medicine, the literature on diagnostic tests has greatly improved in recent years. However, at times it continues to be incomplete and biased. Technologies and knowledge about diagnostic tests evolve, and optimal strategies may change over time. We strongly encourage readers to routinely use the approaches to reading the literature presented in Chapter 4, so that they can better update their own knowledge and that presented in this book with the latest valid information on the value of diagnostic tests and procedures.

Readers should recognize that the quantitative and probabilistic methods used in this book have value in guiding the selection and use of diagnostic tests but are not the only means of accomplishing the goal of rational test use. These methods have limitations and do not address all the important issues that affect ultimate clinical decisions. The bottom line is that clinicians can provide the highest quality care by maximizing their use of various decision-making tools and by integrating information derived from quantitative approaches with their own clinical judgement.

In closing, we particularly want to express our thanks to Paul Griner for his foresight in beginning the efforts that led to this book and for his help as a teacher, mentor, and colleague. We also want to thank our residents, students, and colleagues who have provided us with both positive comments and useful suggestions. We also appreciate the efforts of those who reviewed chapters for this edition or for previous versions. We especially appreciate the assistance and patience of Diane McCabe and Mary Ruff at the American College of Physicians–American Society of Internal Medicine. Brian Haynes of McMaster University deserves thanks for again writing the foreword, continuing the tradition started with McMaster's David Sackett, who wrote the foreword for *Clinical Diagnosis and the Laboratory*. Although word processing software has allowed us to work directly with most of the content of this book, we have been greatly assisted directly and indirectly during its development by our administrative assistants. In particular, we thank Joan Hutton-Steward and Nanette Tiano from the General Medicine Unit in the Department of Medicine at the University of Rochester's Strong Memorial Hospital for their assistance. Finally, we must acknowledge that the time devoted to editing *Diagnostic Strategies for Common Medical Problems* would not have been possible without the understanding and support of our families and colleagues.

Edgar R. Black, MD, FACP
Donald R. Bordley, MD, FACP
Thomas G. Tape, MD, FACP
Robert J. Panzer, MD, FACP

FOREWORD

Evidence-based medicine is defined as the explicit, judicious, and consci-entious use of current best evidence from clinical care research in the man-agement of individual patients (1). *Diagnostic Strategies for Common Medical Problems* provides an important source of useful evidence for making an accurate diagnosis for a wide range of clinical problems in internal medi-cine. It is an invaluable "enabling resource" for practitioners who wish to provide their patients with evidence-based health care.

Sustained investment in medical research since the end of World War II has resulted in astonishing advances in the prospects for maintaining and improving the health of our patients. Sadly, these prospects have been undermined by problems in transferring the new knowledge into practice. At present, it is fair to say that most clinicians do not make use of most of the evidence that has been generated about the diagnostic value of clinical observations, tests, and procedures. Patients frequently receive an inaccurate diagnosis and all too often are subjected to tests that are unnecessary, expensive, or dangerous. The blame for this tragedy and waste lies partly with clinicians but also with inadequacies in the translation of the products of biomedical research into useful resources for clinical practice. This process is a difficult one, requiring both the understanding of clinically important evidence and the collab-oration of the clinicians who are responsible for its application.

During the past decade, important advances have been made in tech-niques for distilling evidence from research and in understanding and applying it to individual patients. We are moving, somewhat haltingly, from intuitive or informal clinical judgments based on the experience of individual practitioners to a more formal, defensible process in which evidence from studies of groups of similar patients augments the judg-ment of practitioners. The publication of *Clinical Diagnosis and the Laboratory*, the predecessor to *Diagnostic Strategies for Common Medical Problems*, was a milestone in clinical decision making. *Clinical Diagnosis and the Laboratory* gave practitioners an approach to the quantitative interpretation of clinical and diagnostic test information for common problems in internal medicine. It also provided a compendium of the information content of a substantial, although still limited, range of tests, so that clinicians who used the book could make wiser use of the avail-able tests and produce more precise quantitative estimates of the likeli-hood of suspected diseases. Before its publication, those of us who were teaching students common sense and scientific guidelines for the critical appraisal of published evidence were often confronted by questions about the practicality of using this approach, given the amount of skill and hard work required to track down and analyze the necessary research reports. These questions were right on the mark at the time: Even those of us who were intent on making decisions based on evidence were hard pressed to come up with the right information at the right time. We welcomed *Clinical Diagnosis and the Laboratory* with great joy and relief: It was the first book that "did it right." The formula included not only quantitative information on laboratory tests but also on clinical findings that provide a basis for estimating pretest probabilities.

The second edition of *Diagnostic Strategies for Common Medical Problems* raises quantitative decision making to new heights. This book is the product of many "people-years" of work and incorporates new evidence from increasingly rigorous clinical research. Readers will acquire greater understanding of the appraisal and interpretation of diagnostic information. They will have access to more and better information on pretest odds and likelihood ratios for continuous and multilevel test results for more and newer diagnostic tests for a broader range of clinical problems than they will find in any other source for internal medicine and adult primary care. Most important, those who use the text in practice will take better care of their patients by making more accurate diagnoses and by sparing them unnecessary tests.

Readers are advised to keep *Diagnostic Strategies for Common Medical Problems* close at hand, to buy extra copies to replace those that will become "missing in action" as co-workers discover them, and to acquire electronic access as soon as it becomes available!

R. Brian Haynes, MD, PhD, FACP
Professor and Chair
Department of Clinical Epidemiology
and Biostatistics
Professor of Medicine
McMaster University
Hamilton, Ontario, Canada

REFERENCE

1. **Sackett DL, Rosenberg WMC, Gray JAM, Haynes RB.** Evidence-based medicine: what it is and what it isn't. BMJ. 1996;312:71–2.

General Issues

Characteristics of Diagnostic Tests and Principles for Their Use in Quantitative Decision Making

1

Edgar R. Black, MD, Robert J. Panzer, MD,
Raymond J. Mayewski, MD, and Paul F. Griner, MD

KEY POINTS

- Each laboratory test has a set of characteristics that reflect the results that are expected in patients with disease as well as those without disease. *Sensitivity* measures the proportion of positive (abnormal) results in patients with disease, and *specificity* measures the percent of negative (normal) results in patients without disease.

- When tests are used for screening, or ruling out, disease, the test with the highest sensitivity is generally preferred.

- When tests are used for confirming, or ruling in, disease, the test with the highest specificity is usually preferred.

- Few tests are perfect. Usually there is an overlap of test results among patients with and without a specific disease. As the cutoff point used to define an abnormal result is made less extreme, test sensitivity improves and specificity deteriorates. Similarly, if the cutoff point is made more extreme, test sensitivity worsens but specificity improves.

- Serial (multiple) tests with results that are all normal tend to rule out disease convincingly, and serial tests with results that are all abnormal tend to confirm disease convincingly.

- Unexpectedly abnormal laboratory results that demand prompt evaluation or prompt treatment should be repeated for confirmation. Spurious factors and human or equipment error probably account for a higher proportion of unexpected significantly abnormal results than do unsuspected disorders.

BACKGROUND

Tests or procedures are performed when the information available from historical review, physical examination, and any previous testing is considered insufficient to address the questions at hand. The decision to obtain a given test or procedure is, therefore, made on the assumption that the results will significantly change the pretest probability that the disease is present or appreciably reduce the uncertainty pertaining to a given question.

The intelligent use of the new information obtained from testing requires that the clinician be aware of the probability of disease that exists before the testing is done (the pretest probability) and of the ability of the proposed test or procedure to modify these probabilities. Furthermore, the clinician must decide what level of certainty is needed before treatment decisions can be made.

USES OF DIAGNOSTIC TESTS

Diagnosis of Disease

The process of diagnosis requires several steps. The initial step is developing diagnostic hypotheses and their associated probabilities. This is followed by attempts to reduce the number of possible diagnoses by progressively ruling out diseases based on the information obtained from the history, physical examination, and laboratory tests. Highly *sensitive* tests are most effective in reducing the probability of disease and ruling out suspected diagnoses. When the results of such tests are normal, the physician can usually confidently exclude the presence of disease. As the list of diagnostic hypotheses becomes shorter, the task shifts to the pursuit of strong clinical suspicions. Highly *specific* tests are most effective in raising the probability of disease and thus ruling in diagnoses. When the results of such tests are abnormal, the physician can confidently confirm the presence of disease.

The intelligent selection of an appropriate laboratory test thus depends on choosing the proper test for the purpose intended. The purpose of the test is determined by the physician's estimate of the likelihood of disease based on an assessment of the available clinical information. The use of a test to exclude or to confirm a diagnosis should indicate that the physician's best estimate regarding the diagnosis, after a careful evaluation of the patient's problem, is either relatively unlikely or probable.

When these principles are followed, the conclusions reached from laboratory test results are likely to be correct and lead to appropriate action. This book focuses primarily on the content and application of these principles in the process of diagnosis.

Screening

The use of laboratory tests to screen asymptomatic patients is a special kind of diagnostic procedure and has several purposes. The primary purpose is to detect those diseases whose morbidity and mortality can be reduced by early detection and treatment. Another benefit of such detection efforts is the reassurance they give to those patients who are found to be free of disease. Yet the extension of these purposes has led to the development of widely applied multiphasic screening procedures. The result has been an increasing tendency to screen for many possible conditions in all patients, leading to unfounded expectations in medicine and an excess demand on both human and technologic resources.

The basic tenets of decision analysis indicate that a particular intervention is undertaken when the relative benefits of that maneuver outweigh its costs, either in terms of dollars, patient risk, or patient discomfort. As with other decisions in clinical practice, the application of these tenets for screening poses no theoretical or conceptual problems. What is often lacking is the empiric evidence on which to make these decisions. Lack of such evidence has made it particularly difficult to outline a rational approach to the evaluation of asymptomatic patients.

Recently numerous attempts have been made to define more clearly the guidelines for the selection of appropriate patients and tests for early disease detection. Ideally, the disease in question should be common enough to justify the attempt to detect it. Secondly, it should be accompanied by significant morbidity or mortality if not treated. Thirdly, effective therapy must exist that will alter its natural history. Finally, detection and treatment in the presymptomatic state should result in benefits beyond those obtained through treatment during the early symptomatic state. Once these criteria are met, then the issue is examined from the standpoint of the availability of tests. An ideal screening test is one whose characteristics are such that its results are abnormal in almost all persons with the disease—that is, it has high sensitivity—and thus provides the physician with confidence that the patient is free of disease when the results are normal. Specificity is also important when one is screening for disease because of the number of false-positive results obtained when a test that is not highly specific is applied to a population composed largely of persons without disease.

In the United States, efforts by task forces have defined sets of health maintenance packages that articulate a series of preventive regimens for patients of different age groups (1). A task force of the Canadian health system has provided similar guidelines and disease prevention packages (2).

Patient Management

Tests or procedures used in patient management are commonly repeated for one or more of the following purposes: 1) to monitor the status of a disease process; 2) to identify and reverse complications of treatment; 3) to ensure therapeutic levels of one or more drugs; 4) to aid in prognosis; and 5) to further evaluate an unexpected test or procedure result. The optimal frequency for monitoring patients with repeat tests or procedures cannot be predicted solely on the basis of knowledge of the disease but requires the application of principles of normal physiology, knowledge of the tests or procedures used to monitor the disease, and awareness of factors other than disease that may influence the test result. Thus, for a hospitalized patient with normal renal function who is receiving intravenous fluids, the practice of ordering daily serum electrolyte measurements for the purpose of aborting electrolyte abnormalities is not consistent with the available knowledge of the role of the kidney in maintaining salt and water homeostasis. Likewise, the practice of repeating chest radiography every 2 to 3 days in a patient with uncomplicated pneumococcal pneumonia whose clinical status is satisfactory overstates the expected rate of radiographic improvement.

OPERATING CHARACTERISTICS OF TESTS AND PROCEDURES

Sensitivity and Specificity

Each laboratory test or diagnostic procedure possesses a set of characteristics that reflect the results expected in patients with the disease in question as well as in those without the disease. These test characteristics answer two fundamental questions: 1) What proportion of those patients *who have the disease* will have an abnormal (i.e., positive) test result? and 2) What proportion of those patients *who do not have the disease* will have a normal (i.e., negative) result? The answer to the first question defines the sensitivity of the test, and the answer to the latter question defines its specificity. These characteristics can be easily displayed by a simple binary table often referred to as a "2 by 2" table, as illustrated in Table 1-1.

The sensitivity of the test is determined by identifying the proportion of patients with disease in whom the test result is positive (i.e., a/a+c). Similarly, the specificity of the test is determined by identifying the proportion of patients without disease in whom the test result is negative (i.e., d/b+d). Each individual cell of Table 1-1 reflects a unique combination of the true situation and the test results as follows: a = true-positive (TP), b = false-positive (FP), c = false-negative (FN), and d = true-negative (TN) results.

Table 1-1. Test Data Display Using a 2 by 2 Table

Test Result	Disease Present	Disease Absent	Total
Positive	a	b	a + b
Negative	c	d	c + d
Total	a + c	b + d	a + b + c + d = N

Table 1-2. Operating Characteristics of the Exercise Tolerance Test in Patients With and Without Coronary Artery Disease

Test Result	CAD Present	CAD Absent	Total
Positive	True-positive n = 815	False-positive n = 115	930
Negative	False-negative n = 208	True-negative n = 327	535
Total	1023	442	1465

Adapted from Weiner DA, Ryan TJ, McCabe CH, et al. Exercise stress testing: correlations among history of angina, ST-segment response and prevalence of coronary artery disease in the coronary artery surgery study (CASS). N Engl J Med. 1979;301:230-5.

The following example illustrates the use of such a table in determining the operating characteristics for any test or procedure. A study of exercise tolerance tests (ETTs) compared study participants with coronary artery disease with those without coronary artery disease (3). The criterion used for the diagnosis of disease was the presence of at least 70% luminal narrowing of one or more major coronary vessels. A positive ETT result was defined as more than 1 mm of horizontal or downward ST-segment depression or elevation for at least 0.08 seconds as compared with the resting baseline recording. Of 1465 men studied, 1023 were found through other testing to have evidence of coronary artery disease. In 815 of these participants, the result of the ETT was positive. Of the 442 men who did not have evidence of coronary artery disease, 115 had a positive test result. Using these data, the 2 by 2 table can be constructed as shown in Table 1-2.

Thus, the sensitivity of the ETT for the presence of coronary artery disease is 815/1023, or 80%, and the specificity is 327/442, or 74%. In this study, for men with proven coronary artery disease, the ETT (using the criteria indicated for a positive test result) reflected the underlying disease 80% of the time. Similarly, in those men without evidence of coronary artery disease, the ETT result was normal in 74%. The test failed to identify the presence of disease in 20% of participants who had disease (208/1023) and yielded a positive result in 26% of participants who did not have disease (115/442). These findings reflect the false-negative and false-positive rates, respectively. The fundamental test characteristics can thus be summarized as follows:

$$\text{Sensitivity} = \frac{\text{True-positive test results}}{\text{Total \# pts. with disease}} = \frac{\text{TP}}{\text{TP+FN}} = \frac{815}{1023} = 80\%$$

$$\text{Specificity} = \frac{\text{True-negative test results}}{\text{Total \# pts. without disease}} = \frac{\text{TN}}{\text{FP+FN}} = \frac{327}{442} = 74\%$$

$$\text{False-negative rate} = \frac{\text{False-negative test results}}{\text{Total \# pts. with disease}} = \frac{\text{FN}}{\text{TP+FN}} = \frac{208}{1023} = 20\%$$

$$\text{False-positive rate} = \frac{\text{False-positive test results}}{\text{Total \# pts. without disease}} = \frac{\text{FP}}{\text{FP+TN}} = \frac{115}{442} = 26\%$$

Once determined among a broad spectrum of patients with and without the disease in question, these four test characteristics tend to be constant and thus are applicable to the study of any given patient. This assumption, however, is only partially true. It requires that the test or procedure not deviate from the method used when the test characteristics were determined, that the population studied remains similar to the types of patients seen in clinical practice (4), and that the same criteria be used to define a positive result. In this study, for example, the sensitivity and specificity of the exercise tolerance test would have been quite different if the criterion for a positive test result had been limited to those participants in whom at least 2 mm of ST-segment changes were observed.

Because the results of many laboratory tests are continuous rather than dichotomous variables, one can often gain important additional diagnostic information by knowing the degree of abnormality (5,6). This is accomplished by calculating a set of likelihood ratios for various ranges of test results and is described in Chapter 3.

Cutoff Points

The ideal test is one for which there is no overlap in the range of results among patients with and without the disease in question. Figure 1-1, *A*, shows a hypothetical distribution of results of such a test. All study participants without the disease have test values lower than those observed among patients with the disease. Line "A" defines the cutoff point, above which the result is 100% sensitive and below which it is 100% specific. There are no false-negative or false-positive test results.

However, with most tests, some overlap of findings is observed among those with and without the disease, as indicated in Figure 1-1, *B*. When a test is developed for clinical use and can be measured ana-

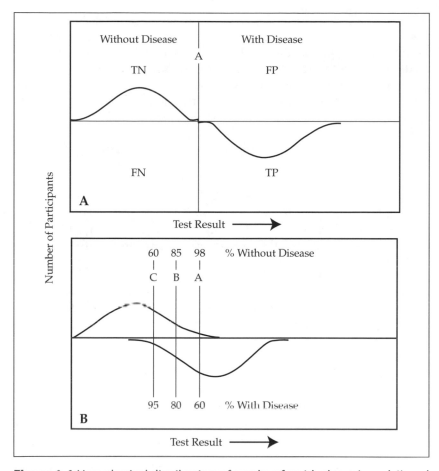

Figure 1-1 Hypothetical distribution of results of an ideal test (panel *A*) and most tests (panel *B*) used in clinical medicine. TN = true-negative; FP = false-positive; FN = false-negative; TP = true-positive.

lytically, it is customary to define the normal range as being limited to two standard deviations from the mean. This range encompasses approximately 95% of the test results among study participants without disease, as described later in this chapter in the section "Normal Ranges for Tests." Approximately 2.5% of participants fall either above or below this arbitrarily defined range. Line "A" indicates this cutoff point in Figure 1-1, *B*. All values that fall to the right of "A" are considered positive; those to the left are negative. The choice of cutoff point "A" for this hypothetical test results in high specificity (98%) but limited sensitivity (60%). Such a cutoff point may be appropriate to confirm a suspected diagnosis but cannot be used to screen for or to exclude disease because of its low sensitivity. To use such a test for these last two purposes, the choice of cutoff point "C" is appropriate because this identifies almost all patients with disease (i.e., the sensitivity is 95%, although the specificity decreases to 60%). Point "B" is intermediate between the two (sensitivity, 80%; specificity, 85%). Each cutoff point thus defines a set of operating characteristics for the test in question. As sensitivity is increased, specificity decreases and vice versa.

To illustrate these principles, consider the following example, which examines the use of the total thyroxine level (T4) in the diagnosis of hypothyroidism (7). In general, the T4 test is not considered adequate for the evaluation of hypothyroidism because in a significant number of patients with hypothyroidism, as determined from elevated TSH levels, the T4 values are in the normal range. Goldstein and Mushlin (7) studied the use of different cutoff points for the T4 value in the diagnosis of hypothyroidism. They showed that when the cutoff point is determined using the conventional (statistically defined) normal range of 4.5 to 11.5 µg/dL, the T4 is a poor test for excluding the diagnosis of hypothyroidism because of its low sensitivity (approximately 65%). However, this range is quite adequate to confirm the presence of suspected disease because of its high specificity (near 100%). They demonstrated that the test's sensitivity could be improved to more than 90% by relaxing the requirement for a positive test (i.e., by defining an abnormal result as a T4 value <7.0 µg/dL). With this change, the specificity decreased, resulting in a greater number of patients with false-positive results (7). However, if the purpose of the test is to rule out disease, then this second cutoff point may be preferable despite the reduction in specificity. This illustrates how a given test may be found useful both for excluding and for confirming a suspected diagnosis by changing the criteria for a positive test result.

The overlap in test results that often occurs between those with and without a disease also illustrates how likelihood ratios can assist in the use of diagnostic information. If instead of using one cutoff point to determine sensitivity and specificity, one determines likelihood ratios for various ranges of test results (see Chapter 3), the diagnostic impact for results markedly above the cutoff point is often increased (5,6). This occurs because results at extreme levels are often associated with a higher relative likelihood of disease than are results closer to the cutoff point.

Receiver Operating Characteristics

A graph can be constructed that correlates true-positive and false-positive rates (sensitivity and [1 – specificity], respectively) for a series of cutoff points for any test. Such a graph is known as the *receiver operating characteristic* (ROC) of a test. The ROC curve can be used to decide the optimal cutoff point based on the purpose of the test. In addition, when two or more tests are available to pursue a diagnosis, a comparison of the ROC curve of each often shows whether one has an advantage over the other.

Consider the example by Swets and colleagues (8) comparing the relative merits of computed tomography (CT) and radionuclide (RN) scanning for the detection of brain tumor, as shown in Figure 1-2. The upper line in Figure 1-2 represents the ROC curve for CT scanning, and the lower line represents the ROC curve for RN scanning. As the criteria for a positive scan are made more stringent, the curves move to the left and down (greater specificity, lower sensitivity). If the purpose of the test is to confirm a strong clinical suspicion, these stringent criteria are appropriate. Conversely, as the criteria for a positive scan are made more liberal, the curves move to the right and up (greater sensitivity, lower specificity). If the purpose of the test is to exclude tumor, the more liberal criteria are appropriate.

A comparison of the two curves also shows that regardless of the purpose of the test, CT is superior to RN scanning. At a sensitivity of 90%, for example, the false-negative rates for CT and RN are 5% and 50%, respectively. Likewise, at a false-positive rate of 10% (specificity, 90%), the comparative sensitivities are 91% and 75%, respectively.

Such comparisons may assist the physician in deciding on the optimal test for a particular purpose (see Chapter 50). It should be obvious,

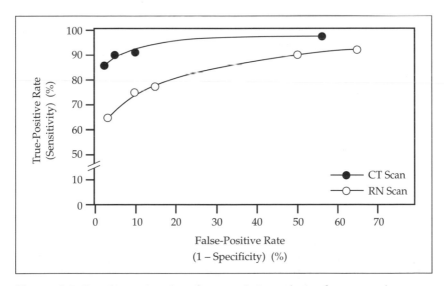

Figure 1-2. Receiver operating characteristic analysis of computed tomography (CT) and radionuclide (RN) scanning for detection of brain tumor. (Data from Swets JA, Pickett RM, Whitehead SF, et al. Assessment of diagnostic technologies. Science. 1979;205:753-9; with permission.)

however, that other factors, including patient risk and cost, may influence the decision for one test over another.

Test Selection According to Operating Characteristics

Knowledge of test characteristics is important in deciding which test to select for a given purpose. If two or more tests are available for the diagnosis of a given disease, the one with the highest sensitivity should generally be selected if it is most important to rule out disease. (If competing tests have similar sensitivities, the test with the higher specificity is preferred to reduce the number of false-positive results.) Conversely, the test with the highest specificity should be selected for use if it is most important to confirm the presence of disease.

Examining the likelihood ratios of tests (Chapter 3) can also be helpful in deciding which of competing tests to use. In general, when one wants to rule out disease, the test with the smallest negative likelihood ratio is preferred, and when ruling in disease, the test with the largest positive likelihood ratio is preferred.

For example, Chapter 40 compares the sensitivity of several measurements (e.g., afternoon plasma cortisol and morning cortisol after a single bedtime dose of dexamethasone) among patients in whom hypercortisolism is suspected. The sensitivities of the tests are calculated to be 83% and 98%, respectively. Thus, determining the morning cortisol level after giving dexamethasone is the preferred test for ruling out Cushing syndrome.

It is important to understand that knowledge of the operating characteristics of a test or procedure cannot, per se, determine the presence or absence of disease unless the test result is always positive when the disease is present (i.e., sensitivity = 100%) or is always negative when the disease is absent (specificity = 100%). Few, if any, such tests have these utopian characteristics. In order to answer the question, "What is the likelihood of the disease when the test is positive or when the test is negative?", knowledge of test characteristics must be coupled with the clinician's estimate of the probability of the disease before the test result was obtained. This integrative process is reviewed in Chapter 2.

Operating Characteristics of Combination Testing

Because relatively few tests are both highly sensitive and highly specific, two or more tests are often used to evaluate a diagnostic possibility. It is thus important to understand the combined operating characteristics of multiple tests (9).

Consider an elderly patient with persistent abdominal or back pain or both and weight loss. When there is no ready explanation for these symptoms, the possibility of carcinoma of the pancreas is frequently considered. Both ultrasonography and CT of the pancreas could be ordered to further pursue this possibility. Table 1-3 presents data from Chapter 19 concerning the operating characteristics of ultrasonography and CT when used individually for this purpose.

If the results of the two tests are independent, the information in Table 1-3 shows the impact on sensitivity and specificity when the criteria for a positive test result are 1) an abnormal finding on either the CT scan or the ultrasonogram compared with 2) an abnormal finding on both. When one or the other test result is positive, the combined sensitivity is higher than the most sensitive of the two, but the specificity is lower. Thus, serial testing that yields only normal results tends to convincingly rule out disease. Conversely, when the criteria for a positive test result are that the results of both ultrasonography and CT scan be positive, the combined specificity is higher than the most specific of the two, but the sensitivity is lower. Thus, serial testing that yields only abnormal results tends convincingly to rule in disease.

THRESHOLDS

In determining diagnostic strategies, clinicians often establish "thresholds" to assist in diagnosis and treatment. When the probability of disease rises above a certain "threshold" level, the diagnosis is confirmed (ruled in) and treatment is given. Similarly, when the probability drops below a specific level, the diagnosis is excluded and the disease is ruled out. Clinicians use the information obtained from the history and physical examination to estimate initial (or pretest) probabilities and then use the results from tests and procedures to modify this probability until the posttest probability is such that the suspected diagnosis is either confirmed or ruled out. This diagnostic process is discussed in detail in Chapter 2.

Table 1-3. Operating Characteristics of Ultrasonography and Computed Tomography of the Pancreas When Done Individually or in Combination for the Diagnosis of Carcinoma of the Pancreas

Test	Sensitivity	Specificity
	←————————— % —————————→	
Ultrasonography	70	85
Computed tomography (CT)	85	90
Ultrasound *or* CT positive*	95	77
Ultrasound *and* CT positive†	60	98

*Combined sensitivity = 100% − (30% × 15% = 5%) = 95%; combined specificity = 85% × 90% = 77%.
†Combined sensitivity = 70% × 85% = 60%; combined specificity = 100% − (15% × 10% = 2%) = 98%.

The approach to diagnosis and treatment uses two thresholds as described by Pauker and Kassirer (10). The first is the "test–no treatment" threshold that is the probability of disease at which there is no difference between the value of withholding treatment and of performing a test. The second is the "test–treatment" threshold that is the probability of disease at which there is no difference between the value of performing a test and of administering treatment. Using this approach, the decision to treat, not treat, or perform tests is based on the estimated pretest probability of disease and the two thresholds. If the estimated disease probability is below the "test–no treatment" threshold, then no further testing is done and no treatment is given. If the probability is above the "test–treatment" threshold, therapy is administered. If the probability is above the "test–no treatment" threshold but below the "test–treatment" threshold, then tests or procedures are used until the post-test probability falls below the "test–no treatment" threshold or rises above the "test–treatment" level (10).

These threshold probabilities vary for different diseases and depend on the characteristics (sensitivity and specificity) of the diagnostic tests being used, the risks of the tests and procedures, and the benefits and risks of treatment. The techniques of decision analysis permit calculation of thresholds (10). When the potential harm caused by missing a diagnosis is great, one asks for a low (e.g., <5%) "test–no treatment" threshold before no further tests are done and the diagnosis is excluded. This may be true in the case of possible myocardial infarction. Similarly, when the harm caused by overdiagnosis is great—for example, with a possible malignancy—then one asks for a high "test–treatment" threshold before accepting the diagnosis and initiating therapy (11).

NORMAL RANGES FOR TESTS

The limits of normal for most analytic tests are determined by measurements performed on a large number of study participants and arbitrarily defined as the range encompassed by two standard deviations from the mean value. Several limitations are inherent in this conventional definition. First, the definition excludes approximately 2.5% of participants whose values lie at the extremes of the distribution curve, rendering them abnormal but presumably not indicative of disease. Second, for most measurable biologic substances, the distribution curve of test results is skewed rather than symmetric and the method used to express the normal range does not precisely define the central 95% of participants (12). This problem is usually "corrected" artificially by plotting the distribution of the logarithm of the test values rather than the values per se. Third, the reference population used to calculate the limits is not necessarily free of disease. It is assumed that with a large enough sample, the impact on patients with disease on determining the normal range will be small. This assumption has been shown to be invalid for many chemistry determinations. As a result, often the normal limits that are reported are too broad (12). Fourth, few laboratories adjust the normal range for the many factors other than disease that may influence the test result. These include the age, sex, weight, diet, time of day, activity, and position of the participant when the specimen is drawn. Finally, and most importantly, the uniform method used to define the normal range does not recognize the multiple purposes that the test may serve. As was noted earlier, this range varies depending on whether the clinician is concerned with confirming a diagnosis, excluding one, or, as Sackett (13) has indicated, identifying a level beyond which treatment should be instituted.

The laboratory values observed in healthy participants tend to be consistent over time. Thus, an abnormal test result, otherwise unexplained, that does not worsen over time can be reassuring. A common example is a patient who has a mild anemia with a normal physical examination, normal erythrocyte indices, normal iron studies, no evidence for occult blood loss, and no change in hematocrit when retested several months later. Such a patient is probably healthy with a hematocrit at the low end of the distribution curve.

FACTORS OTHER THAN DISEASE THAT MAY INFLUENCE TEST RESULTS

Age and Sex
Age and sex have a significant influence on the results of many common tests. An unexpected finding of a blood urea nitrogen (BUN) level of 30 mg/dL that persists on repeat testing usually necessitates further evaluation when observed in a 23-year-old patient. However, the same value in a 75-year-old man without genitourinary symptoms or signs may not call for further action by the clinician, because half of such patients have a BUN above the laboratory's stated range of normal owing to age alone (14). A uric acid level of 7.8 mg/dL in a 40-year-old man with intermittent knee pain and swelling may well indicate gout. A similar value in an apparently healthy pubertal woman is, however, quite normal and does not usually require further study (15).

Body Position
A significant increase in plasma volume is noted in healthy study participants when they move from the standing to the supine position (16). Intermediate increases occur when they move from the sitting to the supine position. Patients whose total body water is increased (i.e., those with congestive heart failure and cirrhosis with ascites) and

patients who have hypertension may show more pronounced changes (17). The net effect of this physiologic phenomenon is to reduce the measured level of nondiffusable substances in the blood when samples are obtained in the supine position compared with the standing or sitting position. It is likely that this phenomenon contributes to the otherwise unexplained variations in day-to-day test results. Thus, a hemoglobin value of 14 g/dL obtained from an edematous, ambulatory patient may be as low as 12.5 g/dL the following morning after the patient had been in bed overnight.

Chance Phenomenon

Because the normal range is limited to 95% of participants, for each test performed, one patient in 20 is expected to have a result above or below the range of normal in the absence of disease. The likelihood of such an event increases in proportion to the number of independent tests performed. Thus, at least one abnormal test result can be expected in 46% of otherwise healthy patients in whom an SMA-12 is performed. With an SMA-20, this probability is 64%. The confusion caused by abnormal results from multichannel autoanalyzers solely owing to this phenomenon is considerable, particularly for those data that were not solicited. When an SMA-6 is performed in an apparently healthy patient primarily for determining the blood glucose and urea nitrogen levels, the likelihood that an accompanying serum potassium level of 3.4 mEq/dL indicates potassium deficiency may be as low as 4%. (This assumes that the prevalence of potassium deficiency in asymptomatic patients not receiving medications is no greater than 1/1000, that the sensitivity and specificity of measuring serum potassium levels are each 97.5%, and that the normal range for potassium is 3.5–5.5 mEq/dL.)

Miscellaneous Factors

The time of day that the blood specimen is drawn, prolonged application of a tourniquet before obtaining the blood specimen, strenuous physical activity, and delay in processing specimens are additional factors that influence test results in some patients (18).

Spurious Abnormality

Whenever a test result is markedly but unexpectedly abnormal and is confirmed on repeat testing, the possibility that it is a spurious abnormality should be considered. In some instances, the abnormal result is caused by the presence of a drug in the serum or urine or by the presence of a coexisting disease. In either case, the test result does not accurately reflect the in vivo concentration of the substance being measured. Several of the more commonly observed spurious abnormalities include hyperkalemia caused by in vitro release of potassium from leukocytes or platelets when counts are very high, as in chronic myelogenous leukemia (19); low serum glucose caused by in vitro glycolysis in patients with very high leukocyte counts (20); hyponatremia from dilutional effects in patients with hyperlipidemia if serum sodium is not determined by an autoanalyzer (21); and falsely positive urine sulfosalicylic acid tests caused by precipitation by reactions with penicillin, semisynthetic penicillin, and intravenous contrast material (22). Failure to consider a spurious cause when confronted with an unexpectedly abnormal test result may lead to inappropriate additional studies or potentially dangerous treatment.

Laboratory Error

Many apparent examples of "laboratory error" are caused by one or more of the factors just mentioned but not recognized by the clinician. True laboratory error may reflect either technical (equipment) or human failure. The latter is more common and is usually caused by one or more of the following problems: The specimen is obtained from the wrong patient; the specimen is mislabeled; or the test result is incorrectly reported.

Clearly, one cannot be aware of all the factors that may influence the results of the many tests that are commonly ordered in the day-to-day practice of medicine. Resources that may be helpful are *Clinical Guide to Laboratory Tests*, edited by Tietz (23); *Effects of Diseases on Clinical Laboratory Tests* by Friedman and colleagues (24); and *Effects of Drugs on Clinical Laboratory Tests* by Young and colleagues (25).

UNEXPECTEDLY ABNORMAL TESTS

Most unexpectedly abnormal test results lie only slightly or moderately outside the normal range. The likelihood that such test results indicate the presence of unsuspected disease is much lower among ambulatory patients than among hospitalized patients, because the prevalence of disease is less in the former group. The most common explanations for these abnormalities are one or more of the nondisease factors just reviewed or an unrecognized association between the abnormal test result and an underlying disorder known to the clinician (26). These observations suggest that the clinician should feel comfortable in repeating the test(s). In at least one third of patients, the result of the follow-up test is normal (26). Unexpected abnormal laboratory results that demand prompt evaluation or treatment or both should be repeated for confirmation while one is preparing to administer the appropriate treatment in the event that the result is true. Spurious factors or human or equipment error probably accounts for a higher proportion of otherwise significant abnormal results than do unsuspected disorders.

REFERENCES

1. Guide to Clinical Preventive Services. Report of the U.S. Preventive Services Task Force. 2nd ed. Baltimore: Williams and Wilkins; 1996.

2. Canadian Task Force on the Periodic Health Examination. The Canadian Guide to Clinical Preventive Health Care. Ottawa: Canada Communication Group-Publishing; 1994.

3. **Weiner DA, Ryan TJ, McCabe CH, et al.** Exercise stress testing: correlations among history of angina, ST-segment response and prevalence of coronary artery disease in the coronary artery surgery study (CASS). N Engl J Med. 1979;301:230-5.

4. **Ransohoff DF, Feinstein AR.** Problems of spectrum and bias in evaluating the efficacy of diagnostic tests and procedures. N Engl J Med. 1978;299:926-30.

5. **Sackett DL, Richardson WS, Rosenberg W, Haynes RB, eds.** Evidence-Based Medicine: How to Practice and Teach EBM. London: Churchill Livingstone; 1997:118-28.

6. **Sackett DL, Straus S.** On some clinically useful measures of the accuracy of diagnostic tests [Editorial]. ACP J Club. 1998;129:A-17-9.

7. **Goldstein BJ, Mushlin AI.** Use of a single thyroxine test to evaluate ambulatory medical patients for suspected hypothyroidism. J Gen Intern Med. 1987;2:20-4.

8. **Swets JA, Pickett RM, Whitehead SF, et al.** Assessment of diagnostic technologies. Science. 1979;205:753-9.

9. **Galen RS, Gambino SR.** Beyond Normality: The Predictive Value and Efficiency of Medical Diagnosis. New York: Wiley; 1975.

10. **Pauker SG, Kassirer JP.** The threshold approach to clinical decision making. N Engl J Med. 1980;302:1109-17.

11. **Sackett DL, Haynes RB, Tugwell P.** Clinical Epidemiology: A Basic Science for Clinical Medicine. Boston: Little, Brown and Company; 1985:97.

12. **Elveback L, Guillier MA, Keating RF.** Health, normality, and the ghost of Gauss. J Am Med Assoc. 1970;211:69-75.

13. **Sackett DL.** Laboratory screening: a critique. Fed Proc. 1975;34:2157-61.

14. **Galen RS.** Beyond normality: an update. In: Benson ES, Rubin M, eds. Logic and Economics of Clinical Laboratory Use. New York: Elsevier/North Holland Biomedical Press; 1978:104.

15. **Walker K.** Commentary. In: Benson ES, Rubin M, eds. Logic and Economics of Clinical Laboratory Use. New York: Elsevier/North Holland Biomedical Press; 1978:150.

16. **Hagan RD, Diaz RJ, Howath SM.** Plasma volume changes with movement to supine and standing positions. J Appl Physiol. 1978;43:414-8.

17. **Brown SS, Mitchell FL, Young DS, eds.** Chemical Diagnosis of Disease. New York: Elsevier/North Holland Biomedical Press; 1979:58.

18. **Statland BE, Winkel P.** Effect of preanalytical factors on the intraindividual variation of analytes in the blood of healthy subjects: consideration of preparation of the subject and the time of venipuncture. Crit Rev Clin Lab Sci. 1977;8:105-44.

19. **Brownson WR.** Pseudohyperkalemia due to release of potassium from white blood cells during clotting. N Engl J Med 1966;274:369.

20. **Field JB, Williams HE.** Artifactual hypoglycemia associated with leukemia. N Engl J Med. 1961;265:946.

21. **Leaf A.** The clinical and physiologic significance of the serum sodium concentration. N Engl J Med. 1962;267:24-30, 77-83.

22. **Line DE, Adler S, Fraley DS, Burns FJ.** Massive pseudoproteinuria caused by nafcillin. JAMA. 1976;235:1259.

23. **Tietz NW, ed.** Clinical Guide to Laboratory Tests. 3rd ed. Philadelphia: WB Saunders; 1995.

24. **Friedman RB, Anderson RE, Entine SM, Hirshberg SB.** Effects of diseases on clinical laboratory tests. Clin Chem. 1980;26:1D-476D.

25. **Young DS, Pestaner LC, Gibberman V.** Effects of drugs on clinical laboratory tests. Clin Chem. 1975;21:1D-432D.

26. **Bradwell AR, Carmalt MKB, Whitehead TP.** Explaining the unexpected abnormal results of biochemical profile investigations. Lancet 1974;II: 1071-4.

Interpretation of Diagnostic Tests and Strategies for Their Use in Quantitative Decision Making

2

Robert J. Panzer, MD, Edgar R. Black, MD, and Paul F. Griner, MD

KEY POINTS
- The selection and interpretation of diagnostic tests is a sequential process with the goal of reducing uncertainty about a patient's diagnosis.
- A test cannot be interpreted properly without considering what the probability of disease was before the diagnostic test or procedure result was obtained.
- Diagnostic tests help revise the probability of disease, and testing is generally continued until either the threshold for treating or not treating the patient is reached.
- When the pretest probability of disease is high, a positive test result tends to confirm the presence of disease, but an unexpectedly negative result is often not sufficiently convincing to rule out disease.
- When the pretest likelihood of disease is low, a normal test result tends to adequately exclude the presence of disease, but an unexpectedly positive result is often not sufficiently convincing to confirm the presence of disease.
- The approach of using a single diagnostic test to diagnose a single disease may be generalized to the use of multiple tests and the diagnosis of multiple diseases in a single patient.

THE SEQUENTIAL PROCESS OF TEST SELECTION AND INTERPRETATION

The selection and interpretation of diagnostic tests is a sequential process with a series of steps that may be repeated several times. The goal is to reduce uncertainty about the patient's diagnosis. The process ideally continues until the diagnosis under consideration is sufficiently certain that the clinician can treat the patient or sufficiently unlikely that the clinician can consider the diagnosis excluded.

The situation becomes more complex when multiple tests and multiple diagnoses are under consideration, but the same principles apply. In the sections that follow, the process is described for a single test and a single diagnosis, after which special issues for multiple tests and multiple diagnoses are presented.

Key steps in a quantitative approach to the diagnostic process include the following:

1. Collection of primary information from a carefully performed history and physical examination, tailored to the task at hand.
2. Development of the differential diagnosis, with estimates of the probability of each diagnosis based on data from the history, physical examination, and already available basic laboratory test results. Both the differential diagnosis and the pretest probability of disease depend on a combination of the patient's characteristics and the epidemiology of disease in the population.
3. Comparison of the estimated probability of disease to the key thresholds discussed in Chapter 1, followed by appropriate actions. If the probability of disease is high and beyond the test–treatment threshold, the patient may be treated without further testing. If the probability of disease is low and is below the test–no treatment threshold, no further testing is needed and the patient may be considered as not having the disease.
4. If the probability is within the testing zone between the two thresholds, selection of the best test for the situation using the principles discussed in Chapter 1.
5. Interpretation of the results of the test using the methods described in subsequent sections, updating the probability of disease with the post-test probability.
6. A return to Step 3 and continuation of the cycle until the likelihood of disease has moved beyond one of the thresholds. If the probability of disease is below the test–treatment threshold but is not low enough that the diagnosis may be considered truly "ruled out" and if there are no useful tests to apply, the best strategy may be to observe the patient over time ("watchful waiting").

Primary Data from the History and Physical Examination

The power of clinical information obtained from the history and the physical examination tends to be underestimated. Yet, in aggregate such information helps define the differential diagnosis for the patient's problem and the relative likelihoods of the various possibilities.

The individual pieces of this clinical information can be considered to have characteristics similar to those of diagnostic tests. In fact, in many of the subsequent chapters in this book, explicit sensitivities and specificities are given for selected items from the history and physical examination. The thoroughness and quality with which each pertinent item is sought modify the sensitivity and specificity that the item would have under ideal circumstances.

Estimating Pretest Probability

The information obtained from the history and physical examination provides what is needed to develop a differential diagnosis with a rough probability for the relevant diagnoses.

Each patient can be considered to present with probabilities of various diseases that reflect the underlying epidemiology of the population from which he or she comes. Basic information such as the age, sex, and chief symptom of the patient modifies these probabilities. Clinical information obtained from the history, physical examination, and already available basic laboratory tests further modifies the probabilities of various diseases, increasing the probability of some diagnoses and decreasing that of other diagnoses on the differential diagnosis list.

Applying Thresholds

The probabilities of various diseases after basic clinical information has been obtained can then be compared with the thresholds for testing described in Chapter 1 (1). The test–no treatment threshold defines the probability at which testing and observing (not treating) the patient for the diagnosis under consideration are equivalent. At higher probabilities, testing is preferred; at lower probabilities, observation is preferred. The test–treatment threshold defines the probability at which testing and treating are equivalent. At higher probabilities, treating is preferred; at lower probabilities, testing is preferred.

The concept of thresholds makes explicit, in quantitative terms, the ideas of "ruling out" and "ruling in" disease, which are equivalent to crossing the two thresholds.

Importantly, basic clinical information may lead to a "pretest" probability that is already beyond one of these thresholds. If so, testing is not necessary because the disease may already be considered "ruled out" or "ruled in." In the chapters that follow, some of the material presented discusses the clinical situations in which testing is or is not appropriate, before addressing the use of tests per se.

Determining the Thresholds for Testing

Explicit methods exist for calculating the disease probabilities corresponding to the test–no treatment and test–treatment thresholds (1).

The risks and costs of false-negative and false-positive diagnoses generally determine how close the thresholds approach 0% and 100%, respectively. For example, with many cancers, false-negative and false-positive diagnoses are both highly undesirable and the two thresholds approach the extremes representing minimal uncertainty. The thresholds are not necessarily equally distant from 0% and 100%. For example, in the initial diagnosis of myocardial infarction, a false-negative diagnosis involves more risk than a false-positive diagnosis. The test–no treatment threshold is quite low in this case, whereas the test–treatment (i.e., patient is admitted for intensive monitoring) threshold may be well under 50%.

The risks and costs of alternative treatments may vary and lead to different thresholds. For example, for a patient with chest pain, the threshold for monitoring the patient for signs of a possible myocardial infarction in the hospital is at one threshold, whereas treating the patient with thrombolytic therapy is at a higher threshold.

The risks and costs of available tests also determine the level of the thresholds. The more risky, more costly, or less accurate the test, the more the thresholds favor not treating the patient or treating the patient without testing (i.e., the thresholds move away from 0% and 100%). Therefore, when multiple tests are available, the threshold for testing may vary for each test.

Selection of Diagnostic Tests

The principles that govern the selection of diagnostic tests are presented in Chapter 1. When this process is conducted with the concepts of *thresholds* in mind, the task can be perceived to be selection of the test(s) that most convincingly and/or most efficiently move the probability of disease past the relevant threshold. The strategies presented in Chapter 4 for finding and interpreting information about diagnostic test performance are important to keeping test selection up-to-date.

The focus on selecting tests with thresholds in mind modifies some of the general principles of test selection. For example, one general principle that is not always correct (2) is that sensitive tests are best at ruling out, and specific tests best at ruling in, disease. However, if the probability of disease is already close to a threshold, the test does not need to be particularly powerful to yield a post-test probability that crosses the threshold: Perhaps this explains the utility of the sedimentation rate in some clinical situations.

Calculating Post-test Probabilities

Knowledge of test characteristics does not, per se, permit accurate interpretation of a test result. Knowledge of sensitivity and specificity tells us what proportion of patients with and without the disease in question have a positive and negative result, respectively. Because the task of the clinician is to determine accurately the presence or absence of the disease, the clinically relevant question is instead: What is the probability that the disease is present if the test is positive or if the test is negative?

The determination of these post-test probabilities requires the integration of knowledge concerning test characteristics with the likelihood of disease before the test was done (prior probability, or pretest probability). This integrative step can easily be demonstrated by referring to a 2 by 2 table of the kind presented in Chapter 1 and looking horizontally across the table, rather than focusing only on the "vertical" characteristics of sensitivity and specificity (Table 2-1).

Let us assume that the question to be addressed is: For a patient referred for an exercise tolerance test (ETT) because of chest pain, what is the likelihood of significant coronary artery disease when the ETT is positive (0.5 mm or more of ST depression), and what is the likelihood when it is negative? We can use information presented in Chapter 5 for the sensitivity and specificity of the procedure for this degree of abnormality. For this example, we will use 86% and 77%, respectively.

Determining post-test probabilities requires that we assign numbers to the 2 by 2 table. These can be derived by combining an estimate of the likelihood of coronary heart disease before the ETT was performed (the pretest probability) with the known operating characteristics of the test.

Suppose that, based on the symptoms, age, and sex of the patient, you consider the likelihood of coronary heart disease to be about 50%. Table 2-2 shows how this pretest clinical estimate is influenced

Table 2-1. Use of the 2 by 2 Table To Determine Post-test Probabilities Given Positive and Negative Test Results

Test Result	Disease Present = Pretest Probability	Disease Absent = 1 – Pretest Probability	
Positive	True-positive a	False-positive b	Post-test probability of disease given a positive result = $a / (a+b)$
Negative	False-negative c	True-negative d	Post-test probability of disease given a negative result = $c / (c+d)$
	Sensitivity = $a / (a+c)$	**Specificity** = $d / (b+d)$	

according to the results of the test. Note that for the sake of simplicity, the pretest probability of coronary heart disease (50%) compared with that of no coronary disease (50%) is expressed in absolute numbers rather than by percentages (i.e., coronary heart disease present, $n = 500$; absent, $n = 500$), by calculating results for 1000 (or some other convenient number) hypothetical patients similar to the patient under consideration.

When the results of the ETT are positive, the combination of the known operating characteristics of the ETT with the pretest probability results in an increase in the likelihood of coronary heart disease from 50% to nearly 80% in this patient. A normal ETT result, on the other hand, reduces the likelihood of disease from 50% to approximately 15% (i.e., the probability of no disease is 85% given a normal ETT result).

Effect of Pretest Probabilities

The impact of the clinician's estimate of the pretest probability of disease on the proper interpretation of the test result can be demonstrated by showing the influence of differing pretest estimates on post-test probabilities. Consider the following examples:

1. A 55-year-old man reports substernal chest discomfort on exertion. The pain radiates into the jaw and down the inner aspect of the left arm. The same degree of activity produces the discomfort repeatedly and is associated with shortness of breath and diaphoresis. The pain is relieved with rest. The findings of the physical examination are unremarkable, and those of the resting electrocardiogram are normal. With this information, the clini-

Table 2-2. Probability That Chest Pain Is Caused By Coronary Heart Disease According to the Results of an Exercise Tolerance Test (ETT) When the Pretest Estimate of Disease Probability Is 50%

ETT Result	Coronary Heart Disease Present $n = 500$	Coronary Heart Disease Absent $n = 500$	
Positive	True-positive $n = 430$	False-positive $n = 115$	Post-test probability of disease given a positive result = 430/545 = 79%
Negative	False-negative $n = 70$	True-negative $n = 385$	Post-test probability of disease given a negative result = 70/455 = 15%
	Sensitivity 86%	**Specificity** 77%	

cian estimates the likelihood of coronary disease to be approximately 90%. Under these circumstances, the post-test probabilities after a positive and a negative ETT result, using the same definitions as in the preceding example, should be as indicated in Table 2-3.

2. A 50-year-old woman with some cardiac risk factors reports recurrent vague chest discomfort after emotional upset. The pain is sharp and lasts for only a few seconds. The findings of the physical examination and electrocardiography are normal. In this example, the clinician's pretest estimate of the likelihood of angina pectoris is 10% or less. The post-test probabilities after a positive and negative ETT result, using the same definitions as in the preceding examples, are indicated in Table 2-4.

These examples illustrate the powerful effects of pretest probability on post-test probabilities. The same positive test result yields post-test probabilities of 97% and 29%, depending on whether the pretest probability is 90% or 10%, respectively. Conversely, the same negative test result yields post-test probabilities of 62% and 2%, depending on whether the pretest probability is 90% or 10%, respectively.

The first example also illustrates the effect of a high pretest probability on the interpretation and usefulness of tests. A positive ETT result causes the likelihood of coronary heart disease to increase from 90% to 97%. The positive test result adds little additional certainty to an already high likelihood of disease that was probably past the test–treatment threshold. Moreover, a negative ETT result does not markedly

Table 2-3. Probability That Chest Pain Is Caused By Coronary Heart Disease According to the Results of an Exercise Tolerance Test (ETT) When the Pretest Estimate of Disease Probability Is 90%

ETT Result	Coronary Heart Disease Present $n = 900$	Coronary Heart Disease Absent $n = 100$	
Positive	True-positive $n = 774$	False-positive $n = 23$	Post-test probability of disease given a positive result = 774/797 = 97%
Negative	False-negative $n = 126$	True-negative $n = 77$	Post-test probability of disease given a negative result = 126/203 = 62%
	Sensitivity 86%	**Specificity** 77%	

Table 2-4. Probability That Chest Pain Is Caused by Coronary Heart Disease According to the Results of an Exercise Tolerance Test (ETT) When the Pretest Estimate of Disease Probability Is 10%

ETT Result	Coronary Heart Disease Present n = 100	Coronary Heart Disease Absent n = 900	
Positive	True-positive n = 86	False-positive n = 207	Post-test probability of disease given a positive result = 86/293 = 29%
Negative	False-negative n = 14	True-negative n = 693	Post-test probability of disease given a negative result = 14/707 = 2.0%
	Sensitivity 86%	Specificity 77%	

reduce the likelihood of disease (pretest compared with post-test probabilities of disease, 90% and 62%, respectively). The usefulness of the test in this instance is marginal because there is only a small confirmatory gain when the test result is positive and a normal result is misleading in about three of five such patients.

In the second example, the utility of the test is also marginal. A negative result contributes little to the process of excluding the disease (i.e., the probability of disease decreases from 10% to 2%), and a positive ETT result still leads the clinician to infer that most such patients (i.e., about three fourths) do not have the disease.

The limited value of the standard ETT in these situations is linked to the increased use of more accurate (more sensitive or more specific or both) tests, such as nuclear imaging with thallium.

Absolute Compared with Relative Changes in Probabilities

When one considers the absolute change in probability after a test, the discriminating ability of a test is greatest and the greatest increments for positive and negative test results occur when the pretest estimates are intermediate, neither very high nor very low. Thus, it seems that the clinician has most to gain from this test when the prior estimate is most uncertain.

On the other hand, when one considers thresholds and the relative odds of disease, it is the relative change in probabilities that matters. That is, a change from 40% to 20% and from 10% to 5% both represent a relative reduction by twofold in disease likelihood. This latter approach to measuring the value of testing is generally more appropriate than one that focuses on absolute changes in probability.

USE OF BAYES' THEOREM TO DERIVE POST-TEST PROBABILITIES

A mathematical model rather than a 2 by 2 table may be used to calculate post-test probabilities for diagnostic tests or procedures. Bayes' theorem is commonly represented in symbols as follows:

$$\text{Post-test probability given a positive result, } P(D+/T+) = \frac{P(D+)\,P(T+/D+)}{P(D+)\,P(T+/D+) + P(D-)\,P(T+/D-)}$$

and

$$\text{Post-test probability given a negative result, } P(D+/T-) = \frac{P(D+)\,P(T-/D+)}{P(D-)\,P(T-/D-) + P(D+)\,P(T-/D+)}$$

where

$P(D+/T+)$	=	probability of disease when test is positive,
$P(D+)$	=	prevalence or clinical estimate (pretest probability) of the likelihood of disease,
$P(T+/D+)$	=	probability that test is positive when disease is present (sensitivity),
$P(T+/D-)$	=	probability that test is positive when disease is absent (false-positive rate or 1 – specificity),
$P(T-/D-)$	=	probability that test is negative when disease is absent (specificity),
$P(D-)$	=	prevalence or clinical estimate (pretest probability) of the likelihood of no disease, and
$P(T-/D+)$	=	probability that test is negative when disease is present (false-negative rate or 1 – sensitivity).

This formula can be more easily expressed as follows:

$$\text{Post-test probability given a positive result} = \frac{\text{True-positives (TP)}}{\text{Total (true + false) positives}}$$

and

$$\text{Post-test probability given a negative result} = \frac{\text{False-negatives (FN)}}{\text{Total (true + false) negatives}}$$

Thus, Bayes' formula simply extrapolates the information gleaned from the horizontal assessment of data from the binary table (Table 2-1):

$$\text{Post-test probability given a positive result} = \frac{a}{a+b} = \frac{TP}{TP+FP} = \frac{P(D+)\,P(T+/D+)}{P(D+)\,P(T+/D+) + P(D-)\,P(T+/D-)}$$

and

$$\text{Post-test probability given a negative result} = \frac{c}{c+d} = \frac{FN}{TN+FN} = \frac{P(D+)\,P(T-/D+)}{P(D-)\,P(T-/D-) + P(D+)\,P(T-/D+)}$$

In this book we use *post-test probability* given positive or negative results rather than *predictive value*. Using *post-test probability* makes interpretation of serial tests much easier for the clinician.

IMPLICATIONS OF ERRONEOUS ESTIMATES OF PRETEST PROBABILITY

A common response when one attempts to learn quantitative decision making by the method just described is: "How can we apply such a method to an individual patient? The test characteristics may be fairly precise, but the estimate of the probability of disease before the test result was obtained is crude at best. What if we think the pretest disease likelihood is 10%, but it is actually 30%, or 70% instead of 90%?" Our response to these questions is threefold: First, it is not possible to interpret the result of a test accurately without fully using the clinical information obtained before the test was performed unless the test's sensitivity and specificity are absolute (i.e., 100%). Second, the well-trained clinician is probably more accurate in estimating the pretest probability of disease than he or she may believe. Third, a moderate error in the pretest estimate of the probability of disease has usually, but not always (3), relatively little effect on test interpretation.

For example, if in the example of the ETT used in Table 2-3 (sensitivity, 86%; specificity, 77%; using a cutoff of 0.5 mm of ST depression), the pretest estimate of 90% should have been 70%, the post-test probability if the test result is positive is not greatly different (i.e., 97% compared with 90%). The post-test probability of disease if the test result is negative also would not be greatly different (i.e., 62% compared with 42%). Similarly, for a pretest estimate of 10% that should have been 30%, the post-test probability of disease if the test result is negative is not greatly influenced (2% compared with 7%, respectively). The post-test probability if the test result is positive seems different (29% compared with 62%) but is probably still in the testing zone.

DIAGNOSTIC VALUE OF THE NORMAL RESULT

A normal test result may accomplish more than simply reducing the probability of a specific disease. If two (or more) diseases are being con-

Table 2-5. Implications of a Normal Test Result When Two or More Diseases Are Considered and the Sensitivity of the Test Is Different for Each

Erythrocyte Indices	Iron Deficiency $n = 500$	Chronic Disease $n = 500$	
Positive	True-positive $n = 450$	False-positive $n = 125$	Post-test probability of iron deficiency given a positive result = 450/575 = 78%
Negative	False-negative $n = 50$	True-negative $n = 375$	Post-test probability of iron deficiency given a negative result = 50/425 = 12%
	Sensitivity for iron deficiency = 90%	Sensitivity for chronic disease = 25%	

sidered, the same test is used for both, and the sensitivity of the test for one is significantly different from that of the other, a normal reading may result in a major revision of the estimates of the probability of each disease. For example, suppose that in a patient with anemia, iron deficiency and chronic disease are considered to be equally plausible explanations for the anemia. If we assume that the erythrocyte indices will be low in 90% of iron-deficient patients with anemia and in 25% of those with the anemia of chronic disease, the finding of normal erythrocyte indices renders the latter diagnosis highly likely (88%), as indicated in Table 2-5. The interested reader is referred to the article by Gorry, Pauker, and Schwartz for a detailed review of the application of this principle (4).

MULTIPLE DIAGNOSES AND MULTIPLE TREATMENTS

In patient care, when investigating a patient problem, the clinician typically considers multiple diagnoses and treatments at once, rather than the single diagnosis and single treatment that much of the previous discussion implies. The same approaches can be applied to consideration of multiple diagnoses and treatments as to single diagnoses and treatments, but there are special issues that arise.

Each diagnosis has its own set of probabilities and thresholds. For any particular diagnosis, each treatment also has its own thresholds. Thus, the diagnostic process can be considered to be the collection of information to move various diagnoses along the probability line, until diagnoses are "ruled in" and are above the test–treatment threshold, or "ruled out" and are below the test–no treatment threshold.

Because each diagnosis and treatment combination has its own thresholds, testing is not necessarily directed only at diagnoses that are at the top of the list of most likely possibilities. For example, take the situation of an elderly patient with the recent onset of persistent back pain (Chapter 35). Findings from the history and physical examination may indicate that the diagnosis of degenerative joint disease without disc protrusion is quite likely and above the test–treatment threshold. However, in an elderly patient, the optimal strategy may still be to perform radiographic studies to address the unlikely possibility of malignancy: The test–no treatment threshold for malignancy in this situation is low, and testing is needed to bring the probability of malignancy below that threshold, "ruling out" the diagnosis. The more likely diagnosis of degenerative joint disease is not "ruled in" until that alternative diagnosis of malignancy is "ruled out." Because multiple diagnoses may coexist, the process may result in more than one diagnosis rising above the test–treatment threshold, as long as these diagnoses are not mutually exclusive.

MULTIPLE TESTS

When multiple tests are applied in sequence using the approaches described earlier in this chapter, each test's post-test probability is derived before the next test (if needed) is selected. At times, the clinician needs to interpret several tests that have already been performed. The straightforward approach to this task is to calculate probabilities after each test using a separate 2 by 2 table, using the post-test probabilities for relevant results of the first test as the pretest probability section of the second table. A method of interpreting multiple tests that is simpler to compute is described in Chapter 3—using likelihood ratios and odds to perform one calculation of the post-test odds after all the tests have been performed. The choice of one method or another is discretionary, because the findings of the calculations will be the same with either method.

TESTS WITH MULTIPLE LEVELS

In this and other chapters, we generally present the likelihood ratio as a method for interpreting diagnostic tests that is equivalent to sensitivity and specificity. However, when a test has multiple levels of abnormality, the likelihood ratio for each category of abnormality carries more discrimination than sensitivity and specificity based on a single cutoff (5). In such situations (e.g., coronary artery disease diagnosis with ETT or pulmonary embolism diagnosis with the V/Q scan), interpretation using likelihood ratios is preferred and is not merely an alternative.

REFERENCES

1. **Pauker SG, Kassirer JP.** The threshold approach to clinical decision making. N Engl J Med. 1980;302:1109-17.

2. **Boyko EJ.** Ruling out or ruling in disease with the most sensitive or specific diagnostic test: short-cut or wrong turn? Med Decis Making. 1994;14: 175-9.

3. **Baron JA.** Uncertainty in Bayes. Med Decis Making. 1994;14:46-51.

4. **Gorry GA, Pauker SG, Schwartz WB.** The diagnostic importance of the normal finding. N Engl J Med. 1978;298:486-9.

5. **Sackett DL, Straus S.** On some clinically useful measures of the accuracy of diagnostic tests. ACP J Club 1998;129:A17-A19.

Odds and Likelihood Ratios   **3**

Anthony L. Suchman, MD, and James G. Dolan, MD

KEY POINTS

- The use of odds and likelihood ratios is an alternate method for determining the quantitative importance of test results.
- This approach is generally more convenient than the 2 by 2 table method, particularly when interpreting sequential tests or single tests with multiple cutoffs.

BACKGROUND

The preceding chapters have shown how a 2 by 2 table is used to calculate a post-test probability, given a pretest probability and the sensitivity and specificity of a diagnostic test. Another method for accomplishing the same task uses odds rather than probabilities and likelihood ratios rather than sensitivity and specificity, and has several advantages over the 2 by 2 table method.

ODDS

An odds expression compares the likelihood that a particular outcome (e.g., a horse winning a race or a disease being present) will occur (i) to the likelihood that it will not occur (j) by means of the expression i:j. A probability can be converted to odds by writing the probability that an event will occur to the left of the colon and the probability that the event will *not* occur (1 – probability of the event) to the right. To obtain more manageable numbers, both sides of the expression can be multiplied or divided by the same number without changing its meaning. For example, a probability of 0.75 (or 75%) becomes odds of 0.75:0.25, which, after dividing both sides by 0.25, becomes 3:1. To convert an odds expression into a probability, the expression to the left of the colon (i) is divided by the sum of the numbers on either side of the expres-

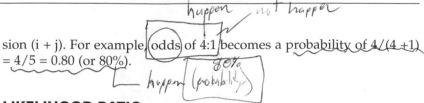

sion (i + j). For example, odds of 4:1 becomes a probability of 4/(4 +1) = 4/5 = 0.80 (or 80%).

LIKELIHOOD RATIO

The likelihood ratio for a test describes the relative odds of an outcome, given a particular test result. Tests with dichotomous results (i.e., positive or negative) will have two likelihood ratios (called the positive and the negative likelihood ratios) that reflect the relative odds of a condition being present after a positive or a negative test, respectively. Like sensitivity and specificity, likelihood ratios are independent of pretest probability in most circumstances.

The positive likelihood ratio (or likelihood ratio for a positive result) is defined as the true-positive rate (sensitivity) divided by the false-positive rate (1 − specificity). In terms of the 2 by 2 table (Table 1-1, p 5, Chapter 1), the positive likelihood ratio can be expressed as follows: [a/(a + c)]/[b/(b + d)]. The negative likelihood ratio (or likelihood ratio for a negative result) is defined as the false-negative rate (1 − sensitivity) divided by the true-negative rate (specificity) and can be expressed as follows: [c/(a + c)]/[d/(b + d)]. Both the positive and negative likelihood ratios represent the rate of the test result (positive or negative) in the *presence of disease* divided by the rate of the test result in the *absence of disease*.

For example, in the diagnosis of coronary artery disease, studies reported that new wall-motion abnormalities on exercise echocardiography had a sensitivity of 81% and a specificity of 89% (Chapter 5). We can then calculate the positive likelihood ratio to be 0.81/(1 − 0.89) = 0.81/0.11 = 7.4 and the negative likelihood ratio to be (1 − 0.81)/0.89 = 0.19/0.89 = 0.21. These ratios indicate that positive results occur 7.4 times as frequently and negative tests occur 0.21 times as frequently in patients with coronary artery disease as they do in those without coronary artery disease.

CALCULATION OF POST-TEST ODDS

From Bayes theorem (1), it can be shown that

Post-test odds = (pretest odds) × (likelihood ratio).

In multiplying the pretest odds by the likelihood ratio, the expression to the left of the colon (i) is multiplied by the likelihood ratio, whereas the expression to the right (j) remains unchanged. This results in a new odds expression, the post-test odds, which then can be converted to the post-test probability, if desired. The conversion to odds, multiplication by the likelihood ratio, and conversion back to probability can also be accomplished by means of a nomogram (Fig. 3-1) (2). A likelihood ratio of 1.0 indicates a test with no predictive power; that is, the post-test odds are the same as the pretest odds. The further the likelihood ratio is from 1.0, the more powerful the test. Likelihood ratios greater than 1 give post-test odds that are greater than pretest

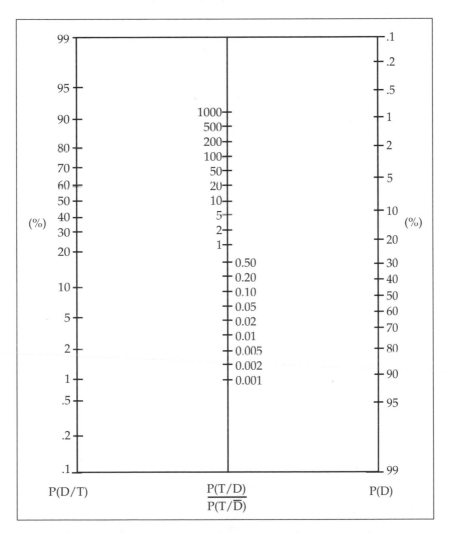

Figure 3-1. Nomogram for calculating post-test probabilities, given probabilities and likelihood ratios (2). To use the nomogram, find the pretest probability on the right-hand scale and the likelihood ratio on the center scale. Connect these two points with a straight line, extending the line to intercept the left-hand scale. Read the post-test probability at this intercept. (Republished with permission from Fagan TJ. Nomogram for Bayes's theorem [Letter]. N Engl J Med. 1975;293:257.)

odds whereas likelihood ratios less than 1 give post-test odds that are less than pretest odds.

For example, a 39-year-old man who presents with a history of exertional chest pressure believed to be typical angina is estimated by his physician to have a probability of coronary artery stenosis of 0.70. If the exercise echocardiography had been done to confirm the diagnosis, the test operating characteristics would be as described in the preceding section. The following calculations show how the post-test probability is determined using either the odds method or the 2 by 2 table method:

> Pretest probability of coronary artery disease = 0.70 (70%)
> Sensitivity = 81%
> Specificity = 89%
> Positive likelihood ratio = 7.4
> Negative likelihood ratio = 0.21

ODDS METHOD

1. Convert prior probability to prior odds: 0.70 becomes 0.70:0.30 = 7:3.
2. Multiply prior odds by likelihood ratio to obtain post-test odds:
   > For a positive test: 7:3 × 7.4 = 52:3 = 17:1
   > For a negative test: 7:3 × 0.21 = 1.47:3 = 0.49:1
3. Convert post-test odds to post-test probability (optionally):
   > For a positive test: 17:1 becomes 17/(17 + 1) = 0.94 (94%)
   > For a negative test: 0.49:1 becomes 0.49/(0.49 + 1) = 0.33 (33%)

2 BY 2 TABLE METHOD

1. Construct a 2 by 2 table (Table 3-1) using a pretest probability of 0.70 (70%) and sensitivity and specificity of 81% and 89%, respectively.
2. Calculate post-test probabilities:
   > For positive test: 567/(567 + 33) = 567/600 = 0.94 (94%)
   > For negative test: 133/(133 + 267) = 133/400 = 0.33 (33%)

In each case, the probability of coronary artery stenosis is estimated to be 0.94 (94%) after a positive test result (new wall-motion abnormalities) and 0.33 (33%) after a negative test result (no new wall-motion abnormalities). It must be remembered that, given the uncertainty of estimates of pretest probability (or pretest odds) and the potential inaccu-

Table 3-1. 2 by 2 Table

Test Result	Disease Present (n = 700)	Disease Absent (n = 300)
Positive	567	33
Negative	133	267

racy of operating characteristics, post-test probabilities (or odds) should be regarded as estimates rather than as precise values.

MULTIPLE CUTOFFS AND SEQUENTIAL TESTS

The results of many laboratory tests are expressed as continuous rather than dichotomous variables. In interpreting these tests, one can gain additional information from knowing the degree of abnormality of the test result as compared with knowing merely whether the test is normal or abnormal. That is, a markedly abnormal result may be more strongly associated with disease than a minimally abnormal finding. This approach can be accomplished by using a set of likelihood ratios determined at several intervals across the range of possible test results: Test results associated with a high likelihood ratio (≥10) may rule in the diagnosis when the pretest odds are at least 1:2, whereas results with a low likelihood ratio (≤0.10) often rule out the disease when the pretest odds are less than 1:2 (3). For example, Guyatt (4) calculated the likelihood ratios at various cutoffs of the serum ferritin assay to help clinicians evaluate patients with possible iron-deficiency anemia (see Chapter 50.)

Using the example of coronary artery disease, Table 3-2 shows the likelihood ratios for several levels of ST-segment depression in exercise electrocardiography (5). Note that 1 mm of ST-segment depression denotes the level below which the likelihood ratios are less than 1 (i.e., post-test odds of coronary artery stenosis will be less than pretest odds) and above which the likelihood ratios are greater than 1 (i.e., the post-test odds will be greater than the pretest odds). If a patient whose pretest probability of coronary artery stenosis is 40% (pretest odds = 2:3) has 2 mm of ST-segment depression, the post-test odds are 2:3 × 11 = 22:3, and the post-test probability is 0.88 (88%). If there is no ST-segment depression, the post-test odds are 2:3 x 0.23 = 0.46:3 and the post-test probability is 0.13 (13%).

Another useful application of the odds method is in sequential testing in which the post-test odds from the first test become the pretest odds for the next test, thereby avoiding the need to construct a series of 2 by 2 tables. Note, however, that this use of Bayes theorem rests on the assumption that the tests in the sequence are conditionally indepen-

Table 3-2. Likelihood Ratios for Coronary Artery Stenosis at Multiple Levels of Nonsloping ST-Segment Depression in Exercise Electrocardiography

ST-Segment Depression (mm)	Likelihood Ratio
>2.50	39
2–2.49	11
1.5–1.99	4.2
1–1.49	2.1
0.50–0.99	0.92
<0.50	0.23

Adapted from Diamond GA, Forrester JS. Analysis of probability as an aid in the clinical diagnosis of coronary-artery disease. N Engl J Med. 1979;300:1350-8.

dent, that is, a particular result of one test is not associated with a particular result of the other.

For example, suppose a 55-year-old woman visits her physician for evaluation of retrosternal fullness felt to be nonanginal. Her physician estimates the prior probability of coronary artery stenosis to be 0.10 (prior odds = 1:9). She undergoes combined exercise electrocardiography and exercise echocardiography. Her exercise electrocardiogram shows 1.5 mm of ST-segment depression (likelihood ratio = 4.2), so her post-test odds are 1:9 × 4.2 = 4.2:9 (probability = 0.32 or 32%). The exercise echocardiogram shows a new wall-motion abnormality (positive likelihood ratio = 7.4). Her revised post-test odds are 4.2:9 × 7.4 = 31:9, representing a post-test probability of 0.78 (78%). As this example illustrates, the sequential calculations can be performed quite easily.

REFERENCES

1. **Weinstein MC, Fineberg HV.** Clinical Decision Analysis. Philadelphia: WB Saunders; 1980:107.

2. **Fagan TJ.** Nomogram for Bayes's theorem [Letter]. N Engl J Med. 1975;293:257.

3. **Sackett DL, Richardson WS, Rosenberg W, Haynes RB, eds.** Evidence-Based Medicine: How To Practice and Teach EBM. London: Churchill Livingstone; 1997:118-28.

4. **Guyatt GH, Oxman AD, Ali M, William A, McIlroy W, Patterson C.** Laboratory diagnosis of iron-deficiency anemia: An overview. J Gen Intern Med. 1992;7:145-53.

5. **Diamond GA, Forrester JS.** Analysis of probability as an aid in the clinical diagnosis of coronary-artery disease. N Engl J Med. 1979;300:1350-8.

Keeping Up to Date with the Best Evidence Concerning Diagnostic Tests

4

R. Brian Haynes, MD, PhD

KEY POINTS

- Keeping up with the medical literature on diagnostic tests is becoming an easier task, with compendia such as this text becoming available. However, keeping up with new tests and new evidence on old tests before they are summarized in compendia requires that clinical users find the pertinent evidence in a timely fashion, using self-service electronic searching of the medical literature, and that they appraise the new evidence critically.

- For clinical use, studies of diagnostic procedures should fulfill at least the following criteria: 1) clearly describe a study setting appropriate to the reader's own clinical practice; 2) assess a sample of patients in whom the disease is suspected but not known to be present; 3) compare the test with a "gold standard" of diagnosis; and 4) offer independent interpretation of both the test and gold standard.

- In addition to the above criteria, studies of clinical prediction rules should also include 1) use of multivariable statistical techniques; 2) use of both a training set and testing set.

BACKGROUND

This book describes principles of diagnostic test interpretation that can be applied to virtually any test. It also applies these principles to many current tests for internal medicine. What it cannot do is assess evidence that does not yet exist or provide a comprehensive assessment of existing tests in internal medicine.

The purpose of this chapter is to provide you with a "tool kit" for dealing with this dilemma of a large and increasing knowledge base about diagnostic tests. Without such tools and their regular application, we all face certain obsolescence of our clinical skills. Our main tools are rapid, typically electronic, access to the medical literature and its burgeoning number of special evidence resources for clinical practice, and rapid critical appraisal of the medical literature.

USING THE MEDICAL LITERATURE TO SOLVE PATIENT PROBLEMS

Studies show that clinicians are not very good at tracking down information as questions arise in clinical practice. For example, Covell and colleagues (1) found that internists left unanswered 70% of the questions that arose when seeing patients and almost never consulted the medical literature for the remaining 30%. Their reasons for failing to do so included lack of time, disorganization of their own journal collection, and not knowing where to look.

The lack-of-time and where-to-look aspects of this problem are now yielding to modern information technology and resources. As Williamson and colleagues (2) found in their survey of physicians, an increasing number are conducting electronic searches of the medical literature from their offices, clinics, and homes. Also, a rapidly increasing number of computerized databases contain evidence about the accuracy of diagnostic tests, information that can often be run on our own microcomputers.

Specialized Resources for Internal Medicine

If the diagnoses and tests you are interested in are in this book, look no further. If not, you can readily broaden your search through one or more of the following American College of Physicians (ACP) resources: *Best Evidence* (3), or the print versions of *Common Diagnostic Tests* (4), and *Common Screening Tests* (5). For example, if you are interested in noninvasive diagnosis for carotid stenosis, start up *Best Evidence*, click with your computer mouse on "Start a Full-Text Search," and type in "carotid and noninvasive tests." You will be instantly rewarded with a systematic review of evidence on noninvasive tests for carotid stenosis (6) abstracted in *ACP Journal Club*. Furthermore, the evidence presented in *Best Evidence* is prescreened for validity and relevance to internal medicine, a matter that we will return to in searching for evidence in other sources.

It is sometimes important to be flexible and creative in doing searches in electronic databases. There is no such thing as a perfect indexing system. For example, in the search above, if you searched instead with the term "carotid ultrasound," an abstract of an original article on duplex Doppler ultrasonography is retrieved (7) but the systematic review is missed even though the review provides useful information on "carotid duplex ultrasonography" and "carotid Doppler ultrasonography." A way to circumvent this problem is to use "wild-cards" in searching, for example, "carotid and ultras*." In this strategy, the "*" allows the computer search to pick up all words that include "ultras," including "ultrasound" and "ultrasonography." Another way to get around the problem is to do a more general search, such as "carotid stenosis," and then look through the titles of the retrieved documents. This list typically includes many studies that are unrelated or that are related but not on target—for example, results of trials of carotid endarterectomy. However, these latter studies are helpful in determining when to assess patients for possible endarterectomy.

General Access to the Medical Literature

In specialized databases such as *Best Evidence*, visual sorting does not take long. For a large database like MEDLINE, however, the retrieval and sorting problems can be substantial and a more sophisticated search strategy is needed. Table 4-1 provides two strategies that have been validated for highly sensitive and highly specific yield for studies of diagnoses. These strategies can be "ANDed" to any clinical topic. For the carotid stenosis example, this would be "carotid stenosis AND Exp Sensitivity a#d Specificity or Predictive (tw) and Value: (tw)." "Exp" here indicates "explode," a special MEDLINE notation that means that several related index terms are automatically searched (8).

The techniques and tools for doing MEDLINE searches yourself have been described elsewhere (8,9). The search for noninvasive diagnostic tests for carotid stenosis using the more specific search strategy in Table 4-1 yielded 91 articles, and the more sensitive search strategy retrieved 840 articles. Both searches retrieved the study by Blakeley and colleagues (6) that was found in *Best Evidence*, but getting to this article involves a great deal more work for the searcher, and deciding which article(s) to use requires critical appraisal of the methods of research (see later in this chapter).

Internet now provides access to MEDLINE, for example, PubMed (www.ncbi.nlm.nih.gov/PubMed/clinical.html), Internet Grateful Med (igm.nlm.nih.gov/), Ovid (www.ovid.com/), and Silverplatter (www.silverplatter.com/), and many other more general information services, including these clinically focused indexes: Medical Matrix (www.kumc.edu/mmatrix/), MedWeb (www.cc.emory.edu/WHSCL/medweb.html), Physician's Guide to the Internet (www.webcom.com/pgi/), and CliniWeb (www.ohsu.edu/cliniweb/). PubMed is free and also provides specialized search strategies for diagnostic tests as point-and-click options on its "Clinical Queries" screen. Unfortunately, most of the information from these sources cannot be assessed for validity because little or no information is provided about research methods. Also, for better or worse, patients have access to this information and may press us to keep up with them. (Try the Web site www.helico.com

to see an example of the types of detailed information—on *Helicobacter pylori* infections in this case—that patients can get that you may not know yet!)

Tracking down answers to clinical questions as they arise will always be a challenge in the fast-paced world of medical care. However, the time barriers are being challenged if not eliminated by new, low-cost, electronic evidence-based resources. Moreover, the value of answers obtained from a quick search, if well done, is high. Not only may the patient benefit, but the educational impact of learning in this way far exceeds that of browsing, after which enough time usually elapses to prevent effective recall.

Most important, if the resources that you use include a credible process for screening research evidence for validity and clinical usefulness, then much of the task of critical appraisal can be streamlined. But at least a working knowledge of the principles of critical appraisal of evidence is needed to enable you to steer clear of research evidence that is not sound or not ready for clinical application. These principles are described in the next section.

CRITICAL APPRAISAL OF EVIDENCE ABOUT DIAGNOSTIC TESTS

Most diagnostic tests are conceived by chemists, physicists, biologists, physiologists, and other "basic" scientists. Once created, tests typically undergo several types of evaluation to define their properties—that is, their operating characteristics. Evaluations begin with bench tests, then

Table 4-1. Sophisticated Strategies for Optimizing MEDLINE Searches for Studies of Diagnostic Tests*

Search Strategy	Sensitivity	Specificity	Precision
Exp Sensitivity a#d Specificity or Predictive (tw) and Value: (tw)	0.55	0.98	0.40
Exp Sensitivity a#d Specificity or Diagnosis& (pe) or Diagnostic Use or Sensitivity (tw) or Specificity (tw)	0.92	0.73	0.09

*Based on data from Haynes RB, Wilczynski NL, McKibbon KA, et al. Developing optimal search strategies for detecting clinically sound studies in MEDLINE. J Am Med Inform Assoc. 1994; 1:447-58. *Sensitivity* is the proportion of all relevant articles that are retrieved, *specificity* is the proportion of irrelevant articles that excluded by the search, and *precision* is the proportion of all retrieved articles that provide evidence concerning the sensitivity and specificity of the test of interest.

preliminary tests among human participants, and finally, proper clinical trials. Usually, only the diagnostic tests that pass the early stages of testing go on to clinical trials. Most fall by the wayside with increasingly rigorous evaluation.

An ideal scenario for the introduction of useful tests into clinical practice would be as follows: In the process of the test's introduction, practitioners would be fully informed of its operating characteristics and would therefore apply it appropriately, using the principles described in earlier chapters. In reality, what happens is not so pristine or there would be no need for this chapter. The literature that appears in clinical journals includes studies from all levels of assessment, requiring careful appraisal by the clinician to obtain a clear message. All too often, a new test is introduced into clinical practice before it has passed all the appropriate evaluations. At the same time, some diagnostic tests that have passed rigorous evaluations are not introduced because they are buried in the literature or because they are not perceived to be needed or affordable. Often there is no evidence available on the utility of a test in comparison with other tests for the same diagnosis or on the cost per accurate diagnosis.

For the purposes of keeping up in clinical practice, only a fraction of studies done on a given test (i.e., the most rigorous clinical trials) are worth paying attention to. This fraction of good clinical trials can be detected by their adherence to a few simple standards (10,11):

1. **Clear description of an appropriate study setting.** The study setting must be clearly delineated (e.g., should specify whether it is primary care or specialty clinic, should describe the types of patients considered and the referral patterns) so that it is obvious to whom the results of the study might apply. Clinicians should determine if the test setting is reasonably appropriate for extrapolation to their own setting. If the match is poor, it is reasonable to carry on the search for a study better suited to the situation of the clinician and his or her patients.

2. **Assessment of a sample of patients in whom the disease is suspected (but not known) to be present.** The test should be put through its paces with patients, preferably a consecutive series, in whom the disease is suspected but who are not known to have it. This emulates the circumstances in which the test will be applied clinically and is far superior to the preliminary stage of testing in which the results are based on a comparison of people who obviously have the disease with "normal" volunteers who clearly do not have the disease. Caution is called for if an article does not indi-

cate how the patients were selected or if patients were selected who were already known to have the disorder of interest. (Selecting patients with known disease does not mean that the study is a "bad" one, merely that it is a preliminary one.)

3. **Comparison with a "gold standard."** The new test must be compared with an accepted standard, usually a complicated or expensive or invasive test, called generically the "gold standard" or "criterion standard." For example, the gold standard for the interpretation of exercise stress tests to detect ischemic heart disease is typically coronary angiography.

4. **Independent interpretation of the test and gold standard.** Initial interpretation of the new test must be made without reference to the gold standard, and vice versa. Without this independent interpretation of the two tests, it is possible that the result of one test will influence or bias the interpretation of the other.

5. **Demonstration of reproducibility of test results.** The test must also be shown to be reproducible in its results. That is, as long as the clinical state of the patient does not change, the result of the test should not change. Similarly, if the test requires subjective interpretation— for example, a diagnostic image—one interpreter should be shown to give the same results as the next.

6. **Demonstration of the clinical utility of the test.** Ideally, the study should indicate the extent to which the new test actually adds useful information to that available from the usual clinical observations and other tests. That is, the incremental value of the test should be ascertained. For example, serum aspartate aminotransferase or lactate dehydrogenase may indicate myocardial infarction with reasonable sensitivity and specificity but provide less information than the creatine kinase MB fraction alone (12) and therefore lack "incremental value." Unfortunately, it is expensive to do studies to assess utility, so they are seldom done.

These guidelines can be used as screening tests to select reports that are believable and that should be incorporated into clinical practice. In fact, most of this process of critical appraisal of the medical literature can be accomplished, quickly and effectively, by applying just the first four of these criteria. In terms of efficiency, it is perhaps easiest for an individual clinician to begin with the first of these: Look into only those investigations in which the setting (in terms of types of patients and level of care) is clearly described and sufficiently similar to one's own that the results of the investigation can be reasonably applied to one's own patients. Studies meeting all four criteria are few and far between. Those that do are well worth reviewing in detail.

Studies of **clinical prediction** may require two additional criteria. These studies often involve evaluating a number of "baseline" clinical variables to determine their ability to predict the subsequent diagnosis, prognosis, or therapeutic responsiveness of a patient. For example, Goldman and colleagues (13) measured the age, sex, past cardiac history, clinical status, electrocardiograms, type of surgery, and so on for patients who were about to undergo surgical procedures and who had been referred to a medical consultation service because of a suspicion of increased risk of cardiac complications during or after surgery. The purpose of this study was to determine if any of the initial clinical observations could predict in which patients cardiac complications were most likely to develop. Statistical procedures were used to "model" the data—that is, to determine the "best fit" between the baseline variables and the subsequent course of the patients. This type of analysis does the best it can with the data. In this example, the statistical model came up with a good match between a small number of baseline variables and the cardiac complications that ensued. However, best statistical fits cannot distinguish between real relations and chance relations that are unlikely to arise again. Thus, the fit must be tested with additional patients in the same setting. Also, the fit may not apply in other settings in which the patients, referral patterns, monitoring procedures, surgeons, internists, and so on are different. Thus, the study should be repeated in other settings, preferably by other investigators. These considerations give rise to two additional criteria for studies of clinical prediction:

1. **Use of multivariable statistical techniques if more than one factor was included in the prediction rule.** These multivariable statistical techniques go by such names as *multiple regression, discriminant function analysis,* and *recursive partitioning.* It is not as important to understand the details of how these tests are performed as it is to ensure that the investigators used one of these approaches to determine the *independent* effect of the variables included in their prediction rule—that is, the extent to which each variable provides additional information to the prediction.

2. **Use of both a training set and testing set.** In the study of Goldman and colleagues, only a training set was provided. Detsky and colleagues (14) tested Goldman's prediction rule, and their own modifica-

> tion of it, at an entirely new setting. In the original
> training set and the subsequent testing set, the predic-
> tion rule performed well, although in the latter study
> a modification of it performed slightly better.

Applying the criteria for critical appraisal can be accomplished most
thoroughly by matching them against statements that appear in the
"Methods" section of articles. Often, however, the task can be easier
than this, as key information appears in the abstract of an article. For
"keeping up to date," it is not necessary to read a study further if it fails
any one of the four major standards discussed above. This might be
termed the "pre-emptive strike mode" of critical appraisal. Often,
flaws can be detected in seconds, sparing reading time for additional
articles or other activities. If no important flaws are found, reading the
complete article is warranted—this may be the time for a change in
your clinical behavior.

  If you are attempting to solve a patient problem, however, the task
becomes a bit more challenging. Here, what is needed is best available
evidence. If no good studies are detected despite vigorous searching,
then the studies available need to be evaluated to find the best ones.
The same principles of appraisal apply, but grading several imperfect
studies takes more time than rapidly eliminating studies that do not
meet all the criteria.

KEEPING UP TO DATE

Browsing through the current medical literature to keep up to date is
an essential activity, but it is not very efficient if it involves personally
perusing the 20 or so journals that publish studies of relevance for
internal medicine and primary care (15). Further, if you do come across
relevant studies, you will likely have forgotten either the studies or
their key details when you see a patient who could benefit from the
information. Recently, the process of regular reading of the medical literature has been made much simpler by publications such as *ACP
Journal Club* and *Evidence-Based Medicine*. These bimonthly "secondary"
journals have research staff and associate editors who prescreen more
than 50 journals for studies that are both valid and ready for clinical
application, then abstract the key information in these studies in a standardized way so that readers can both complete the critical appraisal
from their own practice perspective and discern the key results. It is of
interest that important advances in the broad range of general medical
care can be summarized in fewer than 40 abstracts every two months.
For diagnostic tests, the new information is usually found in fewer
than five articles bimonthly. Thus, the main task of keeping up to date
with new evidence on diagnostic tests is certainly tractable.

REFERENCES

1. **Covell DG, Uman GC, Manning PR.** Information needs in office practice: are they being met? Ann Intern Med. 1985;103:596-9.

2. **Williamson JW, German PS, Weiss R, et al.** Health science information management and continuing education of physicians. Ann Intern Med. 1989;110:151-60.

3. **Haynes RB, ed.** Best Evidence: Linking Medical Research to Practice. Philadelphia: American College of Physicians. Semiannual subscription on computer diskette and CD-ROM.

4. **Sox HC Jr, ed.** Common Diagnostic Tests. Use and Interpretation. 2nd ed. Philadelphia: American College of Physicians; 1990.

5. **Eddy DM, ed.** Common Screening Tests. Philadelphia: American College of Physicians; 1991.

6. **Blakeley DD, Oddone EZ, Hasselblad V, et al.** Noninvasive carotid artery testing: a meta-analytic review. Ann Intern Med. 1995;122:360-7.

7. Duplex Doppler ultrasonography was accurate in determining 60% or greater carotid artery stenosis. ACP J Club. 1996;124:75; Evidence-Based Medicine. 1996;1:122; Best Evidence [CD-ROM]. Philadelphia: American College of Physicians, 1997.

8. **Sackett DL, Richardson SR, Rosenberg W, Haynes RB.** Evidence-Based Medicine: How to Practice and Teach EBM. London: Churchill Livingstone; 1997: Chapter 2.

9. **Haynes RB, Wilczynski NL, McKibbon KA, et al.** Developing optimal search strategies for detecting clinically sound studies in MEDLINE. J Am Med Inform Assoc. 1994;1:447-58.

10. **Jaeschke R, Guyatt GH, Sackett DL, for the Evidence-based Medicine Working Group.** Users' guides to the medical literature. III. How to use an article about a diagnostic test. A. Are the results of the study valid? JAMA. 1994;271:389-91.

11. **Jaeschke R, Guyatt GH, Sackett DL, for the Evidence-based Medicine Working Group.** Users' guides to the medical literature. III. How to use an article about a diagnostic test. B. What are the results and will they help me in caring for my patients? JAMA. 1994;271:703-7.

12. **Grande P, Christiansen C, Pedersen A, Christensen MS.** Optimal diagnosis in acute myocardial infarction: a cost-effectiveness study. Circulation. 1980;61:723-8.

13. **Goldman L, Caldera D, Nussbaum SR, et al.** Multifactorial index of cardiac risk in non-cardiac surgical procedures. N Engl J Med. 1977;197:845-50.

14. **Detsky AS, Abrams HB, McLaughlin JR, et al.** Predicting cardiac complications in patients undergoing non-cardiac surgery. J Gen Intern Med. 1986;1:211-9.

15. **Haynes RB.** Where's the meat in clinical journals? [Editorial]. ACP J Club. 1993 Nov-Dec: A16 (Ann Intern Med. 1993; vol 115, Suppl 3).

Cardiovascular Problems

Coronary Artery Disease   **5**

Nancy M. Bennett, MD, MS, and Mary C. Paris, MPH

KEY POINTS

Pretest Probabilities

- The probability of angiographic coronary artery disease (CAD) can be predicted on the basis of the patient's age and sex, the clinical risk factors, and the characteristics of the chest pain.

Diagnostic Strategies

- In patients with an intermediate pretest probability of CAD and in whom the findings on a resting electrocardiogram (ECG) are normal, ordering an exercise ECG is a logical first step in the evaluation for CAD.

- Both radionuclide and echocardiographic imaging are useful in the initial evaluation of patients in whom the resting ECG shows abnormalities and in the serial testing of patients in whom the probability of CAD remains in an intermediate range after initial exercise ECG testing.

- Currently available noninvasive tests for CAD are not sensitive enough to identify patients with left-main or three-vessel CAD. Markedly abnormal findings on exercise ECG can identify patients with a high probability of these conditions for whom coronary angiography may be worthwhile.

BACKGROUND

Establishing the anatomic presence of coronary artery disease (CAD) has become increasingly important owing to the role of coronary artery bypass grafting (CABG) and percutaneous transluminal coronary angioplasty (PTCA) in the treatment of angina. However, angina or myocardial infarction (MI) may occur in the absence of angiographically proven obstructive coronary lesions and, conversely, coronary obstructions may be asymptomatic and thus have uncertain prognostic significance (1–4).

Some have suggested that a functional evaluation may be more predictive of future cardiac events than anatomy alone (5,6). Others suggest a probabilistic model as an alternative "gold standard"(7–9).

During the evaluation of patients in whom CAD is suspected, it is useful to distinguish high-risk patients who are likely to benefit from aggressive intervention. Anatomically significant left-main CAD (LMCAD) is a widely accepted indication for surgical intervention. Patients with significant three-vessel CAD and left ventricular dysfunction also benefit from coronary artery bypass grafting with improved survival (10–13). Among patients with preserved left ventricular function, those with either two- or three-vessel CAD and proximal left anterior descending artery involvement represent another high-risk subset (14). Conversely, the Coronary Artery Surgery Study (CASS) showed that patients who had mild stable angina or who were asymptomatic after an MI without LMCAD had excellent survival rates with medical therapy (10).

ESTIMATING PRETEST PROBABILITY

The probability of a patient having angiographic CAD can be predicted from clinical data including the patient's age and sex, chest pain symptoms, history of previous MI, and the presence of pathologic Q-waves on the resting ECG (4,11,15–19). The best clinical predictor of angiographic CAD is the character of the patient's chest pain (18). Coronary symptoms can be reliably categorized using three clinical questions (20):

1. Is the patient's chest discomfort substernal?
2. Are the patient's symptoms precipitated by exertion?
3. Does the patient experience prompt (i.e., within 10 minutes) relief with rest or nitroglycerin?

If the patient's symptoms are embraced by all three of these clinical features, the symptoms can be categorized as "typical angina"; having any two of these features suggests "atypical angina"; and if the patient has only one or none of these features, the chest pain is considered nonanginal. Table 5-1 illustrates that the patient's age, sex, and symptom category can define marked differences in the probability of significant CAD, assuming average levels of risk factors (17,21). Integrating data from additional cardiovascular risk factors yields similar results (18,19) but does not significantly refine probabilities of CAD for individual patients (22).

Although increasing or older age, the presence of typical anginal pain, sex (male), and diabetes mellitus have statistically significant correlations with the presence of LMCAD or three-vessel disease

Table 5-1. Pretest Probability of Coronary Artery Disease According to Age, Sex, and Character of Symptoms

Age	Asymptomatic		Nonanginal Chest Pain		Atypical Angina		Typical Angina	
	Men	Women	Men	Women	Men	Women	Men	Women
y	←			%				→
30–39	1.9	0.3	5.2	0.8	21.8	4.2	69.7	25.8
40–49	5.5	1.0	14.1	2.8	46.1	13.3	87.3	55.2
50–59	9.7	3.2	21.5	8.4	58.9	32.4	92.0	79.4
60–69	12.3	7.5	28.1	18.6	67.1	54.4	94.3	90.6

Adapted from Diamond GA, Forrester JS. Analysis of probability as an aid in the clinical diagnosis of coronary artery disease. N Engl J Med. 1979;300:1350-8.

(8,23–25), few, if any, clinical characteristics accurately distinguish patients with left main or three-vessel CAD from those with other forms of CAD (23).

The pretest probability of CAD also varies with the clinical setting; the likelihood of significant disease is much lower in primary care settings than in referral settings (26).

DIAGNOSTIC TESTS

Exercise Electrocardiography

Although exercise testing may be performed for a variety of indications, it is commonly used in the diagnosis of CAD (27,28). The sensitivity and specificity of the exercise test have most often been characterized for ST-segment depression that may occur during exercise-induced myocardial ischemia. Table 5-2 summarizes "average" operating characteristics for different degrees of ST-segment depression (16). Accuracy in identifying CAD is lower in women (29), primarily owing to lower specificity.

Several factors other than ischemia may cause ST changes on exercise ECG and thus reduce its specificity. These include hyperventilation, mitral valve prolapse, left ventricular hypertrophy, left-sided intraventricular conduction delays, Wolff-Parkinson-White syndrome, digoxin, tricyclic antidepressants, abnormalties detected on resting ECG, and vasoregulatory abnormalities (30). Sensitivity decreases if patients are unable to reach 85% of their maximum predicted heart rates, as can occur with beta-blocker therapy.

Recent work has shown that response to exercise may provide information related to prognostic assessment (11). Exercise test find-

Table 5-2. Operating Characteristics of Exercise Electrocardiography for Angiographic Coronary Artery Disease

ST-Segment Depression	Sensitivity*	Specificity*	Likelihood Ratio for Result†
mm	←	% ——→	
<0.5			0.23
0.5–0.99	86	77	0.92
1.0–1.49	65	89	2.1
1.5–1.99	42	98	4.2
2.0–2.49	33	99	11
≥2.5	20	>99	39

Adapted from Diamond GA, Forrester JS. Analysis of probability as an aid in the clinical diagnosis of coronary artery disease. N Engl J Med. 1979;300:1350-8.

*Sensitivity and specificity are calculated for cutoff values greater than or equal to the indicated ranges.

†Likelihood ratios apply only to values within the specified ranges.

ings including marked ST-segment depression of 2.0 mm or greater, exertional hypotension, and diminished exercise capacity have been reported to be relatively specific, but not sensitive, for high-risk coronary anatomies such as LMCAD (23,31–33). Computer-based ECG analysis and multivariate models incorporating exercise data (29,34–43) may improve the diagnostic and prognostic value of exercise ECG compared with conventional analyses using ST-segment changes.

Exercise Myocardial Perfusion Imaging

Myocardial perfusion imaging (MPI) using planar or single photon emission computed tomographic (SPECT) cameras allows comparison of images obtained at rest and during stress. The hallmark of myocardial ischemia is a relative deficit in perfusion during exercise, indicated by an area of diminished tracer uptake, that fills in during a 3- to 5-hour period of recovery. Generally, arterial stenoses ranging from 50% to 85% produce normal MPI images during rest, with stress defects corresponding to ischemic regions supplied by stenosed arteries (15). Although this classic "reversible" perfusion defect has the greatest specificity for CAD, other patterns of abnormalities may occur, including irreversible defects suggestive of previous myocardial injury.

The capacity for three-dimensional visualization and artifact reduction make SPECT more sensitive, although less specific, than planar MPI (14,15). The accuracy of MPI has been further enhanced by the development of computerized quantitative analysis and attenuation correction methods.

The value of MPI in detecting CAD and in prognostic assessment has been well established (44–52). The sensitivity and specificity of exercise SPECT imaging in diagnosing CAD are approximately 90% and 72%, respectively (Table 5-3). However, operating characteristics vary across studies, depending on demographic and methodologic factors such as the proportion of patients with previous infarctions, the percentage of men, the extent of blinding of the interpretations, and the presence of workup bias (53). The number of perfusion defects and the finding of increased pulmonary uptake can be used to estimate the risk of future cardiac events (54).

Although the contrast agent thallium-201 has a longer history of use with MPI, technetium-99m sestamibi (MIBI) confers the advantages of attenuation reduction and left ventricular function assessment. Generally, the two agents are interchangeable in most clinical situations (55).

Exercise Echocardiography

Exercise echocardiography (ECHO) provides comparison of digitized images obtained at rest and during or immediately after exercise and allows imaging of left ventricular chamber size, wall thickness, and motion (15). Qualitative comparison of rest and stress wall motion is used to identify ischemic myocardium, characterized by deterioration of function with stress. Infarction may be identified if a segment is akinetic or dyskinetic at rest. The severity, time of onset, and duration of stress-induced wall motion abnormalities are indicative of the severity of CAD (56).

The limitations of ECHO include the high level of operator and interpreter dependence and difficulties in obtaining adequate windows for viewing all left ventricular walls (57). The rate for nondiagnostic studies ranges from 5% to 10% (15). It is especially difficult to obtain adequate images in patients with lung disease, large body size, or chest wall abnormalities. Training and expertise in acquiring and interpreting images are critical (58).

Pharmacologic Stress Imaging

Pharmacologic stress imaging has been increasingly used in patients who are unable to perform adequate exercise (59). Commonly used agents include the vasodilator, dipyridamole (60), and the beta-sympathomimetic agonist, dobutamine (61). Studies have generally used intravenous dipyridamole, but oral administration results in fewer side effects with minimal changes in operating characteristics (see Table 5-3). Because dobutamine provokes a greater cardiac workload than the vasodilators, it is the predominant agent for stress ECHO (56,62).

Comparison of Common Noninvasive Tests

The advantages of stress imaging modalities compared with exercise ECG include greater accuracy in patients in whom resting ECG or med-

Table 5-3. Operating Characteristics of Common Diagnostic Tests for Angiographic Coronary Artery Disease

Diagnostic Test	Definition of Positive Result	Sensitivity	Specificity	Likelihood Ratio	
				Positive Result	Negative Result
		←——— % ———→			
Exercise ECG	ST-segment depression ≥0.5 mm	86	77	3.7	0.18
	ST-segment depression ≥1.0 mm	65	89	5.9	0.39
Exercise MPI (planar)*	Stress-induced perfusion defect	88	91	9.7	0.13
Exercise MPI (SPECT)	Stress-induced perfusion defect	90	72	3.2	0.14
Pharmacologic MPI (SPECT)	Stress-induced perfusion defect				
Adenosine		89	83	5.2	0.13
Oral dipyridamole		87	75	3.5	0.17
Intravenous dipyridamole		90	78	4.1	0.13
Dobutamine		91	86	6.5	0.10
Exercise ECHO	Stress-induced wall motion deterioration	81	89	7.4	0.21
Dobutamine ECHO	Stress-induced wall motion deterioration	81	83	4.8	0.23

Adapted from O'Keefe JH Jr, Barnhart CS, Bateman TM. Comparison of stress echocardiography and stress myocardial perfusion scintigraphy for diagnosing coronary artery disease and assessing its severity. Am J Cardiol 1995;75:25D-34D.

*Based on studies of thallium-201 only.

ECG = electrocardiography; ECHO = echocardiography; MPI = myocardial perfusion imaging; SPECT = single photon emission computed tomography.

ications make ST-segment analysis unreliable, the ability to localize and estimate the extent of myocardial ischemia, and higher test sensitivity (54). Imaging results are relatively independent of the ECG result and can therefore be applied serially according to Bayesian probability analysis (50,63–66). Some data suggest that stress ECHO is superior to exercise ECG as an initial noninvasive test for women and is a reasonable primary test for patients with uninterpretable ST segments (56,67–69).

The disadvantages of imaging modalities include their relatively limited availability, their greater expense, and their potential for logistic difficulties. Perfusion imaging, in particular, is expensive and time-intensive. Interobserver variability in the subjective interpretation of the images constitutes a serious drawback, especially in borderline cases (15).

Studies directly comparing stress ECHO with stress SPECT show higher overall sensitivity for SPECT in detecting any CAD (83%–96% compared with 73%–85%) and higher specificity for ECHO (64%–83% for SPECT compared with 83%–90% for ECHO) (70,71). A recent meta-analysis of studies published since 1990 showed ECHO to have better specificity than SPECT after adjusting for age, publication year, and inclusion of patients with known CAD (72). ECHO has not been as extensively validated as SPECT MPI for prognostic assessment and is less sensitive in the detection of single vessel disease (54,56,73). Stress SPECT appears superior in the correct identification of multivessel CAD and accurate localization of ischemia (70).

The findings from studies of the sensitivity and specificity of common noninvasive test modalities in detecting angiographic CAD are summarized in Table 5-3. In addition to cost and logistic considerations, selection of an imaging modality should be based on the availability of local expertise, specific information needed for clinical management, and selected patient characteristics (74,75).

Selective Coronary Angiography

Selective coronary angiography remains the "gold standard" for assessing the presence of CAD. However, even the "gold standard" is somewhat tarnished by nonuniform definitions of "significant" CAD, interobserver variability in interpretation (76), and the focus on anatomic structures rather than on physiologic function (77). Intra- and interobserver variability is particularly high and physiologic significance uncertain for midrange (25%–75% luminal diameter narrowing) stenoses (15,70). Some studies suggest that certain noninvasive tests may be better than coronary angiography as long-term predictors of cardiac events (5,73). In response to these widely recognized limitations, new coronary imaging techniques are under development (78).

DIAGNOSTIC STRATEGIES

The first step in diagnosis is to determine the pretest probability of CAD by deciding whether the patient is asymptomatic or whether symptoms are nonanginal, those of atypical angina, or those of typical angina. If the pretest probability is very low (<10%) or very high (>90%), noninvasive testing should usually be avoided, because neither a positive nor a negative test result will adequately change the probability of CAD.

In patients with pretest probabilities greater than 10% and less than 90%, noninvasive testing can lead to a meaningful revision of the probability of CAD (Table 5-4). A single test—for example, exercise ECG—is logical in most patients as a first step. Serial testing, usually with MPI or ECHO, is reasonable if the post-test probability remains at an intermediate level. Generally, if exercise ECG and imaging results are concordant, the diagnosis is fairly certain. In some of these patients—for example, those with resting ECGs showing abnormalities—imaging tests may be used for initial testing.

Currently no noninvasive method definitively excludes critical lesions among those with abnormal test results. Although models have been proposed to predict the probability of LMCAD, the threshold probability at which cardiac catheterization should be performed is set at a low level, given the relative safety of cardiac catheterization and the large benefit of surgery in patients with LMCAD (23). Decision analytic approaches suggest reserving cardiac catheterization for patients with ST-segment depression of 2 mm or more on exercise testing. However, the final decision must be left to the discretion of the individual physician and patient.

Table 5-4. Post-test Probabilities of Coronary Artery Disease Based on Results of Diagnostic Tests

Diagnostic Test	Pre-test Probability		
	20%	50%	80%
	←——————— % ———————→		
Exercise ECG result (ST-depression) (mm)			
<0.5	5	19	44
0.5–0.99	19	48	79
1.0–1.49	34	68	89
1.5–1.99	51	81	94
2.0–2.49	73	92	98
≥2.5	91	98	>99
MPI (SPECT)			
Positive result	44	76	93
Negative result	3	12	36
ECHO			
Positive result	66	88	97
Negative result	5	17	46

ECG = electrocardiography; MPI = myocardial perfusion imaging; SPECT = single photon emission computed tomography; ECHO = echocardiography.

CLINICAL PROBLEMS

Clinical Problem 1
A man aged 50 years or older has typical angina symptoms.

Testing Strategy and Rationale
Noninvasive cardiac testing is rarely necessary in men older than 50 years who have typical anginal symptoms, because the pretest probability of coronary artery disease in these patients is extremely high—that is, greater than 90%. This probability is high enough to justify treatment without a confirmatory test. Neither an exercise ECG nor imaging is sufficiently sensitive for a negative test result to rule out the disease. Therefore, neither positive nor negative test results contribute much to patient management decisions. A decision to recommend cardiac catheterization would depend not on making a diagnosis but on the extent to which the results of angiography would change treatment strategies.

Clinical Example
A 60-year-old man presents with substernal, exertion-induced chest discomfort relieved promptly by rest that is judged to be typical angina. As seen in Table 5-1, for a 60-year-old man with typical angina, the pretest probability of CAD at coronary angiography is 94%. An exercise ECG showing no abnormalities would reduce the probability of significant CAD to about 80%, a probability too high to justify exclusion of CAD. A negative SPECT scintigraphy test result would further reduce the probability of CAD in this patient to about 33%—again, a probability too high to exclude CAD. Therefore, noninvasive tests would not contribute to the exclusion or confirmation of the diagnosis of CAD in this patient.

Clinical Problem 2
A man aged 40 to 70 years or a woman aged 50 to 70 years has nonanginal chest pain.

Testing Strategy and Rationale
Noninvasive testing with exercise ECG or exercise imaging to rule out significant CAD may be appropriate, but there is a significant possibility of false-positive results. In patients in these age groups with nonanginal chest pain, the probability of CAD is relatively low but not sufficiently low to exclude the diagnosis. This probability can readily be estimated using Table 5-1. Noninvasive testing may lower the probability of significant CAD enough to exclude the diagnosis. The individual physician's threshold determines whether a single negative test result is sufficient to rule out CAD.

Continued

However, because a positive test result has a substantial chance of being a false positive, such a test result often requires additional investigation and may lead to coronary angiography in some patients without significant CAD.

Clinical Example
A 53-year-old man presents with a clinical history considered representative of nonanginal chest pain. The pain is left precordial rather than substernal, is not precipitated by exertion but is induced by emotion and stress, and has a typical duration of 30 minutes or more. During an exercise test, he exercises 12 minutes and 54 seconds on a Bruce protocol and has no chest pain or ECG changes. He then asks if additional tests should be done.

This 53-year-old man with nonanginal chest pain has about a 20% probability of significant CAD, according to Table 5-1. An exercise ECG showing abnormalities reduces the probability of his having significant CAD to approximately 5%. If further testing were ordered, a negative SPECT scintigraphy test result would reduce the probability of CAD to approximately 1%.

REFERENCES

1. **Dagenais GR, Rouleau JR, Christen A, Fabia J.** Survival of patients with a strongly positive exercise electrocardiogram. Circulation. 1982;65:452-6.
2. **McNeer JF, Margolis JR, Lee KL, et al.** The role of the exercise test in the evaluation of patients for ischemic heart disease. Circulation. 1978;57:64-70.
3. **Podrid PJ, Graboys TB, Lown B.** Prognosis of medically treated patients with coronary artery disease with profound ST-segment depression during exercise testing. N Engl J Med. 1981;305:1111-6.
4. **Fisher LD, Kennedy JW, Chaitman BR, et al.** Diagnostic quantification of CASS (Coronary Artery Surgery Study) clinical and exercise test results in determining presence and extent of coronary artery disease. A multivariate approach. Circulation. 1981;63:987-1000.
5. **Kaul S, Finkelstein DM, Homma S, et al.** Superiority of Quantitative exercise thallium-201 variables in determining long-term prognosis in ambulatory patients with chest pain: a comparison with cardiac catheterization. J Am Coll Cardiol. 1988;12:25-34.
6. **Wackers FJ, Russo DJ, Russo D, Clements JP.** Prognostic significance of normal quantitative planar thallium-201 stress scintigraphy in patients with chest pain. J Am Coll Cardiol. 1985;6:27-30.
7. **Diamond GA, Rozanski A, Forrester JS, et al.** A model for assessing the sensitivity and specificity of tests subject to selection bias: application to exercise radionuclide ventriculography for diagnosis of coronary artery disease. J Chron Dis. 1986;29:343-55.
8. **Pryor DB, Shaw L, Harrell FE, Jr, et al.** Estimating the likelihood of severe coronary artery disease. Am J Med. 1991;90:553-62.

9. **Pryor DB, Shaw L, McCants CB, et al.** Value of the history and physical in identifying patients at increased risk for coronary artery disease. Ann Intern Med. 1993;118:81-90.

10. **Passamani E, Davis KB, Gillespie MJ, Killip T, CASS Principal Investigators and their associates.** A randomized trial of coronary artery bypass surgery. Survival of patients with a low ejection fraction. N Engl J Med. 1985;312:1665-71.

11. **Pashkow FJ.** Diagnostic evaluation of the patient with coronary artery disease. Cleve Clin J Med. 1994;61:43-8.

12. **European Coronary Surgery Study Group.** Long-term results of prospective randomized study of coronary artery bypass surgery in stable angina pectoris. Lancet. 1982;2:1173-80.

13. **The Veterans Administration Coronary Artery Bypass Surgery Cooperative Study Group.** Eleven-year survival in the Veterans Administration randomized trial of coronary bypass surgery for stable angina. N Engl J Med. 1985;312:1665-71.

14. **Bonow RO, Bohannon N, Hazzard W.** Risk stratification in coronary artery disease and special populations. Am J Med. 1996;101:4A17S-22S.

15. **Patterson RE, Horowitz SF, Eisner RL.** Comparison of modalities to diagnose coronary artery disease. Semin Nucl Med. 1994;24:286-310.

16 **Diamond GA, Forrester JS.** Analysis of probability as an aid in the clinical diagnosis of coronary artery disease. N Engl J Med. 1979;300:1350-8.

17. **Diamond GA, Staniloff HM, Forrester JS, et al.** Computer assisted diagnosis in the noninvasive evaluation of patients with suspected coronary artery disease. J Am Coll Cardiol. 1983;1:444-55.

18. **Pryor DB, Harrell FE Jr, Lee KL, et al.** Estimating the likelihood of significant coronary artery disease. Am J Med. 1983;75:771-80.

19. **Goldman L, Cook EF, Mitchell N, et al.** Incremental value of the exercise test for diagnosing the presence or absence of coronary artery disease. Circulation. 1982;66:945-53.

20. **Diamond GA.** A clinically relevant classification of chest pain. J Am Coll Cardiol. 1983;1:574-5.

21. **Diamond GA.** Bayes' theorem: a practical aid to clinical judgment for diagnosis of coronary artery disease. Practical Cardiology. 1984;10:47-77.

22. **Vliestra RE, Frye RL, Kronmal RA, et al.** Risk factors and angiographic coronary artery disease: a report from the Coronary Artery Surgery Study (CASS). Circulation. 1980;62:254-61.

23. **Lee TH, Cook EF, Goldman L.** Prospective evaluation of a clinical and exercise-test model for the prediction of left main coronary artery disease. Med Decis Making. 1986;6:136-44.

24. **Hubbard BL, Gibbons RJ, Lapeyre AC, et al.** Identification of severe coronary artery disease using simple clinical parameters. Arch Intern Med. 1992;152:309-12.

25. **Conley MJ, Ely RL, Kisslo J, et al.** The prognostic spectrum of left main stenosis. Circulation. 1978;57:947-52.

26. **Sox HC Jr, Hickam DH, Marton KI, et al.** Using the patient's history to estimate the probability of coronary artery disease: a comparison of primary care and referral practices. Am J Med. 1990;89:7-14.

27. **Goldschlager N.** Use of the treadmill test in the diagnosis of coronary artery disease in patients with chest pain. Ann Intern Med. 1982;97:383-8.

28. **American College of Cardiology/American Heart Association Task Force on Assessment of Cardiovascular Procedures.** Guidelines for exercise testing. J Am Col Cardiol. 1986;8:725-38.

29. **Okin PM, Kligfield P.** Gender-specific criteria and performance of the exercise electrocardiogram. Circulation. 1995;92:1209-16.

30. **Friesinger GC, Biern RO, Likar I, Mason RE.** Exercise electrocardiography and vasoregulatory abnormalities. Am J Cardiol. 1972;30:733-40.

31. **Patterson RE, Horowitz SF, Eng C, et al.** Can noninvasive exercise test criteria identify patients with left main or three vessel coronary disease after a first myocardial infarction? Am J Cardiol. 1983;51:361-72.

32. **Evans CH, Karunaratne HB.** Exercise stress testing for the family physician: Part II. Interpretation of the results. Am Fam Physician. 1992;45:679-88.

33. **Morris CK, Ueshima K, Kawaguchi T, et al.** The prognostic value of exercise capacity: a review of the literature. Am Heart J. 1991;122:1423-31.

34. **Morise AP, Diamond GA, Detrano R, Bobbio M.** Incremental value of exercise electrocardiography and thallium-201 testing in men and women for the presence and extent of coronary artery disease. Am Heart J. 1995;130:267-76.

35. **Morise AP, Duval RD, Detrano R, et al.** Comparison of logistic regression and Bayesian-based algorithms to estimate post-test probability in patients with suspected coronary artery disease undergoing exercise ECG. J Electrocardiol. 1992;25:89-99.

36. **Peters RM, Shanies SA, Peters JC.** Fuzzy cluster analysis of positive stress tests, a new method of combining exercise test variables to predict extent of coronary artery disease. Am J Cardiol. 1995;76:648-51.

37. **Richardson MT, Holly RG, Amsterdam EA, Wang MQ.** The value of ten common exercise tolerance test measures in predicting coronary disease in symptomatic females. Cardiology. 1995;86:243-8.

38. **Okin PM, Kligfield P.** Heart rate adjustment of ST segment depression and performance of the exercise electrocardiogram: a critical evaluation. J Am Coll Cardiol. 1995;25:1726-35.

39. **Marcus R, Lowe R III, Froelicher VF, Do D.** The exercise test as gatekeeper. Limiting access or appropriately directing resources? Chest. 1995;107:1442-6.

40. **Deckers JW, Rensing BJ, Simoons ML, Roelandt JR.** Diagnostic merits of exercise testing in females. Eur Heart J. 1989;10:543-50.

41. **Robert A, Melin JA, Detry JMR.** Logistic discriminant analysis improves the diagnostic accuracy of exercise testing for coronary artery disease in women. Circulation. 1991;**83:**1202-9.

42. **Iskandrian AE, Ghods M, Helfeld H, Iskandrian B.** The Treadmill Exercise Score revisited: coronary arteriographic and thallium perfusion correlates. Am Heart J. 1992;124:1581-6.

43. **Yamada H, Do D, Morise A, et al.** Review of studies using multivariable analysis of clinical and exercise test data to predict angiographic coronary artery disease. Prog Cardiovasc Dis. 1997;39:457-81.

44. **Berman DS, Kiat H, Friedman JD, Diamond G.** Clinical applications of exercise nuclear cardiology studies in the era of healthcare reform. Am J Cardiol. 1995;75:3D-13D.

45. **Nallamothu N, Ghods M, Heo J, Iskandrian AS.** Comparison of thallium-201 single-photon emission computed tomography and electrocardiographic response during exercise in patients with normal rest electrocardiographic results. J Am Coll Cardiol. 1995;25:830-6.

46. **Pollock SG, Abbott RD, Boucher CA, et al.** Independent and incremental prognostic value of tests performed in hierarchical order to evaluate patients with suspected coronary artery disease. Validation of models based on these tests. Circulation. 1992;85:237-48.

47. **Beller GA.** Myocardial perfusion imaging with thallium-201. J Nucl Med. 1994;35:674-80.

48. **Mahmarian JJ, Verani MS.** Exercise thallium-201 perfusion scintigraphy in the assessment of coronary artery disease. Am J Cardiol. 1991;67:2D-11D.

49. **Brown KA.** Prognostic value of thallium-201 myocardial perfusion imaging. A diagnostic tool comes of age. Circulation. 1991;83:363-81.

50. **Hachamovitch R, Berman DS, Kiat H, et al.** Exercise myocardial perfusion SPECT in patients without known coronary artery disease: incremental prognostic value and use in risk stratification. Circulation. 1996;93:905-14.

51. **Nallamouthu N, Araujo L, Russell J, et al.** Prognostic value of simultaneous perfusion and function assessment using technetium-99m sestamibi. Am J Cardiol. 1996;78:562-4.

52. **Hachamovitch R, Berman DS, Kiat H, et al.** Effective risk stratification using exercise myocardial perfusion SPECT in women: gender-related differences in prognostic nuclear testing. J Am Coll Cardiol. 1996;28:34-44.

53. **Detrano R, Janosi A, Lyons KP, et al.** Factors affecting sensitivity and specificity of a diagnostic test: the exercise thallium scintigram. Am J Med. 1988;84:699-710.

54. **Allison T, Bardsley WT, Behrenbeck T, et al.** Subspecialty clinics: cardiology-cardiovascular stress testing: a description of the various types of stress tests and indications for their use. Mayo Clin Proc. 1996;71:43-52.

55. **Wackers FJ.** Comparison of thallium-201 and technetium-99m methoxyisobutyl isonitrile. Am J Cardiol. 1992;70:30E-34E.

56. **Marwick T.** Current status of stress echocardiography in the diagnosis of coronary artery disease. Cleve Clin J Med. 1995;62:227-34.

57. **Iliceto S, Galiuto L, Marangelli V, Rizzon P.** Clinical use of stress echocardiography: factors affecting diagnostic accuracy. Eur Heart J. 1994;15:672-80.

58. **Roger VL, Pellikka PA, Oh JK, et al.** Stress echocardiography. Part I. Exercise echocardiography: techniques, implementation, clinical applications, and correlations. Mayo Clin Proc. 1995;70:5-15.

59. **Beller GA.** Pharmacologic stress imaging. JAMA. 1991;265:633-8.

60. **Leppo JA.** Dipyridamole myocardial perfusion imaging. J Nucl Med. 1994;35:730-3.

61. **Gunalp B, Dokumaci B, Uyan C, et al.** Value of dobutamine technetium-99m-sestamibi SPECT and echocardiography in the detection of coronary artery disease compared with coronary angiography. J Nucl Med. 1993;34:889-94.

62. **Madu EC, Ahmar W, Arthur J, Fraker TD Jr.** Clinical utility of digital dobutamine stress echocardiography in the noninvasive evaluation of coronary artery disease. Arch Intern Med. 1994;154:1065-72.

63. **Epstein SE.** Implications of probability analysis on the strategy used for noninvasive detection of coronary artery disease. Am J Cardiol. 1980;46:491-9.

64. **Detrano R, Yiannikas J, Salcedo EE, et al.** Bayesian probability analysis: a prospective demonstration of its clinical utility in diagnosing coronary disease. Circulation. 1984;69:541-7.

65. **Patterson RE, Eng C, Horowitz SF.** Practical diagnosis of coronary artery disease: a Bayes theorem nomogram to correlate clinical data with noninvasive exercise tests. Am J Cardiol. 1984;53:252-6.

66. **Rifkin RD, Hood WB Jr.** Bayesian analysis of electrocardiographic stress testing. N Engl J Med. 1977;297:681-6.

67. **Williams MJ, Marwick TH, O'Gorman D, Foale RA.** Comparison of exercise echocardiography with an exercise score to diagnose coronary artery disease in women. Am J Cardiol. 1994;74:435-8.

68. **Marwick TH, Anderson T, Williams MJ, et al.** Exercise echocardiography is an accurate and cost-efficient technique for detection of coronary artery disease in women. J Am Coll Cardiol. 1995;26:335-41.

69. **Crouse LJ, Kramer PH.** Are there gender differences related to stress of pharmacological echocardiography? Am J Cardiac Imaging. 1996;10:65-71.

70. **O'Keefe JH Jr, Barnhart CS, Bateman TM.** Comparison of stress echocardiography and stress myocardial perfusion scintigraphy for diagnosing coronary artery disease and assessing its severity. Am J Cardiol. 1995;75:25D-34D.

71. **Kisacik HL, Ozdemir K, Altinyay E, et al.** Comparison of exercise stress testing with simultaneous dobutamine stress echocardiography and technetium-99m isonitrile single-photon emission computerized tomography for diagnosis of coronary artery disease. Eur Heart J. 1996;17:113-9.

72. **Fleischmann KE, Hunink MG, Kuntz KM, Douglas PS.** Exercise echocardiography or exercise SPECT imaging: a meta-analysis of diagnostic test performance. JAMA. 1998;280:913-20.

73. **Brown KA.** Prognostic value of cardiac imaging in patients with known or suspected coronary artery disease: comparison of myocardial perfusion imaging, stress echocardiography, and position emission tomography. Am J Cardiol. 1995;75:35D-41D.

74. **Botvinick EH.** Stress imaging. Current clinical options for the diagnosis, localization, and evaluation of coronary artery disease. Med Clin North Am. 1995;79:1025-61.

75. **Kaul S.** Technical, economic, interpretative, and outcomes issues regarding utilization of cardiac imaging techniques in patients with known or suspected coronary artery disease. Am J Cardiol. 1995;75:18D-24D.

76. **Detre KM, Wright E, Murphy ML, Takaro T.** Observer agreement in evaluating coronary arteriography. Circulation. 1975;52:979.

77. **Topol EJ, Nissen SE.** Our preoccupation with coronary luminology. The dissociation between clinical and angiographic findings in ischemic heart disease. Circulation. 1995;92:2333-42.

78. **De Man F, De Scheerder I, Herregods MC, et al.** Role of intravascular ultrasound in coronary artery disease: a new gold standard? An overview. Acta Cardiol. 1994;49:223-31.

Myocardial Infarction　　　　　6

J. Thompson Sullebarger, MD, and Donald R. Bordley, MD

KEY POINTS

Pretest Probabilities

- In most hospitals, approximately 15% of patients who are admitted to the emergency room for evaluation of acute chest pain have an acute myocardial infarction (MI).

- Of patients admitted to coronary care units with acute chest pain, 30% to 50% have acute MI.

- Clinical data are helpful in distinguishing patients with ischemic pain from those with nonischemic pain, but diagnostic tests are required to determine which patients with probable ischemic pain have an infarction.

Diagnostic Strategies

- Patients presenting with chest pain can be divided into high- and low-risk groups based on a careful history, physical examination, and electrocardiography. Initial management decisions can be based on these data.

- Cardiac troponin I (cTn-I) has become the enzyme test of choice to confirm or exclude MI. This test is as sensitive for acute MI as serial creatine kinase, MB isoenzyme (CK-MB) testing for patients presenting within 24 hours of symptom onset and is more sensitive for those who present after 24 hours. Specificity of cTn-I is at least equivalent to that of CK-MB and is superior in patients with skeletal muscle injury and renal failure.

- Serial CK-MB testing has excellent sensitivity and specificity for acute MI in most patients and remains the test of choice where cardiac troponin I is not available.

- In patients in whom onset of chest pain occurred more than 24 hours before presentation, cTn I is the test of choice for MI. If this test is unavailable, a single set of lactate dehydrogenase isoenzymes may aid in the diagnosis.

Continued

> **Risk Stratification**
> - Risk stratification of patients after infarction should include studies for myocardial ischemia and for ventricular dysfunction.
> - Patients who have had infarction who have left ventricular dysfunction, recurrent ischemia, or high-grade arrhythmias are at increased risk for complications.

BACKGROUND

In most hospitals, the prevalence of myocardial infarction (MI) among patients coming to an emergency room with acute chest pain is about 15%. Studies have demonstrated that after evaluation in the emergency room, approximately 30% to 50% of patients admitted to coronary care units for acute chest pain have an acute infarct (1,2). Because the management of these patients involves a significant use of medical resources, strategies to improve early risk stratification are highly desirable to help decide which patients to admit to a coronary care unit. Recent studies suggest that a Bayesian approach to the diagnosis of infarction may help improve diagnostic accuracy and reduce unnecessary coronary care unit admissions and associated costs (1,2).

The diagnosis of MI has traditionally been based on the 1959 World Health Organization criteria of chest pain, the presence of Q waves on electrocardiography, and elevations of serum enzymes. Experience has shown that the use of these criteria leads to both over- and under-diagnosis of infarction (3). Myocardial infarction may present atypically or may be detected incidentally after the acute event (4). In earlier autopsy studies, investigators found that as few as 44% of patients dying of infarction were correctly diagnosed before death (5,6).

Recently, the advent of thrombolytic therapy and coronary angioplasty has allowed more aggressive early management of patients with acute MI. Early intervention to achieve reopening of the infarct-related artery within the first few hours after the onset of chest pain has been shown to improve myocardial function and reduce mortality in selected patients (7). This makes accurate and early diagnosis particularly important because outcomes are better when treatment begins early. The purpose of this chapter is to provide a systematic approach to the diagnosis and management of patients presenting with acute chest pain and possible MI.

ESTIMATING PRETEST PROBABILITY

Although patients with MI may present atypically, elements of the history and physical examination can be useful in distinguishing patients with infarction from those without infarction. The hallmark of myocardial ischemia is discomfort, usually involving the central chest, and often described as a dull sensation of pressure. Previous episodes of similar discomfort, especially if precipitated by exertion, may suggest a previous history of angina. The patient's age, sex, and any previous history of coronary disease, as well as risk factors for atherosclerosis such as smoking, a family history of coronary disease, hypertension, diabetes, and hypercholesterolemia all affect the pretest probability of coronary artery disease (see Chapter 5). Goldman and colleagues (8) found that the patient's age, the timing and duration of the pain, radiation of the pain, associated diaphoresis, previous history of coronary disease, and chest wall tenderness were all significant in distinguishing patients with infarction from those presenting with chest pain. In another study by the same group (9), sharp or stabbing pain, pleuritic or positional pain, absence of previous history of coronary disease, and chest wall tenderness all suggested lower probabilities of infarction. However, although patients with atypical symptoms are less likely to have infarction, those who do are at higher risk for complications than patients who present typically (10). Care should be taken not to dismiss the patient on the basis of atypical presentation alone.

Pozen and colleagues (1) found that the use of a multivariate index using clinical and electrocardiographic criteria helped distinguish ischemic from nonischemic chest pain. Goldman and Lee (11) have described how initial clinical and electrocardiographic information can

Table 6-1. Approximate Probability of Myocardial Infarction Based on Clinical and Electrocardiographic Findings*

Finding	Estimated Probability of MI (%)
New Q waves or ST-segment elevation on ECG suggesting acute MI	80
New ST-segment depression or T-wave inversion suggesting ischemia or strain on ECG	20
No new ECG changes but	
History of MI	15
Pain worse than patient's chronic angina	15
Pain similar to patient's previous MI	15
Pain not worse than patient's chronic angina	5
Pain unlike patient's previous MI	5
Neither new ECG changes nor history of angina or MI	3

Adapted from Goldman L, Lee TH. Chest pain: infarction or not? Acute Care Med. 1975;2:11-8.
*For emergency department setting, where pretest probability of MI is about 15% for patients with a chief symptom of chest pain.
ECG = electrocardiography; MI = myocardial infarction.

be combined to estimate the probability of infarction among patients with chest pain (Table 6-1).

In addition to the character of the pain, other clinical information may help guide decision making for patients in whom infarction is suspected. Fuchs and Scheidt (12) found that most interventions occur in patients with MI who have unrelieved pain, pulmonary rales, or extrasystoles. Gheorgiade and colleagues (13) defined a high-risk group of patients with evidence of heart failure (i.e., Killip Class II or greater, previous history of heart failure, pulmonary rales, jugular venous distention, or S3 gallop) or with hemodynamic compromise (i.e., shock, hypotension, syncope, or coma). Because these patients are at a high risk for life-threatening complications and death, they should be admitted to a coronary care unit. Patients with a normal resting electrocardiogram (ECG) who do not have these risk factors may be candidates for evaluation in a short-stay unit (14).

Table 6-2. Approximate Operating Characteristics of the Most Useful Laboratory Tests for the Diagnosis of Myocardial Infarction

Diagnostic Test	Sensitivity	Specificity	Likelihood Ratio	
			Positive Result	Negative Result
	← % →			
ECG				
New Q waves or new ST-segment elevation	68	94	11	0.34
Any abnormality found on ECG	99	23	1.3	0.04
Enzyme testing (first 24 hours after symptom onset)				
Serial CK-MB testing	99	98	50	0.01
Cardiac troponin I testing (>9 hours after symptom onset)	95	98	47	0.03
Enzyme testing (>24 hours after symptom onset)				
Cardiac troponin I testing	95	98	47	0.03
LD isoenzyme "flip"	81	94	14	0.20
CK-MB testing	55	97	18	0.46

ECG = electrocardiography; CK-MB = creatine kinase, MB isoenzyme.

DIAGNOSTIC TESTS

Electrocardiography

Electrocardiography can be a highly specific test for the early diagnosis of MI (15). The presence of new Q waves has a specificity of 94% (Table 6-2), and in patients presenting with acute chest pain associated with new Q waves or ST elevation, the probability of MI is significantly increased (9,15). However, overall sensitivity of new Q waves in MI is less than 70%, and in one study, only 40% of subendocardial MIs were associated with new Q waves (16). Furthermore, Q waves may not be present early in the course of even a large infarction. In another study, only 29% of patients presenting to the emergency room with infarction had ST elevation (17); and of those with ST elevation, 51% did not have infarction. Left ventricular hypertrophy and left bundle-branch block were the most common noninfarction causes of ST elevation. Patients with acute infarction may also present with ST-segment depression, T wave changes, or bundle-branch block, but these findings have very low specificity (9,18). In the group of patients with these findings, infarction is more likely when more ECG leads are involved or when ST-segment depression is large (18). In patients with pre-existing left bundle-branch block, the ECG diagnosis of ischemia and infarction may be difficult. However, deflection of the J point or ST segment in the direction of the QRS vector, or a finding of at least 5 to 7 mm of ST-segment deflection opposite to the QRS complex may suggest infarction (19,20).

The ECG is also helpful in defining patients with acute chest pain who are at high risk compared with those at low risk for life-threatening complications, independent of the diagnosis of infarction. A normal ECG is highly suggestive of low risk (9,21), whereas increased risk has been associated with the presence of ST-T changes (8,13,22,23), Q waves (8,13,23), left ventricular hypertrophy (22), left bundle-branch block (13,22,23), or paced rhythm (22). Patients with "reciprocal" ECG changes have more angina, exercise tests showing abnormalities, and recurrent infarcts at 6 months after infarction (24), and patients with non–Q wave MIs have recurrent MI more frequently than patients with Q-wave infarctions (25,26). In non–Q wave MI, recent studies suggest that patients with T wave inversion alone have an 80% likelihood of single-vessel disease, whereas those with ST-segment depression tend to have multi-vessel disease (27).

Serum Enzymes

Creatine Kinase

Creatine kinase (CK) is an enzyme found predominantly in myocardial and skeletal muscle, with smaller amounts present in the brain, kidneys, gastrointestinal tract, and spleen (15). Enzyme levels increase at 4 to 8 hours after acute myocardial injury, peak at 12 to 24 hours, and return to normal within 3 days. Creatine kinase has three isoenzymes: CK-MM, CK-BB, and CK-MB. Under normal circumstances, only myocardium has significant amounts of MB isoenzyme (28). However, elevated skeletal muscle MB content may be present in patients with Duchenne dystrophy, myasthenia gravis, and polymyositis (29). Neither intramuscular injection nor cardiac catheterization is associated with significant changes in CK-MB (30,31). Although electrical countershock may increase total serum CK levels, CK-MB levels do not increase unless associated myocardial injury is present (32). False-positive CK-MB test results may also occur when there are large elevations of total CK caused by spillover of the MM band into the zone of the MB band. This artifact can be eliminated by repeating the test after diluting the specimen (33,34).

The value of single CK determinations in decision making is limited. Among all patients with acute chest pain, the sensitivity and specificity of a single total CK measurement are only 38% and 80%, respectively, and of a single CK-MB measurement, only 34% and 88%, respectively. Single measurements are more sensitive after 4 or more hours of pain. Serial CK-MB testing is much more useful, with a sensitivity and specificity of about 99% and 98%, respectively, if used in patients who have had chest pain for less than 24 hours (see Table 6-2) (15,35). Serial CK-MB testing has optimal sensitivity and specificity when three specimens are drawn at 12-hour intervals (15). However, recently some investigators have suggested drawing four specimens at 1-hour intervals for rapid diagnosis (35–37). Although this approach improves sensitivity and specificity somewhat over a single determination and may allow an earlier diagnosis, it is still not sufficiently sensitive to rule out the diagnosis of an infarction.

The interpretation of abnormal CK-MB levels in the presence of normal total CK levels is often unclear. In one study, 16% of patients with elevated CK-MB levels had normal total CK levels. This subgroup had fewer ECG changes and LD isoenzyme "flips" (see discussion in the following section) but in some cases were found to have MI (38). In another study, 65% of patients with elevated MB but normal CK levels had two or more clinical criteria for MI, and 77% had ST-T changes (39). On the other hand, another group reported five cases of positive CK-MB with negative myoglobin as well as no clinical evidence of MI (29).

Recently, a rapid assay for the measurement of CK-MB mass (rather than for the measurement of enzyme activity) has been developed. A single measurement more than 4 hours after the onset of chest pain is more sensitive than single CK or CK-MB activity measurements for the diagnosis of MI (40). However, although it is a modest improvement over the established activity assays, it is probably not sensitive enough (45% sensitivity) for the rapid early exclusion of MI (41,42). Another recently developed assay measures specific isoforms of CK-MB. The advantage of this assay is that certain MB isoforms are completely absent in skeletal muscle (43). CK-MB isoform measurement is highly sensitive (96% sensitivity) and specific (94% specificity) for infarction (44). Its most useful application may be in the diagnosis of MI when associated with skeletal muscle injury from trauma or surgery. However, cTn-I (see discussion in the following section) is also useful in these settings.

Cardiac Troponins

The troponin complex is an important muscular regulatory protein that includes three subunits: an inhibitory subunit, troponin I; a tropomyosin-binding subunit, troponin T; and a calcium-binding subunit, troponin C. Cardiac isoforms of these subunits can be identified by specific immunoassays and can thus be differentiated from skeletal isoforms.

Cardiac troponin I (cTn-I) has emerged as the most useful troponin for the diagnosis of infarction. In comparative studies of patients with chest pain or acute infarction or both (45–49), the sensitivity of cTn-I testing compares favorably with that of CK-MB testing (see Table 6-2). Sensitivity is less than 50% during the first 6 hours after symptom onset, but after 9 to 12 hours, it approaches 95%. A clear advantage of cTn-I over CK-MB testing is apparent in patients who have had symptoms for more than 24 hours. The sensitivity of cTn-I remains over 90% for at least 72 to 96 hours after symptom onset, whereas that of CK-MB falls off rapidly after 24 hours (47,49). Specificity of cTn-I for infarction exceeds 95% and is superior to that of CK-MB for some populations, including those with severe skeletal muscle injury and renal failure.

Cardiac troponin T (cTn-T) is highly sensitive for infarction and may become elevated earlier than both cTn-I and CK-MB (48,50). However, because cTn-T is less specific for myocardium, the risk of false positives limits its usefulness (42).

Myoglobin

Myoglobin is the major oxygen-transporting protein of muscle, and it can be detected in the blood as early as 90 minutes after myocardial injury (51), peaking at 6 to 7 hours after onset of chest pain (52). Of all the currently available assays, measurement of myoglobin yields positive test results the earliest in patients with MI and has a sensitivity of almost 90% 2 to 4 hours after the onset of symptoms (41,48,53). The relatively early increase in serum myoglobin associated with infarction may make single values useful for early decision making (45). However, the assay is not specific for myocardium and may be elevated in the presence of skeletal muscle injury or chronic renal insufficiency.

Lactate Dehydrogenase

Lactate dehydrogenase is a tetrameric enzyme with various combinations of heart (H) and muscle (M) subunits found in five different isoenzymes throughout the body (54). Enzyme levels increase at 8 to 12 hours after myocardial injury, peak at 3 to 6 days, and return to normal after 8 to 14 days. The relatively prolonged elevation of this enzyme level after MI makes it useful in the diagnosis of MI in patients who present more than 24 hours after the episode of chest pain, when other enzymes may have returned to normal. The isoenzymes LD-1 and LD-2 predominate in heart muscle, with greater amounts of LD-1. Because serum LD-2 is usually greater than LD-1, a reversal of this ratio, the so-called LD isoenzyme "flip," may be seen in patients with MI (55). The pattern of erythrocyte LD isoenzymes is similar to that seen in myocardium, and therefore a common cause of false-positive results is hemolysis. False-positive results may also be seen in pregnant women and in patients with myopathy. Where cTn-I is available, it is the preferred test for the late diagnosis of infarction because of its superior sensitivity and specificity (56).

Nuclear Scanning

Perfusion Imaging

Thallium-201 is a heavy metal that is actively taken up by viable myocardial cells. Technetium-99m sestamibi is a nonspecific marker of myocardial perfusion. Scintigraphy using either agent may show a myocardial perfusion abnormality during the first 24 hours after MI, especially if the injury is transmural (57–59). Sestamibi scanning is particularly attractive because the label has a long half-life and because scanning may be performed even hours after the resolution of chest pain, provided that the injection of isotope is given in the acute setting. However, a perfusion abnormality may be absent in cases of spontaneous reperfusion or may be present owing to previous infarction.

Pyrophosphate Scan

Technetium-99m pyrophosphate (TcPP) binds to areas of infarcted myocardium. TcPP uptake depends on the local blood flow, the myocardial calcium content, the degree of myocardial injury, and how much time has elapsed since the infarction. When local blood flow is reduced to 20% to 40% of normal, imaging is optimal. A TcPP scan can detect infarcted myocardium after as much as 5 days (60,61), making this a potentially useful test for patients who present days after the episode of chest pain. False-positive results have been reported that have been caused by the presence of valvular calcium, aneurysms, cardioversion, contusion, and metastases (61). In addition, positive results have been reported in patients with unstable angina without other clinical evidence of infarction (61). The sensitivity and specificity of TcPP scanning depends on whether diffuse, regional, or high-grade regional abnormalities are accepted as diagnostic (60). If diffuse patterns are accepted as positive, sensitivity approaches 94% for transmural infarction but the test has a specificity of only approximately 70%. If only high-grade regional uptake is accepted, specificity is nearly 100% but sensitivity is only about 35%. The difficulties of interpretation, as well as improvements in echocardiography and nuclear perfusion imaging, have led many centers to abandon pyrophosphate scanning.

Radionuclide Angiocardiography (MUGA Scan)
Technetium-99m–radiolabeled blood cell scanning may identify a regional wall motion abnormality in patients with acute chest pain, but in most cases this information may be obtained more rapidly and less expensively by echocardiography. This technique is more commonly used in the evaluation of patients after MI.

Echocardiography
Two-dimensional echocardiography may be used to obtain information about valvular function and global left ventricular function and may detect regional abnormalities of wall motion and thickening associated with ischemia or infarction, but it cannot distinguish between the two (62). However, if echocardiography does not detect a wall motion abnormality, this suggests low risk of life-threatening complications (63).

DIAGNOSTIC STRATEGIES
Patients presenting with acute chest pain and possible MI can be divided into groups according to the probability of infarction and risk from infarction based on the clinical and electrocardiographic data described in the "Estimating Pretest Probability" section. Early clinical decision making, such as whether to admit the patient to a cardiac care unit or whether to use thrombolytic therapy or direct angioplasty, should be based upon these data because other testing may significantly delay appropriate treatment. When in doubt, a serum myoglobin measurement, cTn-T measurement, or immediate echocardiography may aid in risk stratification. Patients with atypical symptoms and a normal or nondiagnostic ECG have a low probability of infarction and are at low risk even if they have an MI. These patients need not be admitted to a coronary care unit, and in many cases, they may be candidates for early or even immediate stress testing. In patients with typical ischemic chest pain and ECG changes, the probability of infarction and complications is higher, and such patients should be admitted to special care units.

Cardiac troponin I testing done more than 9 to 12 hours after the onset of symptoms should be sufficient to rule out or establish a diagnosis of MI. Three sets of serial CK-MB determinations done at 12-hour intervals appear equally effective in most patients. Cardiac troponin I testing is particularly useful in patients with skeletal muscle injury or renal failure or after surgery because of its superior specificity. Myoglobin and cTn-T assays are the tests that yield the earliest positive results after infarction, but the specificity of these tests is poor. Patients presenting with chest pain more than 24 hours after the onset of symptoms may be presenting too late for serial CK-MB testing to be diagnostic. Cardiac troponin I testing, however, yields positive results for 72 to 96 hours after infarction and, where available, is the test of choice in these patients. If cTn-I testing is unavailable, a single set of LD isoenzyme measurements may aid in diagnosis. In most cases this will be sufficient to make the diagnosis. When enzyme testing is nondiagnostic in patients presenting more than 24 hours after the onset of pain, perfusion imaging or a wall motion study using either echocardiography or radionuclide angiocardiography may be helpful in establishing the diagnosis of MI.

Post–Myocardial Infarction Risk Stratification

The most important predictors of risk after MI are recurrent ischemia and ventricular dysfunction (64). Tests capable of detecting residual ischemia and assessing functional capacity and ventricular function give valuable prognostic information. Information about many of the studies commonly used in patients who have had MI is presented in this section.

Stress Testing

Stress testing in patients who have had MI provides useful information about the patient's functional capacity as well as helps to identify recurrent ischemia. A symptom-limited test in stable patients is safe and is more likely to help in the diagnosis than "low-level" protocols (65); even elderly patients may safely undergo exercise testing within 14 days of infarction (66). However, such testing is neither safe nor useful in patients who have had spontaneous ischemic events or serious arrhythmias.

Echocardiography

Resting echocardiography provides an assessment of the heart valves, regional wall motion, and global ventricular function. Exercise or dobutamine stress testing with echocardiography is safe and is reported to have a sensitivity of 86% and specificity of 93% for detecting residual ischemia (67).

Nuclear Imaging

Radionuclide Angiocardiography. Technetium-99m radionuclide angio-cardiography (MUGA scan) provides quantitative information about regional wall motion and global ventricular function, which may have both diagnostic and prognostic value for patients with myocardial ischemia or infarction. Wall motion abnormalities may also be seen in patients who have had previous infarction, myocarditis, and cardiomyopathy (57).

Perfusion Stress Imaging. Perfusion stress imaging with thallium-201 or technetium-99m testing may identify areas of myocardium at risk for recurrent ischemia in patients who have had MI. Electrocardiography-gated scanning with technetium-99m sestamibi also permits regional wall motion assessment with and without stress to identify both areas of ischemia and abnormalities of ventricular function and wall motion (59).

Magnetic Resonance Imaging

Magnetic resonance imaging of the heart is a rapidly developing technique. However, it may be several years before its role in patient management is clearly defined. Studies suggest that it may have sensitivity and specificity comparable to that of echocardiographic and nuclear methods for the assessment of ventricular function and ischemia in patients with coronary artery disease; eventually it may be useful as a noninvasive technique to identify stenotic coronary lesions (67,68).

Cardiac Catheterization

In most cases, patients at high risk for reinfarction or death should undergo cardiac catheterization as a part of their post-MI management, to aid in acute care decisions, and to identify those patients who may benefit from revascularization or surgical repair of valvular or other acquired lesions (69). However, potential risks, including vascular injury, blood loss, allergic reaction, renal injury, arrhythmia, cardiac injury, embolic events, and death should be weighed against the likelihood of benefit to the patient (70). Based on currently available data, routine catheterization of all patients after infarction cannot be justified. Comparison of invasive and conservative strategies has favored the conservative approach after successful treatment with thrombolytics (71,72). The VANQWISH trial, a randomized comparison of early invasive versus conservative approaches in patients with non–Q wave infarctions, may help determine the proper role of catheterization in these patients (25).

Arrhythmia Screening

Holter Monitoring. Although Holter monitoring in patients with infarction may identify spontaneous arrhythmias and ST-segment shifts, it is not useful as a routine test after infarction. All patients who have had MI should have ECG monitoring during the first few days after infarction. Most current systems are capable of automatically identifying and reporting spontaneous arrhythmias. Although ST-segment shifts on Holter monitoring may identify patients at risk (73,74), stress testing with or without imaging is more sensitive and specific for recurrent ischemia.

Signal-Averaged Electrocardiography. A normal signal-averaged ECG may identify patients at low risk for recurrent serious arrhythmias after infarction. However, the predictive value of a positive test result is very low (75). Although this test may be useful in patients who have had serious arrhythmias during the period after infarction, it should not be used routinely.

Electrophysiologic Study. Invasive electrophysiologic testing may be useful for risk stratification, to guide drug therapy, and to determine the need for an implantable cardioverter-defibrillator. Patients who have had MI with left ventricular dysfunction and high-grade arrhythmias may benefit from this testing (76), but electrophysiologic studies should not be used routinely after infarction.

Strategies
Risk stratification of patients who have had MI should include studies that test for myocardial ischemia and for ventricular dysfunction. In patients who do not have spontaneous ischemia, a symptom-limited stress test is indicated. Ventricular function can be assessed using a variety of methods including echocardiography and MUGA scanning. When appropriate post-MI ECG monitoring is used, routine Holter monitoring is not needed for all patients.

Patients who have had MI who are shown to have normal wall motion on ventricular function studies are at low risk for complications. In contrast, patients with left ventricular dysfunction (ejection fraction of less than 50%), recurrent ischemia (spontaneous or provoked by testing), or high-grade arrhythmias are at increased risk for complications and generally should undergo cardiac catheterization.

CLINICAL PROBLEMS

Clinical Problem 1
A patient has chest pain suggestive of myocardial ischemia.

Testing Strategy and Rationale
Electrocardiography should be performed and serum enzyme levels measured. The initial probability of MI in such patients is at least

15%. If new Q waves or ST-segment elevation is detected by ECG, the probability of MI is about 80%; if ST-segment depression or T wave changes are noted, the probability of MI is approximately 20% (see Table 6-1). Depending on the time since onset of symptoms and on the presence of comorbid conditions, either cTn-I or serial CK-MB determination should be used to confirm or exclude the diagnosis.

Clinical Example

A 45-year-old man with a history of hypertension presents with substernal pressure that began 2 hours earlier and is associated with diaphoresis and radiation to the left shoulder. The pain is unrelieved with nitroglycerin and has no sharp, pleuritic, or positional component. Rales are heard at both lung bases. Electrocardiography shows a 2-mm ST elevation in leads V_1 through V_4 with 1-mm ST elevation in leads I, L, and V_5 through V_6. Because the probability of MI is high (80%) and the onset of pain is recent, interventions such as direct angioplasty or thrombolytic therapy should be considered immediately, before the diagnosis is confirmed with enzyme measurement determinations. Appropriately timed cTn-I or serial CK-MB testing should be done. An enzyme study that yields a positive result increases the likelihood of MI to 99% and confirms the diagnosis. If the test result is negative, the probability of MI is reduced to less than 10%.

Clinical Problem 2

The clinical presentation of a patient with chest pain suggests low probability of MI.

Testing Strategy and Rationale

A clinical history should be obtained, and a physical examination and an ECG should be performed. If the pain is sharp, stabbing, pleuritic, or positional, the patient does not have a history of coronary disease, and the findings of the ECG are normal, the probability of MI is low (less than 5%) and no further testing generally is required. If the ECG unexpectedly shows abnormalities such as Q waves or ST-segment elevation, the probability of infarction increases substantially, and measurement of either cTn-I or serial CK-MB testing is necessary to determine the diagnosis.

Clinical Example

A 24-year-old woman with an unremarkable history presents with intermittent sharp left inframammary pain that began 2 days ago and has been constant for the past 2 hours. It is increased by positional changes and reproduced by local palpation. Her ECG is completely normal. This pain is not typical of cardiac ischemia, and a normal ECG effectively rules out MI.

REFERENCES

1. **Pozen MW, D'Agostino RB, Selker HP, et al.** A predictive instrument to improve coronary-care-unit admission practices in acute ischemic heart disease. N Engl Med J. 1984;310:1273-8.

2. **Lee TH, Rouan GW, Weisberg M, et al.** Sensitivity of routine clinical criteria for the diagnosing of myocardial infarction within 24 hours of hospitalization. Ann Intern Med. 1987;106:181-6.

3. **Roberts R.** The two out of three criteria for the diagnosis of myocardial infarction. Is it passe? Chest. 1984;86:511-3.

4. **Paton BC.** The accuracy of the diagnosis of myocardial infarction. Am J Med. 1957;23:761-8.

5. **Zarling EJ, Sexton H, Milnor P.** Failure to diagnose acute myocardial infarction. JAMA. 1983;250:1177-81.

6. **Margolis JR, Kannel WB, Feinleib M, et al.** Clinical features of unrecognized myocardial infarction: silent and symptomatic. Am J Cardiol. 1973;32:1-7.

7. **Braunwald E.** The aggressive treatment of myocardial infarction. Circulation. 1985;71:1087-92.

8. **Goldman L, Weinberg M, Weisberg M, et al.** A computer-derived protocol to aid in the diagnosis of emergency room patients with acute chest pain. N Engl J Med. 1982;307:588-96.

9. **Lee TH, Cook EF, Weisberg M, et al.** Acute chest pain in the emergency room. Arch Intern Med. 1985;145:65-9.

10. **Goldstein RE, Bocuzzi SJ, Cruess D.** Prognosis after hospitalization for acute myocardial infarction not accompanied by typical ischemic chest pain. The Multicenter Diltiazem Postinfarction Trial Research Group. Am J Med. 1995;99:123-31.

11. **Goldman L, Lee TH.** Chest pain: infarction or not? Acute Care Med.1975;2:11-8.

12. **Fuchs R, Scheidt S.** Improved criteria for admission to cardiac care units. JAMA. 1981;246:2037-41.

13. **Gheorgiade M, Anderson J, Rosman H, et al.** Risk identification at the time of admission to cardiac care units in patients with suspected myocardial infarction. Am Heart J. 1988;116:1212-7.

14. **Gaspoz JM.** Cost-effectiveness of a new short-stay unit to "rule out" acute myocardial infarction in low risk patients. J Am Coll Cardiol 1994;24:1249-59.

15. **Lee TH, Goldman L.** Serum enzyme assays in the diagnosis of acute myocardial infarction. Ann Intern Med. 1986;105:221-33.

16. **Uusitupa M, Pyorala K, Raunio H, et al.** Sensitivity and specificity of Minnesota code Q-QS abnormalities in the diagnosis of myocardial infarction verified at autopsy. Am Heart J. 1986;106:753-7.

17. **Otto LA, Aufderheide TP.** Evaluation of ST segment elevation criteria for the prehospital electrocardiographic diagnosis of acute myocardial infarction. Ann Emerg Med. 1994;23:17-24.

18. **Lee HS, Cross SJ, Rawles JM, Jennings, KP.** Patients who present with suspected myocardial infarction who present with ST depression. Lancet. 1993;342: 1204-7.

19. **Fesmire FM.** ECG diagnosis of acute myocardial infarction in the presence of left bundle-branch block in patients undergoing continuous ECG monitoring. Ann Emerg Med. 1995;26:69-82.

20. **Sgarbossa B.** Electrocardiographic diagnosis of evolving acute myocardial infarction in the presence of left bundle-branch block. GUSTO-1 (Global Utilization of Streptokinase and Tissue Plasminogen Activator for Occluded Coronary Arteries) Investigators. N Engl J Med. 1996;334:481-7.

21. **Brush JE, Brand DA, Acampora D, et al.** Use of the initial electrocardiogram to predict in-hospital complications of acute myocardial infarction. New Engl J Med. 1985; 312:1137-41.

22. **Stark, ME, Vacek JL.** The initial electrocardiogram during admission for myocardial infarction. Arch Intern Med. 1987;147:843-6.

23. **Rude RE, Poole K, Muller JE, et al.** Electrocardiographic and clinical criteria for recognition of acute myocardial infarction based on analysis of 3697 patients. Am J Card 1983;52:936-41.

24. **Tzivoni D, Chenzbraun A, Keren A, et al.** Reciprocal electrocardiographic changes in acute myocardial infarction. Am J Cardiol. 1985;56:23-6.

25. **Boden WE.** Non-Q wave myocardial infarction: a prognostic paradox. Hosp Pract. 1992; 27:129-33, 137-8, 140.

26. **Marmor A, Sobel B, Roberts R.** Factors presaging early recurrent myocardial infarction. Am J Cardiol. 1981;48:603-10.

27. **Maeda S.** Different clinical implications for ST segment depression and T wave inversion in non-Q wave myocardial infarction. J Cardiol. 1994;24:357-66.

28. **Roberts R, Gowda KS, Ludbrook PA, Sobel B.** Specificity of elevated serum MB creatine phosphokinase activity in the diagnosis of acute myocardial infarction. Am J Cardiol. 1975;36:433-7.

29. **Adornato BT, Engel WK.** MB-creatine phosphokinase isoenzyme elevation not diagnostic of myocardial infarction. Arch Intern Med. 1977;137:1089-90.

30. **Roberts R, Sobel BE.** Creatine kinase isoenzymes in the assessment of heart disease. Am Heart J. 1978;95:521-8.

31. **Roberts R, Ludbrook PA, Weiss ES, Sobel B.** Serum CPK isoenzymes after cardiac catheterization. Br Heart J. 1975;37:1144-9.

32. **Ehsani A, Ewy G, Sobel B.** Effects of electrical countershock on serum creatine phosphokinase (CPK) isoenzyme activity. Am J Cardiol. 1976;37:12-8.

33. **Smith A.** Separation of tissue and serum creatine kinase isoenzyme on polyacrylamide gel slabs. Clin Chim Acta. 1972;39:351-7.

34. **Ogunro EA, Hearse DJ, Shilingford JP.** Creatine kinase isoenzymes: their separation and quantitation. Cardiovasc Res. 1977;11:94-102.

35. **Hedges JR.** Serial ECGs are less accurate than serial CK-MB results for emergency department diagnosis of myocardial infarction. Ann Emerg Med. 1992;21:1445-50.

36. **Gibler WB, Young GP, Hedges JR, et al.** Acute myocardial infarction in chest pain patients with nondiagnostic ECGs: serial CK-MB sampling in the emergency department. The Emergency Medicine Cardiac Research Group. Ann Emerg Med. 1992;21:504-12.

37. **Marin MM, Teichman SL.** Use of rapid sampling of creatine kinase MB for very early detection of myocardial infarction in patients with acute chest pain. Am Heart J. 1992; 123:354-61.

38. **Dillon MC, Calbreath DF, Dixon AM, et al.** Diagnostic problem in acute myocardial infarction. CK-MB in the absence of abnormally elevated total creatine kinase levels. Arch Intern Med. 1982;142:33-8.

39. **Heller GV, Blaustein AS, Wei JY, Geer D.** Implications of increased myocardial isoenzyme level in the presence of normal serum creatine kinase activity. Am J Cardiol. 1983;51:24-7.

40. **Bakker AJ, Haagen FD.** Contribution of creatine kinase MB mass concentration at admission to early diagnosis of acute myocardial infarction. Br Heart J. 1994; 72:119-24.

41. **deWinter RJ, Koster RW, Sturk A, Sanders GT.** Value of myoglobin, troponin T, and CK-MB mass in ruling out myocardial infarction in the emergency room. Circulation. 1995;92:3401-7.

42. **Bakker AJ, Koelemay MJ, Gorgels JP, et al.** Failure of new biochemical markers to exclude acute myocardial infarction at admission. Lancet. 1993;342:1220-2.

43. **Wu AH, Wang XM, Gornet TG, Ordonez-Llanos J.** Creatine kinase MB isoforms in patients with skeletal muscle injury: ramifications for early detection of acute myocardial infarction. Clin Chem. 1992;38:2396-400.

44. **Puleo PR, Meyer D, Wathen C, Tawa CB, et al.** Use of a rapid assay of subforms of creatine kinase-MB to diagnose or rule out acute myocardial infarction. N Engl J Med. 1994; 331:561-6.

45. **Mair J, Smidt J, Lechleitner P, et al.** A decision tree for the early diagnosis of acute myocardial infarction in nontraumatic chest pain patients at hospital admission. Chest 1995;108:1502-9.

46. **Adams JE 3rd.** Comparable detection of acute myocardial infarction by creatine kinase MB isoenzyme and cardiac troponin I. Clin Chem. 1994;40:1291-5.

47. **Brogan GX, Hollander JE, McCuskey CF, Thode HC, Snow J, Sama A, Bock JL, and the Biomedical Markers for Acute Myocardial Ischemia (BAMI) Study Group.** Evaluation of a new assay for cardiac troponin I vs creatine kinase-MB for the diagnosis of acute myocardial infarction. Acad Emerg Med. 1997;4:6-12.

48. **Tucker JF, Collins RA, Anderson AJ, et al.** Early diagnostic efficiency of cardiac troponin I and troponin T for acute myocardial infarction. Acad Emerg Med. 1997;4:13-21.

49. **Bertinchant J-P, Larue C, Pernel I, et al.** Release kinetics of serum cardiac troponin I in ischemic myocardial injury. Clin Biochem. 1996;29:587-94.

50. **Lindahl B.** Early diagnosis and exclusion of acute myocardial infarction using biochemical monitoring. The BIOMACS Study Group. Biochemical Markers of Acute Coronary Syndromes. Coron Artery Dis. 1995; 6:321-8.

51. **Kilpatrick WS, Wosornu D, McGuiness JB, Glen AC.** Early diagnosis of acute myocardial infarction: CK-MB and myoglobin compared. Ann Clin Biochem. 1993;30:435-8.

52. **Woo J, Lacbawan FL, Sunheimer R, et al.** Is myoglobin useful in the diagnosis of acute myocardial infarction in the emergency room setting? Am J Clin Pathol. 1995;103:725-9.

53. **McComb M, McMaster EA, MacKenzie G, Adgey AAJ.** Myoglobin and creatine kinase in acute myocardial infarction. Br Heart J. 1984;51:189-94.

54. **Hearse DJ, deLeiris J.** Enzymes in Cardiology Diagnosis and Research. New York: Wiley and Sons; 1979.

55. **Vasudevan G, Mercer DW, Varat MA.** Lactic dehydrogenase isoenzyme determination in the diagnosis of acute myocardial infarction. Circulation. 1978;57:1055-7.

56. **Martins JT, Li DJ, Baskin LB, Keffer JH.** Comparison of cardiac troponin I and lactate dehydrogenase isoenzymes for the late diagnosis of myocardial injury. Am J Clin Pathol. 1996;106:705-8.

57. **Berger HJ, Zaret BL.** Nuclear cardiology. N Engl J Med. 1981; 305:799-807, 855-65.

58. **Marzullo P.** Value of the test thallium-201/technetium-99m sestamibi scans and dobutamine echocardiography for detecting myocardial viability. Am J Cardiol 1993;71:166-72.

59. **Flamen P, Dendale P, Bossuyt A, Franken PR.** Combined left ventricular wall motion and myocardial perfusion stress imaging in the initial assessment of patients with a recent uncomplicated myocardial infarction. Angiology. 1995;46:461-72.

60. **Olson HG, Lyons KP, Butman S, Piters KM.** Validation of technetium-99m stannous pyrophosphate myocardial scintigraphy for diagnosing acute myocardial infarction more than 48 hours old when serum creatine kinase-MB has returned to normal. Am J Cardiol. 1983;52:245-51.

61. **Holman BL.** Infarct-avid scintigraphy. Freeman LM, ed. Freeman and Johnson's Clinical Radionuclide Imaging. NewYork: Grune and Stratton; 1984:537-62.

62. **Nieminen S, Parisi AF, O'Boyle JE, et al.** Serial evaluation of myocardial thickening and thinning in acute experimental infarction: identification and quantification using two dimensional echocardiography. Circulation. 1982;66:174.

63. **Horowitz RS, Morganroth J, Parrotto C, et al.** Immediate diagnosis of acute myocardial infarction by two dimensional echocardiography. Circulation. 1982;65:323.

64. **Olona M.** Strategies for prognostic assessment of uncomplicated first myocardial infarction: 5 year follow-up study. J Am Coll Cardiol. 1995;25:815-22.

65. **Jain A, Myers GH, Sapin PM, O'Rourke RA.** Comparison of symptom-limited and low level exercise tolerance tests early after myocardial infarction. J Am Coll Cardiol. 1993;22:1816-20.

66. **Ciaroni S, Delonca J, Righetti A.** Early exercise testing after acute myocardial infarction in the elderly: clinical evaluation and prognostic significance. Am Heart J. 1993;126:304-31.

67. **Dendale P, Franken PR, Waldman GJ, et al.** Low-dosage dobutamine magnetic resonance imaging as an alternative to echocardiography in the detection of viable myocardium after acute infarction. Am Heart J. 1995;130:134-40.

68. **Hundley WG.** Noninvasive determination of infarct artery patency by cine magnetic resonance angiography. Circulation. 1995;91:1347-53.

69. **Ross J, et al.** A decision scheme for coronary angiography after acute myocardial infarction. Circulation. 1989;79:292-303.

70. **Grossman W.** Cardiac Catheterization and Angiography. Philadelphia: Lea and Febiger; 1986.

71. The TIMI Study Group. Comparison of invasive and conservative strategies after treatment with intravenous tissue plasminogen activator in acute myocardial infarction. Results of the Thrombolysis in Myocardial Infarction (TIMI) Phase II trial. N Engl J Med. 1989;320:618-27.

72. **Simoons M, Betriu A, Col J, et al.** Thrombolysis with tissue plasminogen activator in acute myocardial infarction: no additional benefit from immediate percutaneous coronary angioplasty. Lancet 1988;I:197-202.

73. **Stevenson RN, Wilkinson P, Marchant BG, et al.** Relative value of clinical variables, treadmill stress testing, and Holter ST monitoring for postinfarction risk stratification. Am J Cardiol. 1994;74:221-5.

74. **Currie P, Saltissi S.** Significance of ST segment elevation during ambulatory monitoring after acute myocardial infarction. Am Heart J. 1993;125:41-7.

75. **Wong CB, Windle JR.** Clinical applications of signal-average electrocardiography in patients after myocardial infarction. Neb Med J. 1994;79:28-31.

76. **Viskin S, Belhassen B.** Should electrophysiological studies be performed in asymptomatic patients following myocardial infarction? A pragmatic approach. PACE. 1994;17:1082-9.

Secondary Hypertension 7

Eric B. Grossman, MD, and Edgar R. Black, MD

KEY POINTS

Pretest Probabilities

- Secondary hypertension (i.e., hypertension attributable to a specific cause) occurs in 1% to 5% of patients with hypertension.
- Secondary hypertension is most likely present when newly diagnosed hypertension is outside the usual age range for onset of essential hypertension; when there is an acute, unexplained worsening of hypertension; or when hypertension is difficult to treat.
- The most common causes of secondary hypertension in adults are renal artery stenosis and renal insufficiency.
- Alcoholism, obesity, and sleep apnea are common disease entities whose treatment may result in the amelioration or cure of hypertension.

Diagnostic Strategies

- The finding of hypertension should prompt a history and physical examination tailored to elicit the signs and symptoms that differentiate essential from secondary hypertension and that are associated with the various causes of secondary hypertension.
- Owing to the rarity of secondary hypertension, diagnostic evaluation should be pursued only if clinical suspicion is raised by the history, physical examination, or selected laboratory studies such as serum creatinine and serum electrolyte measurements and urinalysis.
- In cases of possible renal artery stenosis, initial testing is best accomplished with the captopril renal scan, or alternatively, by using duplex ultrasonography to evaluate the renal arteries.

BACKGROUND

Hypertension is a common disease, affecting about 50 million people in the United States (1) and accounting for more than 85 million office visits (2). Most (95% or more) hypertension is of the essential, or idio-pathic, type. Treatment is accomplished by lifestyle modifications and medical therapy. Treatment prevents the deleterious consequences of prolonged blood pressure elevation, including cardiac and renal disease and stroke.

Secondary hypertension, comprising 1% to 5% of cases, may be ameliorated or cured with treatment of the underlying disorder, often obviating the need for medical therapy. This chapter discusses the most common causes of secondary hypertension, those factors that should alert the practitioner to its increased likelihood, and approaches to the diagnosis of secondary hypertension.

ESTIMATING PRETEST PROBABILITY

Several factors increase the likelihood that secondary hypertension is present. The onset of essential hypertension usually occurs in patients between the ages of 30 to 55 years, although in African-Americans the onset may commonly be as early as age 20 years. In one study, 7% of those with essential hypertension were found to present after the age of 50 years, and 12% presented at younger than 20 years of age (3). Thus, those presenting with hypertension outside of the expected age range for essential hypertension have an increased chance of having secondary hypertension. Likewise, hypertension that is refractory to treatment or that is accelerated or malignant is more likely to be due to a secondary cause. Similarly, unexplained large increases in blood pressure above previously controlled or baseline values raise concern about a secondary cause. Because essential hypertension is generally asymp-tomatic, the presence of symptoms, especially those commonly associ-ated with types of secondary hypertension, should prompt further investigation.

Diabetes mellitus or a family history of essential hypertension increases the likelihood that the hypertension is essential. The associa-tion between essential hypertension and diabetes is strongest for patients with type II diabetes; approximately 40% of patients with newly diagnosed type II diabetes have essential hypertension (4). Family history of essential hypertension (but not early onset hyperten-sion, as discussed later in the section "Genetic Disorders") significantly increases the risk for essential hypertension. If one first-degree relative has hypertension, the relative risk that a person between 20 and 50 years old will develop essential hypertension is 2.2–2.4 to 1 (odds ratio). If two first-degree relatives were affected, the ratio increases to between 3-4 to 1. However, the ratio is close to 1:1 for those older than 50 years, whether one or two first-degree relatives are affected (5). Thus, for patients older than 50 years, family history does not substantially alter the likelihood that new onset hypertension is essential or secondary.

Although not usually considered reasons for secondary hypertension, obesity, alcoholism, sleep apnea, use of various over-the-counter medications such as nonsteroidal anti-inflammatory drugs, and noncompliance with medical regimen or sodium-restricted diet may result in hypertension or in difficulty treating hypertension. Thus, appropriate attention to these conditions should be considered in the approach to the patient with blood pressure elevation before screening for secondary hypertension.

Determining the prevalence of various secondary causes of hypertension is difficult because of referral bias in many series. A population-based series from the Mayo Clinic found the prevalence of renovascular disease to be 0.18%; pheochromocytoma, 0.04%; and hyperaldosteronism, 0.01% (6). The Cleveland Clinic reported rates of 4.4%, 0.2%, and 0.4%, respectively (7). They also reported coarctation in 0.6% and Cushing syndrome in 0.3% of their sample (7).

Renal Artery Stenosis

In adults, the most common cause of secondary hypertension is renovascular disease. Renal artery stenosis results in hypertension through activation of the renin-angiotensin system and may result from fibromuscular dysplasia or atherosclerosis. The cause of fibromuscular dysplasia is unclear. Fibromuscular dysplasia causes a weakening of the arterial wall, with a characteristic "string of pearls" appearance on angiography. It occurs most commonly in women younger than 30 years of age and is often amenable to treatment by angioplasty of the renal artery. Renal artery stenosis caused by atherosclerosis affects men and women older than 50 years of age. This diagnosis is frequently made when atherosclerosis involves other major arteries. Abdominal or flank bruits will be heard in approximately 40% of patients (8). Hypokalemia should not be used as an indicator for the presence of the disease because it is frequently absent. Acute renal failure or a significant increase in the serum creatinine level after initiation of treatment with an angiotensin-converting enzyme (ACE) inhibitor suggests the presence of renal artery stenosis, although patients with long-standing hypertension may also manifest azotemia with ACE inhibitor therapy.

Renal Disease and Endocrine Causes

Renal disease, hyperaldosteronism, pheochromocytoma, thyroid disease, and hypercortisolism may present at any age and may be associated with hypertension. Renal disease is often initially asymptomatic, but it may be associated early in its course with edema, and later, with the classic symptoms of uremia. Thyroid disease and its manifestations are discussed elsewhere in Chapter 41, but it is important to emphasize that both hyperthyroidism and hypothyroidism may be associated with hypertension. In hyperthyroidism, systolic hypertension is generally observed. In hypothyroidism, the blood pressure elevation is primarily diastolic and results from increased catecholamine secretion. Hypercortisolism (see Chapter 40) causes hypertension both by sodium retention and by effects on peripheral resistance. Bruising, myopathy, and edema may often be found, as well as a variety of metabolic disorders including hypokalemia and glucose intolerance (9).

Hyperaldosteronism is a rare clinical entity, although it may be underdiagnosed. The two main forms of hyperaldosteronism are adrenal adenoma and bilateral adrenal hyperplasia; the adenoma form occurs approximately three times more frequently. The genetic cause of hyperaldosteronism secondary to glucocorticoid-responsive hyperaldosteronism has recently been characterized (see the section "Genetic Disorders" later in this chapter). No specific symptoms are seen at presentation except those associated with hypokalemia, which may not be present, such as muscle weakness, cramping, and polyuria. Trousseau or Chvostek signs may occur in the presence of pronounced alkalosis.

Pheochromocytoma is also a rare disease and presents with sustained or episodic hypertension. Patients with pheochromocytoma often report symptoms of headache, palpitations, or diaphoresis. The combination of all three symptoms is strongly associated with the diagnosis, and their absence makes the diagnosis unlikely (10). Orthostatic hypotension, pallor, anxiety, and weight loss are also frequently seen. Pheochromocytomas usually secrete epinephrine or norepinephrine or both, although some may secrete dopa, dopamine, and other peptide hormones, and the symptoms relate directly to the substances secreted. If associated with multiple endocrine neoplasia type 1 or type 2 (A or B), the characteristic features of those disorders are also present. In both children and adults, more than 15% of these tumors are extra-adrenal, so normal adrenal anatomy should not be used as exclusionary criteria for the diagnosis (11).

Aortic Coarctation

In children, aortic coarctation is the most common cause of secondary hypertension, although it may cause secondary hypertension in adults as well. Because the development of obstruction to outflow has been gradual, the usual presentation in older children and adults is hypertension or systolic murmur, and there is evidence for left ventricular hypertrophy and collateral circulation. A thrill may be appreciated in the suprasternal notch, and more than half of the patients will experience an ejection click signifying an associated bicuspid aortic valve. A blood pressure difference between the arms and the legs of more than 20 mm Hg strongly favors the diagnosis. Involvement of the left subclavian or an anomalous right subclavian artery may produce a diminished left or right brachial pulse, respectively (12).

Genetic Disorders

Recent advances in the understanding and treatment of hypertension have come from the identification of specific genetic disorders that result in blood pressure elevation. These disorders affect very few of those with hypertension, but when hypertension presents during childhood or adolescence, especially in patients with a family history of early onset hypertension, these disorders should be given serious consideration. Although beyond the scope of this chapter, a full discussion of these disorders may be found in the literature (13,14).

Glucocorticoid-remediable aldosteronism is an autosomal dominant trait. Affected persons have early onset hypertension and often have cerebral hemorrhage. The mutation results in primary control of aldosterone secretion by adrenocorticotropic hormone, and treatment is accomplished with glucocorticoid administration or by blocking the action of aldosterone. Apparent mineralocorticoid excess is an autosomal recessive disorder resulting from a defect in the gene encoding 11β-hydroxysteroid dehydrogenase. The enzymatic defect results in elevated levels of cortisol and increased mineralocorticoid activity. Patients present with early moderate to severe hypertension and signs of mineralocorticoid excess, including hypokalemia. Liddle syndrome is an autosomal dominant condition that results from a defect in the gene for the amiloride-sensitive sodium channel. The defect leads to increased salt and water retention by the kidney, independent of aldosterone. Patients often manifest hypokalemia.

DIAGNOSTIC TESTS

The diagnosis of many of the clinical entities that have just been discussed generally requires one or more procedures that are either invasive, costly, or both. The approach to diagnosis therefore usually involves at least one initial test that is used to decide whether to proceed with a more definitive diagnostic procedure.

Renal Artery Stenosis

Initial Tests

Captopril Renal Scanning. In renal artery stenosis, decreased renal perfusion stimulates angiotensin II production, which causes postglomerular (efferent) arteriolar vasoconstriction. The resultant backpressure causes an increase in the glomerular filtration rate toward normal. Captopril (a dose of 25 mg given orally 1 hour before the scan) abrogates this effect by inhibiting ACE and causes a decrease in the glomerular filtration rate, which results in an abnormality shown on the renogram. Some advocate comparing captopril challenge studies with abnormal findings to baseline (i.e., studies without captopril challenge), whereas others do not find this necessary (15,16). Patients should discontinue ACE inhibitors (for 3 days for short-acting agents and for 5 days for long-acting agents) and diuretics (for 3 to 5 days) before the test.

Sensitivity and specificity for this test have been consistently high, generally around 90% for both (Table 7-1). A recent European multicenter study (17) found the test to have 86% sensitivity and 93% specificity, whereas previous representative studies cited values of 90% to 91% and 87% to 92%, respectively (18,19). These values may be lower in the face of renal insufficiency, but the use of a newer radionuclide MAG_3 has ameliorated this problem.

Captopril Test. In renal artery stenosis, overproduction of angiotensin II suppresses renin release. Administration of captopril decreases angiotensin II production, removes its negative feedback effect on renin secretion, and increases plasma renin activity (PRA). For this test, PRA is measured before and 1 hour after the administration of 25 or 50 mg of oral captopril (20); variations of this protocol have also been reported (21). Again, test results appear to be improved if patients discontinue ACE inhibitors and diuretics, although discontinuation of all antihypertensives may also improve results (21).

Different studies have used varying criteria for a positive test. Studies using the criteria devised by Muller (20) have achieved highly variable results: sensitivity of 34% to 76% and specificity of 58% to 93% (22). A prospective study using different criteria (21) achieved excellent sensitivity (96%) but poor specificity (55%). Other reports have also described variable results, with sensitivities ranging from 73% to 91% and specificities ranging from 72% to 89% (22).

Table 7-1. Operating Characteristics of Diagnostics Tests for Renal Artery Stenosis

Diagnostic Test	Sensitivity	Specificity	Likelihood Ratio Positive Result	Likelihood Ratio Negative Result
	←————— % —————→			
Captopril renal scan	86–91	87–93	6.6–13	0.10–0.16
Captopril test	Variable, see text			
Renal artery duplex sonography	88–98	90–99	8.8–98	0.02–0.13
Magnetic resonance angiography	>90	>90	>9	<0.11

Renal Artery Duplex Ultrasonography. This test combines B-mode sonography with color Doppler imaging to measure flow velocity along the renal artery. With this test, peak systolic flow velocity is elevated above normal, or elevated with respect to flow velocity in the aorta, in stenotic segments of the renal artery.

The reported sensitivity and specificity of the technique are quite high: 88% to 98% and 90% to 99%, respectively (23–27). However, this technique is operator dependent, and visualization of the renal artery is difficult in obese patients.

Magnetic Resonance Angiography. The technology used in magnetic resonance angiography (MRA) is rapidly advancing. As a result, there have not been a large number of published reports on any single method nor has any single method gained wide acceptance. However, in recent reports, sensitivity and specificity using various MRA techniques have both had values of more than 90% (28–31). The availability and expertise in using these methods vary depending on the center at which the test is performed. This technique holds promise for becoming the test of choice owing to its noninvasive nature, and it may replace arteriography as the "gold standard" procedure.

Although a structural lesion may be predicted or identified by these tests, the renal captopril scan and the captopril test may also help predict whether correction of a stenotic lesion will result in amelioration of hypertension.

Other Tests. Although we suggest using the tests discussed in the preceding sections, several other tests have been used in the evaluation of possible renal artery stenosis. For the purposes of this chapter, these other tests, along with their operating characteristics, if available, are only mentioned in passing. The random renin level has only fair sensitivity and specificity (57% and 66%, respectively) (32); intravenous pyelography (IVP) (whether rapid sequence or not) has a sensitivity of 59% to 80% and a specificity of 64% to 83% (33,34); conventional renal scan is comparable to IVP (22); intravenous digital subtraction angiography has highly variable sensitivity and specificity, with studies confounded by technical difficulties (35).

Renal size discrepancy, when present, may help indicate the need for further studies but may be absent in about 70% of patients with mild to moderate renal artery stenosis and in 25% of patients with severe renal artery stenosis (33). Renal vein renin measurements have been used to determine the physiologic significance of a stenotic lesion, but although the sensitivity is 92%, the specificity is low (35%) (32). The test is also invasive and may delay intervention.

Definitive Tests

Renal Arteriography. This test remains the "gold standard" in the diagnosis of renal artery stenosis. With the information obtained from renal arteriography, an assessment can be made regarding the presence, degree, and location of a lesion, and a decision can be made about whether to proceed with angioplasty, stent placement, or surgery, or to have no intervention at all. The risks of the procedure are those associated with arteriography in general, including contrast-induced renal failure and atheroembolism (36). The risk of contrast-induced renal failure may be decreased by minimizing the volume of dye administered. Lower renal toxicity may also be observed using the newer technique of carbon dioxide digital angiography, which is becoming more available (37).

Renal Disease

The finding of renal insufficiency may be the first clue to the diagnosis of renovascular disease, or it may itself be the cause of the hypertension. Retention of sodium and water is believed to contribute to blood pressure elevation, although other endothelial, hormonal, or neurohumoral processes may contribute as well. Screening for renal disease as a cause of hypertension is best accomplished by measuring serum creatinine and electrolyte levels and by obtaining a complete urinalysis, including microscopic examination. Although these tests, when combined, are likely to be highly sensitive and specific, one notable exception should be mentioned. Even though the serum creatinine level may be within the normal range, renal function may still be depressed if the patient's muscle mass is decreased. This is most commonly observed in elderly patients, especially women (38).

Hyperthyroidism and Hypothyroidism (See Chapter 41)

Hypercortisolism (See Chapter 40)

Hyperaldosteronism

The diagnosis of hyperaldosteronism is a difficult one in which biochemical, not anatomic, findings are paramount. The best method of diagnosis is controversial, and should probably be pursued by a specialist. Initial testing for hyperaldosteronism is also a matter of controversy but may be attempted before referral. Hypokalemia is not a perfect screening test, because it is present in 55% to 93% of patients in collected series (average, approximately 80%) (39–41). Serum aldosterone is highly variable and dependent on sodium intake, and plasma renin activity (PRA) is low in 25% to 50% of patients with essential hypertension; thus neither is a reliable initial test. As with potential renal artery stenosis, it is important that therapy using diuretics and ACE inhibitors be discontinued for at least 3 days before beginning any of the following initial tests.

Urinary Aldosterone with Salt Loading
For this test, the patient is "salt-loaded" (25 mL/kg of normal saline over a 4-hour period) on 3 consecutive days, after which a 24-hour urine collection is obtained for aldosterone determination. A value greater than 14 µg/24 hours has been found to have a 93% sensitivity for hyperaldosteronism (42).

Urinary Aldosterone Without Salt Loading
An easier method that has been used by established groups (43) but for which sensitivity and specificity data are not available is a 24-hour urine collection for aldosterone, sodium, and potassium without saline loading. The amount of aldosterone excreted may be compared with nomograms of normal secretion for the specific quantities of sodium and potassium present in the collection (44), and if it is above the normal level, further workup should be considered.

Plasma Aldosterone/Renin ratio
Plasma renin activity and plasma aldosterone are measured at 8:00 AM after 2 hours of ambulation. The combination of an aldosterone/PRA ratio greater than 30:1 and a plasma aldosterone value of more than 20 ng/dL results in a sensitivity of 90% and a specificity of 91% (45).

Pheochromocytoma
The approach to the diagnosis of pheochromocytoma is exceedingly controversial. Many approaches may be suggested. However, one point appears to garner general consensus—namely, that biochemical investigations should precede anatomic investigations. This is because of both the high frequency of detecting benign adrenal abnormalities and the difficulty in localizing an extra-adrenal pheochromocytoma.

Biochemical Tests
All biochemical tests are based on the metabolism of the catecholamines secreted by pheochromocytomas, primarily norepinephrine (NE) and epinephrine (E). When catecholamines are determined, generally NE and E are measured, along with their precursor dopamine. Their metabolites, vanillylmandelic acid (VMA), metanephrine, and normetanephrine, may also be measured. The higher the value is above normal, the more likely is the presence of a pheochromocytoma. Newer methods of assaying for these compounds, such as high-performance liquid chromatography (HPLC) and gas-liquid chromatography, seem to improve testing. Various foods and medications may

interfere with the assays and should be reviewed before the tests are ordered (10,46).

The sensitivity and specificity of the tests for pheochromocytoma are summarized in Table 7-2. The variability of the data from study to study is partly the result of the variability in the techniques (HPLC compared with colorimetric assays) used to measure each of the specified compounds. One limitation of all the data is that the reference group consists of patients who are normal or who have essential hypertension, not patients who have disorders that can mimic pheochromocytoma, such as panic disorder and labile essential hypertension.

Positive results from an initial test should be confirmed by repeating the same test or by performing a second test (47). In addition to the assays we have just discussed, another confirmatory test that can be used is the clonidine suppression test: plasma NE and E levels are compared before and 1 and 2 hours after an oral dose of clonidine (0.3 mg). In patients who do not have a pheochromocytoma, NE and E levels are suppressed in response to the clonidine (a decrease in NE + E to < 500 pg/mL and a relative decrease of at least 40%), whereas clonidine fails to suppress the secretion of NE and E from a pheochromocytoma. This test appears to be both sensitive and specific (sensitivity, 97%; specificity, 99%), although these data are from only one study of 102 patients (48). Diuretics and beta-blockers may interfere with the test and should be discontinued before testing.

Table 7-2. Operating Characteristics of Diagnostic Tests for Pheochromocytoma

Tests	Duration	Sensitivity	Specificity	Likelihood Ratio Positive Result	Negative Result
		←———— % ————→			
Urinary tests					
Vanillylmandelic acid (VMA)	24 h	81–98	97	27–33	0.02–0.20
Metanephrine	24 h	82–95	95–98	16–48	0.05–0.19
Metanephrine/ creatinine ratio*	24 h	100	98	50	0
Catecholamines*	24 h	82–88	82–95	4.6–19	0.13–0.22
	overnight	100	98	50	0
Serum tests					
Metanephrine*	spot	100	85	6.7	0
Catecholamines	spot	85–94	82–97	4.7–31	0.06–0.18
Clonidine suppression	0,1,2 h	97	99	97	0.03

*Based on data from a single initial report.

Anatomic Localization Studies

Once biochemical evidence supports the presence of a pheochromocytoma, several imaging techniques are available for localizing the tumor: computed tomography (CT), magnetic resonance imaging (MRI), ^{131}I-meta-iodobenzyl guanidine (MIBG) scanning, and ^{111}In-octreotide scanning. Abdominal CT has a cited sensitivity of 92% and specificity of 80% (47); however, results have been variable, with a reported sensitivity of 80% to 100% and a reported specificity of 29% to 96% (10,49). The major disadvantage of CT is that it may detect "normal" adrenal abnormalities, which are not a pheochromocytoma. Magnetic resonance imaging may be used as an alternative to CT; although a large amount of data is not available on its sensitivity and specificity, one report noted 100% sensitivity and specificity of T2-weighted images (49). Recently, two nuclear medicine techniques have been described, MIBG and octreotide scanning, that use the functional characteristics of a pheochromocytoma for localization. Although MIBG scanning is reported to be more sensitive and specific (sensitivity, 86%–92%; specificity, 100%) (10,50), octreotide scanning may be useful when the results of MIBG scanning are equivocal (50). When biochemical test results are positive and the localization tests do not yield definitive results, sampling along the inferior vena cava may be attempted (51).

Aortic Coarctation

Although chest radiography can demonstrate nonspecific findings of congestive heart failure and left ventricular hypertrophy, the findings may be subtle in older patients. Direct visualization can usually be accomplished with echocardiography or MRI, although the values for sensitivity (43%–86% for echocardiography; 90% for MRI) and specificity (79%–100% for echocardiography; 95% for MRI) are dependent on the techniques used and on the severity of the coarctation (52–54). Selective aortic root or aortic arch angiography with left ventriculography is usually necessary to delineate the type of coarctation, the extent of collaterals, the patency of the ductus arteriosus, and the presence of cardiac defects.

Genetic Disorders

Using genetic tests, diagnosis of the three genetic causes discussed previously (glucocorticoid-remediable aldosteronism, apparent mineralocorticoid excess, and Liddle syndrome) is made with nearly 100% sensitivity and specificity. At this time, these tests are performed on a limited basis only (13).

DIAGNOSTIC STRATEGIES

The diagnosis of hypertension in an individual patient should always prompt a thorough history and physical examination tailored first to determining the magnitude of the problem, including the duration and degree of blood pressure elevation and the extent of end-organ damage and, second, to assessing the likelihood of secondary hypertension. The elements in the history and physical examination that point to secondary hypertension are detailed in the preceding sections on the most common causes. However, no matter what the cause, age of onset or recent changes in symptoms are important clues. In a patient with long-standing hypertension, blood pressure refractory to treatment and a sudden, large increase in blood pressure are also important indications of secondary hypertension.

Because secondary hypertension is uncommon, initial laboratory evaluation should be limited to measurements of serum creatinine and electrolytes (particularly potassium and bicarbonate) and urinalysis, unless suspicion is raised by the history and physical examination. If a specific cause is suggested by the history, physical examination, or initial laboratory screening, identification of that specific cause should be attempted. However, if the patient has a nonspecific presentation indicating secondary hypertension, the patient's age may be the only factor available to guide the selection for potential causes.

When the clinical picture suggests renal artery stenosis, initial testing is best accomplished with captopril renal scanning. The duplex ultrasonography study of the renal arteries is a reasonable alternative, especially if local expertise is available, administration of captopril is contraindicated, or significant renal insufficiency is present. If the results of these studies are positive, definitive diagnosis is made with renal arteriography and therapeutic angioplasty may be done at the same time. If the initial probability of renal artery stenosis is high, arteriography may be the initial test performed.

Identification of intrinsic renal disease as the cause of the hypertension is assessed by performing serum creatinine and serum electrolyte assays and urinalysis.

When hyperaldosteronism is suspected, such as after finding a low serum potassium value, obtaining either a plasma aldosterone/renin ratio or 24-hour urine collection for the measurement of aldosterone, sodium, and potassium is the simplest initial method. Although the clinical reliability of the latter has not been adequately tested, the 24-hour urinary aldosterone collection after sodium loading is a cumbersome test. If results of these tests are abnormal, referral for further evaluation is recommended.

In the evaluation of a possible pheochromocytoma, determination of VMA, metanephrine, or catecholamines in a 24-hour urine collection provides similar reliability (see Table 7-2). However, it is important to review the patient's medications and diet to make sure that interfering substances are not being consumed (10,46). In addition, if the patient has a symptom or a symptom complex (e.g., headaches, palpitations, and diaphoresis), it is preferable to obtain the collection during the occurrence of these symptoms. As discussed earlier, equivocal or positive test results may be confirmed by repeating the same test, a similar test (e.g., a serum level measurement), or the clonidine suppression test. After biochemical screening, imaging studies, such as CT, should be performed to localize the tumor, but if the results are equivocal or negative, MIBG scanning may be done.

For patients with possible aortic coarctation, visualization can be accomplished initially with MRI, although in the presence of significant physical findings echocardiography is likely to be adequate and less expensive. Selective angiography is the definitive test and is usually required before surgical intervention.

CLINICAL PROBLEMS

Clinical Problem 1
A middle-aged woman presents with asymptomatic hypertension.

Diagnostic Strategy and Rationale
A history should be completed and a physical examination should be performed that are tailored to those signs and symptoms that would suggest the possibility of a secondary cause of hypertension. In the absence of such findings, laboratory tests including serum creatinine and serum electrolyte measurements and urinalysis should be ordered. If the results of these tests are normal, the diagnosis of essential hypertension is most likely and no further testing is necessary. Subsequent evaluation for secondary hypertension would be indicated only if new findings suggested a high likelihood of a specific type of secondary hypertension.

Clinical Example
A 45-year-old woman was recently found to have hypertension, with serial blood pressure measurements averaging 150/100 mm Hg. A thorough history reveals no previous history of hypertension, no other medical or surgical problems, and one uncomplicated pregnancy. Family history is significant for hypertension in her mother, with onset occurring when her mother was between 40 and 50 years old. Review of systems is negative aside from rare frontal headaches. Physical examination reveals blood pressure of 150/100 mm Hg, equal in both arms, and is otherwise normal. Laboratory evaluation shows normal serum creatinine and electrolyte levels and normal results of urinalysis. No further testing is ordered. The patient is treated for essential hypertension.

Continued

Clinical Problem 2

A middle-aged or elderly patient with moderate hypertension, which has been under excellent control, presents with a recent increase in blood pressure.

Diagnostic Strategy and Rationale

A sudden exacerbation of hypertension is unusual and suggests that a secondary cause is present. The increase in blood pressure should first be validated by determinations during separate office visits, and recent changes in habits and medications should be sought. If no new contributing factors are identified, a thorough review of systems and a physical examination tailored to identifying the symptoms and signs of secondary hypertension should be completed. If a specific cause is suggested, workup initially should be tailored to its identification. If the results of this workup are negative or if no specific cause is initially suggested, evaluation for other possible causes of secondary hypertension should be considered.

Clinical Example

A 65-year-old man who has had well-controlled hypertension is found to have acute worsening of his blood pressure, with readings averaging 170/110 mm Hg over several days. He also has a history of coronary artery disease. During his evaluation, a right renal artery bruit is heard. Captopril renal scanning is performed, with results that are positive for right renal artery stenosis. This is confirmed by renal arteriography and treated with angioplasty.

REFERENCES

1. **National High Blood Pressure Education Program Working Group.** Report on primary prevention of hypertension. Arch Intern Med. 1993;153:186-208.
2. **Schappert SM.** National Ambulatory Medical Care Survey: 1991 summary. Vital & Health Statistics - Series. 1994;13:Data from the Nation-110.
3. **Maxwell MH.** Cooperative study of renovascular hypertension: current status. Kidney Int. 1975;(Suppl8):S153-60.
4. **Hypertension in Diabetes Study Group.** Hypertension in Diabetes Study (HDS): I. Prevalence of hypertension in newly presenting type 2 diabetic patients and the association with risk factors for cardiovascular and diabetic complications. J Hypertens. 1993;11:309-17.
5. **Williams RR, Hunt SC, Hopkins PN, et al.** Genes, hypertension, and early familial coronary artery disease. In: Laragh JH, Brenner BM, eds. Hypertension: Pathophysiology, Diagnosis, and Management. New York: Raven Press; 1990:127-36.

6. **Tucker RM, Labarthe DR.** Frequency of surgical treatment for hypertension in adults at the Mayo Clinic from 1973 through 1975. Mayo Clin Proc. 1977;52:549-5.

7. **Gifford RWJ.** Evaluation of the hypertensive patient. Chest. 1973;64:336-40.

8. **Albers FJ.** Clinical characteristics of atherosclerotic renovascular disease. Am J Kidney Dis. 1994;24:636-41.

9. **Ross EJ, Linch DC.** Cushing's syndrome—killing disease: discriminatory value of signs and symptoms aiding early diagnosis. Lancet. 1982;2:646-9.

10. **Stein PP, Black HR.** A simplified diagnostic approach to pheochromocytoma. A review of the literature and report of one institution's experience. Medicine. 1991;70:46-66.

11. **Whalen RK, Althausen AF, Daniels GH.** Extra-adrenal pheochromocytoma. J Urol. 1992;147:1-10.

12. **Rao PS.** Coarctation of the aorta. Semin Nephrol. 1995;15:87-105.

13. **Lifton RP.** Molecular genetics of human blood pressure variation. Science. 1996;272:676-80.

14. **Lifton RP.** Genetic determinants of human hypertension. Proc Natl Acad Sci U S A. 1995;92:8545-51.

15. **Bourgoignie JJ, Rubbert K, Sfakianakis GN.** Angiotensin-converting enzyme-inhibited renography for the diagnosis of ischemic kidneys. Am J Kidney Dis. 1994;24:665-73.

16. **Nally JV Jr, Black HR.** State-of-the-art review: captopril renography–pathophysiological considerations and clinical observations. Semin Nucl Med. 1992;22:85-97.

17. **Fommei E, Ghione S, Hilson AJ, et al.** Captopril radionuclide test in renovascular hypertension: a European multicentre study. European Multicentre Study Group. Eur J Nucl Med. 1993;20:617-23.

18. **Setaro JF, Chen CC, Hoffer PB, Black HR.** Captopril renography in the diagnosis of renal artery stenosis and the prediction of improvement with revascularization. The Yale Vascular Center experience. Am J Hypertens. 1991;4:698S-705S.

19. **Dondi M, Fanti S, Monetti N.** Captopril renal scintigraphy: a viewpoint. J Nucl Med. 1993;37:259-63.

20. **Muller FB, Sealey JE, Case DB, et al.** The captopril test for identifying renovascular disease in hypertensive patients. Am J Med. 1986;80:633-44.

21. **Davidson RA, Barri YM, Wilcox CS.** The simplified captopril test: an effective tool to diagnose renovascular hypertension. Am J Kidney Dis. 1994;24:660-4.

22. **Canzanello VJ, Textor SC.** Noninvasive diagnosis of renovascular disease. Mayo Clin Proc. 1994;69:1172-81.

23. **Hansen KJ, Tribble RW, Reavis SW, et al.** Renal duplex sonography: evaluation of clinical utility. J Vasc Surg. 1990;12:227-36.

24. **Hoffmann U, Edwards JM, Carter S, et al.** Role of duplex scanning for the detection of atherosclerotic renal artery disease. Kidney Int. 1991;39:1232-9.

25. **Olin JW, Piedmonte MR, Young JR, et al.** The utility of duplex ultrasound scanning of the renal arteries for diagnosing significant renal artery stenosis [see comments]. Ann Intern Med. 1995;122:833-8.

26. **Stavros AT, Parker SH, Yakes WF, et al.** Segmental stenosis of the renal artery: pattern recognition of tardus and parvus abnormalities with duplex sonography. Radiology. 1992;184:487-92.

27. **Strandness DE Jr.** Duplex imaging for the detection of renal artery stenosis. Am J Kidney Dis. 1994;24:674-8.

28. **Borrello JA, Li D, Vesely TM, et al.** Renal arteries: clinical comparison of three-dimensional time-of-flight MR angiographic sequences and radiographic angiography renal arteries: clinical comparison of three-dimensional time-of-flight MR angiographic sequences and radiographic angiography. Radiology. 1995;197:793-9.

29. **de Haan MW, Kouwenhoven M, Thelissen RP, et al.** Renovascular disease in patients with hypertension: detection with systolic and diastolic gating in three-dimensional, phase-contrast MR angiography. Radiology. 1996;198:449-56.

30. **Fellner C, Strotzer M, Geissler A, et al.** Renal arteries: evaluation with optimized 2D and 3D time-of-flight MR angiography renal arteries: evaluation with optimized 2D and 3D time-of-flight MR angiography. Radiology. 1995;196:681-7.

31. **Grist TM.** Magnetic resonance angiography of renal artery stenosis. Am J Kidney Dis. 1994;24:700-12.

32. **Rudnick MR, Maxwell MH.** Limitations of renin assays. In: Narins RG, ed. Controversies in Nephrology and Hypertension. New York: Churchill Livingstone; 1984:123-60.

33. **Bookstein JJ, Abrams HL, Buenger RE, et al.** Radiologic aspects of renovascular hypertension. 2. The role of urography in unilateral renovascular disease. JAMA. 1972;220:1225-30.

34. **Hricak H, White SS.** Radiologic assessment of the kidney. In: Brenner BM, ed. The Kidney. 5th ed. Philadelphia: WB Saunders; 1996:1175-99.

35. **Distler A, Spies KP.** Diagnostic procedure in renovascular hypertension. Clin Nephrol. 1991;36:174-80.

36. **Rudnick MR, Berns JS, Cohen RM, Goldfarb S.** Nephrotoxic risks of renal angiography: contrast media-associated nephrotoxicity and atheroembolism–a critical review [Review]. Am J Kidney Dis. 1994;24:713-27.

37. **Hawkins IF Jr, Wilcox CS, Kerns SR, Sabatelli FW.** CO2 digital angiography: a safer contrast agent for renal vascular imaging? Am J Kidney Dis. 1994;24:685-94.

38. **Levey AS.** Measurement of renal function in chronic renal disease. Kidney Int. 1990;38:167-84.

39. **Streeten DH, Tomycz N, Anderson GH.** Reliability of screening methods for the diagnosis of primary aldosteronism. Am J Med. 1979;67:403-13.

40. **Weinberger MH, Grim CE, Hollifield JW, et al.** Primary aldosteronism: diagnosis, localization, and treatment. Ann Intern Med. 1979;90:386-95.

41. **Young WFJ, Hogan MJ, Klee GG, et al.** Primary aldosteronism: diagnosis and treatment. Mayo Clin Proc. 1990;65:96-110.

42. **Bravo EL.** Primary aldosteronism: issues in diagnosis and management. Endocrinol Metab Clin North Am. 1994;23:271-83.

43. **Blumenfeld JD, Sealey JE, Schlussel Y, et al.** Diagnosis and treatment of primary hyperaldosteronism. Ann Intern Med. 1994;121:877-85.

44. **Brunner HR, Laragh JH, Baer L, et al.** Essential hypertension: renin and aldosterone, heart attack and stroke. N Engl J Med. 1972;286:441-9.

45. **Weinberger MH, Fineberg NS.** The diagnosis of primary aldosteronism and separation of two major subtypes. Arch Intern Med. 1993;153:2125-9.

46. **Kaplan NM.** Pheochromocytoma. In: Clinical Hypertension. 6th ed. Baltimore: Williams & Wilkins; 1994:367-87.

47. **Pauker SG, Kopelman RI.** Interpreting hoofbeats: can Bayes help clear the haze? N Engl J Med. 1992;327:1009-13.

48. **Bravo EL, Tarazi RC, Fouad FM, et al.** Clonidine-suppression test: a useful aid in the diagnosis of pheochromocytoma. N Engl J Med. 1981;305:623-6.

49. **Peplinski GR, Norton JA.** The predictive value of diagnostic tests for pheochromocytoma. Surgery. 1994;116:1101-9.

50. **Tenenbaum F, Lumbroso J, Schlumberger M, et al.** Comparison of radio-labeled octreotide and meta-iodobenzylguanidine (MIBG) scintigraphy in malignant pheochromocytoma. J Nucl Med. 1995;36:1-6.

51. **Karet FE, Brown MJ.** Phaeochromocytoma: diagnosis and management. Postgrad Med J. 1994;70:326-8.

52. **Carvalho JS, Redington AN, Shinebourne EA, et al.** Continuous wave Doppler echocardiography and coarctation of the aorta: gradients and flow patterns in the assessment of severity. Br Heart J. 1990;64:133-7.

53. **Prince MR, Narasimham DL, Jacoby WT, et al.** Three-dimensional gadolinium-enhanced MR angiography of the thoracic aorta. AJR Am J Roentgenol. 1996;166:1387-97.

54. **Teien DE, Wendel H, Bjornebrink J, Ekelund L.** Evaluation of anatomical obstruction by Doppler echocardiography and magnetic resonance imaging in patients with coarctation of the aorta. Br Heart J. 1993;69:352-5.

Hypertrophic Cardiomyopathy 8

Jules Cohen, MD, and Philip Greenland, MD

KEY POINTS

Pretest Probabilities

- Hypertrophic cardiomyopathy (HCM) is an uncommon disorder of heart muscle that is sometimes difficult to diagnose owing to the wide spectrum of its clinical and hemodynamic presentations.

- The clinical diagnosis of HCM is almost certain in patients who have a fast-increasing arterial pulse, late systolic murmur that is augmented by Valsalva maneuver, and palpable fourth heart sound with left ventricular hypertrophy.

Diagnostic Strategies

- Most suspected HCM can be properly diagnosed based on careful clinical evaluation and echocardiographic studies.

- Some of the echocardiographic criteria, such as asymmetric septal hypertrophy (ASH), initially considered pathognomonic for HCM, occur in other forms of heart disease.

- Echocardiography provides important information concerning the two most serious hemodynamic consequences of HCM: obstruction to left ventricular outflow and impairment of diastolic function.

- Genetic analysis can help confirm the diagnosis in some patients when the usual clinical and imaging methods have not led to a diagnosis.

BACKGROUND

Hypertrophic cardiomyopathy (HCM) is a relatively uncommon cardiac condition characterized by severe myocardial hypertrophy and myofiber disarray (1). The classic condition is characterized by autosomal dominant inheritance and a high degree of penetrance. The first systematic description of the disease in 1958 focused on the anatomic findings observed at necropsy in eight young adults who had died suddenly (2).

It is now generally accepted that the fundamental genetic disturbance in this disease is an abnormality of one or more of the proteins of the contractile apparatus in heart muscle (3). Abnormal gene sequences for beta myosin, tropomyosin, and troponin have all been identified in various patients or families with the disorder. But the precise mechanism by which those abnormalities lead to the specific gross pathologic and histopathologic features of this disease remains uncertain. Further, the precise role played by outflow tract obstruction in the clinical presentation of the disease remains controversial (4,5).

Most authorities now regard HCM as a distinct cardiomyopathy, with a spectrum of clinical, echocardiographic, angiographic, and pathologic features (6,7). Both obstructive and nonobstructive forms exist, and the degree of obstruction is characteristically highly variable in individual patients.

A correct diagnosis is important because treatment of HCM may be quite inappropriate for other cardiac conditions (8,9). However, the diagnosis of HCM may be elusive because there is no gold standard that can be applied to all cases.

Obstruction to left ventricular outflow has probably been over-emphasized in the past. Although true obstruction probably occurs in HCM (10–12) and is hemodynamically important in some patients, impairment of left ventricular filling is likely to be a more functionally important and characteristic feature of HCM and one that is present in nearly all patients (13,14).

The major clinical consequences of impaired diastolic filling are high left ventricular filling pressures leading to dyspnea and to low-output states when left ventricular filling becomes severely compromised (e.g., when atrial fibrillation or other tachyarrhythmias occur).

When both ventricular outflow obstruction and impaired filling are present together, patients may be highly symptomatic. Myocardial ischemia, related to impairment of perfusion of the hypertrophied heart, also may play a role in clinical presentation (15,16).

In recent years, a variant of HCM has been described that is characterized by disproportionate apical hypertrophy. Some patients with the apical form of HCM have clinical features that differ from those seen in the more usual variant of the disorder, confounding diagnosis further (17,18).

ESTIMATING PRETEST PROBABILITY

The diagnosis of HCM is virtually certain when the patient has the following three cardinal physical signs: (1) fast-rising bisferious arterial pulse, (2) late-onset systolic ejection murmur at the left sternal edge and apex that is augmented by Valsalva maneuver, and (3) palpable late diastolic ventricular filling impulse, which is synchronous with atrial contraction and is associated with palpable left ventricular hypertrophy (19).

A family history of hypertrophic cardiomyopathy, with or without obstruction, and other bedside maneuvers that elicit or augment obstruction help support the diagnosis. Pretest probability is high in such patients, well above 50%.

However, many patients do not exhibit characteristic clinical findings. Consequently, diagnostic procedures are required in most patients in whom HCM is suspected. Because HCM is a fairly rare cardiac condition (accounting for < 5% of all cardiac disorders), pretest probability should be considered fairly low (i.e., no more than 5%–10%) in patients who do not have the characteristic physical findings, a convincing family history, or distinctive responses to bedside maneuvers such as Valsalva maneuver or squatting.

DIAGNOSTIC TESTS

Echocardiography

Echocardiography is the primary noninvasive method of evaluating patients in whom HCM is suspected. Certain echocardiographic features such as asymmetric septal hypertrophy (ASH)—(a high ratio of interventricular septum to left ventricular posterior wall thickness), or systolic anterior motion of the mitral valve (SAM) were initially considered pathognomonic for HCM; however, it is now clear that no single echocardiographic finding is 100% specific for HCM, and particularly those based on M-mode studies.

Asymmetric septal hypertrophy, although commonly seen in HCM, has also been reported to occur occasionally in patients with other cardiac conditions, including coronary artery disease (especially in the presence of previous inferior myocardial infarction), pulmonary valve stenosis, primary pulmonary hypertension, acquired aortic valve disease, and systemic hypertension (20). It also has been noted rarely in healthy persons (21). The sensitivity and specificity of ASH greater than 1.3 are both, at best, near 90% in adults. With a stricter cutoff of ASH greater than 1.5, specificity increases to approximately 94%, but sensitivity decreases to less than 80% (Table 8-1) (20). The specificity of ASH is clearly lower in infants, children, and young adults with congenital heart diseases associated with left ventricular hypertrophy.

SAM is observed in approximately 50% of patients with HCM and is believed to be present only in those with obstruction to left ventricular outflow. This finding is considered highly specific (97% in one study) (20). Equally specific (specificity essentially 100%) are findings

Table 8-1. Operating Characteristics of Echocardiography in the Diagnosis of Hypertrophic Cardiomyopathy

Diagnostic Test	Sensitivity	Specificity	Likelihood Ratio	
			Positive Result	Negative Result
	←	%	→	
Asymmetric septal hypertrophy >1.3	~90	~90 (56–90)	9	0.11
Asymmetric septal hypertrophy >1.5	79	94	13	0.22
Systolic anterior motion of the mitral valve	~50 (50–61)	97 (95–97)	17	0.52
Midsystolic closure of aortic valve	~60	99	60	0.40
Decreased interventricular septal amplitude	~70	90	7	0.33
Decreased left ventricular end-systolic dimension	~50	85	3.3	0.59
Interventricular septal thickness >15 mm	~70	99	70	0.30

of midsystolic aortic valve closure and interventricular septal thickness greater than 15 mm (22) (see Table 8-1).

More recent investigations have demonstrated the superiority of two-dimensional echocardiography and Doppler flow studies over M-mode in evaluating patients in whom HCM is suspected (6,23,24). Chamber size and shape as well as septal and free wall dimensions can be more definitively evaluated using two-dimensional methods. Maron and Epstein (20) note that two-dimensional echocardiography improves sensitivity because ASH is absent in the 5% to 18% of patients who have clear-cut asymmetric hypertrophy in left ventricular locations other than the septum. In addition, Martin and colleagues have suggested improvement in specificity using two-dimensional echocardiography because ventricular muscle appears to show a "ground-glass" appearance in HCM that distinguishes it from many other causes of hypertrophy, especially hypertensive cardiomyopathy (25). This distinctive feature, however, may be more characteristic of this disorder in young patients than in older patients (26).

Cardiac Catheterization

Cardiac catheterization is indicated when the clinical suspicion of HCM is high but when the diagnosis remains uncertain after echocardiography. Although angiography and hemodynamic data from catheterization confirm the diagnosis in most cases, even this study may not always permit differentiation of HCM from other forms of cardiac disease (19).

Characteristic angiographic features of HCM include massive hypertrophy of the free wall and especially of the septum, large papillary muscles, obliteration of the left ventricular cavity at end-systole, and starlike projections of contrast medium into the interstices of the trabeculae carneae. In some patients, systolic anterior movement of the mitral valve can be seen on left ventricular angiography. As with echocardiography, few patients have all the angiographic findings necessary for a certain diagnosis, and some of these features are also seen in other forms of heart disease. Consequently, one must recognize that in some patients the diagnosis may remain uncertain even if a pressure gradient can be provoked.

In addition, cardiac catheterization is necessary in patients with HCM in whom surgery is being considered.

Other Tests

Other diagnostic procedures include electrocardiography (ECG), chest radiography, nuclear imaging procedures, computed tomography, magnetic resonance imaging, myocardial biopsy, and genetic analysis.

Electrocardiography is highly sensitive, especially in patients with HCM-related symptoms; however, the specificity of the findings is low. For example, ECG evidence of ST-T segment changes, Q waves, or left ventricular hypertrophy, although commonly present in HCM, are also present in many other cardiac disorders (6,27).

Chest radiography is neither highly sensitive nor highly specific for HCM.

Some recent studies suggest that nuclear imaging procedures can help to define intracardiac anatomy and regional function and to assess the presence and extent of myocardial ischemia (6,15,16,28). Imaging of the heart using computed tomography and magnetic resonance imaging also may help define the anatomy of and contribute to the understanding of regional functional abnormalities (29,30). However, experience with these modalities in patients with HCM remains limited, and both the diagnosis and the precise definition of the anatomy of HCM can usually be made with more readily available and less expensive approaches.

In rare instances, myocardial biopsy may be considered for diagnosis. Testing for myocardial cell disorganization is sensitive for HCM (present in approximately 95% of patients) (31). Testing for extensive myocardial disorganization is nearly 100% specific.

Highly specific genetic analyses have become available in many institutions in recent years. Such analyses provide a useful and, in some cases, critically important addition to the diagnosis of HCM (32). Genetic analyses should be considered when specific confirmation of the diagnosis is required for any reason, but especially when the diagnosis is still in doubt after careful investigation using clinical and imaging methods, particularly in a symptomatic patient. The role of genetic analysis in clinically unaffected family members of patients with confirmed HCM still needs to be defined. Ethical as well as technical considerations need to be carefully examined on an individual case basis before one proceeds with genetic testing in such patients (33,34).

DIAGNOSTIC STRATEGIES

Because HCM is an unusual condition, the pretest probability of this disorder can be considered low unless the distinctive clinical features discussed earlier in this chapter are present, such as a family history of HCM, a systolic murmur that increases with maneuvers that deplete ventricular volume (e.g., Valsalva maneuver), a fast-increasing arterial pulse, and a palpable late-diastolic impulse. When all of these features are present (which is uncommon), the pretest likelihood of HCM is high (>50%) and the diagnosis can often be made with confidence at the bedside. When only a few of the common clinical features are present, other than the distinctive response of the murmur to bedside maneuvers, the pretest probability is much lower.

Echocardiography is the most useful and appropriate test for confirming or excluding a diagnosis of HCM. When clinical suspicion of HCM is high (pretest probability >50%), any of the characteristic echocardiographic signs of HCM can be considered confirmatory. However, when pretest probability of HCM is low, only the more specific findings of SAM, an ASH greater than 1.5, ventricular septal thickness greater than 15 mm, or midsystolic aortic valve closure adequately confirm the diagnosis. The finding of ASH greater than 1.3 (but less than 1.5), however, can be found in many other cardiac conditions; therefore, when the pretest probablitiy of HCM is low, this finding alone should be considered inadequate for a diagnosis of HCM (Table 8-2).

An appreciation of the operating characteristics of the primary noninvasive tests combined with a reasonable estimate of pretest probability generally results in satisfactory classification of patients, obviating the need for more invasive studies. Treatment usually is guided by the presence or absence of symptoms related to the two most serious pathophysiologic consequences of the disease: dynamic outflow obstruction and impaired left ventricular filling. Because echocardiography is useful for identifying these features (11,12,14), treatment can usually be determined on the basis of noninvasive testing even if some diagnostic uncertainty remains. Much has been learned in recent years about the genetic basis for HCM, the pathophysiologic features of the disorder, and the functional cardiac evaluation in patients with the disorder. Except for genetic analysis, however, little new has emerged to supplant the traditional reliance on bedside evaluation supplemented by echocardiography as the most valuable method for arriving at a definitive clinical diagnosis.

Table 8-2. Post-test Probabilities of Hypertrophic Cardiomyopathy Based on Findings

Diagnostic test	Pretest Probability					
	20%		50%		80%	
	Positive Result	Negative Result	Positive Result	Negative Result	Positive Result	Negative Result
	←————————————————— % —————————————————→					
Asymmetric septal hypertrophy >1.3	69	3	90	10	97	31
Asymmetric septal hypertrophy >1.5	77	5	93	18	98	47
Systolic anterior motion of the mitral valve	81	11	94	34	99	67
Midsystolic closure of aortic valve	94	9	98	29	>99	62
Interventricular septal thickness >15 mm	95	7	99	23	>99	55

CLINICAL PROBLEMS

Clinical Problem 1
A patient has a high pretest probability of HCM based on the presence of several characteristic clinical features.

Testing Strategy and Rationale
Echocardiography should be performed. This is the best choice for confirming the diagnosis, because many of the echocardiographic features of HCM are highly specific. Owing to its sensitivity for HCM, if significant ASH cannot be demonstrated by echocardiography, a diagnosis of HCM becomes suspect.

Clinical Example
A 25-year-old woman is referred for evaluation of dyspnea. Her symptoms occur occasionally at rest but more typically with exertion. Her family history is noteworthy for cardiac murmur in her mother and maternal grandfather. Physical examination reveals blood pressure of 120/80 mm Hg and a normal arterial pulse contour. Palpable left ventricular hypertrophy is present. There is a prominent fourth heart sound at the apex and a grade 2/6 systolic ejection murmur that becomes 4/6 during the strain phase of Valsalva maneuver. The murmur decreases with squatting and

increases with standing. Electrocardiography reveals Q waves in V_1–V_3 and left ventricular hypertrophy. The family history, clinical presentation, and murmur characteristics are all highly typical of HCM. Her pretest probability is approximately 80%, despite the relative rarity of HCM overall. An echocardiogram is ordered.

Clinical Problem 2
A patient exhibits clinical findings only somewhat suggestive of HCM.

Testing Strategy and Rationale
Echocardiography should be performed. In a patient with some findings suggestive of HCM, even if the pretest probability is low, it may be important to rule out HCM owing to the risk posed by taking certain drugs if the patient does indeed have HCM. Echocardiography, particularly a two-dimensional study, can reliably rule out HCM if ASH is absent.

Clinical Example
A 67-year-old woman presents with dyspnea and an ECG showing evidence of left ventricular hypertrophy. There is no significant family history of heart disease. The patient may have had "mild hypertension" in the past, but without medication her blood pressure is 120/80 mm Hg. The carotid upstroke is normal, and the apical impulse is not convincing for left ventricular hypertrophy. She has a grade 2/6 systolic ejection murmur at the base of the heart with some radiation to the carotids. No fourth heart sound is present. Valsalva maneuver does not change the murmur.

The clinical picture is not distinctive, and the pretest likelihood of HCM is substantially less than 10%. Echocardiography is probably warranted, however, owing to the clinical findings and the uncertain origin of the left ventricular hypertrophy. If the echocardiogram shows no ASH and no SAM, the diagnosis of HCM is confidently excluded. If concentric left ventricular hypertrophy is present, the specificity of this finding is so low that, with such a low pretest likelihood, the probability of HCM remains very low. If, however, both ASH and SAM are unexpectedly present, the posttest probability of the disorder is high and the diagnosis of HCM is established.

REFERENCES

1. **Maron BJ, Gardin JM, Flack JM, et al.** Prevalence of hypertrophic cardiomyopathy in a general population of young adults: echocardiographic analysis of 4111 subjects in the CARDIA study. Circulation. 1995;92:785-9.

2. **Teare D.** Asymmetrical hypertrophy of the heart in young adults. Br Heart J. 1958;20:1-8.

3. **Roberts R, Marian AJ, Bachinski L.** Molecular genetics of hypertrophic cardiomyopathy. J Card Fail. 1996;2(4 Suppl):587-95.

4. **Maron BJ.** Hypertrophic cardiomyopathy [Review]. Curr Prob Cardiol. 1993;18:639-704.

5. **Criley JM.** Unobstructed thinking (and terminology) is called for in the understanding and management of hypertrophic cardiomyopathy. J Am Coll Cardiol. 1997;29:741-3.

6. **Shaver JA, Salerni R, Curtiss EI, Follansbee WP.** Clinical presentation and noninvasive evaluation of the patient with hypertrophic cardiomyopathy. Cardiovascular Clinics. 1988;19:149-92.

7. **Klues HG, Schiffers A, Maron BJ.** Phenotropic spectrum and patterns of left ventricular hypertrophy in hypertrophic cardiomyopathy: morphologic observations and signficance as assessed by two-dimensional echocardiography in 600 patients. J Am Coll Cardiol. 1995; 26:1699-1708.

8. **Abelmann WH, Lorell BH.** The challenge of cardiomyopathy. J Am Coll Cardiol. 1989; 13:1219-39.

9. **Maron BJ, Bonow RO, Cannon RO III, et al.** Hypertrophic cardiomyopathy: interrelations of clinical manifestations, pathophysiology and therapy. N Engl J Med. 1987;316:780-9, 844-52.

10. **Come PC, Riley MF, Carl LV, Lorell B.** Doppler evidence that true left ventricular-to-aortic pressure gradients exist in hypertrophic cardiomyopathy. Am Heart J. 1988; 116:1253-61.

11. **Sasson Z, Yock PG, Hatle LK, et al.** Doppler echocardiographic determination of the pressure gradient in hypertrophic cardiomyopathy. J Am Coll Cardiol. 1988;11:752-6.

12. **Scheffknecht BH, Bonow RO, Dwyer AJ, Maron BJ.** Functional assessment of left ventricular ejection dynamics by cine magnetic resonance imaging in hypertrophic cardiomyopathy. Am J Cardiol. 1994; 73:981-4.

13. **Goodwin JF.** A current appreciation of cardiomyopathies. Acta Cardiol. 1996;51:189-202.

14. **Bareiss P, Roul G.** Left ventricular diastolic dysfunction in cardiomyopathies. Arch Mal Coeur Vaiss. 1996;89(Spec No. 2):25-31.

15. **O'Gara PT, Bonow RO, Maron BJ, et al.** Myocardial perfusion abnormalities in patients with hypertrophic cardiomyopathy: assessment with Thallium-201 emission computed tomography. Circulation. 1987;76:1214-23.

16. **VonDohlen TW, Prisant LM, Frank MJ.** Significance of positive or negative Thallium-201 scintigraphy in hypertrophic cardiomyopathy. Am J Cardiol. 1989;64:498-503.

17. **Louie EK, Maron BJ.** Apical hypertrophic cardiomyopathy: clinical and two-dimensional echocardiographic assessment. Ann Intern Med. 1987;106:665-70.

18. **Gosselin G, Pasterna A, Lesperance J, et al.** Apical hypertrophic cardiomyopathy: clinical and angiographic characteristics of the first Canadian series. Am J Cardiol. 1988;4:258-61.

19. **Goodwin JF.** Hypertrophic cardiomyopathy: a disease in search of its own identity. Am J Cardiol. 1980;45:177-80.

20. **Maron BJ, Epstein SE.** Hypertrophic cardiomyopathy: recent observations regarding the specificity of three hallmarks of the disease: asymmetric septal hypertrophy, septal disorganization and systolic anterior motion of the anterior mitral leaflet. Am J Cardiol. 1980; 45:141-54.

21. **Wei JY, Weiss JL, Bulkley BH.** The heterogeneity of hypertropic cardiomyopathy: an autopsy and one dimensional echocardiographic study. Am J Cardiol. 1980;45:24-32.

22. **Doi YL, McKenna WJ, Gehrke J, et al.** M mode echocardiography in hypertrophic cardiomyopathy: diagnostic criteria and prediction of obstruction. Am J Cardiol. 1980;45:6-14.

23. **Maron BJ, Gottdiener JS, Epstein SE.** Patterns and significance of distribution of left ventricular hypertrophy in hypertrophic cardiomyopathy: a wide angle, two dimensional echocardiographic study of 125 patients. Am J Cardiol. 1981;48:418-28.

24. **Gardin JM, Daberstani A, Glasgow GA, et al.** Echocardiographic and Doppler flow observation in obstructed and nonobstructed hypertrophic cardiomyopathy. Am J Cardiol. 1985;56:614-21.

25. **Martin RP, Rakowski H, French J, et al.** Idiopathic hypertrophic subaortic stenosis viewed by wide-angle, phased-array echocardiography. Circulation. 1979;59:1206-17.

26. **Vitale DF, Bonow RO, Calabro R, et al.** Myocardial ultrasonic tissue characterization in pediatric and adult patients with hypertrophic cardiomyopathy. Circulation. 1996;94:2826-30.

27. **Ryan MP, Cleland JGF, French JA, et al.** The standard electrocardiogram as a screening test for hypertrophic cardiomyopathy. Am J Cardiol. 1995;76:689-94.

28. **Camici PG, Rosen SD.** Does position emission tomography contribute to the management of clinical cardiac problems? Eur Heart J. 1996;17:174-81.

29. **Casolo GC, Trotta F, Rostagno C, et al.** Detection of apical hypertrophic cardiomyopathy by magnetic resonance imaging. Am Heart J. 1989;117:468-72.

30. **Posma JL, Blanksma PK, vanderWall EE, et al.** Assessment of quantitative hypertrophy scores in hypertrohic cardiomyopathy: magnetic resonance imaging vs echoccardiography. Am Heart J. 1996;132:1020-7.

31. **Maron BJ, Roberts WC.** Quantitative analysis of cardiac muscle cell disorganization in the ventricular septum of patients with hypertrophic cardiomyopathy. Circulation. 1979;59:689-706.

32. **McKenna WJ, Spirito P, Desnos M, et al.** Experience from clinical genetics in hypertrophic cardiomyopathy: proposal for new diagnostic critieria in adult members of affected families. Heart. 1997;77:130-2.

33. **Smart RV, Yu B, Le H, et al.** DNA testing in familial hypertrophic cardiomyopathy: clinical and laboratory implications. Clin Genet. 1996;50:169-75.

34. **Komajda M.** Genetics of hypertrophic cardiomyopathies: what are the clinical perspectives? Arch Mal Coeur Vaiss. 1996;89(Spec. No. 2):11-4.

Deep Venous Thrombosis 9

Rudolph J. Napodano, MD

KEY POINTS

Pretest Probabilities

- The presence or absence of signs and symptoms of deep venous thrombosis does not correlate well with the presence or absence of clots in the veins of the lower extremity. Almost one third of patients with signs suggestive of deep venous thrombosis do not have venographic evidence of clots.
- Deep venous thrombosis is associated with venous stasis (i.e., immobilization) and with various clinical disorders such as neoplasms and hypercoagulable states.

Diagnostic Strategies

- Whenever venous thrombosis is suspected, objective testing is essential.
- Ascending functional venography is the gold standard for proximal or distal deep venous thrombosis.
- When available, ultrasonography is a reasonable noninvasive alternative to venography for identifying proximal deep venous thrombosis. Impedance plethysmography has a lower sensitivity.
- If the results of ultrasonography are negative in a patient in whom a deep venous thrombosis is strongly suspected, either venography or serial ultrasonography is recommended.
- If noninvasive testing is not available or if its accuracy is uncertain, venography is the preferred diagnostic strategy.
- If venography shows only distal disease, the patient may be followed with serial ultrasonography; however, if serial ultrasonography is not available, anticoagulant therapy should generally be started because clinical examination alone cannot determine whether proximal extension of the clot will occur.

BACKGROUND

Deep venous thrombosis, a condition of active thrombosis in the deep venous system of one or both lower extremities, is associated with a high likelihood of extension of the thrombotic process and subsequent embolism. Deep venous thrombosis may occur spontaneously, after prolonged stasis (bedrest), or in association with various clinical disorders, including neoplasms, hypercoagulable states, and disorders associated with estrogen use (1–4).

Lower-extremity deep venous thrombosis is associated with significant morbidity and mortality, principally from the complications of pulmonary embolism and chronic venous insufficiency. More than 90% of pulmonary emboli originate in lower extremity sites. The thrombotic process begins in the deep veins of the calf (5,6). If the process remains confined to the tibial-soleal systems, the chance for subsequent embolic episodes is low; but if such episodes do occur, they usually result in small, asymptomatic pulmonary emboli. However, when thrombi extend into the popliteal and femoral venous systems, the likelihood for further extension and clinically significant embolic events increases markedly.

ESTIMATING PRETEST PROBABILITY

Only half of all patients with active venous thrombosis present with signs or symptoms referable to the involved limb (7–9). In a study of patients with documented pulmonary emboli, deep venous thrombosis was recognized in only 33% of patients before or at the time of the event (10). Conversely, in almost one third of patients with signs suggestive of deep venous thrombosis (e.g., pain, swelling, tenderness, edema), there is no venographic evidence of clots (7). Therefore, the presence or absence of signs and symptoms does not correlate well with the presence or absence of active deep venous thrombosis. Thus, when deep venous thrombosis is considered a reasonable probability, objective testing is necessary.

DIAGNOSTIC TESTS

Venography

Ascending functional venography is the gold standard for the diagnosis of deep venous thrombosis in the lower extremity (11). The procedure is invasive, expensive, and involves risks (e.g., radiocontrast allergy, renal failure, and post-test phlebitis), and it fails to visualize the venous system adequately in 2% to 10% of patients (12–15).

The most specific and reliable venographic criterion for the diagnosis of deep venous thrombosis is an intraluminal filling defect that is consistent in size and shape in all views and visible on several projections. Other criteria, such as the abrupt termination of the opaque column at a constant location in a vein, nonfilling of portions of the deep venous system, and diversion of flow, are much less reliable and may be caused by old venous thrombi or various technical artifacts. Venography fails to visualize the common femoral and iliac veins adequately in approximately 5% to 10% of patients (15), and this is considered an incomplete study.

If the results of venography are normal, the post-test probability of deep venous thrombosis approaches 0% (16). Consecutive patients with signs and symptoms suggesting deep venous thrombosis in whom venography yielded normal results were followed without anticoagulant therapy for several months. Deep venous thrombosis developed within 5 days of venography in only 1.3% of patients, and no deaths or documented episodes of clinical pulmonary embolism occurred. This high level of accuracy is achieved only when proper technique is rigidly adhered to and films are interpreted by experienced clinicians using the criteria discussed earlier (11–16).

Ultrasonography and Impedance Plethysmography

Real-time continuous, compression ultrasonography, Doppler ultrasonography (duplex) with and without color enhancement, and impedance plethysmography are the noninvasive tests used most frequently in a diagnostic workup of symptomatic patients suspected of having proximal deep venous thrombosis (17–44). All of these methods are safe, reliable, rapid, cost-effective, and painless and do not expose a patient to ionizing radiation. However, these methods also require considerable expertise to perform the procedure and to interpret the results, and none are useful in assessing disease localized to the calf.

Real-time compression ultrasonography uses the single criterion of continuous compressibility of a venous segment for the diagnosis of venous thrombosis. Duplex ultrasonography visualizes the veins of the thigh, and color enhancement combines the findings of duplex ultrasonography with color Doppler to detect blood flow and complete filling of a vein. Duplex ultrasonography may also be helpful in distinguishing deep venous thrombosis from other causes of leg pain and swelling—for example, hematoma, muscle tear, or cyst—and in distinguishing acute from chronic deep venous thrombosis.

Impedance plethysmography measures changes in the electrical resistance (impedance) in blood that result from changes in blood volume and from changes in the rate of flow in the deep veins of the leg induced by inflation and deflation of a pneumatic thigh cuff. Recent studies have found plethysmography to have a lower sensitivity for proximal deep venous thrombosis than has been previously reported (45–50). A negative test result does not rule out nonocclusive proximal vein thrombosis. Furthermore, the test does not distinguish acute deep venous thrombosis from other factors affecting venous filling and out-flow, such as arterial insufficiency, right-sided heart failure, compression of the major veins by an external mass, and poor muscle relaxation.

The operating characteristics of the ultrasonography techniques and impedance plethysmography compared with those of ascending functional venography are summarized in Table 9-1. The highest levels of accuracy are achieved only in those centers that are experienced in the technical use of the procedures and in their clinical interpretation.

Combined Testing

Impedance plethysmography may be combined with ultrasound technology or radionuclide scanning using isotopes such as I-125 fibrinogen or technetium-99m HMPAO-labeled platelets (37,38,51). When a test result can be defined as a positive result on either test, combining plethysmography with the I-125 fibrinogen scan results in reported sensitivity and specificity of approximately 92% (37,38). When plethysmography is combined with Doppler ultrasonography, sensitivity and specificity are approximately 96% and 90%, respectively (52).

In some patients with signs and symptoms suggesting deep venous thrombosis and in whom plethysmography and I-125 fibrinogen scanning yielded initially negative results, the results of venography were positive, showing disease localized to the calf (37). When these patients were followed closely for several months without anticoagulant therapy, the frequency of subsequent thromboembolic events was only about 1%.

Table 9-1. Operating Characteristics of Diagnostic Tests for Deep Venous Thrombosis

Diagnostic Test	Sensitivity	Specificity	Likelihood Ratio	
			Positive Result	Negative Result
	←———%———→			
Venography	100	100	∞	0
Real-time compression ultrasonography	95 (83–100)	95 (86–100)	19	0.05
Doppler ultrasonography (duplex)	95 (82–100)	95 (83–100)	19	0.05
Impedance plethysmography	80 (65–100)	95 (77–100)	16	0.21
Combined impedance plethysmography and I-125 fibrinogen scan	92 (90–94)	92 (91–93)	12	0.09
Combined impedance plethysmography and Doppler ultrasonography	96 (90–97)	90 (88–93)	24	0.04

Other Tests

Selected blood tests that are associated with intravascular thrombosis, such as D-dimer, fibrin degradation products, and prothrombin fragments, have been evaluated for use in the identification of deep venous thrombosis (53–58). Testing for D-dimer, a breakdown product of cross-linked fibrin and a marker for acute thromboembolism, is the most promising of these (59–62). In a recent study using D-dimer testing with impedance plethysmography in outpatients in whom a positive test result was defined as an abnormal result on either test, the combination had a sensitivity of 94% and a specificity of 82% for deep venous thrombosis (63). The final word on the utility of D-dimer testing in acute deep venous thrombosis is not yet known; prospective, clinical studies will be needed to clarify this issue.

Magnetic resonance imaging (MRI) and magnetic resonance venography (MRV) are also employed to assess the status of the deep venous system of the lower extremities (64–68). Initial reports show high sensitivity and specificity, at least comparable to those of ultrasonography; however, the test is not always readily available and is expensive. Thus, to date, MRI and MRV have not replaced ultrasonography, impedance plethsymography, and venography in most medical centers. Thrombosis of the iliac-caval system is occasionally detected by computed tomography (CT) of the abdomen.

DIAGNOSTIC STRATEGIES

Objective testing is needed to detect deep venous thrombosis because clinical signs and symptoms have limited discriminating power and because the costs of both false-positive and false-negative results are high. Because proximal deep venous thrombosis is associated with a high incidence of significant thromboembolic events, diagnostic testing focuses on its detection. Venous thrombosis that remains confined to the tibial-soleal system in the calf is rarely associated with clinically significant thromboembolic complications. When there is evidence of such thrombosis, however, follow-up with a reliable noninvasive study is warranted to ensure that proximal extension of the process does not occur (69).

Although ascending functional venography is the most accurate diagnostic test for detecting deep venous thrombosis, the test is invasive and places the patient at risk for significant complications. For the diagnosis of proximal venous thrombosis, noninvasive tests alone or in combination provide reasonable alternatives to venography. Because the accuracy of these tests in centers that perform them frequently may not be replicated everywhere, a good understanding of local operating characteristics is needed. In addition, noninvasive tests often require serial testing.

Continuous and Doppler ultrasonography (duplex), with and without color enhancement, are currently considered more sensitive than impedance plethysmography for detecting proximal deep venous thrombosis of the lower extremity (45–50). Therefore, a suggested diagnostic strategy for symptomatic patients who present with the clinical signs and symptoms suggestive of deep venous thrombosis is as follows:

1. One or more of the ultrasonography methods should be performed on the leg that has the suspected deep venous thrombosis.
2. If the initial ultrasonography findings are positive, anticoagulant therapy should be instituted because deep venous thrombosis is likely.
3. If the initial ultrasonography examination is negative but the pretest probability of disease is high, venography or serial ultrasonography should be performed.
4. If serial ultrasound examinations are normal, it is safe to observe the patient without anticoagulant therapy, because a clinically important deep venous thrombosis is unlikely.
5. If the findings of serial ultrasonography become positive, treatment should be started or the diagnosis confirmed by venography.
6. Impedance plethsymography may be used instead of ultrasonography as the initial noninvasive study. However, the lower sensitivity of this test requires that negative results be interpreted with caution, particularly when the pretest probability of disease is high.

Again, some institutions do not have ultrasonography or impedance plethysmography testing that is as accurate as in reported studies. When local accuracy is unknown or poor, the preferred strategy is to go directly to ascending functional venography for definitive diagnosis.

Because most of the studies supporting the approach that we have just outlined have been completed in symptomatic patients in an ambulatory setting, caution should be observed in applying this strategy to hospitalized patients. Also, this strategy should not be used to screen asymptomatic patients who may be at risk for deep venous thrombosis—for example, patients who have recently undergone surgery or childbirth. In this setting, test characteristics are quite different (50,70–72).

CLINICAL PROBLEM

A patient presents with symptoms or signs suggesting deep venous thrombosis, such as pain, tenderness, swelling, and venous engorgement of one leg.

Testing Strategy and Rationale

If ultrasonography is available and known to be accurate locally, this study should be performed. If it is not available, ascending functional venography should be done. Objective testing is mandatory because clinical signs and symptoms are nonspecific.

Clinical Example

A 26-year-old woman develops acute aching and swelling of the left calf, ankle, and foot. She has no history of trauma or other predisposing factors for deep venous thrombosis. Physical examination reveals discomfort on palpation of the posterior aspect of the left calf, a 2-cm difference in the circumference size of the left leg at midcalf compared with that of the right at midcalf, and no clinical signs of cellulitis. The patient should undergo ultrasonography or ascending functional venography, depending on which testing method is available.

REFERENCES

1. **Juergens JL, Spittell JA, Fairbairn JF.** Peripheral Vascular Diseases. Philadelphia: WB Saunders; 1980:730-821.
2. **Kakkar V.** The diagnosis of deep-vein thrombosis using 125-I fibrinogen test. Arch Surg. 1972;104:152-9.
3. **Coon WW.** Epidemiology of venous thromboembolism. Ann Surg. 1977;186:149-64.
4. **Filip DJ, Eckstein JD, Veltkamp JJ.** Hereditary antithrombin III deficiency and thromboembolic disease. Am J Hematol. 1976;2:343-9.
5. **Hirsh J, Hull R.** Comparative value of tests for the diagnosis of venous thrombosis. World J Surg. 1978;2:27-38.
6. **Moser KM, LeMoine JR.** Is embolic risk conditioned by location of deep venous thrombosis? Ann Intern Med. 1981;94:439-44.
7. **Kakkar VV, Corrigan TP.** Detection of deep-vein thrombosis: survey and current status. Prog Cardiovasc Dis. 1974;17:207-17.
8. **Haeger K.** Problems of acute deep venous thrombosis. Angiology. 1969;20:219-23.
9. **Nicolaides AN, Kakkar VV, Field ES, et al.** The origin of deep-vein thrombosis: a venographic study. Br J Radiol. 1971;44:653-63.
10. Urokinase Pulmonary Embolism Trial Study Group. Urokinase pulmonary embolism trial: phase I results. JAMA. 1970;214:2163-72.
11. **Rabinov K, Paulin S.** Roentgen diagnosis of venous thrombosis in the leg. Arch Surg. 1972;104:134-44.

12. **Benedict KT, Wheeler HB, Patwardhan NA.** Impedance plethysmography correlation with contrast venography. Radiology. 1977;125:695-9.

13. **Comerota AJ, White JV, Katz ML.** Diagnostic methods for deep venous thrombosis: venous Doppler examination, phleborheography, iodine-125 fibrinogen uptake, and phlebography. Am J Surg. 1985;150:14-24.

14. **Redman HC.** Deep venous thrombosis: is contrast venography still the diagnostic "gold standard"? Radiology. 1988;168:277-8.

15. **Athanasoulis CA.** Phlebography for the diagnosis of deep leg venous thrombosis. In: Frantantoni J, Wessler S, eds. Prophylactic Therapy of Deep Vein Thrombosis and Pulmonary Embolism. Bethesda, Maryland: U.S. Department of Health Education and Welfare, National Institutes of Health; 1975:62-76. DHEW publication no. 76-866.

16. **Hull R, Hirsh J, Sackett DL, et al.** Clinical validity of a negative venogram in patients with clinically suspected venous thrombosis. Circulation. 1981;64:622-5.

17. **White RH, McGaham JP, Daschback MM, et al.** Diagnosis of deep-vein thrombosis using duplex ultrasound. Ann Intern Med. 1989;111:297-304.

18. **Sigel B, Felix WR, Popky GL, et al.** Diagnosis of lower limb venous thrombosis by Doppler ultrasound technique. Arch Surg. 1972;104:174-9.

19. **Lensing AW, Levi MM, Buller HR, et al.** Diagnosis of deep-vein thrombosis using an objective Doppler method. Ann Intern Med. 1990;113:9-13.

20. **Strandness DE Jr.** Thrombosis detection by ultrasound, plethysmography and phlebography. Semin Nucl Med. 1977;7:213-8.

21. **Naidich JB, Feinberg AW, Karp-Harman H, et al.** Contrast venography: reassessment of its role. Radiology. 1988;168:97-100.

22. **Markel A, Weich Y, Gaitini D.** Doppler ultrasound in the diagnosis of venous thrombosis. Angiology. 1995;46:65-73.

23. **Cogo A, Lensing AW, Prandoni P, Hirsh J.** Distribution of thrombosis in patients with symptomatic deep-vein thrombosis: implications for simplifying the diagnostic process with compression ultrasound. Arch Intern Med. 1993;153:2777-80.

24. **Quintavalla R, Larini P, Miselli A, et al.** Duplex ultrasound diagnosis of symptomatic proximal deep-vein thrombosis of lower limbs. Eur J Radiol. 1992;15:32-6.

25. **Simons GR, Skibo LK, Polak JP, et al.** Utility of leg ultrasonography in suspected symptomatic isolated calf deep venous thrombosis. Am J Med. 1995;99:43-7.

26. **Savy-Stortz C, Nove-Josserand R, Dubost A, et al.** Venous ultrasonography-coupled with continuous Doppler in the diagnosis of deep venous thrombosis of lower limbs. Evaluation in symptomatic patients. Presse Med. 1995;24:341-4.

27. **Lewis BD, James EM, Welch TJ, et al.** Diagnosis of acute deep venous thrombosis of the lower extremities: prospective evaluation of color Doppler flow-imaging versus venography. Radiology. 1994;192:651-5.

28. **Cogo A, Lensing AW, Prandoni P, et al.** Comparison of real-time B-mode ultrasonography and Doppler ultrasound with contrast venography in the diagnosis of venous thrombosis in symptomatic outpatients. Thromb Haemost. 1993;70:404-7.

29. **Richlie DG.** Noninvasive imaging of the lower extremity for deep venous thrombosis. J Gen Intern Med. 1993;8:271-7.

30. **Montefusco-von Kleist CM, Bakal C, Sprayregen S, et al.** Comparison of duplex ultrasonography and ascending contrast venography in the diagnosis of venous thrombosis. Angiology. 1993;44:169-75.

31. **Wheeler HB, Anderson FA.** Can noninvasive tests be used as the basis for the treatment of deep-vein thrombosis? In: Bernstein EF, ed. Non-Invasive Diagnostic Techniques in Vascular Disease. St. Louis: CV Mosby; 1982:545-59.

32. **Toy PT, Schrier SL.** Occlusive impedance plethysmography: a non-invasive method of diagnosis of deep-vein thrombosis. West J Med. 1978;129:89-93.

33. **Flanigan DP, Goodreau JJ, Burnham SJ, et al.** Vascular laboratory diagnosis of clinically suspected acute deep-vein thrombosis. Lancet. 1978;2:331-4.

34. **Hull R, van Arken WG, Hirsh J, et al.** Impedance plethysmography using the occlusive cuff technique in the diagnosis of venous thrombosis. Circulation. 1976;53:696-700.

35. **Hull R, Taylor DW, Hirsh J, et al.** Impedance plethysmography: the relationship between venous filling and sensitivity and specificity for proximal vein thrombosis. Circulation. 1978;58:898-902.

36. **Cooperman M, Martin EW, Satiani B, et al.** Detection of deep venous thrombosis by impedance plethysmography. Am J Surg. 1979;137:252-4.

37. **Hull R, Hirsh J, Sackett DL, et al.** Replacement of venography in suspected venous thrombosis by impedance plethysmography and I-125 fibrinogen leg scanning. Ann Intern Med. 1981;94:12-5.

38. **Hull R, Hirsh J, Sackett DL, et al.** Cost effectiveness of clinical diagnosis, venography, and noninvasive testing in patients with symptomatic deep-vein thrombosis. N Engl J Med. 1981;304:1561-7.

39. **Hull R, Carter C, Turple AG, et al.** A randomized trial of diagnostic strategies for symptomatic deep-vein thrombosis. Thromb Haemost. 1983;50:160-4.

40. **Hull R, Hirsh J, Carter C, et al.** Diagnostic efficacy of impedance plethysomography for clinically suspected deep-vein thrombosis. Ann Intern Med. 1985;102:21-8.

41. **Huisman MV, Buller HR, ten Cate JW, et al.** Serial impedance plethysmography for suspected deep venous thrombosis in outpatients. N Engl J Med. 1986;314:823-8.

42. **Huisman MV, Buller HR, ten Cate JW, et al.** Management of clinically suspected acute venous thrombosis in outpatients with serial impedance plethysmography in a community hospital setting. Arch Intern Med. 1989;149:511-3.

43. **Wheeler HB.** Ambulatory management of suspected deep-vein thrombosis. Arch Intern Med. 1989;149:501-2.

44. **Chance JF, Abbitt PL, Tegtmeyer CJ, et al.** Real-time ultrasound for the detection of deep venous thrombosis. Ann Emerg Med. 1991;20:494-6.

45. **Kristo DA, Perry ME, Kollef MH.** Comparison of venography, duplex imaging, and bilateral impedance plethysmography for diagnosis of lower extremity deep-vein thrombosis. South Med J. 1994;87:55-60.

46. **Heijboer H, Buller HR, Lensing AW, et al.** A comparison of real-time compression ultrasonography with impedance plethysmography for the diag-

nosis of deep-vein thrombosis in symptomatic outpatients. N Engl J Med. 1993;329:1365-9.

47. **Anderson DR, Lensing AW, Wells PS, et al.** Limitations of impedance plethysmography in the diagnosis of clinically suspected deep-vein thrombosis. Ann Intern Med. 1993;118:25-30.

48. **Kearon C, Hirsh J.** Factors influencing the reported sensitivity and specificity of impedance plethysmography for proximal deep-vein thrombosis. Thromb Haemost. 1994;72:652-8.

49. **Ginsberg JS, Wells PS, Hirsh J, et al.** Reevaluation of the sensitivity of impedance plethysmography for the detection of proximal deep-vein thrombosis. Arch Intern Med. 1994;154:1930-3.

50. **Agnelli G, Cosmi B, Radicchia S, et al.** Features of thrombi and diagnostic accuracy of impedance plethysmography in symptomatic and asymptomatic deep vein thrombosis. Thromb Haemost. 1993;70:266-9.

51. **Honkanen T, Jauhola S, Karppinen K, et al.** Venous thrombosis: a controlled study on the performance of scintigraphy with 99Tcm-HMPAO-labelled platelets versus venography. Nucl Med Commun. 1992;13:88-94.

52. **Naidich JB, Feinberg AW, Karp-Harman H, et al.** Contrast venography: reassessment of its role. Radiology. 1988;168:97-100.

53. **Hirsh J.** Diagnosis of venous thrombosis. Thromb Haemost. 1979;41:450-3.

54. **Rochemaure J, Laaban JP, Achkar A, et al.** Value of the determination of D-dimers in the diagnostic approach of venous thrombo-embolic disorders. Bull Acad Natl Med. 1995;179:299-314, 314-6.

55. **Bouman CS, Ypma ST, Sybesma JP.** Comparison of the efficacy of D-dimer, fibrin degradation products and prothrombin fragment 1+2 in clinically suspected deep venous thrombosis. Thromb Res. 1995;77:225-34.

56. **Tengborn L, Palmblad S, Wojciehowski J, et al.** D-dimer and thrombin/antithrombin III complex—diagnostic tools in deep venous thrombosis? Haemostasis. 1994;24:344-50.

57. **Dale S, Gogstad GO, Brosstad F, et al.** Comparison of three D-dimer assays for the diagnosis of DVT: ELISA, latex and an immunofiltration assay. Thromb Haemos. 1994;71:270-4.

58. **Bounameaux H, de Moerloose P, Perrier A, et al.** Plasma measurement of D-dimer as diagnostic aid in suspected venous thromboembolism: an overview. Thromb Haemost. 1994;71:1-6.

59. **Lee AY, Ginsberg JS.** The role of D-dimer in the diagnosis of venous thromboembolism. Curr Opin Pulm Med. 1997;3:275-9.

60. **Elias A, Aptel I, Huc B, et al.** D-dimer test and diagnosis of deep vein thrombosis: a comparative study of 7 assays. Thromb Haemost. 1998; 76:518-22.

61. **Wildberger JE, Vorwerk D, Kilbinger M, et al.** Bedside testing (SimpliRED) in the diagnosis of deep vein thrombosis: evaluation of 250 patients. Invest Radiol. 1998;33:232-5.

62. **Leroyer C, Escoffre M, LeMoigne E, et al.** Diagnostic value of a new sensitive membrane based technique for instantaneous D-dimer evaluation in patients with clinically suspected deep venous thrombosis. Thromb Haemost. 1997;77:637-40.

63. **Ginsberg JS, Kearon C, Douketis J, et al.** The use of d-dimer testing and plethysmographic examination in patients with clinical indications of deep vein thrombosis. Arch Intern Med. 1997;157:1077-81.

64. **Dupas B, el Kouri D, Curtet C, et al.** Angiomagnetic resonance imaging of iliofemorocaval venous thrombosis. Lancet. 1995;346:17-9.

65. **Carpenter JP, Holland GA, Baum RA, et al.** Magnetic resonance venography for the detection of deep venous thrombosis: comparison with contrast venography and duplex Doppler ultrasonography. J Vasc Surg. 1993;18: 734-41.

66. **Spritzer CE, Norconk JJ Jr, Sostman HD, et al.** Detection of deep venous thrombosis by magnetic resonance imaging. Chest. 1993;104:54-60.

67. **Evans AJ, Sostman HD, Knelson MH, et al.** Detection of deep venous thrombosis: prospective comparison of MR imaging with contrast venography. Am J Roent. 1993;161:131-9.

68. **Spritzer CW, Sussman SK, Blender RA, et al.** Deep venous thrombosis evaluation with limited-flip angle, gradient-refocused MR imaging. Radiology. 1988;166:371-5.

69. **Power LR.** Distal deep venous thrombosis. J Gen Intern Med. 1988;3:288-93.

70. **Agnelli G, Radicchia S, Nenci GG.** Diagnosis of deep-vein thrombosis in asymptomatic high-risk patients. Haemostasis. 1995;25:40-8.

71. **Fongbloets LM, Lensing AW, Koopman MM, et al.** Limitations of compression ultrasound for the detection of symptomless postoperative deep-vein thrombosis. Lancet. 1994;343:1142-4.

72. **Davidson BL, Elliott CG, Lensing AW, et al.** Low accuracy of color Doppler ultrasound in the detection of proximal leg vein thrombosis in asymptomatic high-risk patients. Ann Intern Med. 1992;117:735-8.

Gastrointestinal, Liver, and Pancreatic Problems

Acute Upper Gastrointestinal Bleeding

10

Donald R. Bordley, MD

KEY POINTS

Pretest Probabilities

- Among unselected patients with acute upper gastrointestinal bleeding (UGIB), at least 75% stop bleeding shortly after admission to the hospital and never have recurrence of bleeding.

- Among the 25% of patients with continued or recurrent bleeding, more than 30% require endoscopic therapy or surgery, and 20% to 30% die.

- Advanced age, significant comorbid illness, chronic liver disease, major blood loss, and failure of active bleeding to cease promptly after admission to the hospital are independent predictors of poor outcome.

- In patients who have none of these risk factors, the chance of recurrent bleeding, significant morbidity, or death is less than 5%. In patients who have three or more of these risk factors, risk of further bleeding or other poor outcome exceeds 50%.

- Severe episodes of UGIB are almost always caused by ulcer disease, diffuse erosive gastritis, or varices.

- Malignant disease is a rare cause (2%–4% of cases) of acute UGIB.

Diagnostic Strategies

- Urgent diagnostic evaluation is not necessary for patients whose active bleeding stops within 1 hour after admission and who are at low risk for recurrence based on clinical criteria.

- Urgent esophagogastroduodenoscopy (EGD) is the diagnostic test of choice for patients with persistent or recurrent bleeding and for those in whom the clinical risk of recurrent hemorrhage is high.

- If done within 12 hours of acute bleeding, EGD establishes a diagnosis in 90% of patients and allows proper selection of patients for endoscopic therapy.

Continued

- For patients at low risk for recurrent bleeding whose bleeding episode settles uneventfully, elective diagnostic evaluation should be undertaken only if the result will alter long-term management.
- If a diagnosis is to be pursued after bleeding has settled, EGD remains the test of choice.

BACKGROUND

Acute upper gastrointestinal bleeding (UGIB) is a common problem, resulting in 250,000 to 300,000 hospitalizations annually in the United States. Seventy-five percent of cases are caused by acid peptic disease, divided equally among duodenal ulcer, gastric ulcer, and gastritis. In patients with known or suspected chronic liver disease and portal hypertension, esophageal varices are also a common and potentially lethal cause of UGIB. Most remaining episodes are caused by Mallory-Weiss tears, duodenitis, and esophagitis. Cancer is responsible for no more than 2% to 4% of UGIB. Massive episodes of UGIB are usually caused by ulcer disease, diffuse erosive gastritis, or varices (1–4). Additional less common but important causes of massive bleeding include leiomyomas of the stomach, especially in elderly patients, and aortoenteric fistulas in patients who have previously had aneurysm surgery.

Despite vastly improved therapy for ulcer disease and effective endoscopic treatment for selected patients with bleeding, the mortality associated with acute UGIB remains 5% to 12%. This probably reflects changing epidemiology; an increasing proportion of patients hospitalized for UGIB are older than 60 years old, and in this population, mortality is usually related to cardiovascular complications of bleeding or to other comorbid conditions rather than to the bleeding episode itself (1). In younger patients and even in older patients without significant comorbidity, prompt diagnosis and intervention where appropriate can significantly improve outcomes (5,6).

ESTIMATING PRETEST PROBABILITY

Prognostic Probabilities

Among unselected patients admitted for acute UGIB, at least 75% will stop bleeding shortly after admission and never have recurrence of bleeding. Among patients who continue to bleed or who rebleed, at least 30% require endoscopic therapy or surgery or both and 20% to 30% die (1–3). Predictors of poor outcome include: 1) advanced age; 2) significant comorbid illness; 3) objective evidence of chronic liver disease (jaundice, ascites, or prothrombin time prolongation); 4) evidence of major blood loss (either hypotension or hematocrit <30% on admission);

and 5) failure of active bleeding to cease promptly after admission. In patients who have none of these risk factors, the probability of further bleeding is less than 5%, the probability of needing urgent intervention is only 2%, and the probability of death is less than 1%. As a patient accumulates risk factors, these probabilities steadily increase. In patients with three or more risk factors, probability of further bleeding or other poor outcome exceeds 50% (2,7–10). Regardless of other variables, in patients who develop acute UGIB while hospitalized for another problem, the probability of continued or recurrent bleeding is greater than 30% and the probability of death is greater than 30% (4,10,11).

Time is a valuable prognostic factor in patients whose bleeding stops. In the World Organization of Gastroenterology (OMGE) survey, the initial 23% risk of further bleeding decreased to 13% after 24 hours of observation and to less than 5% after 72 hours. In their low-risk group, the initial 4% risk decreased to 1.6% after 24 hours and to less than 1% after 48 hours (7).

Diagnostic Probabilities

Estimating the pretest probability that a specific lesion is the cause of an episode of UGIB is difficult. Neither expert clinicians nor computer-aided systems can achieve greater than 60% overall diagnostic accuracy based on clinical findings alone. The sole exception occurs in the case of varices. A computer-aided system developed using the OMGE database accurately predicted more than 90% of the varices in a test series of 307 patients (2). In a study of 90 patients with UGIB that included 23 patients with varices, expert clinicians did nearly as well. Their predictions had a sensitivity of 78% and a specificity of 94% for varices (12).

DIAGNOSTIC TESTS

Esophagogastroduodenoscopy

Esophagogastroduodenoscopy (EGD) is the most sensitive diagnostic test for patients with acute UGIB. If studied within 12 hours of bleeding, at least 90% of patients are found to have 1) an actively bleeding lesion; 2) a lesion with evidence of recent bleeding; or 3) a single lesion compatible with the patient's bleeding episode. In the remaining 10% of patients, either no lesion is found or multiple lesions are found, none of which shows evidence of active or recent bleeding (2,3,13–18). Sensitivity of EGD, particularly for active bleeding, falls off after 12 hours (13,14,16).

Specificity of EGD cannot be determined directly in studies of UGIB, because absence of disease is usually defined as negative results of endoscopy (i.e., specificity is presumed to be 100%). Reported specificities of EGD performed for various indications in patients who are not bleeding range from 88% to 100% (17,19).

Endoscopic findings in patients with bleeding ulcer disease have definite prognostic significance. Among patients in prospective trials who did not receive endoscopic therapy, risk of continued or recurrent bleeding was 55% in patients with active bleeding, 43% in patients with a nonbleeding visible vessel, 22% in patients with an adherent clot, 10% in those with a flat pigmented spot, and only 5% in those with a clean ulcer base (20). Furthermore, subsequent trials have demonstrated that for patients with active bleeding or nonbleeding visible vessels, endoscopic therapy can significantly reduce rates of further bleeding, surgery, and mortality (5).

Although EGD is not without risk, in experienced hands and with appropriate patient selection, the risks are very low. In the National American Society for Gastrointestinal Endoscopy (ASGE) Survey of UGIB, 21 complications occurred after 2320 endoscopies (0.9%). Twelve of these were deemed major complications: 5 perforations, 4 aspirations, and 3 hemorrhages; and there were 3 deaths (major complication rate, 0.5%; endoscopy-related mortality rate, 0.1%). Complications tend to occur during emergency procedures or in patients who are older, who have active comorbid disease (especially liver disease), or who have a coagulopathy (21). In the elective setting and in the absence of significant comorbidity, complication and mortality rates are less by an order of magnitude (22).

Barium Contrast Radiography

The sensitivity of barium contrast radiography (BCR) for the evaluation of acute UGIB is only 50% to 70% (14,17,23,24); specificity appears to be about 90% (Table 10-1). Furthermore, BCR does not provide direct visualization, may interfere with subsequent EGD or angiography, requires a cooperative, mobile patient, and offers no options for treatment. Barium contrast radiography is therefore never the test of choice in a patient who is actively bleeding or in whom the risk of rebleeding is high (25). Even for elective evaluation of patients whose episode of acute UGIB stops and does not recur, EGD is superior to BCR. Although a randomized controlled trial comparing EGD with BCR in patients whose bleeding stopped within 6 hours after admission to the hospital demonstrated no outcome difference over 12 months of follow-up (26), a blinded prospective comparison of double-contrast BCR and EGD in the evaluation of 100 patients who were not bleeding demonstrated that BCR had a sensitivity of only 54%, missing 10 of 18 gastric ulcers, 4 of 13 duodenal ulcers, and 1 of 2 gastric carcinomas (19).

Angiography

Angiography has no broad utility in the evaluation of patients with acute UGIB. In the diagnosis of UGIB, its use is limited to patients with persistent bleeding for which EGD is not able to help provide a diag-

Table 10-1. Operating Characteristics of Diagnostic Tests in the Identification of the Causative Lesion of Acute Upper Gastrointestinal Bleeding

Diagnostic Test	Sensitivity	Specificity	Likelihood Ratio	
			Positive Result	Positive Result
	←————— % —————→			
Esophagogastroduodenoscopy	90	95	18.0	0.11
Barium contrast radiography	60	90	6.0	0.44

nosis. For the test result to be positive, the patient must be actively bleeding at the time of angiography. Selective angiography offers treatment options for patients with persistent bleeding caused by diffuse erosive gastritis or for patients with persistent bleeding caused by ulcer disease despite endoscopic therapy who are poor candidates for surgery. In the ASGE survey, angiography was done in only 98 of 2225 patients; the cause of bleeding was identified in only 31 (32.3%) of these 98 patients (11).

Radionuclide Imaging
Like angiography, radionuclide imaging can yield positive results only if the patient is actively bleeding at the time of the study and has utility as a diagnostic test for acute UGIB only when persistent bleeding cannot be diagnosed by EGD. It has the advantage of not being associated with any significant morbidity, but it often provides only inexact information about the source of bleeding. Although it may be useful as a guide to subsequent management by providing the surgeon or angiographer with sufficient localization to direct their efforts (23), some doubt whether it has any usefulness at all in the diagnosis and treatment of acute UGIB (25).

DIAGNOSTIC STRATEGIES
Diagnostic testing is undertaken in patients with acute UGIB for one of two indications: 1) as an aid to management of the acute bleeding episode (i.e., "urgent testing") or 2) as an aid to long-term management after the acute bleeding episode has resolved (i.e., "elective testing"). Each indication requires a separate diagnostic strategy.

Urgent Testing
Esophagogastroduodenoscopy is the test of choice in the urgent setting and establishes the likely source of bleeding in 90% of patients.

However, because at least 75% of patients admitted for acute UGIB and treated only with nonspecific supportive care stop bleeding shortly after admission and never have recurrence of bleeding, urgent testing is not always necessary. Esophagogastroduodenoscopy should be performed urgently in all of the following patients: 1) patients presenting with hypotension; 2) patients who continue to bleed actively for more than 1 or 2 hours after admission despite standard therapy; 3) patients who rebleed; 4) patients who develop UGIB while hospitalized for another problem; and 5) patients with three or more high-risk clinical criteria. This strategy identifies almost all patients with bleeding esophageal varices. It also helps identify the majority of patients with a malignant cause, because more than 50% of such patients rebleed before their discharge from the hospital (2).

Patients who stop bleeding promptly and have no high-risk clinical criteria do not require urgent EGD. Patients with one or two high-risk criteria fall into an intermediate group in which decisions about urgent testing are best made on an individual basis.

Elective Testing

Based on the strategy described in the preceding section, approximately 50% of patients admitted for acute UGIB require urgent testing. Of the remaining patients, those whose hematocrit decreases by more than 25% should be studied at the earliest elective opportunity. Patients with severe gastrointestinal symptoms or any signs or symptoms suggesting malignancy should also be investigated in a timely manner. With this strategy, the risk of missing a treatable malignancy is negligible, because most patients with malignant disease have symptoms or signs other than bleeding.

Appropriate management of clinically low-risk patients with small, self-limited hemorrhages who are either asymptomatic or have only dyspepsia after resolution of the bleeding episode is a subject of some debate. Some would argue that even these patients should undergo endoscopy because the finding of a nonbleeding ulcer with a clean base or other low-risk lesion allows early refeeding and discharge, reducing the duration of the hospital stay and the cost of the episode (27,28). However, because the risk of rebleeding after 24 hours in a clinically low-risk patient is only 1.6%, we believe early discharge is appropriate even without endoscopy. Such patients can reasonably be given therapy for acid peptic disease for 4 to 6 weeks and be studied only for progressive symptoms during therapy or recurrence of symptoms after therapy is withdrawn.

Even in the elective setting, EGD is the test of choice for diagnosis of UGIB in most patients. Its higher sensitivity, when compared with that of BCR, more than outweighs the minimal morbidity and mortality of elective EGD. Although a single EGD is more costly than a single

BCR, a strategy that used BCR as the first test would require that 1) all patients with "suspicious" lesions on BCR undergo EGD for biopsy; and 2) all patients with normal BCR test results and persistent symptoms undergo EGD because of the unacceptably low sensitivity of BCR. The need to do two studies in many patients would, to a great extent, offset the initial savings of the BCR strategy.

In settings in which EGD is not easily available and for patients who are believed to be unsuitable for EGD, double-contrast barium meal is the best available alternative. If this study provides a diagnosis, it is adequate to guide management, because the false-positive rate is only 8% to 10% (19,29). However, if the patient does not respond as expected or if the study is negative and symptoms persist, EGD should be performed.

Response to a Negative Esophagogastroduodenoscopy Test Result
Because more than 95% of patients with UGIB have disease that is within reach of the endoscope, the most likely explanation for a negative EGD test result is that the causative lesion was missed, not that it is elsewhere in the gastrointestinal tract. If a patient's acute bleeding has stopped, a negative result should not prompt additional studies. The patient should be managed empirically for acid peptic disease as described above. In the event of recurrent bleeding, the test of choice is repeat EGD.

A Comment on *Helicobacter Pylori*
Treatment of *Helicobacter pylori*, when present, has reduced the rate of ulcer rebleeding in randomized controlled trials (30,31). Patients with UGIB that is definitely or probably caused by ulcer disease should either be evaluated for the presence of *H. pylori* or should be empirically treated as judged appropriate by the managing physician. Full discussion of the diagnosis of *H. pylori*–related ulcer disease is beyond the scope of this chapter and is provided in Chapter 11.

CLINICAL PROBLEMS

Clinical Problem 1
An otherwise healthy young patient presents with a single self-limited episode of acute upper gastrointestinal bleeding.

Testing Strategy and Rationale
Such patients rarely require diagnostic evaluation. Risk of recurrent hemorrhage is less than 5% to begin with and decreases to less than 1% after 48 hours. In the absence of recurrent hemorrhage,

Continued

such a patient should be studied only for symptoms that are severe or persistent after appropriate therapy.

Clinical Example
A 24-year-old, otherwise healthy man has a single episode of hematemesis after taking eight aspirin daily for several days for a musculoskeletal injury. His only persistent symptom is mild dyspepsia. There is no evidence of major blood loss. No diagnostic testing is necessary either urgently or electively. The patient has either acute mucosal irritation, probably caused by aspirin, or ulcer disease. Aspirin should be discontinued, symptomatic therapy offered, and diagnostic testing pursued only for persistent symptoms.

Clinical Problem 2
A high-risk patient has an episode of acute UGIB that stops shortly after admission to the hospital.

Testing Strategy and Rationale
Patients with multiple risk factors for poor outcome require prompt EGD even if their acute episode stops, because the risk of rebleeding is unacceptably high. Esophagogastroduodenoscopy will secure a diagnosis and, in selected patients, allow therapy.

Clinical Example
A 78-year-old woman is brought by ambulance to the emergency department after an episode of coffee-ground emesis. Initial systolic blood pressure is 80 mm Hg, improving to 105 mm Hg after 1 hour of saline infusion. Nasogastric tube initially returns strongly guaiac(+) coffee-ground material but clears rapidly. General physical examination is unremarkable. Initial hematocrit is 28%. Prothrombin time is normal. Electrocardiography shows evidence of acute ischemia that reverses with correction of her hypotension.

This patient has three high-risk clinical factors: advanced age, evidence of major blood loss (both hypotension and hematocrit <30% on admission), and significant comorbidity in the form of reversible ischemic heart disease. Risk of recurrent hemorrhage is at least 30%; if either EGD or surgery is undertaken in the face of ongoing recurrent hemorrhage, morbidity and mortality are significantly increased. Esophagogastroduodenoscopy should be performed as soon as possible while the patient is stable.

REFERENCES

1. **Friedman LS, Martin P.** The problem of gastrointestinal bleeding. Gastroenterol Clin North Am. 1993;22:717-21.

2. **Morgan AG, Clamp SE.** OMGE international upper gastrointestinal bleeding survey, 1978-1982. Scand J Gastroenterol. 1984;19(Suppl 95):41-58.

3. **Silverstein FE, Gilbert DA, Tedesco FJ, et al.** The national ASGE survey on upper gastrointestinal bleeding. I. Study design and baseline data. Gastrointest Endosc. 1981;27:73-9.

4. **Fleischer D.** Etiology and prevalence of severe persistent upper gastrointestinal bleeding. Gastroenterology. 1983;84:538-43.

5. **Cook DJ, Guyatt GH, Salena BJ, Laine LA.** Endoscopic therapy for acute nonvariceal upper gastrointestinal hemorrhage: a meta-analysis. Gastroenterology. 1992;102:139-48.

6. **Goff JS.** Gastroesophageal varices: pathogenesis and therapy of acute bleeding. Gastroenterol Clin North Am. 1993;22:779-800.

7. **Morgan AG, Clamp SE.** OMGE International upper gastrointestinal bleeding survey, 1978–1986. Scand J Gastroenterol. 1988;23(Suppl 144):51-8.

8. **Bordley DR, Mushlin AI, Dolan JG, et al.** Early clinical signs identify low-risk patients with acute upper gastrointestinal hemorrhage. JAMA. 1985;253:3282-5.

9. **Morgan AG, McAdam WAF, Walmsley GL, et al.** Clinical findings, early endoscopy, and multivariate analysis in patients bleeding from the upper gastrointestinal tract. Br Med J. 1977;2:237-40.

10. **Mueller X, Rothenbuehler J-M, Amery A, Harder F.** Factors predisposing to further hemorrhage and mortality after peptic ulcer bleeding. J Am Coll Surg. 1994;179:457-61.

11. **Silverstein FE, Gilbert DA, Tedesco FJ, et al.** The national ASGE survey on upper gastrointestinal bleeding. II. Clinical prognostic factors. Gastrointest Endosc. 1981;27:80-93.

12. **Ohmann C, Thon K, Stoltzing H, et al.** Upper gastrointestinal tract bleeding: assessing the diagnostic contributions of the history and clinical findings. Med Decis Making. 1986;6:208-15.

13. **Gostout CJ.** Acute gastrointestinal bleeding: a common problem revisited. Mayo Clin Proc. 1988;63:596-604.

14. **Larson DE, Farnell MB.** Upper gastrointestinal hemorrhage. Mayo Clin Proc. 1983;58:371-87.

15. **Lieberman DL.** Gastrointestinal bleeding: initial management. Gastroenterol Clin North Am. 1993;22:723-36.

16. **Silverstein FE, Gilbert DA, Tedesco FJ, et al.** The national ASGE survey on upper gastrointestinal bleeding. III. Endoscopy in upper gastrointestinal bleeding. Gastrointest Endosc. 1981;27:94-103.

17. **Lichtenstein JL.** Accuracy and reliability of endoscopy and x-ray in upper gastrointestinal bleeding. Dig Dis Sci. 1981;26:70S-5S.

18. **Foster DN, Miloszewski KJA, Losowsky MS.** Stigmata of recent haemorrhage in diagnosis and prognosis of upper gastrointestinal bleeding. Br Med J. 1978;1:1173-7.

19. **Dooley CP, Larson AW, Stace NH, et al.** Double-contrast barium meal and upper gastrointestinal endoscopy: a comparative study. Ann Intern Med. 1984;101:538-45.

20. **Laine L, Peterson WL.** Bleeding peptic ulcer. N Engl J Med. 1994;331:717-27.

21. **Gilbert DA, Silverstein FE, Tedesco FJ.** National ASGE survey on upper gastrointestinal bleeding. Complications of endoscopy. Dig Dis Sci. 1981;26:55S-59S.

22. **Katon RM.** Complications of upper gastrointestinal endoscopy in the gastrointestinal bleeder. Dig Dis Sci. 1981;26:47S-54S.

23. **Steer ML, Silen W.** Diagnostic procedures in gastrointestinal hemorrhage. N Engl J Med. 1983;309:646-50.

24. **Herlinger H.** Consensus development conference on endoscopy. Other diagnostic approaches to upper gastrointestinal bleeding: utility of contrast radiology. Dig Dis Sci. 1981;26:76S-7S.

25. **Shapiro MJ.** The role of the radiologist in the management of gastrointestinal bleeding. Gastroenterol Clin North Am. 1994;23:123-81.

26. **Peterson WL, Barnett CC, Smith HJ, Corbett DB.** Routine early endoscopy in upper-gastrointestinal-tract bleeding: a randomized, controlled trial. N Engl J Med. 1981;304:925-9.

27. **Laine L, Cohen H, Brodhead J, et al.** Prospective evaluation of immediate versus delayed refeeding and prognostic value of endoscopy in patients with upper gastrointestinal hemorrhage. Gastroenterology. 1992;102:314-6.

28. **Jiranek GC, Kozarek RA.** A cost-effective approach to the patient with peptic ulcer bleeding. Surg Clin North Am. 1996;76:83-103.

29. Health and Public Policy Committee, American College of Physicians. Endoscopy in the evaluation of dyspepsia. Ann Intern Med. 1985;102:266-9.

30. **Rokkas T, Karameris A, Mavrogeorgis A, et al.** Eradication of *Helicobacter pylori* reduces the possibility of rebleeding in peptic ulcer disease. Gastrointest Endosc. 1995;41:1-4.

31. **Jasperson D, Koerner T, Schorr W, et al.** *Helicobacter pylori* eradication reduces the rate of rebleeding in ulcer hemorrhage. Gastrointest Endosc. 1995;41:5-7.

Peptic Ulcer Disease   **11**

A. Andrew Rudmann, MD

KEY POINTS

Pretest Probabilities

- The probability of finding peptic ulcer disease (PUD) depends on the clinical presentation. The probability is approximately 30% in patients with dyspepsia, 20% in patients with evidence of chronic gastrointestinal blood loss, and 45% in those with acute upper gastrointestinal hemorrhage.

- Age, nonsteroidal anti-inflammatory drugs (NSAIDs), and *Helicobacter pylori* infection are important predictors of peptic ulcer disease in those with dyspepsia. In younger persons with dyspepsia who do not use NSAIDs and lack evidence of *H. pylori* infection, the likelihood of PUD is approximately 1%, whereas in elderly persons who use NSAIDs, the probability is 20% without *H. pylori* infection and 30% with *H. pylori* infection.

Diagnostic Strategies

- When clinical symptoms suggest a high probability of PUD or if certain "alarm" symptoms are present, proceeding directly to esophagogastroduodenoscopy (EGD) is a reasonable approach.

- When the probability of PUD is low or intermediate, several alternative strategies can be pursued, such as initial EGD or empiric therapy. Serologic testing for *H. pylori* may also help guide the diagnostic evaluation, but prospective data are still lacking.

BACKGROUND

Peptic ulcer disease (PUD) is a common medical diagnosis with clinical presentations ranging from belching, bloating, and nausea; to epigastric burning and pain; to anemia and guaiac positive stool; to hematemesis, melena, and hypotension. Definitive diagnosis is made by visualization of ulcers in the stomach or duodenum by upper gastrointestinal endoscopy or barium contrast radiography. Because these procedures are inconvenient, costly, and carry some risk, a clinical diagnosis is often made. Nonsteroidal anti-inflammatory drug (NSAID) use and *Helicobacter pylori* infection are now well-recognized etiologic factors in PUD pathogenesis. *Helicobacter pylori* has complicated the diagnostic approach to PUD somewhat but has revolutionized medical management.

ESTIMATING PRETEST PROBABILITY

More than 250,000 cases of PUD are diagnosed each year in the United States. The lifetime prevalence of PUD is 5% to 10%, and the point prevalence is 1% to 2% (1). Various factors influence the pretest probability of PUD, including presenting signs and symptoms, NSAID use, *H. pylori* infection, and family and medical history.

Men have a one and a half to twofold greater risk of having PUD than women. Having a first-degree relative with PUD increases the risk threefold (1,2). An increased risk of PUD is also seen with several medical conditions, including chronic obstructive pulmonary disease, cirrhosis, and renal insufficiency. Patients with the rare Zollinger-Ellison syndrome have a 90% to 95% lifetime risk of having PUD.

Acute upper gastrointestinal hemorrhage is frequently associated with PUD; 40% to 50% of patients with this condition have PUD (3). Other causes of upper gastrointestinal hemorrhage, as discussed in Chapter 10, include gastritis, esophageal varices, Mallory-Weiss syndrome, esophagitis, and cancer. In contrast, approximately 20% of outpatients presenting with chronic gastrointestinal bleeding and iron deficiency anemia have PUD (4).

Dyspepsia, defined as recurrent or persistent epigastric pain or discomfort, accounts for approximately 5% of visits to primary care practitioners (5–7). In numerous series, less than one third of patients who had dyspepsia were found to have PUD at endoscopy (5,7–11). Other common causes of dyspepsia include functional (nonulcer) dyspepsia (46% to 71%), irritable bowel syndrome (26% to 30%), and gastroesophageal reflux disease (18% to 29%). Less common causes are esophagitis, hiatus hernia, cholelithiasis, gastritis or duodenitis or both, and gastric cancer (5,7,9,12–14).

Age, NSAID use, and *H. pylori* infection further influence the likelihood of PUD in patients with dyspepsia (9,14–16). In patients with dyspepsia who are not infected with *H. pylori* and who do not use NSAIDs the prevalence of PUD is 1% at age 40 years and 3% at age 75 years. NSAID use increases PUD prevalence four- to sevenfold. As a result, the PUD prevalence in patients with dyspepsia who use NSAIDs increases from approximately 5% at age 40 years to 20% or more at age 75 years. *Helicobacter pylori* infection in patients with dyspepsia, including both those who use NSAIDs and those who do not, is associated with a 20% prevalence of PUD at age 40 years and 30% at age 75 years (17).

Several factors do not increase the likelihood of PUD in those with dyspepsia. Classifying dyspepsia as ulcer-like, as opposed to reflux-like or dysmotility-like, and finding epigastric tenderness on physical examination does not define a patient as more likely to have PUD (18,19). Recurrence or persistence of dyspepsia after an empiric trial of antisecretory therapy does not make finding PUD at endoscopy more likely (10).

NSAIDs are an important cause of PUD regardless of symptoms. The use of these agents has been associated with a PUD prevalence of at least 15% to 20% (20–24). The risk of PUD is highest during the first 1 to 3 months of use (25,26), and gastric ulcers (GU) are five times more common than duodenal ulcers (DU) (27). Serious PUD occurs asympto-matically two to four times more often in patients who use NSAIDs (26,28,29). High doses, female sex, advanced age, history of previous gastrointestinal disease, concomitant use of corticosteroids, and *H. pylori* infection are additional factors that increase the risk of NSAID induced PUD (26,30–33). In one study, eradicating *H. pylori* before start-ing naproxen therapy reduced the risk of PUD from 26% to 3% (34).

The ulcerogenic potential of NSAIDs varies in relation to their acidity, cyclooxygenase (COX) selectivity, and other features (35). Anti-inflammatory doses of aspirin are associated with a sixfold increased risk of PUD (36), whereas low doses (<100 mg/d) are asso-ciated with a smaller but still increased risk (33). Older, more COX-1–selective NSAIDs are as much as 20 times more likely to cause PUD than newer, more COX-2–selective agents, such as etodolac and nabumetone, for which the reported incidence of PUD is less than 1% (24,37). However, even highly COX-2–selective agents can inhibit the protective gastrointestinal COX-1 enzyme at recommended therapeu-tic doses and should be used with caution (38). The risk of NSAID-induced PUD can be reduced with misoprostol or omeprazole (22,39). Neither standard-dose H_2-receptor blockers nor sucralfate has been shown to provide effective PUD prophylaxis in the setting of NSAID use (33,40,41).

Helicobacter pylori infection is another important factor in assessing possible PUD. *Helicobacter pylori*–infected persons appear to have a 15% to 20% lifetime risk of PUD compared with 3% for uninfected persons (42). *Helicobacter pylori* infection is associated with more than 80% of GU and more than 95% of DU in those who do not take NSAIDs. Failure to eradicate *H. pylori* in patients with PUD results in a recurrence rate as high as 60% to 100% per year, as compared with less than 15% recur-rence with successful eradication (43). Although *H. pylori* infection is common, in most patients PUD does not develop. The prevalence of *H. pylori* is 10% to 20% at age 25 years, increasing to more than 50% by age 60 years. "Host" characteristics and *H. pylori* strain may influence which individuals will ultimately develop PUD (44).

Smoking does not increase the risk of PUD except in *H. pylori*–seropositive persons in whom the risk is twofold higher (45). Lastly, alcohol, caffeine, stress, and the long-term use of corticosteroids (apart from use with NSAIDs) do not appear to increase the risk of peptic ulcer (20,46).

DIAGNOSTIC TESTS

Gastrointestinal Imaging

Upper gastrointestinal imaging in the diagnosis of PUD is accomplished by esophagogastroduodenoscopy (EGD) or upper gastrointestinal (UGI) barium radiography. In a prospective evaluation of upper gastrointestinal symptoms, EGD was found to be more sensitive than double-contrast UGI series (92% compared with 54%); specificity was excellent for EGD but also quite good for UGI barium radiography (Table 11-1) (47).

Esophagogastroduodenoscopy offers the ability to visualize mucosal lesions directly, to obtain biopsies, to distinguish scarring from ulceration, and to provide therapy. Disadvantages include increased cost, requirement for sedation, and risk of esophageal perforation. Upper gastrointestinal barium radiography permits identification of extrinsic lesions and motility disorders. Indications for EGD include history of

Table 11-1. Operating Characteristics of Diagnostic Tests for Peptic Ulcer Disease and *Helicobacter pylori* Infections

Test	Sensitivity	Specificity	Likelihood Ratio	
			Positive Result	Negative Result
	← % →			
Gastrointestinal imaging				
EGD	92	99	92	0.08
Upper GI Series	54	91	6	0.51
***Helicobacter pylori* testing**				
Rapid urease test	90	100	∞	0.10
Histologic examination				
Warthin-Starry stain	93	99	93	0.07
Chronic inflammation	100	66	3.0	0
Acute inflammation	87	94	15	0.14
Urea breath test	90	96	22	0.10
Serum IgG Antibodies	91	92	11	0.10

EGD = Esophagogastroduodenoscopy.

scarring from operation or ulcer, severe upper gastrointestinal hemorrhage (see Chapter 10), suspected mucosal lesion, and history of gastric cancer. Indications for UGI barium radiography series include severe cardiopulmonary disease and suspected motility disorder (48).

Invasive Tests for *Helicobacter pylori*

The principal clinically useful invasive tests for *H. pylori* are direct urease testing and histologic examination. These require endoscopy and mucosal biopsy. Direct urease testing is accomplished by placing a small piece of gastric mucosa on a pH-sensitive urea-containing substrate. The CLO (*Campylobacter*-like organism) test is a popular commercial urease test. Color change indicates ammonia production from *H. pylori*–associated urease. The sensitivity and specificity are 90% and 100%, respectively (see Table 11-1); although sensitivity is considerably lower in the setting of potent antacid use, anti–*H. pylori* antibiotics, and bismuth-containing compounds (49). For instance, a 35% false negative rate has been observed in the setting of H_2-receptor blocker use (50). Ideally, these agents should be discontinued several days before testing.

Histologic evaluation for *H. pylori* is accomplished by examining at least two hematoxylin and eosin-stained or Warthin-Starry–stained antral mucosal biopsies for organisms or inflammation or both. The presence of spiral rods within the gastric surface constitutes a positive result, with a sensitivity of 93% and specificity of 99%. Chronic inflammation has nearly 100% sensitivity for *H. pylori*; however, specificity is only 66%. Acute inflammation is reported to be 87% sensitive and 94% specific for *H. pylori* infection (49). Although these tests have excellent operating characteristics, results are not always concordant (49).

Culture for *H. pylori* is seldom used because of the fastidiousness of the organism and availability of other diagnostic methods. Culture may become more important if *H. pylori* strains develop resistance to multiple antibiotics (49).

Noninvasive Tests for *Helicobacter pylori*

Urea breath analysis detects active *H. pylori* infection in the upper gastrointestinal tract. Gastric urease activity, which is highly specific for active *H. pylori* infection, converts carbon-labeled urea to labeled carbon dioxide and ammonia. A positive result is defined as the detection of labeled carbon dioxide in the breath. The test must be performed in patients who are taking no medications that suppress *H. pylori* replication, including antibiotics (e.g., amoxicillin, clarithromycin, and metronidazole) and antisecretory agents. If the test is performed in patients taking any of these medications, a high false-negative rate will result. The carbon-14 version exposes participants to a negligible amount of radioactivity but is more convenient to perform than the carbon-13 version that requires mass spectrometry.

Various urea breath test (UBT) kits have been developed and analyzed. The sensitivity and specificity of these tests exceeds 90% (49,51). Because of its noninvasiveness and high sensitivity and specificity for active infection, UBT is ideally suited for assessing *H. pylori* eradication. The UBT is not routinely used for *H. pylori* detection because it is much more inconvenient and more costly than serologic testing; however, it is much less expensive than endoscopy (52).

Anti–*H. pylori* IgG antibodies can be detected in the blood of patients with current or previous infection with *H. pylori*. The sensitivity and specificity of these tests are both approximately 92%. Both quantitative enzyme-linked immunosorbent assays (ELISA) and qualitative assays are available. These tests have limited usefulness in posteradication monitoring because approximately two thirds of successfully treated patients still have positive IgG titers 1 to 2 years after treatment. Although the quantitative test may be used to follow the drop in titer that occurs 4 to 6 months after treatment, acute and convalescent sera must be assayed concurrently because results can vary between assays (49).

Empiric Therapy

Response to empiric therapy could also be considered a diagnostic test for PUD if patients with PUD responded differently to treatment than those with suspected PUD who did not have an ulcer. However, this does not seem to be the case. Most patients with PUD respond symptomatically to appropriate treatment within 2 weeks (2), and at least half of those with nonulcer dyspepsia also improve with empiric antisecretory therapy (53). As noted previously, recurrence or persistence of dyspepsia after an empiric trial of antisecretory therapy does not make finding PUD at endoscopy more likely (10).

DIAGNOSTIC STRATEGIES

The diagnostic approach to patients in whom PUD is suspected varies depending on the patient's age, use of NSAIDs, and severity and type of symptoms. As the relation between *H. pylori* and PUD becomes better defined and testing for *H. pylori* improves, the precise role of evaluating for *H. pylori* in those with suspected PUD will become more clear. Concerns about other serious gastrointestinal disorders, such as malignancy, also influence the diagnostic approach. The strategies presented below are based on currently available information.

When the presenting symptom is high-risk upper gastrointestinal hemorrhage (see Chapter 10) or dyspepsia with certain "alarm" features, such as anemia, anorexia, early satiety, weight loss, age older than 45 years, or a history of chronic symptoms, or if the suspicion for PUD is high because the patient has multiple risk factors, an initial approach using EGD is warranted (54,55). If PUD is found, antral biopsy should be performed for *H. pylori* analysis by direct urease testing and by histologic examination if the results of urease testing are negative. To reduce PUD recurrence, patients with *H. pylori* infections should receive antibiotic treatment. If applicable, NSAIDs should be discontinued whenever possible (44).

When the presenting symptom is uncomplicated dyspepsia, the optimum strategy is controversial. Although upper endoscopy has excellent operating characteristics for the diagnosis of PUD, performing endoscopy as the initial test for PUD is often not recommended because of the costs and inconvenience of using EGD to find the few patients with dyspepsia who have serious diseases. Performing endoscopy on all of these patients results in a large fraction of negative studies. A more cost-effective approach to the accurate diagnosis of active ulcer disease could result from noninvasive testing for *H. pylori* infection.

If the patient with dyspepsia is taking NSAIDs, particularly an older agent, the drug should be discontinued and antisecretory therapy should be initiated, if necessary. The patient should be re-evaluated within 4 to 6 weeks, and EGD may be warranted if symptoms persist. The utility of serologic testing for *H. pylori* infection in the initial evaluation of these patients is not known (56).

If the patient is not taking NSAIDs, several possible strategies may be considered:

1. Initial EGD with *H. pylori* evaluation as noted above
2. Initial *H. pylori* serologic testing followed by EGD, except in patients younger than 45 years old who test negative for *H. pylori*
3. Initial *H. pylori* serologic testing followed by eradication in patients who test positive for *H. pylori*
4. Initial 6-week trial of empiric antisecretory therapy followed by EGD if symptoms persist for 2 weeks during therapy or recur after therapy has been completed
5. Initial empiric antisecretory and anti–*H. pylori* therapy

For all of these strategies, in the event that initial noninvasive management fails, EGD should be performed to exclude a serious disorder. Although UGI may be substituted for EGD in appropriate cases, its sensitivity is much lower.

The first approach may be reasonable when suitable conditions exist, including adequate access to facilities, resources, and expertise, and when there is a high perceived value for a negative endoscopy result. This approach provides early accurate information and precisely guides therapy. However, it is reported to be the most expensive approach in terms of cost per ulcer cured (52).

The second approach employs age and *H. pylori* serologic testing to select patients at the lowest risk for serious disease in whom endoscopy may be safely deferred—that is, those younger than 45 years old who test negative for *H. pylori* (57–59). Adequate prospective data regarding the efficacy of *H. pylori* serologic testing as a screening tool to select patients for endoscopy is not yet available (53).

The third approach uses *H. pylori* serologic testing to identify patients with dyspepsia for whom treatment would cure ulcer disease, if present. With this approach, *H. pylori*–seronegative patients with dyspepsia are considered unlikely to have PUD. As in all initially non-invasive approaches, EGD is reserved for patients whose symptoms persist or recur. Support for this approach comes from decision analysis suggesting that *H. pylori* eradication in seropositive patients with dyspepsia is cost-effective. However, the cost-effectiveness of this approach diminishes over time, because about half of those with nonulcer dyspepsia continue to have symptoms leading to endoscopy (53). This approach has not been studied prospectively and has been criticized because of lack of data showing benefit of eradicating *H. pylori* in patients with nonulcer dyspepsia and because of concerns that antibiotic-resistant organisms may develop with such widespread antibiotic use (60).

The fourth approach, empiric antisecretory therapy without *H. pylori* testing, has been commonly used in clinical practice and has been studied prospectively. In one study, more than half of patients treated with initial empiric therapy experienced symptom relapse that necessitated endoscopy. However, the likelihood of finding important disease was not improved with endoscopy at this point compared with prompt initial endoscopy. Criticisms of this approach are that it does not evaluate for *H. pylori* infection and that failure to detect and treat *H. pylori* infection in the setting of PUD is associated with a high recurrence rate. It has been suggested that restricting this approach to patients younger than 45 years old may be more effective because the prevalence of important disease is lower in these patients (61). The cost-effectiveness of this approach is controversial.

The fifth strategy, empiric antisecretory and anti–*H. pylori* therapy, has been shown to be more cost-effective per ulcer cured than the third and fourth strategies (52). However, with this approach, patients are exposed to antibiotics, many unnecessarily so, raising concerns about antibiotic resistance. The attractiveness of this approach also depends on whether or not eradication of *H. pylori* in seropositive patients with nonulcer dyspepsia improves symptoms, which has not yet been shown (62). In addition, the cost-effectiveness of this strategy assumes a relatively expensive serologic test for *H. pylori*. When the less expensive serologic testing kits become widely available, the third strategy will likely become a more cost-competitive option.

CLINICAL PROBLEMS

Clinical Problem 1
An elderly patient presents with possible peptic ulcer disease (PUD) and also has "alarm" symptoms.

Testing Strategy and Rationale
Risk factors for PUD, such as use of NSAIDs, should be determined, and initial endoscopy should be performed with testing for *H. pylori*. Although the initial approach is uncertain in some cases, when the probability of PUD is high or the patient has "alarm" symptoms, then initial EGD is indicated.

Clinical Example
A 72-year-old man with chronic obstructive pulmonary disease presents with a 3- to 4-month history of dyspepsia, nausea, and fatigue. He intermittently takes prednisone, and he has osteoarthritis, treated with daily naproxen. He reports having had a stomach ulcer several years ago but does not recall the details; he has been taking ranitidine since then. His evaluation also reveals guaiac-positive stools, microcytic anemia, and low serum ferritin level.

Owing to his age, NSAID use, and symptoms, the risk of PUD in this patient is at least 30%, and he also has an "alarm" feature, iron-deficiency anemia. Initial EGD is performed and demonstrates a 2-cm nonbleeding GU and antral gastritis. CLO test for *H. pylori* is positive. Naproxen is discontinued and he receives treatment with antibiotics for *H. pylori* eradication and antisecretory therapy.

Clinical Problem 2
A young woman presents for evaluation of dyspepsia.

Testing Strategy and Rationale
A history and physical examination should be performed to evaluate risk factors for PUD and to assess for "alarm" symptoms. Next, initial endoscopy should be carried out if the pretest probability of PUD is high or if "alarm" symptoms are present. If the pretest probability is low or intermediate, serologic testing for *H. pylori* should be considered. If the result of serologic testing is positive, the patient should receive treatment.

Clinical Example
A 30-year-old healthy woman who is under a great deal of stress at work presents for evaluation of 2 to 3 months of intermittent dys-

Continued

pepsia. She takes ibuprofen (400 mg) only once or twice a month for headaches. She has no "alarm" features such as anemia or weight loss. She has no family history of PUD. In the absence of *H. pylori* infection, the risk of PUD in this patient is less than 5%, whereas the risk would be approximately 20% if the patient were infected with *H. pylori*. Serologic testing is performed, and the results are negative. The patient is treated with a short course of symptomatic therapy, and arrangements for follow-up are made.

REFERENCES

1. **Kurata JH, Haile BM.** Epidemiology of peptic ulcer disease. Clin Gastroenterol. 1984;3:289-307.

2. **Katz PO.** Peptic ulcer disease. In: Barker LR, Burton JR, Zieve PD, eds. Priniciples of Ambulatory Medicine. Baltimore: Williams & Wilkins; 4th ed. 1995: 456.

3. **Silverstein FE, Gilbert DA, Tedesco FJ, et al.** The National ASGE Survey on Upper Gastrointestinal Bleeding. II. Clinical prognostic factors. Gastrointest Endosc. 1981;27:80-93.

4. **McIntyre AS, Long RG.** Prospective survey of investigations in outpatients referred with iron deficiency anemia. Gut.1993;34:1102-7.

5. **Kagevi I, Lofstedt S, Persson LG.** Endoscopic findings and diagnoses in unselected dyspeptic patients at a primary health care center. Scand J Gastroenterol.1989;24:145-50.

6. **Ebell MH, Warbasse L, Brenner C.** Evaluation of the dyspeptic patient: a cost-utility study. J Fam Pract.1997;44:545-55.

7. **Grainger SL, Klass HJ, Rake MO, Williams JG.** Prevalence of dyspepsia: the epidemiology of overlapping symptoms. Postgrad Med J.1994;70: 154-61.

8. **Horrocks JC, DeDombal FT.** Clinical presentation of patients with 'dyspepsia'. Gut. 1978;19:19-26.

9. **Lance P, Gibson-Glubb S, Gazzard JA, Gazzard BG.** Chronic dyspepsia pain in general practice: its causes and diagnosis. Postgrad Med J. 1985; 61:411-3.

10. **Bytzer P, Hansen JM, Schaffalitzky DeMuckadell OB.** Empirical H2-blocker therapy or prompt endoscopy in management of dyspepsia. Lancet. 1994;343:811-6.

11. **O'Riordan TG, Tobin A, O'Morain C.** *Helicobacter pylori* infection in elderly dyspeptic patients. Age Ageing. 1991;20:189-92.

12. **Johannessen T, Petersen H, Kleveland PM, et al.** The predictive value of history in dyspepsia. Scand J Gastroenterol.1990;25:689-97.

13. **Barnes RJ, Gear MWL, Nicol, Dew AB.** Study of dyspepsia in a general practice as assessed by endoscopy and radiology. Br Med J. 1974;41:214.

14. **Talley NJ, Phillips SF.** Nonulcer dyspepsia: potential causes and pathophysiology. Ann Intern Med. 1988;108:865-79.

15. **Williams B, Luckas M, Ellingham JHM, et al.** Do young patients with dyspepsia need investigations? Lancet. 1988:1349-51.

16. **Fraser AG, Ali MR.** Diagnostic tests for *Helicobacter pylori:* can they help select patients for endoscopy? N Z Med J. 1996;109:95-8.

17. **Silverstein MD, Petterson T, Talley N.** Initial endoscopy or empirical therapy with or without testing for *Helicobacter pylori* for dyspepsia: a decision analysis. Gastroenterology. 1996;110:72-83.

18. **Mansi C, Vincenzo S, Sandro Mela G, et al.** Are clinical patterns of dyspepsia a valid guideline for appropriate use of endoscopy? A report on 2253 dyspeptic patients. Am J Gastroenterol. 1993;88:1011-5.

19. **Priebe WM, DaCosta LR, Beck IT.** Is epigastric tenderness a sign of peptic ulcer disease? Gastroenterology. 1982;82:16-9.

20. **Soll AH.** Pathogenesis of peptic ulcer and implications for therapy. N Engl J Med. 1990;322:909-16.

21. **Soll AH, Weinstein WM, Kurata J, McCarthy D.** Nonsteroidal antiinflammatory drugs and peptic ulcer disease. Ann Intern Med. 1991;114:307-19.

22. **Raskin JB, White RH, Jackson JE, et al.** Misoprostol dosage in the prevention of non-steroidal anti-inflammatory drug-induced gastric and duodenal ulcers: a comparison of three regimens. Ann Intern Med. 1995;123:344-50.

23. **Butt JH, Barthel JS, Moore RA.** Clinical spectrum of upper gastrointestinal effects of non-steroidal anti-inflammatory drugs. Am J Med. 1988;84:5-13.

24. **Lanza FL.** Gastrointestinal toxicity of newer NSAIDs. Am J Gastroenterol. 1993;88:1318-23.

25. **Griffin MR, Joyce MP, Daugherty JR, et al.** Nonsteroidal anti-inflammatory drug use and increased risk for peptic ulcer disease in elderly persons. Ann Intern Med. 1991;114:257-63.

26. **Gabriel SE, Jaakkimainen L, Bombardier C.** Risk for serious gastrointestinal complications related to use of non-steroidal anti-inflammatory drugs. Ann Intern Med.1991;115:787-96.

27. **Langman MJS.** Epidemiologic evidence on the association between peptic ulceration and antiinflammatory drug use. Gastroenterology. 1989;96:640-6.

28. **Armstrong CP, Blower AL.** Non-steroidal anti-inflammatory drugs and life threatening complications of peptic ulceration. Gut. 1987;28:527-32.

29. **Savage RL, Moller PW, Ballantyne CL, Wells JE.** Variation in the risk of peptic ulcer complications with nonsteroidal antiinflammatory drug therapy. Arthritis Rheum. 1993;36:84-90.

30. **Piper JM, Ray WA, Daugherty JR, Griffin MR.** Corticosteroid use and peptic ulcer disease: role of nonsteroidal anti-inflammatory drugs. Ann Intern Med. 1991;114:735-40.

31. **Roth SH.** NSAID gastropathy: a new understanding. Arch Intern Med. 1996;156:1623-8.

32. **Li EK, Sung JJ, Suen R, et al.** *Helicobacter pylori* infection increases the risk of pepticulcers in chronic users of non-steroidal anti-inflammatory drugs. Scand J Rheumatol. 1996;25:42-6.

33. **Wallace JL.** Nonsteroidal anti-inflammatory drugs and gastroenteropathy: the second hundred years. Gastroenterology. 1997;112:1000-16.

34. **Chan FK, Sung JJ, Chung SC, et al.** Randomised trial of eradication of *Helicobacter pylori* before non-steroidal anti-inflammatory drug therapy to prevent peptic ulcers. Lancet. 1997;350:975-9.

35. **Roth SH, Tindall EA, Jain AK, et al.** A controlled study comparing the effects of nabumetone, ibuprofen, and ibuprofen plus misoprostol on the upper gastrointestinal tract mucosa. Arch Intern Med. 1993;153:2565-71.

36. **Graham DY, Smith JL.** Aspirin and the stomach. Ann Intern Med. 1986; 104:390-8.

37. **Taha AS, Dahill S, Sturrock RD, et al.** Predicting NSAID related ulcers: assessment of clinical and pathological risk factors and importance of differences in NSAIDs. Gut. 1994;35:891-5.

38. **Cryer B, Feldman M.** Cyclooxygenase-1 and cyclooxygenase-2 selectivity of widely used nonsteroidal anti-inflammatory drugs. Am J Med. 1998;104:413-21.

39. **Ekstrom P, Carling L, Wetterhus S, et al.** Prevention of peptic ulcer and dyspeptic symptoms with omeprazole in patients receiving continuous non-steroidal anti-inflammatory drug therapy: a Nordic multicentre study. Scand J Gastroenterol. 1996;31:753-8.

40. **Feldman M.** Can gastroduodenal ulcers in NSAID users be prevented? [Editorial]. Ann Intern Med. 1993;119:337-9.

41. **Koch M, Dezi A, Ferrario F, Capurso L.** Prevention of non-steroidal anti-inflammatory drug-induced gastrointestinal mucosal injury. Arch Intern Med. 1996;156:2321-32.

42. **Cullen DJE, Collins BJ, Christiansen KJ, et al.** Long term risk of peptic ulcer disease in people with *Helicobacter pylori* infection: community based study [Abstract]. Gastroenterology. 1993;104(Suppl):A60.

43. **Walsh JH, Peterson WL.** The treatment of *Helicobacter pylori* infection in the management of peptic ulcer disease. N Engl J Med. 1995;333:984-91.

44. **NIH Consensus Development Panel on** *Helicobacter pylori* in Peptic Ulcer Disease. JAMA. 1994;272:65-9.

45. **Martin DF, Montgomery E, Dobek A, et al.** *Campylobacter pylori*, NSAIDs, and smoking: risk factors for PUD. Am J Gastroenterol. 1989;84:1268-72.

46. **Conn HO, Poynard T.** Corticosteroids and peptic ulcer: meta-analysis of adverse events during steroid therapy. J Intern Med. 1994:236:619-32.

47. **Dooley CP, Larson AW, Stace NH, et al.** Double-contrast barium meal and upper gastrointestinal endoscopy: a comparative study. Ann Intern Med. 1984;101:538-45.

48. **Colin-Jones DG.** Endoscopy or radiology for upper gastrointestinal symptoms? Lancet. 1986;1:1022-3.

49. **Cutler AF.** Testing for *Helicobacter pylori* in clinical practice. Am J Med. 1996;100(5A):35S-41S.

50. **Deltenre M, Glupczynski Y, De Prez C, et al.** The reliability of urease tests, histology and culture in the diagnosis of *Campylobacter pylori* infection. Scand J Gastroenterol. 1989;24(Suppl 160):19-24.

51. **Faigel DO, Childs M, Furth EE, et al.** New noninvasive tests for *Helicobacter pylori* gastritis: comparison with tissue-based gold standard. Dig Dis Sci. 1996;41:740-8.

52. **Fendrick AM, Chernew M, Hirth RA, Bloom BS.** Alternative management strategies for patients with suspected peptic ulcer disease. Ann Intern Med. 1995;123:260-8.

53. **Ofman JJ, Etchason J, Fullerton S, et al.** Management strategies for *Helicobacter pylori* seropositive patients with dyspepsia: clinical and economic consequences. Ann Intern Med. 1997;126:280-91.

54. **Soll AH.** Medical treatment of peptic ulcer disease: practice guidelines. JAMA.1996;275:622-9.

55. **Graham DY, Rabeneck L.** Patients, payers and paradigm shifts: what to do about *Helicobacter pylori*. Am J Gastroenterol. 1996;91:188-91.

56. **Publig W, Wustinger C, Zandl C.** Non-steroidal anti-inflammatory drugs cause gastrointestinal ulcers mainly in *Helicobacter pylori* carriers. Wien Klin Wochenschr. 1994;106:276-9.

57. **Sombala GM, Crabtree JE, Pentith JA, et al.** Screening dyspepsia by serology to *Helicobacter pylori*. Lancet. 1991;338:94-6.

58. **Tham TCK, McLaughlin N, Hughes DF, et al.** Possible role of *Helicobacter pylori* serology in reducing endoscopy workload. Postgrad Med J. 1994;70:809-12.

59. **Vyas SK, Sharpstone D, Treasure J, et al.** Pre-endoscopy screening using serodiagnosis of *Helicobacter pylori* infection. Eur J Gastroenterol Hepatol. 1994;6:783-7.

60. **Sonnenberg A.** Cost-benefit analysis of testing for *Helicobacter pylori* in dyspeptic subjects. Am J Gastroenterol. 1996;91:1773-7.

61. **Mansi C, Savarino V, Mela GS, Celle G.** Optimum timing for endoscopy in management of dyspepsia. Lancet. 1994;343:1501-2.

62. **Talley NJ.** A critique of therapeutic trials in *Helicobacter pylori*-positive functional dyspepsia. Gastroenterology. 1994;106:1174-83.

Colon Cancer

12

Ann Butler Nattinger, MD, MPH

KEY POINTS

Pretest Probabilities

- The frequency of undiagnosed colorectal cancer and adenomas increases with age. In persons 60 to 69 years old, the prevalence of cancer is approximately 0.5% and that of adenomas 0.5 cm or larger is approximately 18%.

- Persons 40 to 59 years old who have one first-degree relative with colon cancer have a relative risk of 1.7 for developing this disease, and persons with two or more first-degree relatives with the disease have a relative risk of 2.75.

Screening Strategies

- There is good evidence that beginning at the age of 50 years, average-risk patients should undergo screening with flexible sigmoidoscopy, fecal occult blood testing (FOBT), or both. Indirect evidence supports an alternative strategy of total colon examination every 10 years by colonoscopy or by air-contrast barium enema (ACBE) for those at average risk.

- Positive FOBT results necessitate follow-up with total colon examination by colonoscopy or by ACBE plus sigmoidoscopy. Persons in whom sigmoidoscopy shows adenomas also require colonoscopy.

- Persons with one or more first-degree relatives with colon cancer should start receiving screening by the age of 40 years. Total colon examination may be the best test in such patients, owing to the elevated risk for development of colorectal cancer.

- Symptomatic persons and those at extremely high risk (e.g., those who have long-standing ulcerative colitis, hereditary polyposis, or nonpolyposis colon cancer syndromes) require total colon examination as part of the routine management of these conditions.

BACKGROUND

Colorectal cancer is quite common, with an estimated 136,000 new cases and 55,000 deaths occurring in 1998 (1). Most colon cancers are believed to develop from adenomas, but only 5% to 40% of adenomas progress to cancer (2). Potential approaches to the control of colon cancer include screening for and removing benign adenomatous polyps (primary prevention) and screening for and removing early cancers in time to allow cure (secondary prevention).

As discussed in Chapter 1, the decision to screen for a disease depends on the availability of methods that detect disease early enough to effect a cure, the sensitivity and specificity of the available tests, and the attributes of the tests in terms of risks, costs, and patient acceptability. This chapter discusses colon cancer screening strategies, as well as the studies required when the results of screening tests are positive.

ESTIMATING PRETEST PROBABILITIES

The prevalence of colon cancer and adenomas increases with age. In those 60 to 69 years old, the prevalence of undiagnosed colorectal cancer at autopsy is approximately 0.5% (3), and the prevalence of unsuspected adenomatous polyps is approximately 36%, with about 18% of persons having one or more polyps that are 0.5 cm or larger (4,5).

Persons at very high risk of colorectal cancer include those with the familial syndromes of hereditary polyposis and hereditary nonpolyposis colorectal cancer and persons with ulcerative colitis of more than 10 years' duration. Those with a family history of colon cancer are at moderately increased risk In a recent large study, persons with a first-degree relative with colon cancer had a relative risk of colon cancer of 1.7, and persons with two or more affected relatives had a relative risk of 2.75 (6). However, this excess risk was confined to persons aged 40 to 59 years. By the age of 60 years, the relative risk had decreased to baseline.

Patients with a personal history of colon cancer or large adenomas are at moderately increased risk for the disease. Women with a personal history of endometrial, ovarian, or breast cancer also are at slightly increased risk for colon cancer.

DIAGNOSTIC TESTS

Fecal Occult Blood Testing

Fecal occult blood testing (FOBT) detects blood, which is a surrogate marker of the real outcome of interest—neoplasm. Most FOBT depends on the peroxidase-like activity of heme, although an immunologic test for heme is also now available (7). The sensitivity of these tests in asymptomatic average-risk persons is unknown because this determination would require total colon examinations in several asymptomatic persons with negative FOBT results. Instead, the sensitivity figures are generally derived from studies of persons with known polyps or colon cancer (8) or by determining the number of persons who are diagnosed with colon cancer within 1 to 2 years after negative FOBT results (7,9). Both of these methods for determining the sensitivity of the testing tend to overestimate the true sensitivity for early, potentially curable tumors in asymptomatic persons.

In studies using varying FOBTs and differing study designs, the sensitivity of FOBT for colon cancer has ranged from about 30% to 92% (with most studies reporting values of 40% to 60%) and the specificity has ranged from 87% to 99% (7,9–13) (Table 12-1). The sensitivity of FOBT for adenomas is low, approximately 10% to 30% (14–16). Rehydrated Hemoccult II has been reported to have a higher sensitivity than the standard nonrehydrated Hemoccult II (9), but this is associated with a substantial decrease in specificity. It is not clear that the HemoQuant test improves on the sensitivity of Hemoccult II (11,17). In a recent study, HemeSelect (an immunochemical test) and a combination of Hemoccult II Sensa (another guaiac test) followed by HemeSelect each provided better sensitivity than Hemoccult II while maintaining specificity of 94% to 97% (7).

One randomized controlled trial conducted in the United States of the effect of FOBT on colorectal cancer mortality has been reported (9). In this trial of 46,551 participants aged 50 to 80 years, those randomly assigned to receive annual FOBT using rehydrated Hemoccult II had a 33% reduction in cumulative colorectal cancer mortality over 13 years. This reduction was not observed in the group that was randomly assigned to receive biennial FOBT. The use of rehydrated Hemoccult slides led to a 9.8% rate of positive FOBT results, and 38% of those

Table 12-1. Operating Characteristics of Diagnostic Tests for Colon Cancer

Diagnostic Test	Sensitivity for Cancer	Sensitivity for Adenoma	Specificity (Any Neoplasia)
	←————————— % —————————→		
Three-day fecal occult blood test (in asymptomatic patient)	40–60	10–30	87–99
Flexible sigmoidoscopy (60-cm scope)	40–65	65–75	100
Air-contrast barium enema	82–92	50	95
Colonoscopy	94	94	100

screened annually underwent at least one colonoscopy. Based on this information, other authors have questioned whether as much as half of the mortality reduction may have been attributable to "chance" selection for colonoscopy (18).

More recently two European randomized trials of FOBT have been reported (19,20). In one city in Denmark, 61,933 persons aged 45 to 75 years were randomly assigned to receive biennial screening with Hemoccult II (up to four screens) compared with usual care. Approximately 67% of the group that received screening actually underwent one or more screenings, and a colorectal cancer mortality reduction of 18% was observed in these patients (19). In a British study, approximately 150,000 persons aged 45 to 74 years were randomly assigned to receive biennial Haemoccult screening (up to six screens) compared with usual care (20). Of the group that received screening, all screening was completed in 38.2% and at least one screen was completed in 59.6%. A colorectal cancer mortality reduction of 15% was observed. In these two European studies, neither of which used rehydration, only about 4% of the participants who received screening underwent colonoscopy, presumably making "chance" selection for colonoscopy an unlikely explanation for the observed results.

Flexible Sigmoidoscopy

Sigmoidoscopy is quite sensitive within the range of examination, but the overall sensitivity of this test for colorectal cancer depends on the length of the scope. The 60-cm sigmoidoscope can detect 65% to 75% of colonic polyps and 40% to 65% of colorectal cancers (21–23) (Table 12-1). The specificity of flexible sigmoidoscopy is in the range of 97% for cancer and approaches 100% for any neoplasia. However, one must recognize that, because most polyps do not progress to cancer, flexible sigmoidoscopy detects many polyps that would never have become clinically significant within the patient's lifetime (23). Because it cannot be determined in advance which polyps would eventually prove to be clinically significant, some persons undergo biopsies, polypectomies, and follow-up colonoscopies that are not truly beneficial for these patients because those polyps were never destined to progress to malignancy.

A recent case–control study found that exposure to sigmoidoscopic screening within the preceding 10 years was associated with a 60% to 70% reduction in the risk of fatal colorectal cancer within the reach of the sigmoidoscope (24,25). The protective association was limited to the distal colon and not found in the proximal colon, which would seem to make bias an unlikely explanation of the findings.

Colonoscopy

The sensitivity of colonoscopy is approximately 94% for both cancers and adenomatous polyps (26). The specificity approaches 100%.

Air-Contrast Barium Enema

The sensitivity of air-contrast barium enema (ACBE) for cancer is approximately 82% to 92% (27). Although the overall sensitivity for adenomatous polyps is lower, the sensitivity for polyps greater than 1 cm is about 90% (28). The specificity of ACBE is 90% to 95% (23).

Other Tests

Hydrocolonic ultrasonography does not appear sensitive enough for colorectal cancer screening (29). Research is ongoing to attempt to identify markers that might be detectable before the development of frank carcinoma (8), but these are not yet clinically useful.

SCREENING STRATEGIES

Average-Risk and Asymptomatic Patients

Colorectal screening for average-risk patients should begin at the age of 50 years. At a minimum, screening should consist of FOBT, flexible sigmoidoscopy, or both.

When FOBT is used, samples should not be rehydrated (30). A recommendation for the use of FOBT must carry the caveat that the reduction in colorectal cancer mortality may be modest, and that although FOBT itself is inexpensive and noninvasive, subsequent evaluations that result from the use of this test are both expensive and invasive. A positive FOBT result should preferably be followed up by colonoscopy or by ACBE with sigmoidoscopy (30). If the test result is positive, repeating FOBT is unnecessary, because total colon examination will be needed regardless of the result of the repeated test. An upper gastrointestinal series is not necessary unless symptoms are present.

The evidence supporting the use of flexible sigmoidoscopy as a screening modality is convincing (25). Flexible sigmoidoscopy probably reduces colorectal cancer mortality by primary prevention through polypectomies as well as by early detection, thus enhancing the attractiveness of this strategy. The major problems with this technique are the inherent lack of sensitivity for right-sided colon lesions, the fact that too many colonoscopies are performed when all adenomatous polyps are followed up with colonoscopy, and the relatively poor acceptability of the test to patients.

Currently there is much support for screening for colorectal cancer. For example, the report of the U.S. Preventive Services Task Force recommends sigmoidoscopy, annual FOBT, or both for all persons 50 years of age or older.

Evidence has been shown that if only small (<1 cm) tubular adenomas are found during sigmoidoscopy and are removed, then the risk of subsequent colon cancer is low and follow-up colonoscopy may be unnecessary (31). Confirmation of this finding would be helpful, because it implies that flexible sigmoidoscopy may be used for risk stratification as well as for screening. In the absence of such confirmation, colonoscopy is recommended for the follow-up of adenomatous polyps, with continued surveillance every 3 to 5 years (32,33).

Colonoscopy or ACBE at 10-year intervals has been recommended by some as a screening strategy (34,35), although there has not been direct evidence to support this strategy. In particular, the appropriateness of the 10-year interval and the cost-effectiveness of this approach are uncertain. Total colon examination every 3 to 5 years presently appears impractical to recommend as a national strategy (25).

Symptomatic and High-Risk Patients

Neither the FOBT nor flexible sigmoidoscopy has sufficient sensitivity for colorectal cancer to be used in ruling out the disease. Therefore, patients who are symptomatic require a total colon examination with either colonoscopy or ACBE plus sigmoidoscopy.

Families with hereditary polyposis or nonpolyposis colon cancer syndromes require total colon screening beginning at an early age; testing for genetic abnormalities can help to identify those at risk (36). Persons with ulcerative colitis of 10 years' duration also require total colon screening, preferably with colonoscopy.

Asymptomatic patients with an isolated first-degree relative with colon cancer have a moderately elevated risk of colon cancer and may develop the disease earlier than members of the general population. Although direct evidence is not available, clinicians may wish to consider total colon examination. Whether total colon examination is used or not, some type of screening should probably be instituted by the time the patient is 40 years old. For persons with two or more first-degree relatives with colon cancer, clinicians may strongly consider total colon examination, based on the indirect evidence available.

CLINICAL PROBLEMS

Clinical Problem 1

A patient with a family history of colon cancer inquires about screening.

Testing Strategy and Rationale

In patients with one or two first-degree relatives with colon cancer, the relative risk for developing the disease is 1.7 to 2.7. In most of these patients, the excess risk is highest between the ages of 40 to 59 years. These patients should receive FOBT, which should be followed by flexible sigmoidoscopy if the results of FOBT are nega-

Continued

tive. However, total colon examination is also a reasonable alternative, owing to its greater sensitivity. If total colon examination is elected, FOBT is unnecessary.

Clinical Example
A 48-year-old asymptomatic woman presents at the office of her primary care physician. Her father died of colon cancer 5 years ago, and a cousin has recently been diagnosed with colon cancer. Given the increased relative risk for this patient, colonoscopy is arranged.

Clinical Problem 2
A patient has a positive FOBT result.

Testing Strategy and Rationale
Total colon examination is recommended. Colonoscopy is preferred, but ACBE with sigmoidoscopy is an acceptable alternative. Repeat FOBT is unnecessary, because tumors may bleed only intermittently and a negative result on repeat testing would not change the need for total colon examination. An upper gastrointestinal evaluation is also unnecessary unless symptoms are present.

Clinical Example
A 65-year-old asymptomatic man is followed for hypertension. He received FOBT routinely provided to average-risk patients; for one sample, the results are positive for occult blood. After discussion with the patient, colonoscopy is scheduled.

REFERENCES

1. **Landis SH, Murray T, Bolden S, Wingo PA.** Cancer statistics, 1998. CA Cancer J Clin. 1998;48:6-29.
2. **Muto T, Bussey HJR, Morson BC.** The evolution of cancer of the colon and rectum. Cancer. 1975;36:2251-70.
3. **Berg TW, Downing A, Lukes RJ.** Prevalence of undiagnosed cancer of the large bowel found at autopsy in different races. Cancer. 1970;25:1076-80.
4. **Arminski TC, McLean DW.** Incidence and distribution of adenomatous polyps of the colon and rectum based on 1000 autopsy examinations. Dis Colon Rectum. 1964;7:249-61.
5. **Blatt LJ.** Polyps of the colon and rectum: incidence and distribution. Dis Colon Rectum. 1961;4:277-82.
6. **Fuchs CS, Giovannucci E, Colditz GA, et al.** A prospective study of family history and the risk of colorectal cancer. N Engl J Med. 1994;331:1669-74.
7. **Allison JE, Tekawa IS, Ransom LJ, Adrain AL.** A comparison of fecal occult-blood tests for colorectal-cancer screening. N Engl J Med. 1996;334:155-9.

8. **Weinberg DS, Strom BL.** Screening for colon cancer: a review of current and future strategies. Semin Oncol. 1995;22:433-47.

9. **Mandel JS, Bond JH, Church TR, et al.** Reducing mortality from colorectal cancer by screening fecal occult blood. N Engl J Med. 1993;328:1365-71.

10. **Winawer SJ, Flehinger BJ, Schottenfeld D, Miller DG.** Screening for colorectal cancer with fecal occult blood testing and sigmoidoscopy. J Natl Cancer Inst. 1993;85:1311-8.

11. **Ahlquist DA, Wieland HS, Moertel GC, et al.** Accuracy of fecal occult blood screening for colorectal neoplasia: a prospective study using hemoccult and hemoquant tests. JAMA. 1993;269:1262-7.

12. **Kewenter J, Bjorck S, Hagland E, et al.** Screening and rescreening for colorectal cancer: a controlled trial of fecal occult blood testing in 27,700 subjects. Cancer. 1988;3:645-51.

13. **Hardcastle JD, Chamberlain J, Sheffield J, et al.** Randomized, controlled trial of fecal occult blood screening for colorectal cancer. Results for the first 107,349 subjects. Lancet. 1989;1:1160-4.

14. **Demers RY, Stawick LE, Demers P.** Relative sensitivity of the fecal occult blood test and flexible sigmoidoscopy in detecting polyps. Prev Med. 1985;14:55-62.

15. **Robinson MHE, Kronborg O, Williams CB, et al.** Faecal occult blood testing and colonoscopy in the surveillance of subjects at high risk of colorectal neoplasia. Br J Surg. 1995;82:318-20.

16. **Yoshinaga M, Motomura S, Takeda H, et al.** Evaluation of the sensitivity of an immunochemical fecal occult blood test for colorectal neoplasia. Am J Gastroenterol. 1995;90:1076-9.

17. **St John DJB, Young GP, McHutchison JG, et al.** Comparison of the specificity and sensitivity of Hemoccult and HemoQuant in screening of colorectal neoplasia. Ann Intern Med. 1992;117:376-82.

18. **Lang CA, Ransohoff DF.** Fecal occult blood screening for colorectal cancer: is mortality reduced by chance selection for screening colonoscopy? JAMA. 1994;271:1011-3

19. **Kronborg O, Fenger C, Olsen J, et al.** Randomised study of screening for colorectal cancer with faecal-occult-blood test. Lancet. 1996;348:1467-71

20. **Hardcastle JD, Chamberlain JO, Robinson MHE, et al.** Randomised controlled trial of faecal-occult-blood screening for colorectal cancer. Lancet. 1996;348:1472-7

21. **Lieberman DA, Smith FW.** Screening for colon malignancy with colonoscopy. Am J Gastroenterol. 1991;86:946-51.

22. **Johnson DA, Gurney MS, Volpe RJ, et al.** A prospective study of the prevalence of colonic neoplasms in asymptomatic patients with age-related risk. Am J Gastroenterol. 1990;85:969-74.

23. **U.S. Preventive Services Task Force.** Guide to Clinical Preventive Services. 2nd ed. Baltimore: Williams and Wilkins; 1996.

24. **Selby JV, Friedman GD, Quesenberry CPJ, Weiss NS.** A case-control study of screening sigmoidoscopy and mortality from colorectal cancer. N Engl J Med. 1992;326:653-7.

25. **Ransohoff DF, Lang CA.** Sigmoidosocopic screening in the 1990s. JAMA. 1993;269:1278-81.

26. **Hogan WJ, Stewart ET, Geenen JE, et al.** A prospective comparision of the accuracy of colonoscopy versus air-barium contrast examination for detection of colonic polypoid lesions. Gastrointest Endosc. 1977;23:230.

27. **Leiwicke JL, Dodds WJ, Hogan WJ, Stewart ET.** A comparison of colonoscopy and roentgenography for detecting polypoid lesions of the colon. Gastrointest Radiol. 1977;2:125-8.

28. **Fort FT.** Reliability of routine double contrast examination of the large bowel: a prospective study of 2590 patients. Gut. 1983;24:672-7.

29. **Chui DW, Gooding GAW, McQuaid KR, et al.** Hydrocolonic ultrasonography in the detection of colonic polyps and tumors. N Engl J Med. 1994;331:1685-8.

30. American College of Physicians. Suggested technique for fecal occult blood testing and interpretation in colorectal cancer screening. Ann Intern Med. 1997;126:808-10.

31. **Atkin WS, Morson BC, Cuyick J.** Long-term risk of colorectal cancer after excision of rectosigmoid adenomas. N Engl J Med. 1992;326:658-62.

32. **Winawer SJ, Zauber AG, O'Brien MJ, et al.** Randomized comparison of surveillance intervals after colonoscopic removal of newly diagnosed adenomatous polyps. N EnglJ Med. 1993;328:901-6.

33. **Bond JH for the American College of Gastroenterology.** Polyp guideline: diagnosis, treatment, and surveillance for patients with nonfamilial colorectal polyps. Ann Intern Med. 1993;119:836-43.

34. **Byers T, Levin B, Rothenberger D, et al.** American Cancer Society guidelines for screening and surveillance for early detection of colorectal polyps and cancer: update 1997. CA-Cancer J Clin. 1997;47:154-60.

35. **Winawer SJ, Fletcher RH, Miller L, et al.** Colorectal cancer screening: clinical guidelines and rationale. Gastroenterology. 1997;112:594-642.

36. **Giardiello FM.** Genetic testing in hereditary colorectal cancer. JAMA. 1997;278:1278-81.

Acute Diarrhea

13

Benson T. Massey, MD

KEY POINTS

Pretest Probabilities

- More than 95% of cases of acute diarrhea are self-limited and require no specific diagnostic testing or therapy.
- Certain clinical symptoms (bloody diarrhea, fever, cramps), signs (fecal leukocytes, fecal occult blood, anemia, eosinophilia), and settings (hospitalization, antibiotic use, foreign travel) increase the likelihood of identifying a causative pathogen in 10% to 20% of cases.
- Nosocomial diarrhea essentially never results from enteroinvasive bacteria or parasites. *Clostridium difficile* is a frequent (10%–20%) causative agent in this setting.

Diagnostic Strategies

- For most patients with mild episodes of diarrhea, no diagnostic testing is indicated.
- Patients with severe symptoms or with concomitant debilitating disease require stool culture for the identification of invasive bacterial pathogens and special studies for *Escherichia coli* O157:H7.
- In certain clinical settings, including those involving issues of public health, the risks to the individual and community are high enough to warrant diagnostic testing, including studies for parasites and *C. difficile*, even if the illness is mild.
- One stool specimen for bacterial pathogens is sufficient. At least two stool specimens are required to detect *C. difficile* and parasites with a 90% certainty.
- Endoscopic examination of the bowel is unnecessary in most cases and should be deferred until the results of stool studies to identify pathogens are shown to be negative.

BACKGROUND

Acute diarrhea, defined as symptoms of diarrhea for less than 2 weeks, is a common clinical problem, with adults in Western countries averaging one episode per year (1,2). Most of these episodes are mild and self-limited, and most do not come to medical attention. The differential diagnosis of acute diarrhea is long and includes both infectious and noninfectious causes. Although among patients seeking treatment, some are persons with severe illness caused by treatable infections, most patients will require only symptomatic care. Diagnostic testing of every episode of acute diarrhea would be costly and would yield few treatable findings. The principal reasons for diagnostic testing in acute diarrhea are to identify organisms that require specific therapy, to institute appropriate infection control measures for communicable organisms, and to detect and control emerging endemics or epidemics of acute diarrheal illness. Stool cultures are ordered for approximately 5% of all episodes of diarrhea (1) or 25% of patients presenting to a physician with acute enteric illness (3).

ESTIMATING PRETEST PROBABILITY

In most patients presenting with acute diarrhea, a specific pathogen is not found, even when tests are performed to look for agents for which no specific treatment would be given, such as rotavirus. In studies from different settings, only 2% to 12% of stool cultures (4–9) and 0.4% to 7% of stool examinations for ova and parasites (5,6,10,11) yielded positive results for enteric pathogens. These figures likely overestimate the pretest probability, because most of these series reflect the yield of selected testing based on clinical features rather than testing of every patient presenting with diarrhea. Certain clinical settings raise the pretest probability for specific causative agents and thus increase the yield of diagnostic testing. Other clinical settings are known to have a low incidence of some pathogens; thus, testing in these settings can be avoided.

Patients with enteroinvasive organisms, such as *Campylobacter, Salmonella, Yersinia,* and *Shigella* species, or enterohemorrhagic strains of *Escherichia coli,* such as O157:H7, are more likely to have a clinical course marked by frequent, bloody stools and abdominal cramping and tenderness. These features are approximately three times more likely in patients with stool specimens that yield positive results for these pathogens compared with patients with stool studies with negative results (9). About 20% of patients with visibly bloody stools have one of these pathogens (9). Compared with the other pathogens, patients with O157:H7 are more likely to have bloody diarrhea and abdominal tenderness but are less likely to have fever (9).

Homosexual men (both those who test positive for HIV and those who test negative) who present with diarrhea are reported to have a high rate of bacterial, protozoal, and viral infections (12). As many as 85% of patients with the acquired immunodeficiency syndrome (AIDS) with diarrhea may have identifiable opportunistic infections (13), although not all such infections may be amenable to therapy.

Diarrhea associated with antibiotic administration has been associated with *Clostridium difficile* infection in 15% to 25% of cases (14). Only a small minority of patients with *C. difficile*–associated diarrhea have evidence of pseudomembranous colitis. Among patients who are hospitalized or in extended care facilities, *C. difficile* is the cause of 10% to 20% of nosocomial diarrhea (6,15–18). Hospitalized patients with previous use of antibiotics, prolonged hospital stay, or the finding of fecal leukocytes are more likely to have diarrhea that is caused by *C. difficile* (16–19). However, except in endemic areas or during outbreaks, diarrhea that is acquired during hospitalization is essentially never caused by enteroinvasive bacterial or protozoan infections (5,7,20).

DIAGNOSTIC TESTS

Stool Examination for Leukocytes and Occult Blood
Invasive bacterial and parasitic pathogens, such as *Shigella*, *Entamoeba histolytica*, and enterohemorrhagic *Escherichia coli* generally cause an inflammatory mucosal response that leads to exudation of leukocytes and blood into the stool. However, studies have found widely varying sensitivities (20%–90%) and specificities (20%–90%) for both fecal blood and fecal leukocytes when stool culture has been used as the gold standard for an enteroinvasive infection (Table 13-1) (8,21–24). Hence, the findings on these tests cannot be used to select patients for further testing to find a specific causative agent.

Stool Examination for Ova and Parasites
Stool examination for ova and parasites (O&P) is the standard method for detecting parasitic infections, primarily *Giardia lamblia* and *E. histolytica*, that can cause diarrhea. This test relies on the skill of the examiner. Proficiency testing has found parasitology laboratories to have a sensitivity of 80% to 90% and a specificity of 80% to 90% (25). This may in part explain why sensitivity for a single specimen appears to be about 80% (26,27). The use of multiple, purged, and fresh specimens increases the yield of O&P testing. Contamination of the stool specimens with barium, antacids, or polyethylene glycol lavage solutions is reported to hamper testing. Previous antibiotic administration can also prevent some parasites from being recovered. *Cryptosporidium* requires acid-fast staining of stool specimens for identification (28).

More recently, direct fluorescent antibody (DFA) and enzyme immunoassay (EIA) techniques to examine stool specimens for both *Giardia* and *Cryptosporidium* have become commercially available. These offer improved sensitivity (90%–99%) and high specificity (95%–100%) compared with standard microscopic techniques (29), and sensitivity increases with submission of multiple specimens (30). However, evaluation of stool specimens using only these antibody assays will cause other parasites to be missed.

Stool Culture for Enteroinvasive and Enterohemorrhagic Bacteria

Stool culture is generally used as the gold standard in the diagnosis of diarrhea caused by bacterial infections. However, epidemiologic studies suggest that the sensitivity may decline if cultures are obtained late in the course of diarrhea (9,31). *Escherichia coli* O157:H7 is not detected on routine stool culture and requires special isolation techniques.

Stool Culture and Toxin Assays for *Clostridium difficile*

Stool culture for *C. difficile* has a sensitivity and specificity of about 95% (see Table 13-1), because some asymptomatic patients carry a non–toxin–producing strain (32). The cytotoxin tissue culture assay has a sensitivity of approximately 67% and is highly specific (99%). New EIAs for the A and B cytotoxins have reported sensitivities ranging from 70% to 95% and specificities ranging from 95% to 100%, using the cytotoxin tissue culture assay as the gold standard. At least two stool specimens should be sent for cytotoxin EIA to obtain a sensitivity of 90% (16).

Endoscopy

Quantitative information on the utility of endoscopic examination of the large and small bowel is lacking. None of the mucosal changes associated with invasive infections are pathognomonic, and all such infections can at times cause mucosal changes that are indistinguishable from those of idiopathic inflammatory bowel disease. The presence of pseudomembranous mucosal changes strongly suggests infection with *C. difficile*, although such changes are not pathognomonic (33). Immunocompromised patients are at risk for diarrhea caused by infections, such as cytomegalovirus, not found by the usual stool examinations. Endoscopy with biopsy is necessary to identify these pathogens.

DIAGNOSTIC STRATEGIES

Because most acute diarrheal episodes are self-limited and the laboratory effort to screen for all potential infections would be considerable, clinicians should use a selective strategy in evaluating acute diarrhea. A careful history should include details of the frequency, onset, and severity of gastrointestinal and systemic symptoms and inquiry into food intake, recent travel and potential exposure to specific agents. This information combined with the physical examination may raise the pretest likelihood of some causative agents but may also identify those patients in whom the severity of the illness mandates an aggressive approach. Many patients with invasive intestinal infections have a mild illness that requires only supportive therapy. An aggressive diagnostic approach should therefore be taken only in patients in whom there is evidence of a severe illness, with findings such as significant abdominal pain or tenderness, bloody stools, or fever. In such cases, stool specimens should be sent for bacterial culture, including *E. coli* O157:H7. It is expected that the results of most cultures will be negative. Consideration should also be given to culturing the stool in those patients who are at increased risk from an enteroinvasive infection and bacteremia or who may not manifest the typical signs of such infections (e.g., patients who are immunocompromised, have severe organ system disease, have an implanted prosthetic device, or are elderly).

Patients with travelers' diarrhea and severe symptoms who have negative stool cultures should have a stool examination for ova and parasites if symptoms persist. Male homosexual patients with diarrhea should be tested for the presence of enteric pathogens and ova and parasites. If the patient has persistent symptoms at least two specimens should be submitted for O&P examination and use of one of the newer antibody-labeling techniques for *Giardia* should be considered. Severely immunocompromised patients, including those with AIDS, require specific studies to identify *Cryptosporidium*. Persistent symptoms in these patients despite negative stool study results should prompt endoscopic examination of the bowel with biopsy.

Patients who are nursing home residents, patients who have recently been or who currently are hospitalized, or patients who have previously received antibiotic therapy should have stool specimens submitted for *C. difficile* cytotoxin assay or culture. If the EIA is used, the test should be repeated if the results of the first test are negative and symptoms persist. When symptoms persist in this setting after two negative EIA results, consideration should be given to performing an endoscopic examination of the colon to look for pseudomembranes. Routine stool cultures and examination for ova and parasites should not be performed in patients who develop diarrhea during hospitalization.

Certain clinical situations warrant further diagnostic testing, even when the illness appears to be mild. For public health purposes, one could consider evaluating those who handle food, day care workers, and health care workers for communicable pathogens. Community outbreaks of diarrhea or possible episodes of food poisoning should

Table 13-1. Operating Characteristics of Diagnostic Tests for Acute Diarrhea

Diagnostic Test	Sensitivity	Specificity	Likelihood Ratio	
			Positive Result	Negative Result
	← % →			
Enteroinvasive infection				
Fecal leukocytes	20–90	20–90	0.25–9.0	0.11–4.0
Fecal occult blood	20–90	20–90	0.25–9.0	0.11–4.0
Parasitic infection				
O&P examination	80–90	80–90	4.0–5.0	0.10–0.20
EIA or DFA	90–95	95–99	18–95	0.05–0.11
Clostridium difficile				
Stool culture	95	95	19	0.05
Cytotoxin tissue culture assay	67	99	67	0.33
EIA	70–95	95–99	14–95	0.05–0.32

*EIA = enzyme immunoassay, DFA = direct fluorescent antibody.

prompt more extensive testing of some of the affected persons to help identify the cause of the outbreak and thus contain it. In addition to the above studies, diarrhea associated with raw seafood consumption warrants specific stool culture for *Vibrio* species.

In patients with diarrhea that persists for more than 2 weeks, even if mild, further diagnostic evaluation is required. However, the approach to these patients is beyond the scope of this chapter.

CLINICAL PROBLEMS

Clinical Problem 1
A previously healthy adult has persistent diarrhea and systemic symptoms that developed during travel abroad (e.g., during a trip to Mexico).

Testing Strategy and Rationale
Stool culture for identifying bacterial pathogens should be performed. If the results of this test are negative and symptoms persist, a stool specimen should be submitted for O&P examination. Although this patient has no underlying disease and a short duration of illness, the presence of systemic symptoms raises the likelihood that a bacterial pathogen is the causative agent, warranting specific treatment. The yield of stool O&P testing in this setting

would be expected to be low, but *Giardia* can be a coinfection, and the morbidity resulting from missing a severe *E. histolytica* infection could be significant.

Clinical Example

A previously healthy, heterosexual 22-year-old male college student is on vacation in Mexico when he contracts acute diarrhea. He takes no antibiotics. Over the next 48 hours, tenesmus, fever, severe abdominal pain, and bloody stools develop. When he arrives home, he reports directly to the emergency room. On physical examination he appears ill, with a fever of 38 °C. He has diffuse tenderness on abdominal examination and hyperactive bowel sounds. The stool is grossly bloody. A stool specimen is sent for enteric pathogen culture. *Campylobacter jejuni* is identified.

Clinical Problem 2

A nursing home resident develops frequent diarrhea after a recent hospitalization for treatment of an infection.

Testing Strategy and Rationale

A stool specimen should be submitted for *C. difficile* toxin assay or culture. Such patients are at increased risk for *C. difficile*–associated diarrhea, and the probability of *C. difficile* is at least 20% to 25%. If the results of the first assay are negative and symptoms persist, a repeat specimen should be submitted. In a patient with severe symptoms and signs suggesting toxic megacolon (e.g., fever, distended abdomen, bloody stools, and dilated colon on abdominal radiography), sigmoidoscopy may be useful as an initial test, because if pseudomembranes are found by this testing, culture for other bacterial pathogens would be unnecessary. However, in most patients, negative results of testing with sigmoidoscopy do not rule out *C. difficile* as the cause of diarrhea.

Clinical Example

A 70-year-old nursing home resident presents with diarrhea and fecal incontinence. He had been hospitalized 3 weeks ago for pneumonia, for which he was initially treated with a third-generation cephalosporin followed by 1 week of treatment with cephalexin. Two other residents in his ward had episodes of pseudomembranous colitis during the previous month. On examination, he is found to be afebrile with no abdominal tenderness and with normal bowel sounds. The results of examination of stool are negative for gross or occult blood. *Clostridium difficile* cytotoxin EIA yields negative test results. Repeat testing is performed because the patient's symptoms persist. The results of the repeat testing are positive.

REFERENCES

1. **Feldman RA, Banatvala N.** The frequency of culturing stools from adults with diarrhoea in Great Britain. Epidemiol Infect. 1994;113:41-4.

2. **Guerrnat RL, Shields DS, Thorson SM, et al.** Evaluation and diagnosis of acute infectious diarrhea. Am J Med. 1985;78(Suppl 6B):91-8.

3. **Thomas MEM, Tillett HE.** Diarrhea in general practice: a sixteen-year report of investigations in a microbiology laboratory, with epidemiological assessment. J Hygiene. 1975;74:183-94.

4. **Koplan JP, Fineberg HV, Ferraro MJB, Rosenberg ML.** Value of stool cultures. Lancet. 1980;2:413-6.

5. **Siegel DL, Edelstein PH, Nachamkin I.** Inappropriate testing for diarrheal diseases in the hospital. JAMA. 1990;263:979-82.

6. **Bowman RA, Bowman JM, Arrow SA, Riley TV.** Selective criteria for the microbiological examination of faecal specimens. J Clin Pathol. 1992;45: 838-9.

7. **Barbut F, Leluan P, Antoniotti G, et al.** Value of routine stool cultures in hospitalized patients with diarrhea. Eur J Clin Microbiol Infect Dis. 1995;14:346-9.

8. **Chitkara YK, McCasland KA, Kenefic L.** Development and implementation of cost-effective guidelines in the laboratory investigation of diarrhea in a community hospital. Arch Intern Med. 1996;156:1445-8.

9. **Slutsker L, Ries AA, Greene KD, et al.** *Escherichia coli* O157:H7 diarrhea in the United States: clinical and epidemiologic features. Ann Intern Med. 1997;126:505-13.

10. **Massey BT, Black ER.** Clinical parameters associated with a positive stool ova and parasite (O&P) exam in medical inpatients. Gastroenterology. 1989;96:A325.

11. **Morris AJ, Wilson ML, Reller LB.** Application of rejection criteria for stool ovum and parasite examinations. J Clin Microbiol. 1992;30:3213-6.

12. **Laughon BE, Druckman DA, Vernon A, et al.** Prevalence of enteric pathogens in homosexual men with and without acquired immunodeficiency syndrome. Gastroenterology. 1988;94:984-93.

13. **Smith PD, Lane HC, Gill VJ, et al.** Intestinal infections in patients with the acquired immunodeficiency syndrome (AIDS). Ann Intern Med. 1988;108: 328-33.

14. **Bartlett JG.** Pseudomembranous enterocolitis and antibiotic-associated colitis. In: Sleisenger MH, Fordtran JS, eds. Gastrointestinal Disease: Pathophysiology, Diagnosis, Management. Philadelphia: WB Saunders; 1993:1174-89.

15. **McFarland LV, Surawicz CM, Stamm WE.** Risk factors for *Clostridium difficile* carriage and *C. difficile*-associated diarrhea in a cohort of hospitalized patients. J Infect Dis. 1990;162:678-84.

16. **Manabe YC, Vinetz JM, Moore RD, et al.** *Clostridium difficile* colitis: an efficient clinical approach to diagnosis. Ann Intern Med. 1995;123:835-40.

17. **Katz DA, Lynch ME, Littenberg B.** Clinical prediction rules to optimize cytotoxin testing for *Clostridium difficile* in hospitalized patients with diarrhea. Am J Med. 1996;100:487-95.

18. **Barbut F, Corthier G, Charpak Y, et al.** Prevalence and pathogenicity of *Clostridium difficile* in hospitalized patients: a French multicenter study. Arch Intern Med. 1996;156:1449-54.

19. **Cooper GS, Lederman MM, Salata RA.** A predictive model to identify Clostridium difficile toxin in hospitalized patients with diarrhea. Am J Gastroenterol. 1996;91:80-4.

20. **Yannelli B, Gurevich I, Schoch PE, Cunha BA.** Yield of stool cultures, ova and parasite tests, and *Clostridium difficile* determinations in nosocomial diarrheas. Am J Infect Control. 1988;16:246-9.

21. **Stoll BJ, Glass RI, Banu H, et al.** Value of stool examination in patients with diarrhoea. Br Med J. 1983;286:2037-40.

22. **Siegel D, Cohen PT, Neighbor M, et al.** Predictive value of stool examination in acute diarrhea. Arch Pathol Lab Med. 1987;111:715-8.

23. **Huicho L, Sanchez D, Contreras M, et al.** Occult blood and fecal leukocytes as screening tests in childhood infectious diarrhea: an old problem revisited. Pediatric Infect Dis J. 1993;12:474-7.

24. **Singh T, Verma M, Chhatwal J, et al.** Predictive utility of clinical and stool parameters in bacterial diarrhoea in children. Indian J Med Sci. 1995;49: 285-90.

25. **Smith JW.** Identification of fecal parasites in the special parasitology survey of the College of American Pathologists. Am J Clin Pathol. 1979;72: 371-3.

26. **Thomson RB, Haas RA, Thompson JH.** Intestinal parasites: the necessity of examining multiple stool specimens. Mayo Clin Proc. 1984;59:641-2.

27. **Massey BT, Black ER.** The stool examination for ova and parasites: reasons for suboptimal utilization in medical inpatients. Gastroenterology. 1989;96:A326.

28. **Wolfson JS, Richter JM, Waldron MA, et al.** Cryptosporidiosis in immunocompetent patients. N Engl J Med. 1985;312:1278-82.

29. **Garcia LS, Shimizu RY.** Evaluation of nine immunoassay kits (enzyme immunoassay and direct fluorescence) for detection of *Giardia lamblia* and *Cryptosporidium parvum* in human fecal specimens. J Clin Microbiol. 1997;35:1526-9.

30. **Addiss DG, Mathews HM, Stewart JM, et al.** Evaluation of a commercially-available enzyme-linked imunosorbent assay for *Giardia lamblia* antigen in stool. J Clin Microbiol. 1991;29:1137-42.

31. **Tarr PI, Neill MA, Clausen CR, et al.** *Escherichia coli* O157:H7 and the hemolytic uremic syndrome: importance of early cultures in establishing the etiology. J Infect Dis. 1990;162:553-6.

32. **Peterson LR, Olson MM, Chanholtzer CJ, Gerding DN.** Results of a prospective, 18-month clinical evaluation of culture, cytotoxin testing, Culturette brand (CDT) latex testing in the diagnosis of *Clostridium difficile*-associated diarrhea. Diagn Microbiol Infect Dis. 1988;10:85-91.

33. **Franco J, Massey BT, Komorowski R.** Cytomegalovirus infection causing pseudomembranous colitis. Am J Gastroenterol. 1994;89:2246-8.

Cholelithiasis and Acute Cholecystitis

14

Eric A. Richard, MD, and Robert A. Greene, MD

KEY POINTS

Pretest Probabilities

- Gallstones are highly prevalent. They are found in 20% of women and 8% of men. Most patients with gallstones are asymptomatic.

- Approximately 40% of patients presenting with signs and symptoms suggesting biliary colic have cholelithiasis.

- Approximately 30% of patients evaluated for symptoms suggesting acute cholecystitis have the disease.

- Fewer than 10% of patients with symptomatic cholelithiasis have common bile duct stones.

Diagnostic Strategies

- Real-time ultrasonography (RTUS) is the imaging technique of choice for detecting gallstones and for evaluating acute right upper quadrant pain.

- Although cholescintigraphy is the single best test for the diagnosis of acute cholecystitis, RTUS also has very good operating characteristics for this disease and provides more information about other causes of right upper quadrant pain. Cholescintigraphy is most useful when the clinical suspicion of cholecystitis remains high despite negative or nondiagnostic ultrasonography.

- Endoscopic retrograde cholangiopancreatography is currently the study of choice for those patients with a high likelihood of choledocholithiasis.

BACKGROUND

Gallstones are highly prevalent in the United States, being found in 10% to 20% of adult autopsies (1). Women with gallstones outnumber men 2 to 1. The prevalence in both sexes increases with age; a prospective study from Denmark (2) estimated that prevalence increases 3%

every 5 years. However, symptomatic disease attributable to gall-stones is much less common. It is estimated that symptoms develop in only 2% to 5% of those with gallstones each year. Diagnostic tests must be carefully selected to differentiate other, more common, caus-es of abdominal symptoms from gallstone-related disease and to dif-ferentiate the various forms of gallstone-related disease from each other.

Biliary colic is the most common form of symptomatic disease. Acute cholecystitis and choledocholithiasis are less common. In the case of choledocholithiasis, diagnosis is sought in two different situa-tions. First, patients with acute symptoms and signs suggesting chole-docholithiasis must be promptly evaluated and closely monitored for the development of ascending cholangitis, a potentially lethal compli-cation of common duct stones. Second, common duct stones must be excluded in patients undergoing cholecystectomy.

A small number of patients develop acute cholecystitis without evi-dence of a stone. These cases of acalculous cholecystitis generally occur in the setting of sepsis, burns, trauma, or recent surgery. Because imag-ing studies are not as reliable for the diagnosis of acalculous disease, a high level of suspicion is important. The diagnosis of acalculous dis-ease is not discussed further in this chapter.

ESTIMATING PRETEST PROBABILITY

Cholelithiasis
Classic biliary colic is characterized by a steady, severe aching in the epigastrium or right upper quadrant, frequently radiating to the inter-scapular area or the right scapula. This pain usually begins suddenly, persists for 1 to 3 hours, and often leaves residual discomfort after sub-siding (1). Unfortunately, many patients with gallstones do not have classic symptoms or signs. Among patients who undergo real-time ultrasonography (RTUS) for suspected biliary colic, nearly 40% have stones; about twice the prevalence in the general population (3). This value provides a rough pretest probability for gallstones in a typical patient undergoing diagnostic evaluation.

Acute Cholecystitis
Most patients with acute cholecystitis have a history of previous episodes of biliary colic. The attack of acute cholecystitis may begin similarly but does not remit and is associated with fever, leukocytosis, and a mild elevation of liver function tests. In prospective evaluations of patients referred for imaging because of symptoms and signs con-sistent with acute cholecystitis, between 14% and 46% were found to have the disease, with an average of approximately 30% (4–8).

Choledocholithiasis

Fewer than 10% of patients with symptomatic gallstones will have choledocholithiasis (9). Like cholelithiasis, the pain associated with choledocholithiasis is usually in the right upper quadrant or epigastrium; however, some patients have no pain. Patients with stones in their common bile duct may also present with elevated liver function tests indicative of cholestasis (typically elevated alkaline phosphatase and bilirubin) or with signs of pancreatitis. When these patients are referred for imaging studies of their common bile ducts, 50% are found to have common bile duct stones (10–12).

DIAGNOSTIC TESTS

Real-time Ultrasonography of the Gallbladder

Cholelithiasis

Real-time ultrasonography has become the standard of evaluation for patients in whom gallstone disease is suspected (13). The procedure is painless and virtually risk-free, without ionizing radiation. The preparation requires a 6-hour fast, but the test itself takes only 15 minutes to perform. More than 95% of patients have a technically adequate study. The study may be limited by obesity, bandages, and large wounds.

The two major criteria for diagnosis of gallstones by ultrasonography are echogenic densities that cast an acoustic shadow and nonvisualization of the gallbladder (13). Nonvisualization with shadowing in the gallbladder fossa is highly specific and probably indicates a fibrotic gallbladder filled with small stones. Results from a meta-analysis estimated the sensitivity of RTUS in detecting gallstones to be 89% and estimated the specificity to be 97% (14) (Table 14-1).

Acute Cholecystitis

The ultrasonographic criteria that indicate acute cholecystitis are the presence of gallstones along with signs of gallbladder inflammation (13). These signs include sonographic Murphy's sign (tenderness of gallbladder when palpated during the sonographic examination), gallbladder enlargement greater than 5 cm, fluid around the gallbladder, and gallbladder thickening. Real-time ultrasonography for the diagnosis of acute cholecystitis is sensitive but not specific because gallbladder thickening can also be seen in other conditions such as ascites, hypoalbuminemia, hepatitis, congestive heart failure, and renal failure (15). Results from the meta-analysis (14) estimate the sensitivity of ultrasonography to diagnose acute cholecystitis at 91% and specificity at 79% (Table 14-1).

Table 14-1. Operating Characteristics of Diagnostic Tests in the Diagnosis of Cholelithiasis, Acute Calculous Cholecystitis, and Choledocholithiasis

Diagnostic Test	Sensitivity	Specificity	Likelihood Ratio	
			Positive Result	Negative Result
	←——— % ———→			
For cholelithiasis				
RTUS	89	97	30	0.11
OCG	75	96	19	0.26
CT	79	99	79	0.21
For acute cholecystitis				
RTUS	91	79	4.3	0.11
Cholescintigraphy	97	90	9.7	0.03
For choledocholithiasis				
RTUS	~25	~95	5	0.79
ERCP	90	99	90	0.1
MRI	88	92	11	0.13
EUS	93	97	31	0.07
CT	75	94	13	0.27
Helical CT	88	97	29	0.12

RTUS = real-time ultrasonography; CT = computed tomography; MRI = magnetic resonance imaging; OCG = oral cholecystography; ERCP = endoscopic retrograde cholangiopancreatography; EUS = endoscopic ultrasonography.

Choledocholithiasis

Real-time ultrasonography is often performed as part of the diagnostic evaluation for right upper quadrant abdominal pain or elevated liver function tests. The main criterion to diagnose choledocholithiasis with RTUS is visualization of stones in the common bile duct; however, finding a dilated common bile duct may suggest the presence of stones. Real-time ultrasonography is particularly insensitive for small (<1 cm) stones (16). On average, ultrasonography has a sensitivity of only 22% to 25% and a specificity of 92% to 100% in the diagnosis of choledocholithiasis (9,16).

Oral Cholecystography

Oral cholecystography (OCG) assesses gallbladder anatomy and function and may help diagnose cholelithiasis but not acute cholecystitis or choledocholithiasis (1,13). An iodine-containing contrast material is ingested the night before the test, along with a fatty meal. Normally, the contrast material is concentrated in the gallbladder. Adequate images are obtained in 90% of patients, but as many as 15% to 25% require a second dose. Abnormality as demonstrated by the test is defined as stones in the gallbladder or inability to visualize the gallbladder after two doses. The sensitivity of oral cholecystography in diagnosing gallstones is approximately 75% and the specificity is 96% (14) (see Table 14-1).

Approximately 25% of patients have side effects, including diarrhea, nausea, dysuria, and skin rash. Rarely, a more severe reaction such as severe diarrhea or renal failure occurs. The test does use radiation and the preparation may take as long as 2 days. The test is not available at all centers.

Cholescintingraphy

During cholescintigraphy or "HIDA" scanning (1,13), the liver extracts an injected technetium 99m–labeled iminodiacetic acid derivative from the bloodstream and excretes it into the bile. The patient must fast for 2 to 4 hours before the study. Images are obtained every 10 to 15 minutes for the first hour. The normal filling sequence is the gallbladder, then the common bile duct, and finally the duodenum. Abnormality as demonstrated by the study is defined as visualization of the tracer in both the common bile duct and the duodenum but not in the gallbladder. Because the gallbladder fills if the cystic duct is patent, the test cannot determine the presence of gallstones. The sensitivity of cholescintigraphy for acute cholecystitis is 97%, and the specificity is 90% (14) (see Table 14-1). Even in the absence of acute cholecystitis, some gallbladders do not "fill" after 1 hour. Although many advocate the use of prolonged (i.e., up to 4–24 hours) imaging to improve specificity, a recent meta-analysis (14) suggests that delayed imaging does not improve the diagnostic characteristics of the test. Common causes of false-positive test results (nonvisualization) include ethanol abuse, prolonged fasting, total parenteral nutrition, pancreatitis, and hepatitis. Cholescintigraphy is essentially risk-free with very slight radiation.

Several trials have examined the incremental value of the intravenous administration of morphine sulfate (0.04–0.10 mg/kg) if the gallbladder has not been visualized by cholescintigraphy at 1 hour (5–7,17,18). Morphine sulfate contracts the sphincter of Oddi, with a subsequent increase in biliary duct pressures. This increased pressure augments the flow into the cystic duct if the duct is patent. Imaging is then usually performed for an additional hour. In one study that directly compared delayed imaging with morphine augmentation, the sensitivity and specificity of morphine sulfate augmentation (77% and 98%) was similar to that of delayed imaging (77% and 92%) (6).

Endoscopic Retrograde Cholangiopancreatography

Endoscopic retrograde cholangiopancreatography (ERCP) is usually reserved for those patients in whom common bile duct stones are suspected who present with elevated total bilirubin and elevated alkaline phosphatase levels, increased diameter of common bile duct on ultrasonography, or concurrent evidence of acute pancreatitis (10). The main complications of ERCP include pancreatitis, cholangitis, and aspiration pneumonia. The sensitivity of ERCP in detecting common bile duct stones is approximately 90%, and the specificity is almost 100% (12,19). The sensitivity is not perfect, because small stones may be missed. In cases in which a stone is visualized and within reach, stone removal is a potential added benefit of ERCP. The procedure may not be technically feasible in approximately 5% of patients.

Magnetic Resonance Imaging

Magnetic resonance imaging (MRI) has gained some popularity in the diagnosis of common bile duct stones. Multiplanar views can be obtained without radiation exposure or use of contrast material; however, the procedure requires a special multicoil device that is not always available. The image quality is distorted by surgical clips and air in the biliary tree. Early studies, which have not always included "blinded" interpretation, show a sensitivity of 81% to 95% and a specificity of 85% to 98% (20,21). Additional studies are needed to define the role of MRI in the evaluation of these patients.

Endoscopic Ultrasonography

Endoscopic ultrasonography is an emerging technique that may be useful in the diagnosis of common bile duct stones. With a transducer attached to an endoscope, RTUS can be performed. Initial studies reported sensitivity and specificity to be more than 90% (16,22). Using sphincterotomy and common bile duct exploration as a gold standard, one well-designed study showed this procedure to have a sensitivity of 93% and a specificity of 97% (12). However, the test is expensive and operator dependent, and in some settings, general anesthesia is used.

Computed Tomography

Computed tomography (CT) is less sensitive (79%) than ultrasonography in detecting cholelithiasis but is equally specific (99%) (14). For choledocholithiasis, CT has a sensitivity of 75% and a specificity of 94% (16). Results with newer helical CT scans show an increased sensitivity of approximately 88% and a specificity of 97% (23), but these are not available at most centers.

Other Procedures

Only 10% to 20% of all gallstones are calcified and thus apparent on plain abdominal radiographs. A recent retrospective study (24) showed no differences in the appearance of radiographs in patients with symptomatic gallbladder disease and those without. Intravenous cholangiography is insensitive, potentially harmful, and not helpful in diagnosing cholelithiasis (25).

DIAGNOSTIC STRATEGIES

Cholelithiasis

For the detection of gallstones, RTUS is the procedure of choice. The operating characteristics (see Table 14-1) are superior to those of oral cholecystography. This procedure is fast and convenient, requires minimal preparation time, and is free of side effects. Imaging is adequate in more than 95% of patients. Furthermore, RTUS can provide information about nongallbladder causes of abdominal pain. Other imaging studies, such as oral cholecystography, may be used when ultrasonography is technically difficult or when the post-test probability remains high after ultrasonography yields negative findings. (Comparative data for the two tests over a range of pretest probabilities are displayed in Table 14-2.)

Neither of these tests addresses the question of whether stones, when present, are actually the cause of the patient's symptoms.

Acute Cholecystitis

The single best diagnostic test for acute cholecystitis is cholescintigraphy (13,14). However, in actual practice, when a patient presents with right upper quadrant pain and fever, the physician is often considering many possible diagnoses in addition to cholecystitis. Compared with cholescintigraphy for the diagnosis of cholecystitis, RTUS has operating characteristics that are not quite as good, but RTUS will also provide a diagnosis in an additional 20% of patients with typical symptoms who do not have acute cholecystitis (26).

At moderate-to-high pretest probability, the post-test probability of acute cholecystitis when the results of RTUS are positive is similar to that when the results of cholescintigraphy are positive (Table 14-2). Conversely, in patients with a low-to-moderate pretest probability, negative RTUS results have nearly the same predictive value as negative cholescintigraphy results. Therefore, patients who present with right upper quadrant pain and fever should initially have imaging with RTUS. Cholescintigraphy can be used when the RTUS is not diagnostic or when the RTUS is negative in the setting of a high pretest probability.

This approach has been studied in outpatients presenting with acute right upper quadrant pain. However, in hospitalized patients, especially those in whom acute acalculous cholecystitis is suspected, both RTUS and cholescintigraphy may be less accurate.

Table 14-2. Post-test Probabilities for Diagnostic Tests in the Diagnosis of Cholelithiasis, Acute Calculous Cholecystitis, and Choledocholithiasis

Diagnostic Test	Pretest Probability					
	20%		50%		80%	
	Positive Result	Negative Result	Positive Result	Negative Result	Positive Result	Negative Result
	←			%		→
For cholelithiasis						
RTUS	88	3	97	10	99	31
OCG	83	6	95	21	99	51
CT	95	5	99	17	100	46
For acute cholecystitis						
RTUS	52	3	81	10	95	31
Cholescintigraphy	71	1	91	3	97	11
For choledocholithiasis						
ERCP	96	2	99	9	100	29
MRI	73	3	92	12	98	34
EUS	89	2	97	7	99	22
CT	76	6	93	21	98	52
Helical CT	88	3	97	11	99	32

RTUS = real-time ultrasonography; CT = computed tomography; MRI = magnetic resonance imaging; OCG = oral cholecystography; ERCP = endoscopic retrograde cholangiopancreatography; EUS = endoscopic ultrasonography.

Choledocholithiasis

Endoscopic retrograde cholangiopancreatography is the test of choice when suspicion of choledocholithiasis is high in patients who are acutely ill. The sensitivity and specificity of this procedure are superior to any other easily available test (see Table 14-1), and ERCP also offers the benefit of potential stone removal.

The strategy for excluding choledocholithiasis in patients in whom cholecystectomy is planned depends on clinical suspicion. Before the advent of laparoscopic surgery, in patients who underwent open cholecystectomy the surgeon would perform common bile duct (CBD) exploration and/or these patients would undergo an interoperative cholangiography to rule out choledocholithiasis. However, with the use of laparoscopic cholecystectomy, alternative diagnostic approaches are needed to identify the 10% of patients with cholelithiasis who have coincident choledocholithiasis. Clinical information obtained during the patient's evaluation is useful. One study found that a CBD diameter of less than 5 mm as found on RTUS, normal liver enzymes, and no history of acute cholecystitis, jaundice, or pancreatitis confidently ruled out common bile duct stones (27). Another study found common duct stones to be more prevalent in patients older than 55 years who presented with elevated bilirubin levels and positive RTUS findings (e.g., a dilated CBD or a stone or both) (11).

Patients in whom the probability of choledocholithiasis is low based on clinical information or studies or both done during the evaluation for cholelithiasis or acute cholecystitis probably do not require additional preoperative studies for CBD stones. When the preoperative probability of a CBD stone is moderate to high and a laparoscopic approach is planned, the patient should be referred for a preoperative ERCP and stone extraction if the test is positive. If stone extraction is unsuccessful, either open cholecystectomy or laparoscopic stone removal should be performed (27). Alternatively, if a stone is detected at the time of surgery and cannot be removed laparoscopically, the patient could be referred for postoperative ERCP.

Endoscopic ultrasonography, MRI, and helical CT are emerging as studies that have operating characteristics similar to those of ERCP (12,20,21). These approaches have less morbidity and mortality than ERCP; however, they are not available at all centers. Furthermore, these diagnostic studies offer no potential therapeutic benefit. As additional experience is gained, these studies may be used more, particularly in patients in whom the pretest probability of choledocholithiasis is intermediate.

CLINICAL PROBLEMS

Clinical Problem 1

A middle-aged woman has recurrent pain in the right upper quadrant of the abdomen.

Testing Strategy and Rationale

Real-time ultrasonography of the abdomen should be done. The operating characteristics of RTUS are better than than those of OCG, with a higher percentage of adequate studies, fewer side effects, and easier preparation for the patient.

Clinical Example

A 43-year-old, moderately overweight woman reports three to four episodes of relatively severe pain below the right rib cage. The pain is steady in nature, lasts for up to 1 hour, and recurs over a period of months. She does not associate the discomfort with meals. Physical examination yields no abnormal findings. The clinician estimates that the likelihood that the discomfort is caused by gallstones to be approximately 40%. If the results of the RTUS are positive, the post-test probability of stones is approximately 95%, whereas if the results are negative, the post-test probability is about 7%. Oral cholecystography would be useful only if the RTUS were technically inadequate.

Clinical Problem 2
A middle-aged woman with a history suggestive of biliary colic presents with acute right upper quadrant abdominal pain and fever.

Testing Strategy and Rationale
First, RTUS of the abdomen should be performed. The test has reasonable operating characteristics for acute cholecystitis and provides a diagnosis in as many as 20% of patients who have right upper quadrant pain and fever from another cause. If RTUS provides a diagnosis, further testing does not need to be done. If RTUS is nondiagnostic and the suspicion of acute cholecystitis remains high, then cholescintigraphy should be performed.

Clinical Example
A 48-year-old woman reports having symptoms of moderate-to-severe right upper quadrant pain for the past 6 hours, which began soon after she ate a hamburger. She has had similar episodes of pain after meals in the past. However, no episodes lasted more than an hour, and the pain was not as intense. She has mild abdominal discomfort and has a temperature of 38.3 °C. Moderate tenderness just to the right of the epigastrium is noted, as is a positive Murphy sign. The clinical likelihood of acute cholecystitis is at least 30%. An RTUS study confirms the presence of gallstones and detects no other process to explain the patient's symptoms. In addition, sonographic Murphy sign is positive, and fluid around the gallbladder is seen. These findings on RTUS, when combined with the clinical presentation, raise the probability of acute cholecystitis to at least 65% to 70%. Under most circumstances, this is a sufficient level of probability to guide management. Further testing with cholescintigraphy is indicated only if an alternative diagnosis that would significantly change management is under consideration.

REFERENCES

1. **Johnston DE, Kaplan MM.** Pathogenesis and treatment of gallstones. N Engl J Med. 1993;328:412-21.
2. **Jensen KH, Jorgensen T.** Incidence of gallstones in a Danish population. Gastroenterology. 1991;100:790-4.

3. **Diehl AK, Sugarek NJ, Todd KH.** Clinical evaluation for gallstone disease: usefulness of symptoms and signs in diagnosis. Am J Med. 1990;89:29-33.

4. **Johnson H, Cooper B.** The value of HIDA scans in the initial evaluation of patients for cholecystitis. J Natl Med Assoc. 1995;87:27-32.

5. **Flancbaum L, Choban PS, Sinha R, et al.** Morphine cholescintigraphy in the evaluation of hospitalized patients with suspected acute cholecystitis. Ann Surg. 1994;220:25-31.

6. **Kim CK, Tse KKM, Juweid M, et al.** Cholescintigraphy in the diagnosis of acute cholecystitis: morphine augmentation is superior to delayed imaging. J Nucl Med. 1993;34:1866-70.

7. **Fink-Bennett D, Balon H, Robbins T, Tsai D.** Morphine-augmented cholescintigraphy: its efficacy in detecting acute cholecystitis. J Nucl Med. 1991;32:1231-3.

8. **Flancbaum L, Alden SM.** Morphine cholescintigraphy. Surg Gynecol Obstet. 1990;171:227-32.

9. **Koo KP, Traverso LW.** Do preoperative indicators predict the presence of common bile duct stones during laparoscopic cholecystectomy? Am J Surg. 1996;171:495-9.

10. **Cisek PL, Greaney GC.** The role of endoscopic retrograde cholangiopancreatography with laparoscopic cholecystectomy in the management of choledocholithiasis. Am Surg. 1994;60:772-6.

11. **Barkun AN, Barkun JS, Fried GM, et al.** Useful predictors of bile duct stones in patients undergoing laparoscopic cholecystectomy. Ann Surg. 1994;220:32-9.

12. **Prat F, Amouyal G, Amouyal P.** Prospective controlled study of endoscopic ultrasonography and endoscopic retrograde cholangiography in patients with suspected common-bile duct lithiasis. Lancet. 1996;347:75-9.

13. **Marton KI, Doubilet P.** How to image the gallbladder in suspected cholecystitis. Ann Intern Med. 1988;109:722-9.

14. **Shea JA, Berlin JA, Escarce JJ, et al.** Revised estimates of diagnostic sensitivity and specificity in suspected biliary tract disease. Arch Intern Med. 1994;154:2573-81.

15. **Raghavendra BN, Feiner HD, Subramanyan BR, et al.** Acute cholecystitis: sonographic-pathologic analysis. AJR Am J Roentgenol. 1981;137:327-32.

16. **Amouyal P, Amouyal G, Levy P, et al.** Diagnosis of choledocholithiasis by endoscopic ultrasonography. Gastroenterology. 1994;106:1062-7.

17. **Flancbaum L, Choban PS.** Use of morphine cholescintigraphy in the diagnosis of acute cholecystitis in critically ill patients. Intens Care Med. 1995;21:120-4.

18. **Kistler AM, Ziessman HA, Gooch D, Bitterman P.** Morphine-augmented cholescintigraphy in acute cholecystitis: a satisfactory alternative to delayed imaging. Clin Nucl Med. 1991;16:404-6.

19. **Frey CF, Burbige EJ, Meinke WB, et al.** Endoscopic retrograde cholangiopancreatography. Am J Surg. 1982;144:109-14.

20. **Chan Y, Chan ACW, Lam WWM, et al.** Choledocholithiasis: comparison of MR cholangiography and endoscopic retrograde cholangiography. Radiology. 1996;200:85-9.

21. **Guibaud L, Bret PM, Remhold C, et al.** Bile duct obstruction and choledocholithiasis: diagnosis with MR cholangiography. Radiology. 1995;197: 109-15.

22. **Palazzo L, Girollet P, Salmeron M, et al.** Value of endoscopic ultrasonography in the diagnosis of common bile duct stones: comparison with surgical exploration and ERCP. Gastrointest Endosc. 1995;42:225-31.

23. **Neitlich JD, Topazian M, Smith RC, et al.** Detection of choledocholithiasis: comparison of unenhanced helical CT and endoscopic retrograde cholangiopancreatography. Radiology. 1997;203:753-7.

24. **Rothrock SG, Goorhuis H, Howard RM.** Efficacy of plain abdominal radiography in patients with biliary tract disease. J Emerg Med. 1990;8:271-5.

25. **Goodman MW, Ansel HJ, Vennes JA, et al.** Is intravenous cholangiography still useful. Gastroenterology. 1980;79:642-5.

26. **Laing FC, Federle MP, Jeffrey RB, Brown TW.** Ultrasonic evaluation of patients with acute right upper quadrant pain. Radiology. 1981;140:449-55.

27. **Voyles CR, Sanders DL, Hogan R.** Common bile duct exploration in the era of laparoscopic cholecystectomy: 1050 cases later. Ann Surg. 1994;219:744-52.

Obstructive Jaundice   **15**

James P. Corsetti, MD, PhD, and Dean A. Arvan, MD

KEY POINTS

Pretest Probabilities

- In adults, approximately 30% of patients presenting with jaundice as the primary symptom have extrahepatic biliary obstruction.

- Obstructive jaundice can be differentiated from hepatocellular jaundice in approximately 85% of cases by using clinical information and first-line biochemical tests.

Diagnostic Strategies

- Confirmation of the diagnosis of obstructive jaundice and determination of its site or cause require the use of imaging procedures such as ultrasonography (US), computed tomography (CT), endoscopic retrograde cholangiopancreatography (ERCP), or percutaneous transhepatic cholangiography (PTC).

- Ultrasonography is usually chosen as the initial imaging test because it is noninvasive, relatively inexpensive, and commonly available, even though CT is slightly more sensitive and specific than US in identifying extrahepatic obstruction.

- Endoscopic retrograde cholangiopancreatography and PTC are more sensitive and specific than US or CT and have greater precision in locating the site and cause of obstruction but are more costly and are associated with more complications.

- Either US or CT is the procedure of choice for excluding obstructive jaundice when the pretest probability of disease is low. At high pretest probability of obstruction, or when the patient has had previous biliary surgery, proceeding directly to ERCP or PTC should be considered.

BACKGROUND

Obstructive jaundice results from obstruction to the flow of bile from the liver to the duodenum. The underlying cause may be an intrahepatic process, such as primary biliary cirrhosis or drug-induced cholestasis, or an extrahepatic obstructive process. Among adults presenting with jaundice as the primary symptom, the various causes of extrahepatic obstructive jaundice, which is the focus of this chapter, accounts for approximately one third of cases (1–7). The most common causes are tumors of the extrahepatic biliary tract, pancreas, and ampulla of Vater; tumors metastatic to the biliary tract; choledocholithiasis; pancreatitis; cholangitis; and iatrogenic strictures of the biliary tract.

Differentiation between extrahepatic and intrahepatic causes of obstructive jaundice is clinically important because the therapeutic modes are quite different; operative drainage and alleviation of the obstruction constitute the primary treatment for extrahepatic biliary obstruction, whereas nonoperative medical management is the treatment "rule" for intrahepatic processes.

ESTIMATING PRETEST PROBABILITY

Overall, in approximately 30% of adult patients presenting with jaundice as the first disease manifestation, the cause is an extrahepatic obstruction (1–4). The remaining patients may have obstructive jaundice related to an intrahepatic cause; hepatocellular (parenchymal) disease, such as viral hepatitis or cirrhosis; other liver diseases such as Gilbert syndrome; or hemolysis. Age is an important variable in further refining pretest probability, because patients with an extrahepatic obstructive process tend, on average, to be older than those with parenchymal liver disease (2,5). The presence of abdominal pain increases the pretest probability of obstruction from approximately 30% to 50%. The finding of a palpable gallbladder is virtually pathognomonic of extrahepatic obstruction, but it lacks sensitivity, as is demonstrated by the fact that it is found in no more than 30% of these cases (Table 15-1) (2). Symptoms considered by many as useful in differentiating obstruction from parenchymal liver disease, such as nausea, pruritus, distaste for tobacco, or duration of jaundice, give no clear aid in distinguishing between the two diseases (2,5,7,8). On the other hand, clinical history and signs commonly found in patients with parenchymal liver disease, such as alcoholism, poor nutrition, spider angiomata, palmar erythema, and ascites, are highly specific for parenchymal disease. When present, these factors markedly reduce the probability of extrahepatic obstruction.

Table 15-1. Operating Characteristics of Clinical Findings and Biochemical Tests in the Diagnosis of Obstructive Jaundice

Diagnostic Finding	Sensitivity	Specificity	Likelihood Ratio	
			Positive Result	Negative Result
	←——— % ———→			
History of abdominal pain	70	68	2.2	0.44
Relief of pain by flexion	20	98	10	0.82
Palpable gallbladder*	30	100	∞	0.70
Direct-reading bilirubin >50%	95	32	1.4	0.16
Alkaline phosphatase measurement >three times upper limit of normal	85	65	2.4	0.23

*Assumes the ability to differentiate accurately a distended gallbladder from other right upper quadrant masses.

DIAGNOSTIC TESTS

Biochemical Tests

Despite some limitations, obstructive and parenchymal jaundice can be differentiated in about 85% of patients, using a combination of clinical and biochemical findings (5–12).

Bilirubin

The fractionation of bilirubin into conjugated (direct-reacting) and unconjugated (indirect-reacting) levels is the classic method used in attempts to differentiate parenchymal from obstructive jaundice. Elevation of direct-reacting bilirubin levels to greater than 50% of total bilirubin is believed to indicate obstructive disease, whereas lower fractions are thought to be more indicative of parenchymal jaundice. The overlap is considerable, however, and direct bilirubin fractions in the 40% to 60% range may be seen in either entity (13). Thus, bilirubin fractionation has little or no value in this differential diagnosis (6,7,13,14); however, it can be helpful in identifying jaundice caused by hemolysis or by certain liver diseases such as Gilbert syndrome.

Alkaline Phosphatase and Related Enzymes

Alkaline phosphatase has long been touted as a good test for discriminating between parenchymal and obstructive jaundice. With complete obstruction of the biliary tract, alkaline phosphatase levels are usually elevated to three to eight times the upper limit of normal and at times may be even higher. Incomplete or intermittent obstruction is often accompanied by more modest elevations. A cutoff point of three times the upper limit of normal results in good sensitivity for obstruction (85%), but specificity is lower (60%–70%) because elevations in this range are common in patients with parenchymal liver disease, particularly those with prominent intrahepatic cholestasis (2,14–16) (see Table 15-1). Thus, this test is somewhat more helpful in determining a reduced probability of obstructive disease when the alkaline phosphatase levels are normal or only moderately elevated than it is in confirming obstruction when they are elevated. Alkaline phosphatase is of no help in the differential diagnosis of intrahepatic cholestasis compared with extrahepatic cholestasis (9).

The serum gamma glutamyl-transpeptidase (GGT) level changes in liver diseases in ways similar to the alkaline phosphatase level, but unlike the alkaline phosphatase level, does not change with bone disease. Thus the GGT is helpful, as is fractionation of alkaline phosphatase into bone and liver fractions, in confirming that an alkaline phosphatase elevation is caused by liver disease.

Aminotransferases (Transaminases)
Serum aspartate aminotransferase (AST) and alanine aminotransferase (ALT) levels tend, on average, toward modest elevation in obstructive jaundice (<200 U/L) (7,9,14,16). Higher levels (>200 U/L) are more typical of patients with parenchymal liver disease (see Chapter 16). However, overlap exists because AST levels may be elevated only slightly in parenchymal disease, and a few patients with obstructive jaundice show very high AST values (7,10,17). Unless markedly elevated or near normal, transaminase levels are not very discriminating.

Imaging Tests
Ultrasonography, computed tomography (CT), endoscopic retrograde cholangiopancreatography (ERCP), and percutaneous transhepatic cholangiography (PTC) have well-established roles in diagnostic confirmation of obstructive jaundice, in localizing the site of obstruction, or in identifying the cause of obstruction (5–8,10,18–20). For diagnostic purposes, a positive result for each test is a finding of dilated extrahepatic bile ducts or the demonstration of a specific obstructive lesion. The gold standard against which each test's efficacy is measured is confirmation of obstruction by biopsy, surgery, autopsy, or extended clinical follow-up. Radionuclide scintigraphy plays only a limited role in the diagnosis of obstructive jaundice (5,6,8). As noted below, the use of magnetic resonance imaging in the evaluation of patients with obstructive jaundice is being studied.

Ultrasonography
Ultrasonography (US) is noninvasive and the least costly imaging technique available for the evaluation of obstructive jaundice. The sensitiv-

ity and specificity of US in detecting dilated biliary ducts are estimated to be 85% (range, 55%–91%) and 90% (range, 81%–97%), respectively, as reviewed by Lucas and Chuttani (7) (Table 15-2). Because the diagnosis of obstruction using US relies on finding dilated ducts, conditions in which the ducts are not dilated may give rise to false-negative results. Such conditions include sclerosing cholangitis and stones that partially obstruct the common bile duct. The most common cause of false-negative results is the presence of stones in the distal common bile duct (7), possibly because ductal dilatation has not yet occurred (21). Ultrasonography is further limited by its relative ineffectiveness in identifying the site or cause of obstruction (7). This is particularly true in patients who have had previous biliary tract surgery (cholecystectomy) (22) and in patients with choledocholithiasis because visualization of the distal common bile duct is often obscured by bowel gas. To minimize the effect of bowel gas, US should be done with the patient in the fasting state.

Computed Tomography

Computed tomography also relies on the identification of dilated ducts to diagnose obstruction. It is both more sensitive (90%; range, 63%–93%) and specific (95%; range 93%–100%) than US in detecting extrahepatic biliary obstruction (7). The ability to determine the site or cause of obstruction, including choledocholithiasis, is also greater with CT scanning than with US (6–8). Radiation exposure and increased expense are disadvantages of CT imaging. Newer CT techniques may prove to have improved operating characteristics.

Table 15-2. Operating Characteristics of Imaging Tests in the Diagnosis of Obstructive Jaundice

Diagnostic Test	Definition of Positive Result	Sensitivity	Specificity	Likelihood Ratio Positive Result	Negative Result
		← % →			
Ultrasonography	Detection of dilated bile ducts	85	90	8.5	0.17
Computed tomography	Detection of dilated bile ducts	90	95	18	0.11
Endoscopic retrograde cholangio-pancreatography	Detection of dilated bile ducts or a stenosis of bile or pancreatic ducts	95	99	95	0.05
Transhepatic cholangiography	Detection of dilated bile ducts	95	99	95	0.05

Endoscopic Retrograde Cholangiopancreatography

Endoscopic retrograde cholangiopancreatography is performed by endoscopic insertion of radio-opaque contrast into the ampulla of Vater coupled with standard radiographic visualization of the ducts. It requires a skilled endoscopist. The typical success rate ranges from 90% to 95% (7). Endoscopic retrograde cholangiopancreatography has a complication rate of approximately 2%, with the major complications being pancreatitis and cholangitis. The overall sensitivity and specificity of ERCP are 95% (range, 75%–99%) and 99% (range, 90%–100%), respectively (20,23). The ability of ERCP to give specific diagnostic information concerning site and cause is approximately 85% (23) and is better than US or CT (7). Advantages of ERCP are the ability to provide direct inspection of the stomach, duodenum, and ampulla of Vater and that it enables the clinican to obtain biopsy specimens and to perform various therapeutic maneuvers. Disadvantages include invasiveness, need for sedation, and relative expense (7).

Transhepatic Cholangiography

Percutaneous transhepatic cholangiography is done by inserting a fine needle through the liver into a biliary radicle, injecting radio-opaque material, and visualizing the biliary tract by standard radiography. The procedure also allows therapeutic intervention through temporary biliary drainage if an obstruction is found. The success rate, the ability to complete the procedure with interpretable results, which is heavily dependent on the presence of dilated ducts (7), is approximately 90% to 95%, slightly lower than that for noninvasive procedures (20,24). The sensitivity and specificity of the completed procedure are very high (95%; range, 88%–99%; and 99%; range, 90%–100%), respectively (20,25). The ability of PTC to determine the site and cause of obstruction is significantly higher than that of US and CT (24,26,27). As an invasive procedure, PTC has risks. Major complications occur in 3% to 5% of patients and include pain, sepsis (1%–2%), bile leakage (1%–2%), intraperitoneal hemorrhage (0%–0.5%), cholangitis, and occasionally death (0.2%) (20,28). The patient must be considered a good candidate for surgery because subsequent surgery may be required.

Recent Developments

Endoscopic ultrasonography uses an endoscope with a transducer. The technique has been shown to be potentially useful for detecting common bile duct stones (29) and small masses (30) and may be useful for detecting and staging biliary system–associated neoplasms (6,8). However, the technique has limitations, and its role in this area awaits further work (31).

Magnetic resonance imaging has been shown to be at least as good as US and CT in detecting dilated bile ducts (7). Development of fast MRI pulse sequences with breath-hold imaging along with the use of contrast agents shows potential for its use in the detection of hilar cholangiocarcinomas (32). In addition, newer techniques allow three-dimensional imaging of fluid in bile ducts (magnetic resonance cholangiopancreatography), enabling detection of dilated bile ducts on a par with ERCP (7,33,34). The specific role of MRI in evaluating patients with possible obstructive jaundice will be clarified as larger case series are reported.

DIAGNOSTIC STRATEGIES

The diagnostic approach to adults presenting with jaundice is usually straightforward. The physician must first determine if the jaundice is caused by obstruction, liver disease, or other causes, such as hemolysis. The history and physical examination help modify pretest probability; in particular, right upper quadrant pain is seen more commonly in patients with jaundice caused by bile duct (extrahepatic) obstruction. The relative increases in alkaline phosphatase and AST levels are also of considerable help in differentiating jaundice caused by extrahepatic obstruction from that caused by parenchymal liver disease.

Most patients then require imaging tests to confirm the diagnosis and investigate the site and cause of the obstruction. Although US does not have the best operating characteristics, it is the most widely used initial technique because it is noninvasive, is relatively inexpensive, does not use ionizing radiation, and is commonly available (5–8). Computed tomography is used when the results of US are normal but there is still a strong clinical suspicion of obstruction, or when the results of US are unsatisfactory. Endoscopic retrograde cholangiopancreatography or PTC or both are used as follow-up tests when US or CT is not definitive or does not determine the site or cause of obstruction (6,8). They can also be used as therapeutic modalities. When the pretest probability of obstruction is high or when the patient has had previous biliary surgery such as cholecystectomy, slightly higher overall precision is obtained with the initial use of ERCP or PTC (Table 15-3). This precision is, in part, owing to the lower sensitivity of US (9,19) and to the ability of ERCP and PTC to provide more information about the site and cause of the obstruction (5–8).

Distinguishing intrahepatic cholestasis from extrahepatic biliary obstruction is a problem that cannot be solved by biochemical tests alone. When medical history, physical examination, and laboratory test findings lead the clinician to have a high suspicion of intrahepatic cholestasis and thus cause the pretest probability of extrahepatic obstruction to be low, imaging studies may still be needed. In such cases, normal findings (i.e., no dilated biliary ducts) would provide further evidence against the diagnosis of extrahepatic obstruction. Confirmation of intrahepatic cholestasis may require liver biopsy.

Table 15-3. Post-test Probabilities for Tests and Procedures in the Diagnosis of Obstructive Jaundice

Diagnostic Test	Pretest Probability					
	20%		50%		80%	
	Positive Result	Negative Result	Positive Result	Negative Result	Positive Result	Negative Result
	←———————————————— % ————————————————→					
Alkaline phosphatase (>3 times normal)	38	5	71	19	91	48
Ultrasonography (dilated ducts)	68	4	89	15	97	40
Computed tomography (dilated ducts)	82	3	95	10	99	31
Endoscopic retrograde cholangiopancrea-tography (dilated, narrowed or stenotic ducts)	96	1	99	5	>99	17
Pancreatic transhepatic cholangiography (dilated ducts)	96	1	99	5	>99	17

CLINICAL PROBLEM

An elderly patient presents with jaundice and abdominal pain.

Testing Strategy and Rationale

Total bilirubin, AST, and alkaline phosphatase levels should be measured. Depending on the results, the next testing should be US or CT. In an older patient who does not consume alcohol, jaundice caused by parenchymal disease is less common than that caused by extrahepatic obstruction. The history and physical examination should focus on signs or symptoms of hepatocellular disease and on any abnormalities in the right upper quadrant of the abdomen. Measurement of AST and alkaline phosphatase levels is sufficient for the initial laboratory evaluation. In patients with jaundice, measuring ALT and GGT levels is of little additional value in cases in which the hepatic origin of AST or alkaline phosphatase elevation is not in doubt, because changes in these enzymes generally parallel the AST and alkaline phosphatase levels, respectively. The higher the alkaline phosphatase level, the greater is the probability of

Continued

obstructive jaundice. The reverse is true for AST. If the probability of extrahepatic obstruction remains high, then imaging tests should be performed to confirm the diagnosis and to help determine its cause.

Clinical Example

A 65-year-old man presents with a 3-week history of vague abdominal pain and increasing yellowness of the skin and eyes. His urine has been somewhat darker than usual. He has no history of alcohol use or of exposure to hepatitis. He is taking no medications. Other than the presence of icterus and mild abdominal discomfort, physical examination yields no abnormal findings. Based on these findings, the probability of obstructive jaundice is estimated to be 50%.

Initial laboratory tests show a total bilirubin level of 8.0 mg/dL; AST level of 110 U/L (normal, 10–36 U/L); and alkaline phosphatase level of 700 U/L (normal, 53–120 U/L). Based on the test characteristics shown in Table 15-1, the revised probability of obstruction is approximately 70%. Ultrasonography of the right upper quadrant is then done. If the results are positive, the revised likelihood of obstructive jaundice would be approximately 95%. If negative, the post-test probability would still be relatively high (about 30%). If CT had been ordered first, the post-test probability with a positive test result would be slightly higher than with US, and the probability with a negative test result would be lower (approximately 20%). A negative US result coupled with a negative CT result would reduce the probability of extrahepatic obstruction from approximately 70% to approximately 5%.

REFERENCES

1. **Knill-Jones RP, Stern RB, Girmes DH, et al.** Use of sequential Bayesian model in diagnosis of jaundice by computer. Br Med J. 1973;1:530-4.

2. **Schenker S, Balint J, Schiff L.** Differential diagnosis of jaundice: report of a prospective study of 61 proved cases. Am J Dig Dis. 1962;7:449-63.

3. **Malchow-Moller A, Matzen P, Bjerregaard B, et al.** Causes and characteristics of 500 consecutive cases of jaundice. Scand J Gastroent 1981;16:1-6.

4. **Malchow-Moller A, Bjerregaard B, Hilden J.** Computer-assisted diagnosis in gastroenterology. Scand J Gastroenterol Suppl. 1996;216:225-33.

5. **McKnight JT, Jones JE.** Jaundice. Am Fam Phys. 1992;45:1139-48.

6. **Banerjee B.** Extrahepatic biliary tract obstruction. Postgrad Med. 1993;93:113-8.

7. **Lucas WB, Chuttani R.** Pathophysiology and current concepts in the diagnosis of obstructive jaundice. Gastroenterologist. 1995;3:105-18.

8. **Hulse PA, Nicholson DA.** Investigation of biliary obstruction. Br J Hosp Med. 1994;52:103-7.

9. **O'Connor KW, Snodgrass PJ, Swonder JE, et al.** A blinded prospective study comparing four current non-invasive approaches in the differential diagnosis of medical versus surgical jaundice. Gastroenterology. 1983;84:1498-504.

10. **Ginsberg AL.** Very high levels of SGOT and LDH in patients with extrahepatic biliary tract obstruction. Dig Dis. 1970;15:803-7.

11. **Siegel JH, Yatto RP.** Approach to cholestasis. Arch Intern Med. 1982;142:1877-9.

12. **Thomas MJ, Pellegrini CA, Way LW.** Usefulness of diagnostic tests for biliary obstruction. Am J Surg. 1982;144:102-8.

13. **Fevery J, Claes J, Heirwegh CK, DeGroote J.** Hyperbilirubinemia: significance of the ratio between direct-reacting and total bilirubin. Clin Chim Acta. 1967;17:73-9.

14. **Rosalki SB, Dooley JS.** Liver function profiles and their interpretation. Br J Hosp Med. 1994;51:181-6.

15. **Gutman AB, Olson KB, Gutman EB, Flood CA.** Effect of disease of the liver and biliary tract upon the phosphatase activity of the serum. J Clin Invest. 1940;19:129-52.

16. **Neuschwander-Tetri BA.** Common blood tests for liver disease. Postgrad Med. 1995;98:49-63.

17. **Gregory PB, Cooney DP.** Misleading SGOT values in obstructive jaundice due to pancreatic carcinoma. Dig Dis. 1976;21:509-11.

18. **Hadid A.** Distinction between obstructive and non-obstructive jaundice by sonography. Clin Radiol. 1980;31:181-7.

19. **Fischer MG, Gelb AM, Weingarter LA.** Cholestatic jaundice in adults. JAMA. 1981;245:1945-8.

20. **Richter JM, Silverstein MD, Schapiro R.** Suspected obstructive jaundice: a decision analysis of diagnostic strategies. Ann Intern Med. 1983;99:46-51.

21. **Pasanen PA, Partanen K, Pikkarainen P, et al.** Diagnostic accuracy of US, CT, and ERCP in the detection of obstructive jaundice. Scand J Gastroenterol. 1991;26:1157-64.

22. **Gross BA, Harter LP, Gore RM, et al.** Ultrasonic evaluation of common bile duct stones: prospective comparison with endoscopic retrograde cholangiopancreatography. Radiology. 1983;146:471-4.

23. **Gregg JA, McDonald DG.** Endoscopic retrograde cholangiopancreatography and gray-scale abdominal ultrasound in the diagnosis of jaundice. Am J Surg. 1979;137:611-5.

24. **Gold RP, Casarella WJ, Stern G, Seaman WB.** Transhepatic cholangiography: the radiologic method of choice in suspected obstructive jaundice. Radiology. 1979;133:39-44.

25. **Raval B, Lamki N, Bandali K.** Radiologic investigation of suspected extrahepatic biliary obstruction. Can Med Assoc J. 1982;127:1191-4.

26. **Vas W, Salem S.** Accuracy of sonography and transhepatic cholangiography in obstructive jaundice. J de L'Assoc Can des Rad. 1981;32:111-3.

27. **Wild SR, Cruikshank JG, Fraser GM, et al.** Gray-scale ultrasonography and percutaneous transhepatic cholangiography in biliary tract disease. Br Med J. 1980;281:1524-6.

28. **Harbin WP, Mueller PR, Ferrucci JT.** Transhepatic cholangiography: complications and use patterns of the fine-needle technique. Radiology. 1980;135:15-22.

29. **Palazzo L, Girollet PP, Salmeron M, et al.** Value of endoscopic ultrasonography in the diagnosis of common bile duct stones: comparison with surgical exploration and ERCP. Gastrointest Endosc. 1995;42:225-31.

30. **Snady H, Cooperman A, Siegel J.** Endoscopic ultrasonography compared with computed tomography with ERCP in patients with obstructive jaundice or small peripancreatic mass. Gastrointest Endosc. 1992;38:27-34.

31. **Mehta SN, Barkun A.** The role of endoscopic ultrasonography in biliary tract disease: obstructive jaundice. Gastrointest Endosc. 1996;43:534-5.

32. **Low RN, Sigeti JS, Francis IR, et al.** Evaluation of malignant biliary obstruction: efficacy of fast multiplanar spoiled gradient-recalled MR imaging vs. spin-echo MR imaging, CT, and cholangiography. Am J Roentgenol. 1994;162:315-23.

33. **Meakem TJ III, Schnall MD.** Magnetic resonance cholangiography. Gastroenterol Clin North Am. 1995;24:221-38.

34. **Lee MG, Lee HJ, Kim MH, et al.** Extrahepatic biliary diseases: 3D MR cholangiopancreatography compared with endoscopic retrograde cholangiopancreatography. Radiology. 1997;202:663-9.

Acute Viral Hepatitis

16

James P. Corsetti, MD, PhD, and Dean A. Arvan, MD

KEY POINTS

Pretest Probabilities

- More than 90% of patients with acute viral hepatitis or other forms of hepatocellular necrosis report anorexia, malaise, and nausea. More than 90% of these patients have hepatomegaly or hepatic tenderness or both.
- In the United States, more than 95% of cases of acute viral hepatitis are caused by hepatitis A, B, or C.

Diagnostic Strategies

- Serum transaminase levels (aspartate aminotransferase [AST] or alanine aminotransferase [ALT]) are sensitive tests for acute viral hepatitis when a positive result is defined as any level above the upper limit of normal.
- At a higher cutoff point (more than ten times the upper reference limit), AST and ALT determinations have high specificity (>95%) but low sensitivity (about 50%) for acute viral hepatitis.
- In patients with clinical and laboratory evidence of acute hepatitis, serologic testing should be obtained for the most likely agent(s). If, however, no one agent seems likely, then the following four serologic tests should be obtained: IgM-specific antibody to hepatitis A virus (IgM anti-HAV), hepatitis B surface antigen (HBsAg), IgM-specific antibody to hepatitis B core antigen (IgM anti-HBc), and antibody to hepatitis C (anti-HCV).
- Positive IgM anti-HAV indicates acute HAV infection.
- Positive IgM anti-HBc with or without positive HBsAg indicates acute HBV infection. Negative IgM anti-HBc with positive HBsAg indicates chronic HBV infection.
- Positive anti-HCV indicates HCV infection that may be either acute or chronic. For suspected false-negative results in early infection, a test to detect HCV RNA can be ordered.

BACKGROUND

Patients with clinically apparent acute viral hepatitis present most often with a prodrome of anorexia, malaise, and fatigue, which is followed by nausea, vomiting, fever, and jaundice (1,2). Several different viruses cause hepatitis, including hepatitis A (HAV); hepatitis B (HBV); hepatitis D (HDV), a defective virus that requires coinfection with HBV; hepatitis C (HCV); hepatitis E (HEV); hepatitis G (HGV); Epstein-Barr virus; and cytomegalovirus. Viral hepatitis must be differentiated from hepatic injury caused by drugs, alcohol, or other toxins; chronic hepatitis; and obstructive jaundice. It is important to establish the cause of viral hepatitis so that proper precautions, preventive measures, and prognostic considerations may be undertaken.

ESTIMATING PRETEST PROBABILITY

Although acute viral hepatitis is uncommon in the general population, several groups are at increased risk. Table 16-1 gives routes of transmission and risk factors for the viral hepatitides (1,3,4). Although the incidence of post-transfusion HBV has decreased, it remains the most common cause of acute viral hepatitis (3). Distribution of causes for acute hepatitis in the United States shows HAV at 32%, HBV at 43%

Table 16-1. Routes of Transmission and Risk Factors for Viral Hepatitis

Virus	Routes of Transmission	Risk Factors
Hepatitis A	Fecal-oral	Water and food contamination
		International travel
		Person-person contact
		Day care workers and attendees
Hepatitis B Hepatitis D	Contact with infected body fluids	Sexual contact
		Blood product transfusions
		Intravenous drug use
		Health care workers
		Hemodialysis
Hepatitis C	Parenteral Direct percutaneous exposure to blood	Intravenous drug use
		Contact with blood products
		Sexual contact
Hepatitis E	Fecal-oral	Contaminated drinking water
		Poor sanitation in undeveloped countries

(4% with concurrent HDV), HCV at 21%, and non-ABCDE at 4%, with HEV transmission not yet identified in the United States (3). Historical features consistent with acute hepatitis include anorexia, malaise, and nausea, which are present in more than 90% of patients with acute hepatocellular necrosis from any cause (5,6). Patients with hepatitis who smoke often describe a distaste for cigarettes; however, this symptom lacks specificity. A history of alcohol abuse or exposure to drugs or chemicals known to be associated with liver cell injury argues against the diagnosis of viral hepatitis, as does a history of a chronic disease (e.g., malignancy or sarcoidosis) that may involve the liver.

At the physical examination, at least 90% of patients with viral hepatitis are found to have either hepatomegaly or hepatic tenderness or both (7). Such findings are helpful in the diagnosis because, when these findings are absent, hepatitis is unlikely. Except for jaundice, no other physical findings are commonly seen. Enlarged lymph nodes and a palpably enlarged spleen in a patient with presumed hepatitis should raise the suspicion of cytomegalovirus or Epstein-Barr virus infection.

DIAGNOSTIC TESTS

Serum Aminotransferases

Serum alanine aminotransferase (ALT) and aspartate aminotransferase (AST) levels are sensitive markers of hepatocellular damage. Elevated serum transaminase levels are often considered a defining characteristic of acute hepatitis (8). Although normal values are believed to effectively rule out a diagnosis of acute viral hepatitis (9), recent studies suggest that in acute and chronic HCV infection there can be a fluctuating pattern of transaminase levels to normal or near normal values (10,11). Specificity for the diagnosis of hepatitis increases with the degree of enzyme elevation, and levels more than ten times the upper reference limit are unusual in patients with liver disease with any cause other than viral hepatitis (specificity, approximately 99%), particularly if ingestion of toxins such as alcohol or hypotensive or hypoxic episodes can be excluded (2,9,12). More moderate elevations in transaminase levels occur in patients with liver cell injury due to various causes and are thus not as helpful in differentiating viral hepatitis from other causes of liver cell damage, as shown in Table 16-2 (12,13).

The AST/ALT ratio has also been used in the differential diagnosis of hepatocellular damage. A ratio greater than 2 is highly suggestive of alcohol-induced injury, whereas a value less than 1 is suggestive of viral hepatitis (2,12,14). According to one study, in the diagnosis of viral hepatitis the ratio had a sensitivity and specificity of 90% and 77%, respectively (14). However, because these test characteristics apply only to the ratio noted at peak ALT values, serial determinations are

Table 16-2. Operating Characteristics of Serum Aspartate Aminotransferase Levels in the Diagnosis of Acute Viral Hepatitis*

Definition of Positive Result	Sensitivity	Specificity	Likelihood Ratio for Result
	←——— % ———→		
Normal	—	—	0.1
Abnormal, but			
<200 U/L	99	81	0.4
201–400 U/L	73	98	1.0
401–600 U/L	57	99	~7
601–1000 U/L	50	>99	~20
>1000 U/L	28	100	⮆

*Control (nondisease) patients used to calculate specificity were patients with obstructive jaundice. The sensitivity and specificity are calculated for cutoff values greater than or equal to the indicated ranges. Likelihood ratios are for values only within the specified ranges.
Adapted from Clermont RJ, Chalmers TC. The transaminase tests in liver disease. Medicine. 1967;46:197-207.

required. For this reason and because of the relatively mediocre operating characteristics of the ratio, use of the AST/ALT ratio probably adds little to the diagnostic accuracy of the individual tests.

Other Liver Function Tests

The diagnostic accuracy of other standard liver function tests in acute viral hepatitis is poor; measurement of neither the total nor the fractionated bilirubin level is helpful in distinguishing patients with viral hepatitis from those with other causes of liver cell damage. However, serial measurements of bilirubin are often useful in following the clinical course. Mild elevations of alkaline phosphatase, up to 2.5 times the normal value, are seen in patients with acute viral hepatitis, whereas much greater increases are common in patients with obstructive jaundice. Thus, the increase in transaminase levels relative to the increase in alkaline phosphatase can be helpful in distinguishing patients with hepatitis from those with obstructive jaundice. Elevations in transaminase level to more than six times normal with an elevation in alkaline phosphatase level less than 2.5 times the normal value is highly suggestive of hepatitis. In contrast, an elevation in transaminase level less than six times the normal value with an alkaline phosphatase level more than 2.5 times normal is highly suggestive of obstructive jaundice. However, the usefulness of these cutoffs is limited because fewer than 40% of patients with jaundice have these combinations of laboratory findings. Additionally, multivariate approaches using AST, alka-

Table 16-3. Operating Characteristics of Serologic Tests in the Diagnosis of Acute Viral Hepatitis

Diagnostic Test	Sensitivity	Specificity	Likelihood Ratio	
			Positive Result	Negative Result
	←	%	→	
Hepatitis A serologic test				
Anti-HAV	99	84	6.2	0.01
IgM anti-HAV	99	99	99	0.01
Hepatits B serologic test				
HBsAG	80	97 (95–99)	27	0.2
IgM anti-HBc	90	98	45	0.1
Hepatitis C serologic test				
Anti-HCV	90	99	90	0.1

Anti-HAV = antibody to hepatitis A virus; IgM anti-HAV = IgM-specific antibody to hepatitis A virus; HBsAg = hepatitis B surface antigen; IgM anti-HBc = IgM antibody to hepatitis B core antigen; anti-HCV = antibody to hepatitis C virus.

line phosphatase, bilirubin, and other tests of hepatic function have not resulted in significantly better diagnostic accuracy in this setting (15,16). Thus, it is essential to correlate the patient's clinical findings with laboratory test results to arrive at an accurate diagnosis.

Hepatitis A Serologic Tests

Immunoassays are available for determining both total hepatitis A antibody (anti-HAV) and IgM-specific antibody to hepatitis A virus (IgM anti-HAV). Both tests have almost uniformly positive results in patients with acute symptomatic hepatitis A (sensitivity, 99%), but the IgM anti-HAV assay is more specific (99% compared with 84%) (Table 16-3), and as such, it is the test of choice for active HAV infection. A negative result for either test effectively rules out a diagnosis of HAV. With resolution of active infection, total anti-HAV becomes almost entirely IgG anti-HAV, lasts throughout life, and serves as a marker of past infection (12,17).

Hepatitis B and Hepatitis D Serologic Tests

Two serologic tests are performed in testing for acute HBV: hepatitis B surface antigen (HBsAg) and IgM antibody to hepatitis B core antigen (IgM anti-HBc) (17). A positive HBsAg result indicates HBV infection. The anti-HBc helps distinguish acute infection from chronic infection. If the results of the IgM anti-HBc are negative, the infection is considered chronic; if the anti-HBc is positive, the infection is acute. The combination of a negative HBsAg result and a positive IgM anti-HBc result also indicates acute hepatitis B. The results of the HBsAg test are positive in at least 80% of patients eventually shown to have acute HBV, and the test has a high specificity (95%–99%) (see Table 16-3) (16–19). The results of the IgM anti-HBc test are positive in 90% to 100% of patients with acute HBV (18–20), but the appearance of IgM anti-HBc tends to lag behind that of HBsAg by about 1 week. After acute infection, IgM anti-HBc remains elevated for variable periods, with the test results of 15% of patients remaining positive for more than 1 year. False-positive results often occur in patients with rheumatoid arthritis (18). False-negative results may occur in immunosuppressed patients (21).

Other available serologic tests are less helpful in the diagnosis of HBV infection. The e antigen of the B virus (HBeAg) may play a role in the development of tolerance to the virus by the host (12), but the test has little value in establishing the initial diagnosis of hepatitis B. Viral replication as monitored by circulating HBV DNA levels using a variety of molecular diagnostic approaches is also currently available (17,22), but again, it currently has no role in the initial evaluation for acute hepatitis B.

The defective virus, hepatitis D, requires HBV for replication to supply HBsAg for its envelope (22). Infection with HDV may occur as acute coinfection with HBV, acute infection in an HBV carrier, or chronic infection with HBV. The diagnostic test for acute HDV infection is IgM anti-HDV (17,22).

Hepatitis C Serologic Tests

Second-generation immunoassays for determining hepatitis C antibody (anti-HCV) are available. There is, however, a lag period of approximately 3 months between onset of symptoms and detectable serologic response (12,17). False-positive results can occur in patients with autoimmune diseases, hypergammaglobulinemia, and immune globulin therapy. A second-generation recombinant immunoblot assay (RIBA II) should be done to confirm or refute the diagnosis in such patients (12,22,23). False-negative results can occur in patients who receive testing early in the clinical course, and in patients with immunosuppression, chronic renal failure, and hemodialysis (12). Sensitivity and specificity of second-generation anti-HCV testing is estimated to be approximately 90% and 99%, respectively (24). To make the diagnosis of acute hepatitis C early in the course of the disease when the results of antibody tests may be negative, HCV RNA can be determined by molecular diagnostic approaches including polymerase chain reaction (12,17,22).

Hepatitis E Serologic Tests

Travelers returning from countries where the virus is endemic have been the only confirmed cases of hepatitis E in the United States (1,3). Immunoassays for IgG and IgM anti-HEV and molecular diagnostic approaches for HEV RNA are being developed and evaluated (17,25,26).

Testing for Non-ABCDE Hepatitis

The diagnosis of non-ABCDE hepatitis is made by exclusion. Because infectious mononucleosis and cytomegalovirus infection can cause hepatitis, these illnesses must be excluded by appropriate testing before a diagnosis of non-ABCDE hepatitis is made. Evidence of additional hepatitis agents has been presented (27,28). These agents include hepatitis F virus, hepatitis G virus, and the GB viruses. The importance of these agents in human hepatitis remains to be determined.

DIAGNOSTIC STRATEGIES

The clinical history is important in determining the cause of acute hepatocellular necrosis. Exposure to viral hepatitis, known hepatotoxic agents, alcohol, illicit drugs, or recent transfusion changes the pretest probability of hepatitis and may suggest a cause. Regardless of the cause, patients with hepatocellular damage are likely to have anorexia, nausea, malaise, dark urine, jaundice, hepatomegaly, and right upper quadrant tenderness.

Next, the serum transaminase (AST or ALT) and alkaline phosphatase levels should be measured. If the AST or ALT level is normal, acute hepatitis can usually be excluded (Table 16-4). However, the fluctuations in transaminase levels to normal or near normal levels in HCV infection should be kept in mind. If the transaminase levels are abnormal, then the higher the level is above 200 U/L, the more likely the diagnosis of acute hepatitis becomes. The relative elevations of the AST, ALT and alkaline phosphatase levels can help distinguish acute hepatitis from obstructive jaundice.

Definitive diagnosis of acute viral hepatitis is made by demonstrating the presence of relevant serologic markers. When the likelihood of exposure to certain hepatitis agents is high, initial testing should be for that virus only. If, however, no exposure is likely, then a reasonable strategy is to order the following four tests: HBsAg, IgM anti-HBc, IgM anti-HAV, and anti-HCV (1). A positive IgM anti-HAV result indicates acute HAV infection. Acute HBV infection is indicated by positive IgM anti-HBc with or without positive HBsAg. Chronic HBV infection is indicated by negative IgM anti-HBc results and positive HbsAg results. A positive anti-HCV result in patients who do not have any supporting clinical history can be evaluated with a RIBA II.

Table 16-4. Post-test Probabilities for Diagnostic Tests in the Diagnosis of Acute Viral Hepatitis

Diagnostic Test	Pretest Probability					
	20%		50%		80%	
	Positive Result	Negative Result	Positive Result	Negative Result	Positive Result	Negative Result
	←			%		→
Aspartate aminotransferase						
Normal	—	2	—	9	—	29
Abnormal, but						
<200 U/L	9	—	29	—	62	—
201–400 U/L	20	—	50	—	80	—
401–600 U/L	64	—	88	—	97	—
601–1000 U/L	83	—	95	—	99	—
>1000 U/L	>99	—	>99	—	>99	—
Hepatitis B serologic test						
HBsAg	87	5	96	17	99	45
IgM- anti-HBc	92	2	98	9	99	29
Hepatitis A serologic test						
Anti-HAV	61	<1	86	1	96	5
IgM anti-HAV	96	<1	99	1	>99	4
Hepatitis C serologic test						
Anti-HCV	96	2	99	9	>99	29

Anti-HAV = antibody to hepatitis A virus; IgM anti-HAV = IgM-specific antibody to hepatitis A virus; HBsAg = hepatitis B surface antigen; IgM anti-HBc = IgM antibody to hepatitis B core antigen; anti-HCV = antibody to hepatitis C virus.

Negative results with anti-HCV should be interpreted with caution because of the relatively late appearance of anti-HCV in the clinical course of the disease. Thus, if HCV infection is strongly suspected, repeat anti-HCV should be performed later in the course of disease or the presence of HCV RNA should be determined. Evaluation with these four tests can also indicate if simultaneous acute infection with more than one agent is present.

Other types of acute viral hepatitis may be identified in the future when more effective tests for specific markers of infection with these agents become available. The hepatitis associated with infectious mononucleosis can be confirmed by appropriate tests discussed in Chapter 20. Generally, the diagnosis of hepatitis caused by toxins is made either by obtaining an appropriate history or by exclusion. When acute liver disease is evident but the results of all aforementioned marker studies are negative, testing strategies for other diagnoses such as chronic hepatitis, biliary obstruction, and cholestasis need to be pursued.

CLINICAL PROBLEMS

Clinical Problem 1
An ambulatory patient has signs and symptoms suggestive of liver disease.

Testing Strategy and Rationale
Serum bilirubin, AST (or ALT), and alkaline phosphatase levels should be measured. If values are abnormal with a pattern suggesting hepatitis, then appropriately selected hepatitis markers should be measured. If the initial tests findings are normal, a diagnosis of acute viral hepatitis can be effectively ruled out unless there is a high suspicion of HCV infection. Early in the course of viral hepatitis, the bilirubin level may be normal or show minimal elevation. High transaminase levels increase substantially the probability of hepatocellular damage. The alkaline phosphatase level may help in discriminating between obstructive jaundice and acute hepatitis. If the probability of acute hepatitis is sufficiently high at this point, proceed with the selection of the four hepatitis markers: HBsAg, IgM anti-HBc, IgM anti-HAV, and anti-HCV. When the suspicion for HCV infection is high but the results of anti-HCV testing are negative (as can occur early in the clinical course of the disease), testing for HCV RNA should be done.

Clinical Example
A 25-year-old woman has a history of fatigue, anorexia, nausea, and distaste for cigarettes. She has no history of previous liver disease, blood transfusion, drug use, or exposure to toxins or to patients with known hepatitis. She recalls eating poorly cooked steamed clams about a month ago. At examination, she is not jaundiced but has a slightly enlarged liver and tenderness in the right upper quadrant. The probability of acute hepatitis is estimated to be 50%. The bilirubin level is 1.6 mg/dL; the AST level is 450 U/L; and the alkaline phosphatase level is minimally elevated. The likelihood ratio for this AST level for acute hepatitis is approximately 7, and the post-test probability of acute hepatitis is now approxi-

Continued

mately 85%. Owing to the history (i.e, of eating clams), testing should begin with the IgM anti-HAV.

Clinical Problem 2

An ambulatory homosexual man has jaundice and a previous history of hepatitis.

Testing Strategy and Rationale

Measurements of AST (or ALT) and alkaline phosphatase levels and hepatitis screen should be done, as in Clinical Problem 1. In a patient with obvious liver disease and for whom the pretest probability of viral hepatitis is reasonably high, the AST determination is likely to increase further the probability of this diagnosis. Hepatitis B is the most prevalent form of hepatitis in homosexual men. When the patient has a history of liver disease at the time of presentation, the key question may be whether the patient's current problem is acute hepatitis or reactivation of chronic hepatitis. Results from the hepatitis screen can help with this assessment.

Clinical Example

A 30-year-old homosexual man has a history of fatigue and anorexia. He is jaundiced. He has no history of blood transfusion, toxin exposure, shellfish ingestion, or known exposure to patients with hepatitis. He states that he has had an episode of hepatitis in the past but that he was not hospitalized. Physical examination shows a moderately enlarged tender liver but no palmar erythema, spider angiomata, or splenomegaly. Because symptoms and signs are consistent with acute viral hepatitis and because there are no findings suggesting chronic liver disease, the probability of acute viral hepatitis is estimated to be approximately 50%. The alkaline phosphatase level is slightly elevated, and the AST value is 510 U/L. The estimated likelihood ratio for the AST at this level is about 7 (see Table 16-2). On the basis of these findings, the revised probability of viral hepatitis is approximately 85%. Hepatitis B is considered to be the most likely diagnosis. A positive IgM anti-HBc result from the hepatitis screen would confirm the suspected diagnosis.

REFERENCES

1. **Becherer PR.** Viral hepatitis. Postgrad Med. 1995;98:65.
2. **Moseley RH.** Evaluation of abnormal liver function tests. Med Clin North Am. 1996;80:887-906.
3. **Alter MF, Mast EE.** The epidemiology of viral hepatitis in the United States. Gastroenterol Clin North Am. 1994;23:437-55.

4. **Kuhns MC.** Viral hepatitis. Lab Med. 1995;26:650-9.

5. **Hoofnagle JH.** Acute non-A, non-B hepatitis: clinical course and diagnosis. In: Geretz RJ, ed. Non-A, Non-B Hepatitis. New York: Academic Press; 1982:24.

6. **Koff RS, Galambos JT.** Viral hepatitis. In: Schiff L, Schiff ER, eds. Diseases of the Liver. Philadelphia: JB Lippincott; 1982:530.

7. **DeRitis F, Giusti G, Piccinino F, et al.** Statistical analysis of clinical and laboratory data recorded in a sample of 893 patients hospitalized with acute viral hepatitis. Acta Hepato-Gastroenterol. 1973;20:371.

8. **Bader TF.** Viral Hepatitis: Practical Evaluation and Treatment. Seattle: Hogrefe & Huber; 1995:1.

9. **Rosalki SB, Dooley JS.** Liver function profiles and their interpretation. Br J Hosp Med. 1994;51:181-6.

10. **Gretch D, Lee W, Corey L.** Use of aminotransferase, hepatitis C antibody, and hepatitis C polymerase chain reaction RNA assays to establish the diagnosis of hepatitis C virus infection in a diagnostic virology laboratory. J Clin Microbiol. 1992;30:2145-9.

11. **Cordoba J, Camps J, Esteban JI.** The clinical picture of acute and chronic hepatitis C. Curr Stud Hematol Blood Transfus. 1994;61:69-88.

12. **Neuschwander-Tetri BA.** Common blood tests for liver disease. Postgrad Med. 1995;98:49-56, 59, 63.

13. **Clermont RJ, Chalmers TC.** The transaminase tests in liver disease. Medicine. 1967;46:197-207.

14. **Cohen JA, Kaplan MM.** The SGOT/SGPT ratio: an indicator of alcoholic liver disease. Dig Dis Sci. 1979;24:835-8.

15. **Winkel P, Ramshoc K, Lyngbye J, et al.** Diagnostic value of routine liver tests. Clin Chem. 1975;21:71-5.

16. **Sher P.** Diagnostic effectiveness of biochemical liver function tests as evaluated by discriminant function analysis. Clin Chem. 1977;23:627-30.

17. **Sjogren MH.** Serologic diagnosis of viral hepatitis. Med Clin North Am. 1996;80:929-56.

18. **Lemon SM, Gates N, Sims E, et al.** IgM antibody to hepatitis B core antigen as a diagnostic parameter of acute infection with hepatitis B virus. J Infect Dis. 1981;143:803-9.

19. **Perrillo RP, Chau KH, Overby LR, et al.** Anti-hepatitis B core immunoglobulin M in the serologic evaluation of hepatitis B virus infection and simultaneous infection with type B, Delta agent, and non-A, non-B viruses. Gastroenterology. 1983;85:163-7.

20. **Tsuda F, Naito S, Takai E, et al.** Low molecular weight (7) immunoglobulin M antibody against hepatitis B core antigen in the serum for differentiating acute from persistent hepatitis virus infection. Gastroenterology. 1984;87:159-64.

21. **Vergani D, Masera G, Moroni G, et al.** Histological evidence of hepatitis - B virus infection with negative serology in children with acute leukemia who develop chronic liver disease. Lancet. 1982;1:361-4.

22. **Hu KQ, Vierling JM.** Molecular diagnostic techniques for viral hepatitis. Gastroenterol Clin North Am. 1994;23:479-98.

23. **Bhandari BN, Wright TL.** Hepatitis C: an overview. Annu Rev Med. 1995;46:309-17.

24. **Whyte G, Beal R.** Screening—sensitivity, specificity and hepatitis C. Med J Australia. 1995;163:63-4.

25. **Bradley DW.** Hepatitis E virus: a brief review of the biology, molecular virology, and immunology of a novel virus. J Hepatology. 1995;22(Suppl 1):140-5.

26. **Mast EE, Alter MJ, Holland P, Purcell RH.** Evaluation of assays for antibody to hepatitis E virus by a serum panel. Hepatology. 1998;27:857-61.

27. **Bowden DS, Moaven LD, Locarnini SA.** In the alphabet? Med J Australia. 1996;164:87-9.

28. **Tepper ML, Gully PR.** Viral hepatitis: know your D, E, F and G's. Can Med Assoc J. 1997;156:1735-6.

Hepatic Metastases 17

Robert J. Panzer, MD

KEY POINTS

Pretest Probabilities

- A minority of patients who undergo surgery for primary colorectal neoplasms have palpable hepatic metastases on examination or at laparotomy; hepatic imaging is generally necessary to identify metastases accurately before initiating therapy or determining prognosis.

- The frequency of hepatic metastases in patients with breast or lung cancer at the time of diagnosis is much lower than in patients with colon or pancreatic cancer.

- Pancreatic cancer is commonly associated with hepatic metastases, which are usually already addressed by tests to diagnose the primary cancer when pancreatic cancer is suspected.

- The presence of hepatomegaly, jaundice, or a painful liver increases the likelihood of hepatic metastases, but only a minority of patients have these signs.

- Most patients have no overt clinical evidence of their hepatic metastases. Clinical features correlating with a poorer prognosis in colorectal cancer reflect the effects of both local disease extension and metastases.

Diagnostic Strategies

- Blood tests such as liver function tests and the various antigen assays do not effectively identify cancer patients who have hepatic metastases.

- Liver radionuclide scanning has a limited diagnostic role, because it is less sensitive (especially for small lesions) and less specific than other available tests.

- Ultrasonographic studies lack sensitivity for small lesions and suboptimal studies reduce overall sensitivity. Ultrasonography does have high specificity and is effective at confirming disease at high pretest probabilities.

- Computed tomography is more sensitive than other imaging tests for smaller hepatic metastases and has high specificity. It is generally the test of choice for evaluating patients for hepatic metastases at any but high pretest probabilities.

BACKGROUND

Detection of occult hepatic metastases is most often considered during the preoperative evaluation of patients with suspected colorectal cancer, one of the most common cancers in both men and women. It is also considered in patients with primary breast, lung, or pancreatic cancer. Patients found to have hepatic metastases may often be spared the morbidity of surgical procedures aimed at cure, and some may be offered surgery directed at excising limited hepatic metastasis. Establishing the diagnosis in either setting requires a testing strategy that results in high post-test probabilities after positive test results have been obtained, given the high cost of a false-positive result.

Direct palpation of the liver at the time of laparotomy was long considered the diagnostic standard for establishing the presence or absence of hepatic metastases. However, support for this idea was mainly based on older autopsy studies (1,2). Studies with long-term follow-up found that only about half of lesions were palpable at the time of surgery (3,4). With more routine hepatic imaging using accurate tests able to screen out many patients by determining that they have incurable disease, the frequency of palpable lesions at surgery is even lower today.

With colorectal cancer, laparotomy is often performed even if preoperative studies suggest hepatic metastases. In this case, tests should be evaluated for the amount of information that they add to direct palpation of the liver. In cases in which laparotomy is deferred in abdominal malignancy and when breast or lung surgery are contemplated, the discriminating power of the isolated test is more critical. The accuracy of imaging tests may vary with the type of primary cancer. For example, metastases from breast cancer, which must pass through the pulmonary circulation, may be smaller and more diffuse than those from colon cancer (5). This chapter focuses on testing to diagnose metastases to the liver and does not directly address the diagnosis of hepatocellular carcinoma or preoperative evaluation of patients considered for surgical resection of metastases to the liver.

ESTIMATING PRETEST PROBABILITY

In the past, between 15% and 30% of patients who underwent surgery for resection of primary colorectal neoplasms had palpable hepatic metastases at laparotomy (6). Perhaps an equal number had truly occult disease detectable by long-term follow-up (3) or by meticulous liver palpation guided by preoperative imaging studies (7). As patients more routinely have accurate hepatic imaging preoperatively and, in some cases, have palliative chemotherapy instead of surgery, the proportion of patients with palpable disease at the time of surgery decreases.

The frequency with which breast or lung cancer is associated with isolated hepatic metastases at the time of diagnosis is much lower (10% or less). Although pancreatic cancer is commonly associated with hepatic metastases, usually the tests performed during the evaluation of the primary tumor (e.g., computed tomography [CT]) already have adequately evaluated the liver for metastatic disease. The presence of hepatomegaly, jaundice, or a painful liver increases the likelihood of hepatic metastases and often indicates an untreatable late stage of disease. However, only a minority of patients have these signs.

Most patients with hepatic metastases and colorectal cancer have no overt clinical evidence of hepatic involvement. Clinical features correlating with a poorer prognosis relate more to the presence of locally extensive disease (Dukes Class C) than to the presence of distant metastases; such features include bowel obstruction or perforation, ulcerating or circumferential lesions, distal tumor sites, and younger age. Patients with these clinical features include those patients most likely to benefit from aggressive surgery as well as those most likely to have occult hepatic metastases, which would make surgery fruitless. Patients without symptoms, with bleeding alone, or with proximal lesions have a better prognosis. In patients with poor prognostic indicators, the likelihood of hepatic metastases is probably 40% to 50% as opposed to perhaps 10% to 20% in those who have good prognostic indicators.

DIAGNOSTIC TESTS

Blood Tests

Liver function tests and antigen assays lack adequate sensitivity and specificity to serve as screening tests for hepatic metastases in patients with colorectal or other cancer. For example, measurement of the alkaline phosphatase had a sensitivity and specificity of approximately 65% for hepatic metastases (7).

As an example of the limitations of antigen assays, the CEA assay has only slightly better characteristics (Table 17-1). Elevated CEA levels do correlate with prognosis, but as noted earlier, poorer prognosis is associated both with locally extensive disease, potentially curable by aggressive surgery, and with distant hepatic metastases, in cases in which palliative or no surgery may be more appropriate (8–10).

Attempts to improve test characteristics by altering test cutoff points or by combining tests have met with limited success (7). High sensitivity can be achieved only with major decreases in specificity, and vice versa (see Table 17-1).

Periodically, new blood tests for colon cancer are proposed for use in diagnosis. However, these tests generally suffer from the same prob-

Table 17-1. Operating Characteristics of Diagnostic Tests for Hepatic Metastases

Diagnostic Test	Definition of Positive Result	Sensitivity	Specificity	Likelihood Ratio	
				Positive Result	Negative Result
		← % →			
Alkaline phosphatase	Abnormal	65 (50–77)	65 (59–75)	1.9	0.54
	>135 IU/L	54	90	5.4	0.51
Gamma GT	Abnormal	75	45	1.4	0.56
CEA by RIA	Abnormal	86	60	2.2	0.23
	>5 ng/dL	80	72	2.9	0.28
	>10 ng/dL	70	87	5.4	0.34
Liver scanning	Abnormal	~90 (82–94)	~70 (67–76)	~3	~0.14
	Focal	~80 (68–86)	~90 (81–99)	~8	~0.22
Ultrasonography					
all	Focal	~70 (61–80)	~90 (83–94)	~7	~0.33
adequate	Focal	~80	~90	~8	~0.22
Computed tomography	Focal	~90 (76–96)	~90 (88–89)	~9	~0.11
Helical CT		>90	>90	>9	<0.11

GT = glutamyl transferase; CEA = carcinoembryonic antigen; RIA = radioimmunoassay; CT = computed tomography.

lems as other blood tests—they correlate with the total burden of disease rather than with hepatic or other metastases. Consequently, they tend not to distinguish between curable and incurable disease.

Radionuclide Scanning

The reported test characteristics of technetium liver scanning varied widely depending on the requirements for a positive test result and on the diagnostic gold standard. When nonfocal abnormalities were included as positive results for hepatic metastases, technetium liver scanning was sensitive (approximately 90%) but less specific (approximately 70%) than the other imaging studies (see Table 17-1). Diffuse small defects caused by hepatocellular disease were the most common cause of false-positive results. When the presence of focal defects was required for a positive test result, the specificity improved to approximately 90% but the sensitivity decreased to about 80% (see Table 17-1) (4).

Liver scanning had a low sensitivity for smaller lesions, approximately 30% for 1- to 2-cm lesions (8) and only about 10% for nonpalpable hepatic metastases (3). As a result, radionuclide liver scanning must be superceded by other tests for the diagnosis of hepatic metastases.

Ultrasonography

Ultrasonography has good specificity (90%) for hepatic metastases but appears to be less sensitive overall (70%) (see Table 17-1) (8). Suboptimal studies owing to bowel gas or obesity may occur in as many as 25% of patients (11) and account for some of the apparent lack of sensitivity. Among adequate studies, ultrasonography is as sensitive (80%) as liver scanning in detecting palpable hepatic metastases and larger individual lesions, but similarly is not highly sensitive for smaller lesions (8) or disease that is not palpable at laparotomy (less than 50% in one study) (3). The sensitivity of ultrasonography for occult small lesions may improve as technical improvements enhance its discriminating ability (12,13). The main reason to pay attention to the operating characteristics of ultrasonography is that the test is often done during the evaluation of symptoms or signs such as jaundice before cancer is diagnosed and before hepatic metastases are suspected. Once suspected, the probability of hepatic metastases and any ultrasound findings need to be addressed.

Ultrasound loses accuracy in the presence of cirrhosis. In one study of patients with both primary and metastatic tumors, ultrasound had a sensitivity of only 50%, though its specificity was 98% (14).

Computed Tomography

Contrast abdominal CT is more expensive than most older tests for hepatic metastases, but it also has better sensitivity (85%–90%) than either the liver scan or an adequate ultrasound study (8,15). Furthermore, CT is much more sensitive for small nonpalpable lesions, detecting approximately 60% to 80% of such lesions (3,8) in early studies. The specificity of CT for hepatic metastases is also quite good (90%). Although not high enough to rule in disease at low pretest probabilities, its specificity is at least as good as and possibly better than that of liver scanning or ultrasonography. Unless contraindicated, contrast-enhanced CT is preferred over noncontrast studies.

Computed tomography accuracy declines in the presence of cirrhosis. One study, including both primary and metastatic tumors, showed contrast CT to have only 68% sensitivity and 81% specificity, with noncontrast CT being even less accurate (16).

Helical CT permits more rapid acquisition of images, reducing the adverse effects of respiration on the image. According to the published literature, this increases both the apparent sensitivity and specificity of CT, although no large published studies in usual settings are available to determine precise operating characteristics. Sensitivity and specificity likely increase to more than 90% with these techniques. Similar improvements in accuracy occur with scanning during preoperative staging for potential resection in which helical scanning can be linked to arterial portography (17,18).

For resection of hepatic metastases, the relevant unit of analysis is the lesion rather than the patient; this reduces both sensitivity and specificity given the need for correct classification of small lesions (14). At the lesion level, helical CT was 91% sensitive for lesions over 1 cm and 56% sensitive for lesions less than 1 cm, giving an overall sensitivity of 81% (19).

Magnetic Resonance Imaging

Magnetic resonance imaging (MRI) of the liver may be the most sensitive and specific test available for hepatic metastases, with contrast-enhanced MRI providing the greatest accuracy (20,21). However, MRI is more expensive than CT, and head-to-head comparisons with CT alternatives in usual care settings are limited. Prospective blinded, unbiased comparisons with CT in large numbers of study participants are needed to determine the true operating characteristics of MRI. Such limitations apply to various newer techniques or modifications of older techniques (22).

Fine-Needle Biopsy

Hepatic biopsy is less frequently included in routine evaluations for hepatic metastases, because the identification of the primary tumor usually makes the interpretation of hepatic lesions clear. When biopsy is needed, fine-needle biopsy of the liver guided by ultrasonography is successful in more than 90% of attempts, with a sensitivity and specificity for hepatic metastases of 84% to 93% and 99% to 100%, respectively (23,24).

Other Tests

Hepatic angiography, given its invasiveness, now has a limited role in the diagnosis of hepatic metastases. However, it has uses in the differentiation of hemangiomas from other lesions and in surgical planning.

DIAGNOSTIC STRATEGIES

The clinical setting helps define the pretest probability of hepatic metastases. In patients with no evidence of metastases after the basic clinical evaluation, hepatic metastases is found more commonly in those with colon or pancreatic cancer than in those with breast or lung cancer.

Liver function tests are both insensitive and nonspecific for hepatic metastases. Except for extremely abnormal results, findings from these tests should be interpreted with caution.

The CEA and similar tests are of little use in the initial diagnosis of hepatic metastases. However, these tests may have a role in the management of patients with colon cancer who do not have metastases,

Table 17-2. Post-test Probabilities of Hepatic Metastases Based on the Results of Diagnostic Tests

Diagnostic Test	Pretest Probabilities					
	20%		50%		80%	
	Positive Result	Negative Result	Positive Result	Negative Result	Positive Result	Negative Result
	←——————————————————— % ——————————————————→					
Alkaline phosphatase abnormal	32	12	65	35	88	68
Gamma GT abnormal	25	12	58	36	85	69
CEA by RIA > 5 ng/dL	42	6	74	22	92	53
Liver scanning						
Abnormal	43	3	75	13	92	36
Focal	67	5	89	18	97	47
Ultrasonography						
Focal—all	64	8	88	25	97	57
Focal—adequate only	67	5	89	18	97	47
Computed tomography	69	3	90	10	97	31

GT = glutamyl transferase; CEA = carcinoembryonic antigen; RIA = radioimmunoassay.

because serial determinations may identify recurrent disease in patients whose CEA levels decrease perioperatively.

The optimal diagnostic strategy for detection of hepatic metastases changed several years ago (25). Accurate identification of the location and number of individual lesions has become more important in certain cases, such as in those in which resection of metastases is a consideration.

Contrast CT has the best combination of operating characteristics (26). Liver scanning is no longer a primary test for hepatic metastases, because it is sensitive only for larger lesions and is nonspecific. Ultrasonography is specific, but the frequency of technically suboptimal studies contributes to a lack of sensitivity and it is therefore not a primary test for hepatic metastases.

Contrast CT appears to be the test of choice when accurately identifying hepatic metastases will significantly affect disease management, such as when the extent of colorectal surgery would be affected or when resection of isolated hepatic metastases for cure is a consideration. It is also the most accurate test for tracking the effects of treatment. Helical CT offers improved sensitivity and specificity by reducing the effects of respiration on image quality.

Ultrasonography is an alternative when the pretest probability of hepatic metastases is high, given its high specificity. Many patients have already had unexpected hepatic metastases identified by ultrasonographic studies performed earlier in the evaluation of problems such as obstructive jaundice or abdominal pain. Clear-cut positive findings on ultrasonography may not require confirmation, unless ultrasonography indicates that the patient may be a candidate for surgical resection of isolated metastases, in which case CT would also be performed owing to its sensitivity for smaller occult lesions.

The literature and reviews of newer modalities tend not to provide blinded comparisons of alternative imaging tests in large numbers of patients in whom the disease of interest is suspected. In addition, it is likely that local availability and experience will increase or decrease operating characteristics from general experience in typical care settings. Clinicians should be aware of this variation and adopt newer approaches as their imaging services become skilled and experienced with those approaches.

CLINICAL PROBLEMS

Clinical Problem 1
A patient with colon cancer but no overt signs of hepatic metastases presents for preoperative evaluation.

Testing Strategy and Rationale
Computed tomography is the test of choice to detect hepatic metastases, especially those that are small. It has the highest sensitivity and specificity of the available tests.

Clinical Example
A 68-year-old man is found to have guaiac positive stools on screening. A barium enema shows a cecal lesion. The findings of a thorough history, physical examination, and basic laboratory studies (including liver function tests) are normal except for the finding of mild anemia.

The probability of hepatic metastases is approximately 10%. A CT scan with negative findings would reduce the probability of hepatic metastases to less than 2%, and the clinician and patient could proceed with plans for curative surgery.

Clinical Problem 2
A patient has overt clinical findings suggesting a high probability of hepatic metastases.

Testing Strategy and Rationale

Ultrasonography of the liver should be performed, followed by CT if the the findings of ultrasonography are unexpectedly negative. Ultrasonography is as specific as CT and, because of its lower cost, is preferable for confirming strongly suspected hepatic metastases. However, it is not sufficiently sensitive to exclude the diagnosis at high pretest probabilities, especially when suboptimal studies are considered. Thus, unexpected results should be followed by additional evaluation.

Clinical Example

A 55-year-old woman finds a lump in her breast during a self- examination that displays malignant characteristics on mammography. Her liver is moderately enlarged on physical examination and the alkaline phosphatase level is elevated to five times normal. Hepatic metastases would be suspected, with a probability of perhaps 80%. If ultrasonography is performed, a positive result would increase the probability of hepatic metastases to more than 96% and the diagnosis would be established with confidence. However, an unexpectedly negative result would give a post-test probability of close to 50% (see Table 17-2, p 199), and additional evaluation, such as with CT, would be required.

REFERENCES

1. **Hogg L, Pack CT.** Diagnostic accuracy of hepatic metastases at laparotomy. Arch Surg. 1966;72:251-2.

2. **Goligher JC.** The operability of carcinoma of the rectum. Br Med J. 1941; 2:393-7.

3. **Finlay IG, Meek DR, Gray HW, et al.** Incidence and detection of occult hepatic metastases in colorectal carcinoma. Br Med J. 1982;284:803-5.

4. **Christensen M, Ingeberg S, Brochner-Mortensen J, et al.** Variable interpretation of liver scintigraphy in malignancy as an aid in clinical decision making. Acta Med Scand. 1982;211:23-6.

5. **Alderson PO, Adams DF, McNeil BJ, et al.** Computed tomography, ultrasound, and scintigraphy of the liver in patients with colon or breast carcinoma: a prospective comparison. Radiology. 1983;149:225-30.

6. **Foster JH, Lundy J.** Liver metastases. Curr Probl Surg. 1981;28:160-202.

7. **Kemeny MM, Sugarbaker PH, Smith TJ, et al.** A prospective analysis of laboratory tests and imaging studies to detect hepatic lesions. Ann Surg. 1982;195(2):163-7.

8. **Tartter PI, Slater G, Gelernt I, et al.** Screening for liver metastases from colorectal cancer with carcinoembryonic antigen and alkaline phosphatase. Ann Surg. 1981;193:357-60.

9. **Aburana T, Tonami N, Hisada K.** Radioimmunoassay for carcinoembryonic antigen as an adjunct to liver scan in the detection of liver metastases from digestive tract cancer. J Nucl Med. 2979;20:232-5.

10. **Szymendera JJ.** Serial CEA assays and liver scintigraphy for the detection of hepatic metastases from colorectal carcinoma. Dis Colon Rectum. 1982;25:191-7.

11. **Smith TJ, Kemeny MM, Sugarbaker PH.** A prospective study of hepatic imaging in the detection of metastatic disease. Ann Surg. 1982;195:486-91.

12. **Leen E, Angerson WJ, Wotherspoon H, et al.** Detection of colorectal liver metastases: comparison of laparotomy, CT, US, and Doppler perfusion index and evaluation of postoperative follow-up results [see Comments]. Radiology. 1995;195:113-6.

13. **Shuman WP.** Liver metastases from colorectal carcinoma: detection with Doppler US-guided measurements of liver blood flow--past, present, future [Editorial; Comment]. Radiology. 1995;195:9-10.

14. **Dodd GD III, Miller WJ, Baron RL, et al.** Detection of malignant tumors in end-stage cirrhotic livers: efficacy of sonography as a screening technique. AJR Am J Roentgenol. 1992;159:727-33.

15. **Freeny PC, Marks WM, Ryan JA, Bolen WJ.** Colorectal carcinoma evaluation with CT: preoperative staging and detection of post-operative recurrence. Radiology. 1986;158:347-53.

16. **Miller WJ, Baron RL, Dodd GD III, Federle MP.** Malignancies in patients with cirrhosis: CT sensitivity and specificity in 200 consecutive transplant patients. Radiology. 1994;193:645-50.

17. **Strotzer M, Gmeinwieser J, Schmidt J, et al.** Diagnosis of liver metastases from colorectal adenocarcinoma: comparison spiral-CTAP combined with intravenous contrast-enhanced spiral-CT and SPIO-enhanced MR combined with plain MR imaging. Acta Radiol. 1997;38:986-92.

18. **Soyer P, Bluemke DA, Hruban RH, et al.** Hepatic metastases from colorectal cancer: detection and false-positive findings with helical CT during arterial portography. Radiology. 1994;193:71-4.

19. **Kuszyk BS, Bluemke DA, Urban BA, et al.** Portal-phase contrast-enhanced helical CT for the detection of malignant hepatic tumors: sensitivity based on comparison with intraoperative and pathologic findings. AJR Am J Roentgenol. 1996;166:91-5.

20. **Fretz CJ, Stark DD, Metz CE, et al.** Detection of hepatic metastases: comparison of contrast-enhanced CT, unenhanced MR imaging, and iron oxide-enhanced MR imaging. AJR. 1990; 155:763-70.

21. **Hagspiel KD, Neidl KF, Eichenberger AC, et al.** Detection of liver metastases: comparison of superparamagnetic iron oxide-enhanced and unenhanced MR imaging at 1.5 T with dynamic CT, intraoperative US, and percutaneous US. Radiology. 1995;196:471-8.

22. **Semelka RC, Schlund JF, Molina PL, et al.** Malignant liver lesions: comparison of spiral CT arterial portography and MR imaging for diagnostic accuracy, cost, and effect on patient management. J Magn Reson Imaging. 1996;6:39-43.

23. **Bognel C, Rougier P, Leclere J, et al.** Fine needle aspiration of the liver and pancreas with ultrasound guidance. Acta Cytol. 1988;32:22-6.

24. **Fornari F, Civardi G, Cavanna L, et al.** Ultrasonically guided fine-needle aspiration biopsy: a highly diagnostic procedure for hepatic tumors. Am J Gastroenterol. 1990;85:1009-13.

25. **Ferrucci JT.** Liver tumor imaging: current concepts. AJR. 1990;155:473-84.

26. **Pasanen PA, Partanen KP, Pikkarainen PH, et al.** A comparison of ultrasound, computed tomography and endoscopic retrograde cholangiopancreatography in the differential diagnosis of benign and malignant jaundice and cholestasis. Eur J Surg. 1993;159:23-9.

Acute Pancreatitis 18

James P. Corsetti, MD, PhD, and Dean A. Arvan, MD

KEY POINTS

Pretest Probabilities

- Estimating the likelihood of acute pancreatitis on the basis of clinical findings alone is limited because such findings lack specificity.

- Plain films of the abdomen may show localized findings, such as a "sentinel" loop or duodenal distention. Although such findings increase the probability that a patient has pancreatitis, they are neither sensitive nor specific.

Diagnostic Strategies

- Serum amylase and lipase levels are sensitive and specific tests in the diagnosis of acute pancreatitis. When improved lipase assays and optimum cutoffs are used, the lipase level is both more sensitive and more specific than the amylase level.

- Serum lipase is the preferred determination when there is a delay between the onset of symptoms and patient evaluation, because lipase levels remain elevated longer than amylase levels.

- Simultaneous determination of both serum amylase and lipase offers little benefit in the evaluation of a patient in whom pancreatitis is suspected.

BACKGROUND

Acute pancreatitis is defined pathologically by the presence of gross and microscopic inflammatory changes within the pancreas. These changes include edema, hemorrhage, and necrosis of the gland, often in association with fat necrosis. The clinician, however, must define acute pancreatitis on the basis of clinical and laboratory findings. Except in situations in which the diagnosis of acute pancreatitis is clear-cut—that is, when patients have known risk factors together with a characteristic history and markedly abnormal laboratory or radiographic results—the diagnostic accuracy of combined clinical and laboratory information cannot be precisely determined because of the lack of a practical gold standard.

ESTIMATING PRETEST PROBABILITY

Acute pancreatitis is more common in men in their thirties and forties and women in their fifties and sixties. These peaks correlate with the two most common predisposing factors, alcohol abuse and biliary tract disease. Most studies of patients with acute pancreatitis show that approximately half have alcoholism, one third have gallstones, and the next largest group have an idiopathic form (1). Recently, most idiopathic cases have been shown to be caused by occult biliary microlithiasis and biliary sludge (2). Other risk factors include abdominal surgery, trauma, pancreatic carcinoma, hyperlipidemia, systemic infection, use of certain drugs (e.g., thiazide diuretics and sulfonamides), hyperparathyroidism, posterior penetrating peptic ulcer, diabetes mellitus, uremia, and a family history of pancreatitis. More recent additions to this list include organ transplantation and medications used in the treatment of patients with human immunodeficiency virus infections including pentamidine, sulfamethoxazole-trimethoprim, and didanosine.

Table 18-1 shows clinical findings commonly seen in patients with acute pancreatitis. Abdominal pain, the cardinal symptom, is usually sudden in onset and increases in severity over a period of hours. It is often described as radiating to the back, a nonspecific finding. Painless

Table 18-1. Frequency of Various Symptoms and Signs in Patients with Acute Pancreatitis*

Symptom	Sensitivity (%)
Abdominal pain	95
Pain radiating to the back	50
Anorexia	85
Nausea, vomiting	75
Decreased bowel sounds	60
Fever	60
Abdominal guarding	50
Shock	15
Icterus	15
Hematemesis	10
History of alcoholism	$\cong 50$
Biliary tract disease	$\cong 30$

*Specificity of each finding is unknown.

pancreatitis is uncommon (3). Other common symptoms and signs include anorexia, nausea, vomiting, fever, and decreased bowel sounds. Few patients have findings indicating the severe pancreatic necrosis associated with acute hemorrhagic pancreatitis; such findings include shock, anemia, and hypocalcemia. Reasonable estimates of pretest probability of pancreatitis are difficult to make because many of the clinical findings associated with pancreatitis are seen in patients with other acute abdominal disorders, such as gastritis, ischemic bowel, or ectopic pregnancy.

Elevations in the leukocyte count and blood glucose level are commonly seen. Less frequently observed are increases in serum triglyceride, bilirubin, alkaline phosphatase, and transaminase levels. These findings lack specificity and are therefore more helpful in suggesting the presence of an intra-abdominal inflammatory process than in defining its cause. Reductions in hemoglobin or hematocrit and in calcium levels tend to occur later in the course of the disease and correlate more strongly with the development of early complications (4).

Plain films of the abdomen show localized abnormalities in approximately one third of patients with acute pancreatitis. These abnormalities include localized ileus (i.e., a "sentinel" loop of jejunum), isolated distention of the transverse colon, or duodenal distention with air fluid levels. Although such localized findings are not highly sensitive or specific, they increase the probability of a patient's having pancreatitis.

DIAGNOSTIC TESTS

Because none of the primary clinical or laboratory findings associated with acute pancreatitis are specific, pancreatitis is assessed primarily by measuring pancreatic enzymes. Imaging techniques, such as ultrasonography and computed tomography, are generally used in assessing complications or determining the cause of acute pancreatitis rather than as part of the initial diagnostic approach.

Amylase

Measurement of serum amylase has long been viewed as essential to the diagnosis of pancreatitis (5). Large amounts of amylase are found in salivary glands and pancreas and lesser amounts are found in other organs. Elevated serum amylase levels (i.e., false-positive results) may be seen in patients with mumps, acute salivary gland inflammation, bowel necrosis, ectopic pregnancy, severe burns, cerebral or other trauma, opiate administration, diabetic ketoacidosis, biliary tract disease, renal insufficiency, and rarely, some types of malignancy (6,7). Increased serum amylase is also found in patients with macroamylasemia, a condition characterized by accumulation of amylase bound to immunoglobulins leading to reduced renal clearance. Normal serum amylase values (i.e., false-negative results) may be seen in patients with extensive parenchymal destruction (patients with pancreatic calcification or diabetes mellitus), in those with relatively rapid normalization of amylase levels (8), and in some patients with hyperlipidemia for whom accuracty in measuring amylase values requires serial dilution of serum before testing. To overcome biases in previous studies, which have used the amylase level in identifying patients with disease, recent investigations of the operating characteristics have used independent criteria to make the diagnosis (8–13). Typical results (Table 18-2) from such studies show sensitivity of 73% to 87% and specificity of 84% to 92% when cutoff levels are optimized (12,14,15).

In spite of earlier claims that measurement of urinary amylase concentration or clearance has greater sensitivity and specificity than that of serum amylase in diagnosing acute pancreatitis (16), more recent studies refute these claims, indicating no role for these measurements (8,11,12).

Amylase Isoenzymes

Two amylase isoenzymes exist, P-type from the pancreas, which comprises approximately 40% of total serum amylase, and S-type from the salivary gland and other organs, especially the fallopian tubes, which comprises about 60% of total serum amylase. Amylase isoenzyme fractionation has not gained wide acceptance because of its greater complexity, limited availability, and only marginal improvement in operating characteristics over serum amylase and lipase (17).

Lipase

The pancreas is the major source of serum lipase, but serum lipase is also found in the stomach, tongue, and liver (17). Lipase levels are elevated in patients with acute pancreatitis generally more than five times the upper reference limit. However, smaller elevations, generally less than three times the upper reference limit, can be seen in patients with ruptured aortic aneurysms, cholelithiasis, choledo-

Table 18-2. Operating Characteristics of Serum Amylase and Lipase Levels in the Diagnosis of Acute Pancreatitis

Diagnostic Test	Sensitivity	Specificity	Likelihood Ratio	
			Positive Result	Negative Result
	←———— % ————→			
Serum amylase measurement	82	91	9.1	0.20
Serum lipase measurement	94	96	24	0.06

cholithiasis, small bowel obstruction, nephrolithiasis, and macroli-pasemia (18). As reviewed by Gumaste (17), recent data suggest that serum lipase is more sensitive and specific in diagnosing acute pancreatitis than serum amylase. Typical sensitivity and specificity values using optimized cutoffs are 94% and 96%, respectively (see Table 18-2). Another advantage of lipase measurement over amylase measurement is seen in patients with "late" presentation, because serum lipase levels normalize more slowly than amylase levels (8). Additionally, the methodologic difficulties previously associated with serum lipase determinations have been largely resolved, resulting in assays that are rapid and inexpensive and that ensure high selectivity for pancreatic lipase.

New Diagnostic Tests

Serum human pancreas-specific protein, urinary trypsinogen-2, and serum trypsin-2/α_1-antitrypsin complex have demonstrated great potential in preliminary studies as markers of acute pancreatitis (19–21). However, further work needs to be done to validate the use of these assays.

Severity and Etiologic Assessment

After the diagnosis of acute pancreatitis, the severity of the disease must be assessed. Amylase and lipase elevations may not correlate with disease severity. Disease severity can be assessed using a combination of biochemical and clinical criteria such as the Ranson criteria, the Glasgow system, and the Acute Physiology and Chronic Health Evaluation (APACHE) II system (22–24). Elevations in other markers have also been demonstrated to correlate with clinical outcome (22); the most well known of these is the acute phase protein, C-reactive protein (CRP). Other markers include interleukin 6 (IL-6), polymorphonuclear elastase, trypsinogen activation peptide, and phospholipase A_2. Additional, more recent potential markers of severity include pancreatitis-associated protein (25), IL-8 and β_2-microglobulin (26), trypsin-2/α_1-antitrypsin complex (21), and trypsinogen-2 (20). At present, only the CRP assay is widely available. The potential clinical utility of these markers remains to be determined.

Appropriate clinical management of acute pancreatitis is aided by the knowledge of its causes. This is especially true for gallstone pancreatitis. In general, amylase levels are markedly elevated in gallstone pancreatitis and only moderately elevated in alcoholic pancreatitis, whereas the relation is reversed for lipase (17). Gumaste has proposed the lipase/amylase ratio with a cutoff value of two to distinguish alcoholic from gallstone pancreatitis; although subsequent studies have not supported this cutoff value, the general trend seems to be established (17). Elevations in serum alanine aminotransferase have also been reported to be highly diagnostic of gallstone pancreatitis (27).

DIAGNOSTIC STRATEGIES

When clinical findings suggest acute pancreatitis, the testing strategy is straightforward. A serum lipase determination is the initial test of choice. An elevated level is presumptive evidence of acute pancreatitis (Table 18-3); the higher the level, the greater the certainty of the diagnosis. A negative assay for lipase virtually excludes the diagnosis, except when the pretest probability of disease is high.

Except when the lipase assay is unavailable or when information about the cause of the pancreatitis is sought, there seems little reason to measure serum amylase in the evaluation of patients in whom acute pancreatitis is suspected. If it is used, however, caution should be exercised, especially in patients who may be well into the clinical course of the disease before diagnosis, owing to the decreasing sensitivity of amylase levels over time (8). Hyperamylasemia in the presence of vague clinical symptoms may be indicative of macroamylasemia rather than of pancreatitis, particularly when sequential samples fail to show the expected decline. In this instance, measurement of the amylase/creatinine ratio may be useful, with lower than normal ratios associated with macroamylasemia.

Because of the ready availability of simple, rapid, and relatively inexpensive serum amylase and lipase assays, one may question whether ordering both tests simultaneously is advantageous. One study showed that combining amylase and lipase results using an "AND" or an "OR" rule is not helpful in discriminating acute pancreatitis from other causes of abdominal pain (12). Another study showed that combining the tests using discriminant functions resulted in only marginal improvement in operating characteristics compared with

Table 18-3. Post-test Probabilities for Diagnostic Tests in the Diagnosis of Acute Pancreatitis

Diagnostic Test	Pretest Probability					
	20%		50%		80%	
	Positive Result	Negative Result	Positive Result	Negative Result	Positive Result	Negative Result
	←——————————————— % ———————————————→					
Amylase	69	5	90	17	97	44
Lipase	85	1	96	6	99	19

using the lipase assay alone (15). Therefore, no clear advantage is gained by simultaneously ordering both tests.

Imaging techniques, especially ultrasonography and computed tomography, are second-level tests that are most useful for the staging and assessment of the complications of acute pancreatitis.

CLINICAL PROBLEMS

Clinical Problem 1

A patient with gallstones develops persistent abdominal pain suggestive of pancreatitis.

Testing Strategy and Rationale

The pretest probability of acute pancreatitis in a patient with gallstones and abdominal pain radiating to the back is significant and consistent with the well-known etiologic relation between the two. A serum lipase determination is the preferred test, because the amylase level may be normal if the patient presents after the acute symptoms begin to subside.

Clinical Example

A 65-year-old woman who has recently had a myocardial infarction is admitted with right upper quadrant pain radiating to the back. In the course of multiple recent admissions, including several for jaundice, the patient was found to have gallstones. Surgery had been postponed because of the recent myocardial infarction. A serum lipase assay was ordered at admission and was found to be elevated at 1500 U/L (normal range, 0 to 208 U/L). The lipase level is followed and returns to normal within 3 days, which is consistent with acute pancreatitis.

Clinical Problem 2

A patient who has sustained a traumatic injury has an elevated amylase level.

Testing Strategy and Rationale

An elevated serum amylase level is expected in a patient with significant trauma, owing to the wide tissue distribution of amylase (e.g., salivary glands, fallopian tube). To rule out traumatic pancreatitis, a lipase assay should be ordered because of its higher specificity for acute pancreatitis.

Clinical Example

A 31-year-old woman with no history of pancreatic disease is admitted with multiple injuries, including head injuries, which were sustained when she was involved in a motorcycle collision. She is semiconscious and reports that she has severe abdominal pain but is otherwise stable. She is found to have an ethanol level of 185 mg/dL and an amylase level of 261 U/L (normal, 0 to 110 U/L). Her lipase level is 1031 U/L (normal, 0 to 208 U/L). Monitoring and treatment for pancreatitis are instituted. A normal lipase level would have indicated that organs other than the pancreas were the source of the elevated amylase level.

REFERENCES

1. **Steinberg W, Tenner S.** Acute pancreatitis. N Engl J Med. 1994; 330:1198-210.

2. **Marshall JB.** Acute pancreatitis: a review with emphasis on new developments. Arch Intern Med. 1993;153:1185-98.

3. **Read G, Braganza JM, Howat NT.** Pancreatitis: a retrospective study. Gut. 1976;17:945-52.

4. **Jacobs ML, Daggett WM, Civetta JM, et al.** Acute pancreatitis: analysis of factors influencing survival. Ann Surg. 1977;185:43-51.

5. **Elman R, Arneson N, Graham E.** Value of blood amylase estimation in the diagnosis of pancreatic disease: a clinical study. Arch Surg. 1929;19:943-67.

6. **Salt WB, Scherber S.** Amylase: its clinical significance: a review of the literature. Medicine. 1976;55:269-89.

7. **Howat HT, Braganza JM.** Assessment of pancreatic dysfunction in man. In: Howat HT, Surle H, eds. The Exocrine Pancreas. Philadelphia: WB Saunders; 1979:129-75.

8. **Gwozdz GP, Steinberg WM, Werner M, et al.** Comparative evaluation of the diagnosis of acute pancreatitis based on serum and urine enzyme assays. Clin Chim Acta. 1990;187:243-54.

9. **Lott JH, Patel ST, Sawhney AK, et al.** Assays of serum lipase: analytical and clinical considerations. Clin Chem. 1986;32:1290-302.

10. **Lott JA, Ellison EC, Applegate D.** The importance of objective data in the diagnosis of pancreatitis. Clin Chim Acta. 1989;183:33-40.

11. **Werner M.** Strategies to integrate laboratory information into the clinical diagnosis of hepatic and acute pancreatic disease. Prog Clin Biochem Med. 1989;8:175.

12. **Werner M, Steinberg WM, Pauley C.** Strategic use of individual and combined enzyme indicators for acute pancreatitis analyzed by receiver-operator characteristics. Clin Chem. 1989;35:967-71.

13. **Ventrucci V, Pezzilli R, Gullo L, et al.** Role of serum pancreatic enzyme assays in diagnosis of pancreatic diseases. Dig Dis Sci. 1989;34:39-45.

14. **Steinberg WM, Goldstein SS, Davis ND, et al.** Diagnostic assays in acute pancreatitis. Ann Intern Med. 1985;102:576-80.

15. **Corsetti JP, Cox C, Schulz TJ, Arvan DA.** Combined serum amylase and lipase determinations for diagnosis of suspected acute pancreatitis. Clin Chem. 1993;39:2495-99.

16. **Levitt MD, Johnson SG.** Is the CAm/Ccr ratio of value for the diagnosis of pancreatitis. Gastroenterology. 1978;75:118-9.

17. **Gumaste VV.** Diagnostic tests for acute pancreatitis. Gastroenterologist. 1994;2:119-30.

18. **Gumaste VV, Roditis N, Mehta D, Dave P.** Serum lipase levels in non-pancreatic abdominal pain versus acute pancreatitis. Am J Gastroenterol. 1993;88:2051-5.

19. **Pezzilli R, Billi P, Plate L, et al.** Human pancreas-specific protein/procarboxypeptidase B: a useful serum marker of acute pancreatitis. Digestion. 1994;55:73-7.

20. **Hedstrom J, Sainio V, Kemppainen E, et al.** Urine trypsinogen-2 as marker of acute pancreatitis. Clin Chem. 1996;42:685-90.

21. **Hedstrom J, Sainio V, Kemppainen E, et al.** Serum complex of trypsin-2 and alpha-1-antitrypsin as diagnostic and prognostic marker of acute pancreatitis: clinical study in consecutive patients. BMJ. 1996;313:333-7.

22. **Formela LJ, Galloway SW, Kingsnorth AN.** Inflammatory mediators in acute pancreatitis. Br J Surg. 1995;82:6-13.

23. **Larvin M, McMahon MJ.** APACHE-II score for assessment and monitoring of acute pancreatitis. Lancet. 1989;2:201-5.

24. **Wilson C, Heath DI, Imrie CW.** Prediction of outcome in acute pancreatitis: a comparative study of APACHE II, clinical assessment and multiple factor scoring systems. Br J Surg. 1990; 77:1260-4.

25. **Iovanna JL, Kein N, Norback I, et al.** Serum levels of pancreatitis-associated protein as indicators of the course of acute pancreatitis. Gastroenterology. 1994;106:728-34.

26. **Pezzilli R, Billi P, Miniero R, et al.** Serum interleukin-6, interleukin-8, and β_2-microglobulin in early assessment of severity of acute pancreatitis. Dig Dis Sci. 1995;40:2341-8.

27. **Kazmierczak SC, Catrou PG, Van Lente F.** Enzymatic markers of gallstone-induced pancreatitis identified by ROC curve analysis, discriminant analysis, logistic regression, likelihood ratios, and information theory. Clin Chem. 1995;41:523-31.

Pancreatic Masses 19

Robert J. Panzer, MD

KEY POINTS

Pretest Probabilities

- With acute pancreatitis, the differential diagnosis for a possible pancreatic mass is dominated by the pancreatic pseudocyst, with abscess and hemorrhage being less common complications.

- Major complications, primarily pancreatic pseudocysts, occur in approximately 10% of cases of acute pancreatitis but are clinically overt in fewer than 5%.

- Of patients with clinical evidence suggesting a mass complicating acute pancreatitis, nearly 50% have a complication, most often a pseudocyst.

- Ten to twenty percent of major complications of acute pancreatitis are pancreatic abscesses. Abscesses are more common in clinically severe acute pancreatitis.

- For findings consistent with chronic pancreatic disease, the differential diagnosis of a possible pancreatic mass is dominated by pancreatic cancer and chronic pancreatitis.

- Symptoms, signs, and basic laboratory tests do not routinely identify pancreatic cancer at an early stage. The prognosis of the disease is poor, even for patients with apparently resectable disease who are to undergo surgery.

- The findings of both a history of excessive alcohol intake and pancreatic calcification on a plain abdominal radiograph may obviate the need for further testing in some patients where chronic pancreatitis is highly suspected.

Diagnostic Strategies

- Pancreatic imaging studies are not necessary in every case of uncomplicated acute alcoholic pancreatitis.

- Ultrasonography is the test of choice for patients in whom complications are not evident but in whom the cause of uncomplicated acute pancreatitis is uncertain, making it necessary to rule out gallstones.

Continued

- Contrast computed tomography (CT) is the test of choice for identifying significant pancreatic pseudocysts or infections in clinically severe or otherwise complicated pancreatitis.

- Follow-up studies for pancreatic pseudocysts should be guided by the fact that pseudocysts that spontaneously resolve usually do so within 3 to 6 weeks after onset.

- Contrast CT is the most sensitive and specific noninvasive test for detection of pancreatic cancer.

- Endoscopic retrograde cholangiopancreatography is also sensitive and specific for pancreatic cancer, but because of its technical difficulty and invasiveness the most appropriate role of this test is the evaluation of equivocal CT findings and for patients needing only confirmation of chronic pancreatitis.

- Ultrasonography lacks sufficient sensitivity to serve as an initial test for pancreatic cancer, but in jaundiced patients and in patients in whom the probability of pancreatic cancer is high, it may be used as an alternative to CT. However, additional testing is needed in most patients for whom the results of ultrasonography are positive and in many for whom the results are negative. Endoscopic ultrasonography adds sensitivity and specificity, but this study is invasive, adding cost and time to the procedure.

BACKGROUND

In patients with acute pancreatitis, a variety of early changes commonly develop that generally have a benign prognosis: extrapancreatic fluid, pancreatic edema, or pancreatic phlegmon (1,2). More severe complications include hemorrhagic pancreatitis, pancreatic pseudocyst, and pancreatic infection including abscess, infected pseudocyst, or infected pancreatic necrosis. Such infections account for most deaths due to pancreatitis (3).

Pancreatic pseudocysts are the most frequent important complication of acute pancreatitis and are associated with high rates of morbidity and mortality. Any of the causes of pancreatitis (excessive alcohol intake, biliary tract diseases, or trauma) may result in pseudocyst formation. The common feature is disruption of a pancreatic duct, with leakage of pancreatic enzymes, causing pancreatic debris, secretions, and fluid to accumulate in the lesser sac or within the pancreas itself. The term "pseudocyst" refers to the fact that these collections do not have an epithelium-lined wall and therefore are not true cysts.

Pseudocysts result in death or serious morbidity through the occurrence of further complications: rupture, abscess formation, or hemorrhage. In older reported studies, such complications occurred in 30% or more of patients who had persistent pseudocysts that were treated without surgery (4,5). A series of similarly untreated patients would be difficult to assemble today, with operative or percutaneous drainage procedures more widely applied to known pseudocysts.

However, improved imaging tests show smaller and less symptomatic pseudocysts that are more likely to resolve than the large symptomatic pseudocysts that comprise most of those included in earlier studies. Pseudocysts that resolve usually do so by 3 weeks after onset, whereas spontaneous resolution is uncommon beyond 6 weeks (6).

For patients with chronic abdominal pain or unexplained weight loss, the possibility of pancreatic cancer arises in the differential diagnosis of such symptoms as chronic pancreatitis. The incidence of pancreatic cancer has been slowly rising; it became responsible for approximately 5% of cancer-related deaths by the beginning of the 1990s (7). The likelihood of pancreatic cancer increases with age, with most cases occurring after the age of 50 years and with the peak incidence in the seventh decade of life. It is somewhat more common in men and in black persons (8).

The evaluation of nonjaundiced patients with symptoms or signs suggestive of pancreatic cancer is included in this chapter, along with the differentiation of chronic pancreatitis from pancreatic cancer. See Chapter 15 for discussion of the approach to patients with obstructive jaundice. The diagnosis of functioning islet cell (usually benign) neoplasms is not directly addressed in this chapter.

The diagnostic approach to pancreatic cancer is dominated by its dismal prognosis. At the time of diagnosis, more than half of patients with ductal carcinoma have evidence of distant metastases and one fourth have evidence of locally invasive disease or lymph node involvement. Of those who appear to be candidates for surgical resection, at most about one third have truly resectable disease, of which only one third of cases are curable. Five-year survival rates in patients who have undergone surgery for cure have been low. The less common cystadenocarcinomas have a better prognosis (9). In contrast, cancer of the body and tail of the pancreas (one third of the total) is almost always unresectable owing to local or distant spread.

The goals of diagnostic testing for most patients in whom pancreatic cancer is suspected are to establish whether cancer is present and, if so, whether it is resectable. In some patients, the differential diagnosis includes chronic pancreatitis, and ruling in or ruling out this diagnosis is an important additional goal of testing. When the primary focus is on chronic pancreatitis, testing may be directed toward understanding anatomic changes, primarily to explain chronic pain and its possible treatment, or toward understanding functional changes, to explain endocrine (i.e., insulin) or exocrine (pancreatic enzyme) deficiency.

ESTIMATING PRETEST PROBABILITY

Clinically apparent pseudocysts occur in fewer than 5% of cases of acute pancreatitis. However, use of abdominal ultrasonography and similar tests show a true prevalence of about 10%, not including patients with early and less significant findings such as extrapancreatic fluid or pancreatic edema (4,6).

Of patients with signs and symptoms suggesting a complication of acute pancreatitis, 35% to 50% are actually found to have a complication (4,10). Most of these complications are pseudocysts, but about 10% to 20% of such clinically complicated cases involve a pancreatic abscess (6).

Clinical criteria that each identify patients with acute pancreatitis in whom the probability of pseudocyst is higher (as much as 50%) include 1) a palpable abdominal mass, 2) no clinical improvement within 1 week, 3) a persistent elevation of pancreatic enzyme levels, 4) displacement anteriorly of the stomach as detected on upper gastrointestinal barium series, or 5) evidence of intra-abdominal infection (4).

The symptoms and signs of pancreatic cancer are often nonspecific (11). The late stage of disease that is typical at the time of diagnosis suggests that clinical findings are absent or subtle during the early stages of the disease. The diagnosis should be suspected in patients older than age 50 years who have unexplained persistent abdominal pain or back pain, anorexia with loss of 10% of body weight, or jaundice. Although the approach to jaundice is discussed in Chapter 15, it should be noted that although approximately 50% of patients with pancreatic cancer are jaundiced at the time of diagnosis, less than one fourth have jaundice as the initial manifestation of the disease.

Of those patients reported in the literature who have been evaluated for suspected pancreatic disease (chronic symptoms rather than acute pancreatitis), approximately 15% to 25% (10,12,13) are found to have pancreatic cancer. In highly selected populations, this rate increases to 40% or higher (11,14). An additional 10% to 15% have a nonpancreatic abdominal malignancy (14,15). Ten to thirty percent of the population have chronic pancreatitis (10,13,16) as the cause of their suspicious symptoms. A picture of acute pancreatitis does not exclude the possibility of pancreatic cancer, because the two conditions coexist (17) in approximately 1.5% of patients with acute pancreatitis, primarily older patients with unexplained disease (18).

Once the possibility of chronic pancreatic disease has been suggested, clinical findings do not discriminate well between patients having pancreatic cancer, other abdominal malignancies, chronic pancreatitis, or other diseases. Anorexia, fatigue, light-colored stools, pruritus, weight loss, abdominal pain, or a change in bowel habits can occur in all these conditions (11). A history of pancreatitis is found in approximately 50% of patients with chronic pancreatitis, and as such, may increase the probability of this disease (11). However, the risk of pancreatic cancer is increased in patients with chronic pancreatitis; approximately 4% of patients evaluated for pancreatic disease and in whom abdominal radiography shows pancreatic calcification have had coexisting pancreatic carcinoma (19).

DIAGNOSTIC TESTS

Numerous tests are available to evaluate the pancreas. Many of these, such as measurement of serum enzymes, pancreatic function tests, and pancreatic radionuclide scanning, address primarily the question of whether pancreatic disease is present but not the specific nature of that disease (20). Some tests identify pancreatic masses but do not routinely determine whether pancreatic cancer is present or whether an apparent pancreatic cancer is resectable. Tests also vary in their ability to identify chronic pancreatitis. Athough newer approaches such as helical CT and endoscopic ultrasonography are reported to have higher sensitivity and specificity, accurate test characteristics from large, unbiased studies comparing different modalities in the same population are lacking in the published literature (21,22).

Blood Tests

The diagnosis of acute pancreatitis using measurement of serum enzymes (primarily the serum lipase and amylase assays) is discussed in Chapter 18.

Simple blood tests are rarely helpful in determining whether pancreatic cancer is present, although liver function tests are of some help in raising the possibility of hepatic metastases (see Chapter 17).

The serum amylase and lipase are normal in most patients with either pancreatic cancer or chronic pancreatitis, and abnormal results indicate probable pancreatic disease without differentiating among the possibilities.

Several assays have been suggested as helpful in identifying pancreatic cancer—for example, carcinoembryonic antigen (CEA) (11,15,23), carbohydrate antigen 19-9 (CA 19-9) (23), galactosyl transferase isoenzyme II (15), CA 50, and CA 242 (24). However, all of these tests have been studied primarily in patients with advanced cancer and have poor sensitivity (60%–80%), while having uncertain specificity because their evaluation usually lacks a sufficient range of patients in whom cancer is suspected but who are found not to have cancer on long-term follow-up.

For example, the results of the CEA assay are abnormal in one third to half of patients with pancreatic cancer (11,15), mostly those with more advanced cases. The results are positive in a large percent of patients without cancer, especially in patients who smoke, and in many patients with nongastrointestinal cancer. The results are also positive in patients with nonpancreatic gastrointestinal cancer as often as they are positive in patients with pancreatic cancer (15).

Tests of pancreatic secretion, stimulated or unstimulated, are of some value in measuring pancreatic function. However, these functional tests correlate poorly with the presence or absence of early disease and thus are of limited use in the early diagnosis of chronic pancreatitis or in the differentiation of chronic pancreatitis from pancreatic cancer (25).

Computed Tomography

Computed tomography is substantially more sensitive and specific than ultrasonography in detecting complications of acute pancreatitis (10,26). It also has a low rate of technically inadequate studies (27). Routine contrast CT (oral and intravenous) maximizes sensitivity and specificity. Computed tomography has a sensitivity of approximately 95% and a specificity of about 90% for pseudocysts (Table 19-1). Obesity tends to enhance accuracy, whereas in thin patients the lack of fat planes has the opposite effect.

Although not well quantified because of the lack of an independent standard, CT appears to identify a variety of pancreatic abnormalities other than pseudocyst more accurately than ultrasonography: pancreatic edema, intrapancreatic and extrapancreatic fluid collections, phlegmon, necrosis, abscess, and hemorrhage (28). Computed tomography can also guide needle aspiration of fluid collections to identify abscesses, infection of pseudocysts, or infection of pancreatic necrosis.

The sensitivity of CT for all pancreatic masses in general is at least 85%, and, unlike that of ultrasonography, this sensitivity is maintained in the identification of pancreatic cancer (10). Computed tomography is substantially more sensitive than ultrasonography for smaller lesions. Similarly, specificity is high (≥90%) (Table 19-2). Contrast-enhanced CT appears to have even higher sensitivity than the sensitivity of noncontrast CT in early studies—near 95% (29).

Computed tomography is the most appropriate initial test when carcinoma of the body or tail of the pancreas is suspected, as may be the case with many nonjaundiced patients in whom pancreatic cancer is suspected.

Computed tomography also is more sensitive for pancreatic calcifications than plain radiography, an advantage when chronic pancreatitis is part of the differential diagnosis. In one study, plain abdominal radiographs demonstrated calcifications in only half as many patients with chronic pancreatitis (18%) as did CT (36%) (30).

Helical CT allows more rapid acquisition of the CT image data. As a result, distortion caused by respiratory variation is reduced and higher levels of contrast during the imaging sequence occur, giving better visualization of blood vessels. This enhancement will likely allow CT

Table 19-1. Operating Characteristics of Imaging Tests for Pancreatic Pseudocysts

Diagnostic Test	Sensitivity	Specificity	Likelihood Ratio Positive Result	Negative Result
	← % →			
Ultrasonography				
Technically adequate	95	90	9.5	0.06
All studies	75	85	5.0	0.29
Computed tomography	95	90	9.5	0.06

Table 19-2. Operating Characteristics of Imaging Tests in the Diagnosis of Pancreatic Cancer

Diagnostic Test	Sensitivity	Specificity	Likelihood Ratio Positive Result	Negative Result
	← % →			
Ultrasonography	70 (67–90)	85 (78–96)	4.7	0.35
Computed tomography	85 (78–96)	90 (88–98)	8.5	0.17
ERCP (technically adequate)	95 (73–100)	97 (80 100)	32	0.05
Angiography	75 (72–83)	80 (68–95)	3.8	0.31

ERCP = endoscopic retrograde cholangiopancreatography.

to remain superior to other methods that have undergone their own improvements, such as endoscopic ultrasonography and evolving magnetic resonance imaging (MRI) (31).

Computed tomography sensitivity and specificity are much lower in determining resectability—in one study, 77% and 50%, respectively—when the unit of analysis is the lesion rather than the patient (32).

Ultrasonography

Technically adequate ultrasonography studies detect clinically important mass complications of acute pancreatitis with a sensitivity of more than 95% and a specificity of 80% to 90% (see Table 19-1) (6,10,26). However, ultrasonography less reliably determines whether the abnormality is a pancreatic pseudocyst, phlegmon, abscess, or area of necrosis. In addition, it misses many cases with lesser complications such as pancreatic edema or a small pseudocyst.

Ultrasonography has two advantages in the initial evaluation of patients with severe or apparently complicated acute pancreatitis: 1) it can identify gallstones in patients with pancreatitis not caused by excessive alcohol intake, and 2) a negative ultrasonography finding makes the presence of a clinically important pseudocyst unlikely.

An important limitation of ultrasonography is a high rate of inadequate or incomplete studies, with its usual 15% failure rate increasing to as much as 40% in cases of acute pancreatitis. This high failure rate is related both to the location of portions of the pancreas posterior to the stomach or large intestine and to the frequent occurrence in pancreatitis of ileus with increased intestinal gas. Most false-negative studies may be categorized as technically inadequate. If such technically inadequate studies are not further evaluated, the overall sensitivity of this test is only about 75% (28).

Technically adequate ultrasonography studies have a sensitivity of approximately 70% and a specificity of approximately 85% for the detection of pancreatic masses in patients evaluated for chronic symptoms possibly consistent with malignancy (10,14–16) (see Table 19-2). However, as with acute pancreatitis, 5% to 25% of studies are technically inadequate for a variety of reasons, such as obesity or excessive bowel gas (10,16).

Ultrasonography can both detect a pancreatic mass and correctly classify it as a probable carcinoma only 60% of the time (10,15). Thus, the test is unable to rule out pancreatic cancer reliably when that diagnosis is suspected. The lack of sensitivity is especially important when small, possibly resectable lesions are present.

The false-positive rate for ultrasonography is also substantial (approximately 15%), making it necessary for many positive findings to be confirmed by another imaging test. Despite its problems, certain ultrasonography results, such as the finding of both a pancreatic mass and apparent hepatic metastases, are sufficiently convincing to justify proceeding directly to a histologic diagnosis of cancer via biopsy.

Because of its role in evaluating the biliary tree, at present ultrasonography may be the initial test of choice in cases of suspected pancreatic cancer in which the patient presents with obstructive jaundice (see Chapter 15).

Ultrasonography may have fairly good sensitivity (85%–90%) and specificity (near 100%) for chronic pancreatitis when measured against endoscopic retrograde cholangiopancreatography (ERCP) as the gold standard, but studies of its accuracy for this purpose are small and imperfect (33).

Endoscopic ultrasonography can better image the pancreas than normal abdominal ultrasonography, but published experience and evaluation of this technique compared with other techniques is limited (34). Although invasive, it may serve as an alternative to angiography in imaging blood vessel involvement and may offer value in the preoperative staging of patients who are being considered for resection.

Endoscopic Retrograde Cholangiopancreatography

Endoscopic retrograde cholangiopancreatography is a highly sensitive and specific test for the diagnosis of pancreatic duct abnormalities, such as those seen with pancreatic cancer or chronic pancreatitis. It is also accurate in identifying pseudocysts, but it has little to offer as an initial test in cases of acute pancreatitis with a suspected pseudocyst, because it is invasive with potential infectious complications and has a significant rate of test failure. See Chapters 14 and 15 for further discussion of ERCP in the evaluation of biliary tract disease.

Technically successful ERCP has a high sensitivity (approximately 95%) and specificity (approximately 97%) for pancreatic cancer (see Table 19-1), because most such cancers are of ductal origin and it is the anatomy of pancreatic ducts that ERCP defines (13–15,35,36). This test is also sensitive for smaller, more curable cancers (37). However, ERCP is expensive, invasive, and technically difficult to perform, with failure rates of 5% to 25% (13–15,32). It may precipitate acute pancreatitis in 2% to 5% of patients (38). Also, it cannot determine the full extent of disease and thus, unlike CT, does not address the issues of whether metastases are present or whether a lesion is resectable. The test may be most appropriate when CT has failed to identify the site or nature of disease in nonjaundiced patients or when evaluation is focused on identifying ductal abnormalities in cases of highly suspected chronic pancreatitis.

Percutaneous Fine-Needle Biopsy

Percutaneous pancreatic fine-needle biopsy is a highly specific test for pancreatic cancer but is insensitive when rates of success in obtaining tissue are taken into account (39–42). With ultrasonography guidance, sensitivity is approximately 70% to 80% (43–45). Computed tomography–guided biopsy also improves accuracy. It is an important confirmatory procedure in many patients with ultrasonography- or CT-demonstrated masses of the body or tail of the pancreas. However, overt evidence of a pancreatic mass and hepatic metastases may eliminate the need for histologic confirmation in some patients.

Plain Abdominal Radiography

Plain abdominal radiography does not directly address the issue of pancreatic cancer. However, the finding on abdominal radiography of pancreatic calcifications may obviate the need for further testing in some patients by confirming a highly suspected diagnosis of chronic pancreatitis. The finding of pancreatic calcification is considered specific for chronic pancreatitis; 1.5% of patients with pancreatic cancer have calcification, giving a specificity of 98.5% (18,46). However, it is not sensitive: CT detects calcification in twice as many patients as does plain radiography, and approximately 50% of patients with alcohol-related chronic pancreatitis and even more with gallstone-related chronic pancreatitis lack calcifications (13,31). Pancreatic calcification also correlates poorly with the presence and degree of pancreatic insufficiency (47).

Other Tests

Upper gastrointestinal barium x-ray studies provide limited direct information about the possibility of a pancreatic pseudocyst or cancer. The finding of a mass effect (e.g., anterior displacement of the stomach) is an insensitive indicator of a pancreatic mass (sensitivity <50%). Nevertheless, in some patients the diagnosis of pancreatic cancer becomes unlikely through the ruling in of an alternative explanation of the patient's symptoms (e.g., a posterior penetrating ulcer).

Angiography now has a limited role because it is not as specific for pancreatic cancer as biopsy and because it is no more sensitive overall than the less invasive CT for answering initial questions about resectability (48,49) (see Table 19-2). It does address more directly the issue of blood vessel involvement with a cancer that may be important to surgical planning for patients evaluated for resection.

As yet, MRI does not have a primary role in the evaluation of patients with possible pancreatic pseudocyst or cancer for either diagnosis or determination of resectability (32). Its operating characteristics are likely close to those of CT but at higher cost (50).

Positron-emission tomography (PET) is not widely available and has not been studied in this population in broad-based studies. Early studies in limited numbers of patients suggest that PET may be equal or superior to CT (51,52).

DIAGNOSTIC STRATEGIES

Because clinically important pancreatic pseudocysts occur in only about 10% of patients with acute pancreatitis and because most of those that are significant are evident using basic clinical information, routine pancreatic imaging to detect pseudocyst formation is not necessary. Imaging is appropriate in uncomplicated cases if the cause is in doubt, as in patients with a first episode of pancreatitis or in those with no history of alcohol abuse when gallstones have not been excluded. Recurrences not clearly related to alcohol abuse do require evaluation.

Although ultrasonography is less accurate than CT in evaluating unselected pancreatic masses, the sensitivity and specificity of a technically adequate ultrasonographic study for clinically important pseudocysts are excellent (approximately 95% and 90%, respectively).

Ultrasonography is, therefore, the test of choice for patients with a suspected uncomplicated pseudocyst. For those patients found to have a pseudocyst, a follow-up study 3 to 6 weeks later can determine whether spontaneous resolution is likely.

When the etiology of pancreatitis is in doubt, ultrasonography can also simultaneously evaluate (with high sensitivity and specificity) patients for gallstones (see Chapter 14).

Computed tomography offers the greatest accuracy in discriminating between the various complications of acute pancreatitis. This issue becomes important in the assessment of severely ill patients with shock and possible hemorrhagic pancreatitis, or in the evaluation of patients with delayed fever and possible pancreatic abscess, infected pseudocyst, or infected pancreatic necrosis.

Computed tomography is also appropriate for pursuing the diagnosis of pseudocyst when ultrasonography is nondiagnostic owing to excess bowel gas or is otherwise technically inadequate (Table 19-3).

The diagnostic evaluation of a patient with chronic symptoms or signs of possible pancreatic cancer has several goals. Determining whether pancreatic disease is present is only a first step: Testing must establish whether a pancreatic mass is present, whether a mass represents pancreatic cancer, and whether a cancer is likely to be resectable.

Clinical symptoms, signs, and blood tests are both insensitive and nonspecific. Therefore, imaging tests are required to evaluate virtually all patients with clinically suspected pancreatic cancer.

For nonjaundiced patients considered to have possible pancreatic cancer, CT offers the best diagnostic yield after the basic clinical evaluation has been performed. It is sufficiently sensitive to identify many

Table 19-3. Post-test Probabilities of Pancreatic Pseudocysts Based on the Results of Imaging Tests

Diagnostic Test	Pretest Probabilities					
	20%		50%		80%	
	Positive Result	Negative Result	Positive Result	Negative Result	Positive Result	Negative Result
	←			%		→
Ultrasonography						
Technically adequate	70	1	90	5	97	18
All studies	56	7	83	23	95	54
Computed tomography	70	1	90	5	97	18

(but not all) small cancers, some of which may be curable. Its overall specificity is high (see Table 19-2), and some findings are virtually diagnostic (e.g., the combination of a pancreatic mass and evidence of hepatic metastases). For these reasons, it is the test of choice at low and intermediate probabilities of pancreatic cancer. However, the high cost of false-positive diagnoses in some situations suggests that confirmation of the diagnosis is still needed after many positive CT results (Table 19-4). Percutaneous fine-needle biopsy of the pancreas can provide histologic proof of the nature of isolated pancreatic masses, and ERCP can confirm the presence of a ductal carcinoma suggested by more subtle CT findings.

Ultrasonography has a limited role in diagnosis of pancreatic cancer. It is insensitive, especially for smaller lesions, and cannot rule out disease at low or intermediate pretest probabilities (see Table 19-4). At very high pretest probabilities, such as cases with a palpable mass or overt hepatic metastases, it may suffice to confirm already strong impressions.

Endoscopic retrograde cholangiopancretography has the best operating characteristics for determining the presence or absence of ductal carcinoma. However, it is invasive with a significant complication rate, and has a technical failure rate ranging widely from less than 5% to more than 25%. In addition, unlike CT, it does not uniformly address resectability. It is highly accurate in diagnosing chronic pancreatitis and may be the test of choice when the differential diagnosis is limited to chronic pancreatitis compared with pancreatic cancer and plain abdominal radiography has not demonstrated pancreatic calcifications, or when the simultaneous existence of both chronic pancreatitis and pancreatic cancer is a possibility.

Table 19-4. Post-test Probabilities of Pancreatic Cancer Based on the Results of Imaging Tests

Diagnostic Test	Pretest Probabilities					
	20%		50%		80%	
	Positive Result	Negative Result	Positive Result	Negative Result	Positive Result	Negative Result
	←		%			→
Ultrasonography	54	8	82	26	95	59
Computed tomography	68	4	89	14	97	40
ERCP	89	1	97	5	99	17
Angiography	48	7	79	24	94	56

ERCP = endoscopic retrograde cholangiopancreatography.

CLINICAL PROBLEMS

Clinical Problem 1
A patient with acute pancreatitis has a prolonged course, a palpable abdominal mass, persistent pancreatic enzyme elevation, or other indications of a possible pseudocyst.

Testing Strategy and Rationale
Abdominal ultrasonography should be performed; if a pseudocyst is demonstrated, this study should be repeated in 3 to 6 weeks. If the ultrasonography is technically inadequate, CT should be done. Among patients with clinical findings suggesting a pseudocyst, approximately 50% are found to have one. Most such clinically important masses are readily detectable by ultrasonography. However, in the setting of acute pancreatitis, suboptimal ultrasonographic studies are common and should be followed by CT if diagnostic issues are not clearly answered by the available information from ultrasonography.

Clinical Example
A 40-year-old man presents with severe abdominal pain a few days after a prolonged drinking binge. The serum lipase level is markedly elevated, as had occurred with his last episode of pancreatitis 2 years earlier. After 7 days, he still has abdominal pain and an elevated pancreatic enzyme level. The probability of a pseudocyst in this patient is approximately 40% to 50%, and abdominal ultrasonography should be performed.

CLINICAL PROBLEM 2
An elderly patient has symptoms suggesting the possibility of pancreatic cancer.

Testing Strategy and Rationale
If basic laboratory testing is not helpful by identifying an alternative diagnosis, the possibility of pancreatic cancer should be pursued with contrast abdominal CT and further testing should be individualized. Of all patients evaluated for possible chronic pancreatic disease, approximately 15% to 25% are found to have pancreatic cancer. In patients whose symptoms are nonspecific, the likelihood of pancreatic cancer is probably at best near this range. Computed tomography has good sensitivity and specificity for pancreatic cancer (see Table 19-2).

Clinical Example
A 70-year-old man presents with a 3-month history of midabdominal pain unrelated to eating and a weight loss of 15 lb. He has

Continued

never been a heavy alcohol consumer. Physical examination is unremarkable. Laboratory studies show minimal anemia but normal liver and thyroid function. Earlier, treatment with an H_2 blocker had not affected his abdominal pain, and plain abdominal radiography did not show pancreatic calcifications.

The probability of pancreatic cancer is estimated to be low but significant (approximately 20%), given the presence of only nonspecific symptoms. Computed tomography is the test of choice for identifying whether a pancreatic mass is present and, if so, whether the patient has hepatic metastases. Guided percutaneous needle biopsy would be appropriate for histologic identification of any masses found at a site that could be biopsied.

REFERENCES

1. **Hunter TB, Habor K, Pond GD.** Phlegmon of the pancreas. Am J Gastroenterol. 1982;77:949-52.
2. **Siegelman SS, Copeland BE, Saba GP, et al.** CT of fluid collections associated with pancreatitis. AJR. 1980;134:1121-32.
3. **Lumsden A, Bradley EL.** Secondary pancreatic infections. Surg Gynecol Obstet. 1990;170:459-67.
4. **Bradley EL, Gonzalez, AC, Clements JL Jr.** Acute pancreatic pseudocysts: incidence and implications. Ann Surg. 1976; 184:734-7.
5. **Sankaran S, Walt AJ.** The natural and unnatural history of pancreatic pseudocysts. Br J Surg. 1975;62:37-44.
6. **Bradley EL, Clements JL, Gonzalez AC.** The natural history of pancreatic pseudocysts: a unified concept of management. Am J Surg. 1979;137:135-41.
7. **Silverberg E, Lubera JA.** Cancer statistics, 1989. CA Cancer J Clin. 1989;39: 3-20.
8. **McMahon B.** Risk factors for cancer of the pancreas. Cancer. 1982;50:2676-80.
9. **Cubilla AL, Fitzgerald PJ.** Cancer of the exocrine pancreas: the pathologic aspects. CA Cancer J Clin.1985;35:2-18.
10. **Hessel SJ, Siegelman SS, McNeil BJ, et al.** A prospective evaluation of computed tomography and ultrasound of the pancreas. Radiology. 1982; 143:129-33.
11. **Fitzgerald PJ, Fortner JG, Watson RC, et al.** The value of diagnostic aids in detecting pancreas cancer. Cancer. 1978;41:868-79.
12. **Freeny PC, Ball TJ.** Rapid diagnosis of pancreatic carcinoma. Radiology. 1978;127:627-33.
13. **Moss AA, Federle M, Shapiro, HA, et al.** The combined use of computed tomography and endoscopic retrograde cholangiopancreatography in the assessment of suspected pancreatic neoplasm: a blind clinical evaluation. Radiology. 1980;134:159-63.
14. **Mackie CR, Cooper MJ, Lewis MH, Moossa AR.** Non-operative differentiation between pancreatic cancer and chronic pancreatitis. Ann Surg. 1979; 189:480-7.

15. **Podolsky DK, McPhee MS, Albert E, et al.** Galactosyltransferase isoenzyme II in the detection of pancreatic cancer: comparison with radiologic, endoscopic, and serologic tests. N Engl J Med. 1981;304:1313-8.

16. **Cotton PB, Lees WR, Vallon AG, et al.** Gray-scale ultrasonography and endoscopic pancreatography in pancreatic diagnosis. Radiology. 1980;134:453-9.

17. **Bansal P, Sonnenberg A.** Pancreatitis is a risk factor for pancreatic cancer. Gastroenterology. 1995;109:247-51.

18. **Lin A, Feller ER.** Pancreatic carcinoma as a cause of unexplained pancreatitis: report of ten cases. Ann Intern Med. 1990;113:166-7.

19. **Ring EJ, Eaton SB, Ferrucci JT, Short WF.** Differential diagnosis of pancreatic calcification. Am J Roentgenol. 1973;117:446-52.

20. **Dimagno EP, Malagelada JR, Taylor WF, Go VLW.** A prospective comparison of current diagnostic tests for pancreatic cancer. N Engl J Med. 1977; 297:737-42.

21. **Riker A, Libutti SK, Bartlett DL.** Advances in the early detection, diagnosis, and staging of pancreatic cancer. Surg Oncol. 1997;6:157-69.

22. **Moossa AR, Gamagami RA.** Diagnosis and staging of pancreatic neoplasms. Surg Clin North Am. 1995;75:871-90.

23. **Satake K, Kanazawa G, Kho I, et al.** Evaluation of serum pancreatic enzymes, carbohydrate antigen 19-9, and carcinoembryonic antigen in various pancreatic diseases. Am J Gastroenterol. 1985;80:630-6.

24. **Pasanen PA, Eskelinen M, Partanen K, et al.** Receiver operating characteristic (ROC) curve analysis of the tumour markers CEA, CA 50 and CA 242 in pancreatic cancer: results from a prospective study. Br J Cancer. 1993;67:852-5.

25. **Boyd EJS, Wormsley KG.** Laboratory tests in the diagnosis of the chronic pancreatic diseases. Part I and II. Int J Pancreatol. 1987;2:137-48, 211-21.

26. **Williford ME, Foster WL Jr, Halvorsen RA, et al.** Pancreatic pseudocyst: comparative evaluation by sonography and computed tomography. Am J Roentgenol. 1983;140:53-7.

27. **VanSonnenberg E, Casola G, Varney RR, Wittich GR.** Imaging and interventional radiology for pancreatitis and its complications. Radiol Clin North Am. 1989;27:65-72.

28. **Block S, Maier W, Bittner R, et al.** Identification of pancreas necrosis in severe acute pancreatitis: imaging procedures versus clinical staging. Gut. 1986;27:1035-42.

29. **Freeny PC.** Radiologic diagnosis and staging of pancreatic ductal adenocarcinoma. Radiol Clin North Am. 1989;27:121-8.

30. **Ferrucci JT, Wittenberg J, Black EB, et al.** Computed body tomography in chronic pancreatitis. Radiology. 1979;130:175-82.

31. **Zeman RK, Silverman PM, Ascher SM, et al.** Helical (spiral) CT of the pancreas and biliary tract. Radiol Clin North Am. 1995;33:887-902.

32. **Megibow AJ, Zhou XH, Rotterdam H, et al.** Pancreatic adenocarcinoma: CT versus MR imaging in the evaluation of resectability: report of the Radiology Diagnostic Oncology Group. Radiology. 1995;195:327-32.

33. **Jones SN, Lees WR, Frost RA.** Diagnosis and grading of chronic pancreatitis by morphological criteria derived by ultrasound and pancreatography. Clin Radiol. 1988;39:43-8.

34. **Nakaizumi A, Uehara H, Iishi H, et al.** Endoscopic ultrasonography in diagnosis and staging of pancreatic cancer. Dig Dis Sci. 1995;40:696-700.

35. **Ralls PW, Halls J, Renner I, Juttner H.** Endoscopic retrograde cholangiopancreatography (ERCP) in pancreatic disease. Radiology. 1980;134:347-52.

36. **Freeny PC, Ball TJ.** Evaluation of endoscopic retrograde cholangiopancreatography and angiography in the diagnosis of pancreatic carcinoma. AJR Am J Roentgenol. 1978;130:683-91.

37. **Ariyama J, Shirakabe H, Ikenobe H, et al.** The diagnosis of the small resectable pancreatic carcinoma. Clin Radiol. 1977;28:437-44.

38. **Stanten R, Frey CF.** Pancreatitis after endoscopic retrograde cholangiopancreatography. Arch Surg. 1990;125:1032-5.

39. **Wittenberg J, Mueller PR, Ferrucci JT, et al.** Percutaneous core biopsy of abdominal tumors using 22 gauge needles. AJR Am J Roentgenol. 1982;139:75-80.

40. **Beazley RM.** Needle biopsy diagnosis of pancreatic cancer. Cancer. 1981;47:1685-7.

41. **Sundaram M, Wolverson MK, Heiberg E, et al.** Utility of CT-guided abdominal aspiration procedures. AJR Am J Roentgenol. 1982;139:1111-5.

42. **Harter LP, Moss AA, Goldberg HI, Gross BH.** CT-guided fine-needle aspirations for diagnosis of benign and malignant disease. AJR Am J Roentgenol. 1983;140:363-7.

43. **Bret PM, Nicolet V, Labadie M.** Percutaneous fine-needle aspiration biopsy of the pancreas. Diagn Cytopathol. 1986;2:221-7.

44. **Bognel C, Rougier P, Leclere J, et al.** Fine needle aspiration of the liver and pancreas with ultrasound guidance. Acta Cytol. 1988;32:22-6.

45. **Athlin L, Blind PJ, Angstrom T.** Fine-needle aspiration biopsy of pancreatic masses. Acta Chir Scand. 1990;156:91-4.

46. **Paulino-Netto A, Dreiling DA, Baronofsky ID.** The relationship between pancreatic calcification and cancer of the pancreas. Ann Surg. 1960;151:530-7.

47. **Lankisch PG, Otto J, Erkelenz I, Lembcke B.** Pancreatic calcifications: no indicator of severe exocrine pancreatic insufficiency. Gastroenterology. 1986;90:617-21.

48. **Mackie CR, Lu CT, Noble HG, et al.** Prospective evaluation of angiography in the diagnosis and management of patients suspected of having pancreatic cancer. Ann Surg. 1979;189:11-7.

49. **Jafri SZ, Aisen AM, Glazer GM, Weiss CA.** Comparison of CT and angiography in assessing resectability of pancreatic carcinoma. AJR Am J Roentgenol. 1984;142:525-9.

50. **Bluemke DA, Fishman EK.** CT and MR evaluation of pancreatic cancer. Surg Oncol Clin North Am. 1998;7:103-24.

51. **Inokuma T, Tamaki N, Torizuka T, et al.** Evaluation of pancreatic tumors with positron emission tomography and F-18 fluorodeoxyglucose: comparison with CT and US. Radiology. 1995;195:345-52.

52. **Hawkins RA.** Pancreatic tumors: imaging with PET [Editorial; Comment]. Radiology. 1995;195:320-2.

Infectious Disease Problems

Sore Throat and Acute Infectious Mononucleosis in Adult Patients

20

Anthony L. Komaroff, MD

KEY POINTS

Pretest Probabilities

- In adults with sore throat, when neither fever, nor tonsillar exudate, nor anterior cervical adenopathy is present, the probability of streptococcal pharyngitis is very low (i.e., <3%).

- When all three of these findings are present, the probability of streptococcal pharyngitis is at least 40%.

- In patients with a culture or rapid strep test results that are negative for group A streptococci but who have persistent sore throat, or in patients with a culture that is positive for group A streptococci but who do not respond to antibacterial therapy, one should suspect infection with other potentially treatable pathogens, such as non–group A streptococci, *Mycoplasma pneumoniae*, *Chlamydia pneumoniae*, *Haemophilus influenzae*, and the gonococcus.

- Many patients with sore throat have a variety of viral infections that do not respond to any currently practical forms of antiviral therapy; and in 15% to 40% of patients, no viral or bacterial agent is identified despite exhaustive study.

- The full-blown acute infectious mononucleosis syndrome, usually caused by new infection with Epstein-Barr virus (EBV), can generally be distinguished on the basis of clinical findings from bacterial and other viral forms of pharyngitis. However, many cases of new EBV infection present as "common cold" syndromes with pharyngitis but without the classic findings of mononucleosis.

Continued

> ### Diagnostic Strategies
>
> - When the probability of streptococcal pharyngitis is very low, neither throat culture nor rapid streptococcal antigen testing is required unless special risk factors are present.
> - When the probability of streptococcal pharyngitis is high (e.g., >40%), immediate antibiotic treatment can be justified without performing culture or rapid strep tests.
> - At intermediate pretest probabilities of streptococcal infection, throat cultures and rapid strep tests are useful in guiding therapy.
> - Full throat culture, not restricted to only the recognition of beta-hemolytic streptococci, is preferred because it may identify other potentially treatable pathogens.
> - Rapid heterophil antibody tests and differential leukocyte counts are valuable when acute infectious mononucleosis is suspected, but antibody testing for EBV is generally unnecessary.

BACKGROUND

Clinical findings can be used to predict the presence or absence of pharyngitis caused by streptococcal infection or new Epstein-Barr virus (EBV) infection, with considerable accuracy. By estimating the probability of either of these infectious causes of pharyngitis in this manner, the clinician can be aided in making decisions about the use of diagnostic laboratory tests and in prescribing therapy.

The clinician traditionally has believed that the principal goal in caring for patients with a sore throat is to distinguish patients with streptococcal pharyngitis from all other patients—who have been assumed to have various forms of viral pharyngitis. Recent studies suggest, however, that several other forms of bacterial pharyngitis may occur frequently enough that the clinician should always keep them in mind. Infection with *Mycoplasma pneumoniae* and chlamydial organisms (particularly *Chlamydia pneumoniae*, formerly called the *TWAR agent*) may cause 5% to 30% of cases of pharyngitis (1,2). *Hemophilus influenzae* (3) and *Neisseria gonorrhoeae* (4) may each be the cause of pharyngitis in 1% to 2% of adult patients seeking primary care for a sore throat.

Studies of these potentially treatable forms of pharyngitis have not been nearly as extensive as studies of group A streptococcal pharyngitis. Therefore, discussion of clinical findings and diagnostic strategies related to these types of pharyngitis does not rest on the same solid ground as the discussion of group A streptococcal pharyngitis. Moreover, it has not been proved that antibacterial treatment speeds the resolution of symptoms and signs of any of these types of non-streptococcal pharyngitis, although the recognition of gonorrheal infection under any circumstances warrants immediate therapy.

ESTIMATING PRETEST PROBABILITY

Group A Streptococcal Pharyngitis

With the caveats to be noted subsequently, we define streptococcal pharyngitis as present in any patient with sore throat from whom group A streptococci are isolated. Several studies have demonstrated that group A streptococci are isolated on throat culture in 9% to 15% of adult patients seeking primary care for a sore throat (5–11). The frequency may be as high as 35% in children (5). During the 1980s, group A streptococcal infections in the United States became more virulent than they had been during the previous 30 years (12), but that phenomenon may now be on the wane.

Several prospective studies have evaluated the sensitivity and specificity of individual clinical findings in the diagnosis of streptococcal pharyngitis in adult patients (6–9). For most of the predictors, the findings of these studies are remarkably consistent. The combination of three findings—fever (>37.7 °C), tonsillar exudate, and anterior cervical adenopathy—does a good job of stratifying adult patients with suspected streptococcal pharyngitis. As summarized in Table 20-1, the probability of streptococcal isolation was only 3% in patients without any of the three findings, 14% in those with any one of the findings, and 42% in patients with all three findings. However, these post-test probability estimates would be increased or decreased in settings in which the prevalence (pretest probability) of streptococcal pharyngitis is higher or lower than the average of 9% to 15% reported in most studies.

Table 20-1. Probability of Group A Streptococcal Pharyngitis in Adult Patients Based on Clinical Findings

Clinical Findings	Probability* (%)
No anterior cervical adenopathy, no tonsillar exudate, and no temperature >37.7 °C	3
Either anterior cervical adenopathy or tonsillar exudate or temperature >37.7 °C	14
Anterior cervical adenopathy and tonsillar exudate and temperature >37.7 °C	42

*Presumes a prior probability (prevalence) of group A streptococcal infection to be 9%.
From Komaroff AL (unpublished data).

Another way of dealing with combinations of predictors is to perform a multivariate analysis and create a weight for individual findings. Such a streptococcal pharyngitis risk score has been developed (9) and is summarized in Table 20-2. It can be used to predict the likelihood of a positive culture for group A streptococci in adults using the nomogram shown in Figure 20-1.

Non–Group A Streptococcal Pharyngitis

Because non–group A streptococci only rarely produce nonsuppurative complications such as acute rheumatic fever or glomerulonephritis, they have traditionally been dismissed as "unimportant" when identified by throat culture from a patient with pharyngitis. However, non–group A streptococci are isolated more frequently than are the group A streptococci in adults with pharyngitis (13,14). Moreover, the isolation rate of non–group A streptococci among patients with symptomatic pharyngitis is much higher than among patients of comparable age and sex seeking medical care at the same medical facilities at the same time for conditions other than pharyngitis (14). Group C streptococci are most solidly established as pharyngeal pathogens (15,16). Furthermore, strong anecdotal experience, not yet confirmed by a controlled clinical trial, suggests that patients with pharyngitis from whom non–group A streptococci are isolated respond to antibacterial therapy.

Mycoplasmal and Chlamydial Pharyngitis

Mycoplasmal or chlamydial pharyngitis are two common forms of pharyngitis. Both should be considered in patients with a persistent sore throat with a negative culture for group A streptococci or in patients with a positive culture who do not respond to antibiotic treatment.

Table 20-2. Probability of Group A Streptococcal Pharyngitis Based on the Strep Score

Clinical Findings	Strep Score
Marked tonsillar exudate	+2
Pinpoint tonsillar exudate	+1
Enlarged tonsils	+1
Tender anterior cervical adenopathy (adenitis)	+1
Myalgia	+1
Positive throat culture in the past year	+1
Itchy eyes	−1

Adapted with permission from Komaroff AL, Pass TM, Aronson MD, et al. The prediction of streptococcal pharyngitis in adults. J Gen Intern Med. 1986; 1:1-7.

It has long been recognized that *M. pneumoniae* often causes pharyngitis at the same time it produces lower respiratory tract infection. In recent years, it has become clear that this organism can also produce a respiratory syndrome characterized predominantly by pharyngitis (1). Unfortunately, diagnostic testing for *M. pneumoniae* is difficult.

A recently discovered organism, *C. pneumoniae* (originally called *TWAR*), is an important respiratory tract pathogen in adults (17) that may explain 9% of cases of pharyngitis in adults (2). As with mycoplasmal

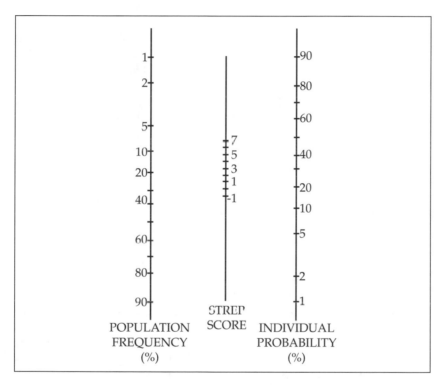

Figure 20-1. To use the nomogram, determine the overall frequency of positive cultures among all adult patients presenting with sore throat at the site. Second, add the "strep score" points based on the clinical findings to arrive at a score for an individual patient. Third, place a ruler on the figure so that it crosses the left line at the site frequency rate and the center line at a strep score value. The point where the ruler crosses the right line is the probability of a positive culture for that patient. As an example, if 20% of adult patients with sore throat at a site typically have positive cultures, and a patient in this group has a strep score of 5, then a straight line connecting 20% on the left line with 5 points on the center line crosses the right line at value of 55%, the likelihood of a positive culture for that patient. (Republished with permission from Komaroff AL, Pass TM, Aronson MD, et al. The prediction of streptococcal pharyngitis in adults. J Gen Intern Med. 1986;1:1-7.)

pharyngitis, patients with chlamydial pharyngitis often have concomitant bronchopulmonary symptoms. Infection may prove very difficult to eradicate, even with antibacterial agents to which the organism is sensitive in vitro (18).

Other Bacterial Pharyngitis

Hemophilus influenzae pharyngitis may cause 1% to 2% of cases of pharyngitis in adults (3,19). It should be suspected in patients with concomitant symptoms or signs of otitis media or cough. It probably also should be suspected in patients with persistent sore throat.

Neisseria gonorrhoeae may be the cause of pharyngitis in 1% of adult patients seeking primary care for a sore throat (4), although gonococcal infection of the pharynx is more often asymptomatic than symptomatic. Gonococcal pharyngitis should be suspected when the patient is a homosexual man, has associated symptoms of urogenital infection, is a woman who has practiced fellatio with a man with current genital gonorrhea (4,20), or has persistent sore throat and has been unresponsive to treatment for presumptive streptococcal pharyngitis. Pharyngeal gonorrhea, when symptomatic, may be mild to severe, with a protracted pharyngitis characterized by pain, fever, and pharyngeal exudate. Care must be exercised in obtaining cultures (21). The value of new polymerase chain reaction tests for gonococcal nucleic acids has not been established in pharyngitis.

Several other bacteria have been identified as occasional causes of pharyngitis: *Moraxella catarrhalis* and *Streptococcus pneumoniae* (11), *Neisseria meningitidis* (22), *Yersinia enterocolitica* (associated with a milk-borne epidemic) (23), and *Corynebacterium haemolyticum* (24); in pharyngitis caused by the latter bacterium, there may be an associated scarlatiniform rash indistinguishable from that occasionally seen with group A streptococcal infections. Diphtheria remains rare in the United States (25) and produces only a mild pharyngitis beneath its characteristic pseudomembrane. Another rare cause of pharyngitis in immunocompetent adults is fusospirochetal infection (Plaut-Vincent angina). Pharyngeal and oral candidiasis raise the possibility of infection with human immunodeficiency virus.

Supraglottitis/Epiglottitis

In adults presenting with sore throat, along with associated odynophagia, hoarseness, and stridor or tachypnea, the practitioner must always be alert to the possibility that the patient has supraglottitis or epiglottitis. The inflamed and enlarged epiglottis protrudes up into the hypopharynx, sometimes called the "rising sun sign." Attempts to swab the posterior pharynx to obtain a culture can provoke laryngospasm. Because obstruction of the airway may become life threatening with dramatic suddenness, the patient with epiglottitis must be observed in a hospital setting where an airway can be established immediately, if necessary.

In adults, conservative therapy under observation is sufficient in most cases, but tracheostomy may become necessary (26). *Hemophilus influenzae*, the most common cause of supraglottitis in children, is less common in adults: Other responsible organisms in adults are *Streptococcus pneumoniae, Streptococcus pyogenes*, and *Staphylococcus aureus*.

Acute Infectious Mononucleosis

The full-blown acute infectious mononucleosis ("mono") syndrome is characterized by a triad of clinical, hematologic, and serologic findings. The clinical presentation is typified by the development over several days of malaise, fever, sore throat, and marked adenopathy, particularly evident in the cervical lymph nodes. On physical examination, marked adenopathy is virtually always present and is most specific for mononucleosis when the posterior cervical or posterior auricular nodes are involved. Splenomegaly, an exudative pharyngitis with prominent tonsillar swelling, palatine petechiae, and a gelatinous uvula are often noted. The classic hematologic findings are an absolute lymphocyte count greater than 4000/mm^3 or a relative lymphocyte count greater than 50% and "atypical" morphologic features in more than 10% of the lymphocytes. The characteristic serologic finding is heterophil antibody.

Because infectious mononucleosis is a viral illness that has not been shown to improve more rapidly with antiviral (acyclovir) therapy (27), why bother to try to diagnose it? The disorder should be diagnosed for several reasons. First, the prominent adenopathy may sometimes suggest a neoplastic process; a positive diagnosis of mononucleosis is thus reassuring. Second, the duration of illness is typically longer than pharyngitis with other viral causes, and the diagnosis thus gives prognostic information. Third, patients with mononucleosis may sometimes have tonsillar swelling sufficient to compromise the airway seriously, necessitating emergent steroid therapy and even the establishment of an airway. Fourth, patients with mononucleosis often have splenomegaly and should be advised to avoid any activity that could lead to abdominal trauma and splenic rupture. Finally, there are a host of rare multisystem complications of mononucleosis, and establishing the diagnosis can alert the clinician to the possibility of these complications.

Most often, mononucleosis is caused by new primary infection with EBV. Less often, it is caused by cytomegalovirus or human herpesvirus 6 (28–30). New EBV infection may be the cause of pharyngitis in 1% to 6% of young adults. It only rarely is the cause of pharyngitis in adults older than 40 years of age (31). Only one fourth of patients with new EBV infection seeking medical care for pharyngitis manifest the complete infectious mononucleosis syndrome: Most are clinically indistinguishable from patients with other forms of viral pharyngitis and have a similarly brief and benign clinical course (31). Therefore, nothing is lost by failing to test for and recognize new EBV infection in such patients.

DIAGNOSTIC TESTS

Throat Culture for Group A Streptococci

Like any test, throat cultures are imperfect. A single-swab throat culture has a sensitivity of approximately 85% to 90%, as defined by isolation of group A streptococci on a second swab (32,33). A throat culture can also be falsely positive for a true infection: Some patients with a culture positive for group A streptococci may be only uninfected carriers, as defined by their failure to exhibit a fourfold increase in antistreptococcal antibodies. Among adults (1) and children (34) seeking medical care for a sore throat, test specificity may be as low as 50% to 70% because of patients who do not exhibit serologic evidence of infection.

Rapid Tests for Group A Streptococcus

Recently, various rapid tests that detect group A streptococcal antigen ("rapid strep tests") have been developed and become widely used. Early studies reported that the specificity of these rapid strep tests was as high as 99%, whereas the sensitivity ranged from 80% to 95% (35). However, more recent studies found the tests to have lower sensitivity (30%–50%) and specificity (80%–90%) (36,37). Furthermore, the specificity of a rapid strep test is defined as its ability to predict a positive culture for group A streptococcus; if one defined the specificity of a rapid strep test as its ability to predict not just a positive culture but also a true infection, as contrasted to a carrier state, the specificity would be considerably less.

The obvious value of the rapid strep tests is that their results are available before the results of a throat culture. Indeed, some give results within 30 minutes and can be used to make therapeutic decisions before the patient leaves the office. A positive rapid strep test result probably should be grounds for prescribing antistreptococcal therapy, except when the pretest probability of streptococcal infection is low. However, we would not recommend obtaining a rapid strep test when the pretest probability of streptococcal infection is low.

The biggest problem with the rapid strep test is that a negative test result may lead the clinician automatically to refrain from considering antibacterial therapy. Not only is the rapid strep test relatively insensitive, but other, potentially treatable bacterial organisms may be causing the patient's pharyngitis.

Heterophil Antibody Testing

The horse-cell agglutination test for heterophil antibody is practical and is as accurate as the original Paul-Bunnell sheep cell test (38). The most frequently used horse cell test is the Monospot® test. The results of the horse cell test can be falsely negative until 7 to 14 days after the onset of symptoms. The horse cell test results also may stay positive for much longer than the sheep cell test; thus, it can produce false-positive results in future episodes of pharyngitis caused by other organisms. Heterophil antibody is not a specific antibody directed at antigens of EBV; however, it is reliably elevated in full-blown infectious mononucleosis. Therefore, it is generally unnecessary to perform specific antibody testing for EBV. Such testing rarely provides more information than does the heterophil test, takes several days to receive results, is expensive, and is not performed reliably by all laboratories.

Testing for Other Agents

Full throat culture may identify other potentially treatable infectious agents. Diagnostic testing for M. pneumoniae is difficult: Special culture techniques are required; cold agglutinin tests lack sensitivity and specificity; and serologic testing is of no value in acutely ill patients. A rapid test for mycoplasmal nucleic acid is not yet widely used. Testing for C. pneumoniae is impractical for the physician in office practice, because isolation of the organism requires cell culture.

DIAGNOSTIC STRATEGIES

The diagnostic approach to adult patients with sore throat involves looking for clinical evidence that will increase or decrease the pretest probability of each illness on the differential diagnosis list (Table 20-3) and obtaining laboratory tests accordingly.

As shown in Tables 20-1 and 20-2, clinical findings can be used to estimate the probability of group A streptococcal pharyngitis. Probably, although not solidly established yet, these same findings apply to the probability of infection with non–group A streptococci.

Patients for whom the probability of streptococcal pharyngitis is low based on clinical findings require neither a throat culture nor a rapid strep test. This strategy is based on the observation that both tests can be falsely positive (i.e., can indicate a carrier state), and penicillin treatment prescribed on the basis of a falsely positive culture may produce more suffering than it is expected to eliminate. This strategy should be avoided, however, when patients are at special risk from undiagnosed and untreated streptococcal infection, such as those with a history of acute rheumatic fever, patients with documented strep exposure in the past week, patients who live in a community with a current strep epidemic, or those who are diabetic or otherwise immunocompromised. In such cases, the clinician should have a lower threshold for diagnosing and treating group A streptococcal pharyngitis.

Conversely, immediate antibacterial treatment is justified in patients with a relatively high probability of streptococcal pharyngitis (i.e., >40%), because a throat culture can be falsely negative. As shown in Tables 20-1 and 20-2, clinical findings can identify these patients.

When clinical findings suggest an intermediate probability of streptococcal infection, treatment must be individualized. In general, it is appropriate to obtain a culture in such circumstances; a rapid strep test may be used initially in some situations.

When group C streptococci are isolated on culture, treatment is indicated. When other non–group A streptococci are isolated on repeated cultures in a patient with a persistent sore throat, treatment is also indicated.

Currently, there are no practical tests to identify mycoplasmal or chlamydial pharyngitis. Therefore, the decision to treat must be based on clinical grounds. There is evidence that patients with pharyngitis who do not have group A streptococci may benefit from erythromycin therapy (39); however, the value of treating specifically diagnosed mycoplasmal or chlamydial pharyngitis has not yet been established.

Table 20-3. Clinical Findings That Suggest Various Forms of Non-Streptococcal Pharyngitis

Suspected Infection	Clincal Findings
Hemophilus influenzae	Cough and otitis media
Neisseria gonorrhoeae	Homosexual male
	Associated urogenital symptoms
	Woman practicing fellatio with man who has current urogenital symptoms
	Persistent sore throat unresponsive to treatment with penicillin
Moraxella catarrhalis	Chronic lung disease
Streptococcus pneumoniae	Cough productive of purulent sputum
Corynebacterium hemolyticum or group A streptococcus	Scarlatiniform rash
Supraglottitis/epiglottitis	"Rising sun sign"
Acute infectious mononucleosis	Marked adenopathy (especially if involving posterior cervical or auricular nodes)
	Splenomegaly
	Palatine petechiae
	Gelatinous uvula

When the clinical findings increase the pretest probability of gonococcal infection, cultures should be obtained on New York City or Thayer-Martin media and treatment should be offered to any patient with a positive culture. As summarized above and in Table 20-3, other forms of bacterial pharyngitis must be kept in mind. Many of these organisms will be isolated on throat culture.

When the clinical presentation is consistent with full-blown mononucleosis, differential leukocyte count and heterophil antibody (horse cell test) should be obtained for confirmation.

CLINICAL PROBLEMS

Clinical Problem 1
A middle-aged patient has a mild sore throat but no abnormal physical findings.

Testing Strategy and Rationale
No tests are indicated. The probability of an infection requiring diagnosis or specific treatment is very low in this clinical situation.

Clinical Example
A healthy 46-year-old man reports having a mild sore throat for the past 3 days. He has had no other symptoms. Physical examination does not uncover any abnormalities such as adenopathy or fever.

In the absence of any historical or physical findings to support the diagnosis of a bacterial infection or any other infection that should be definitively diagnosed (e.g., EBV infection), no further study is necessary. The patient may be treated with simple supportive measures.

Clinical Problem 2
A young adult presents with sore throat, fever, and neck swelling.

Testing Strategy and Rationale
A rapid slide test for heterophil antibody should be obtained, followed by throat culture if the results of the rapid test are negative. In a young adult, the findings of pharyngeal exudate, fever, or cervical adenopathy, particularly anterior cervical adenopathy, are seen commonly in both infectious mononucleosis and streptococcal pharyngitis. The probability of streptococcal pharyngitis in this situation is at least 40% if anterior cervical adenopathy is present (see Table 20-1); if posterior cervical or posterior auricular adenopathy is present, new EBV infection is relatively more likely. Although it would be unusual for the lymphadenopathy associated with mononucleosis to be

Continued

limited to the anterior cervical region, in young adults, this diagnosis should be evaluated before the throat is cultured and treatment is given for a presumptive diagnosis of streptococcal pharyngitis.

Clinical Example

An 18-year-old man presents with a temperature of 38.8 °C, an exudate covering the tonsils, and multiple enlarged, tender anterior cervical lymph nodes. No other lymph nodes are palpable, the spleen is not enlarged, and no palatal petechiae are present. The patient indicates that his girlfriend had similar symptoms some weeks ago, did not seek medical treatment, and her symptoms resolved spontaneously.

If a monospot test is obtained and the results are negative, the diagnosis of infectious mononucleosis would be unlikely. Treatment would be started for probable group A streptococcal pharyngitis.

REFERENCES

1. **Komaroff AL, Aronson MD, Pass TM, et al.** Serologic evidence of chlamydial and mycoplasmal pharyngitis in adults. Science. 1983;222:927-9.
2. **Huovinen P, Lahtonen R, Ziegler T, et al.** Pharyngitis in adults: the presence and coexistence of viruses and bacterial organisms. Ann Intern Med. 1989;110:612-6.
3. **Bridger RC.** *Haemophilus influenzae*: the relationship to upper respiratory tract infection. N Z Med J. 1974;80:19-22.
4. **Komaroff AL, Aronson MD, Pass TM, Ervin CT.** Prevalence of pharyngeal gonorrhea in general medical patients with sore throat. Sex Transm Dis. 1980;7:116-9.
5. **Glezen WP, Clyde WA, Senior RJ.** Group A streptococci, mycoplasmas, and viruses associated with acute pharyngitis. JAMA. 1967;202:455-60.
6. **Walsh BT, Bookheim WW, Johnson RC, Tompkins RK.** Recognition of streptococcal pharyngitis in adults. Arch Intern Med. 1975;135:1493-7.
7. **Crawford G, Brancato F, Holmes KK.** Streptococcal pharyngitis: diagnosis by Gram stain. Ann Intern Med. 1979;90:293-7.
8. **Centor RM, Witherspoon JM, Dalton HP, et al.** The diagnosis of strep throat in adults in the emergency room. Med Decis Making. 1981;1:239-46.
9. **Komaroff AL, Pass TM, Aronson MD, et al.** The prediction of streptococcal pharyngitis in adults. J Gen Intern Med. 1986;1:1-7.
10. **Evans AS, Diete EC.** Acute pharyngitis and tonsillitis in University of Wisconsin students. JAMA. 1964;190:699-708.
11. **Heald A, Auckenthaler R, Borst F, et al.** Adult bacterial nasopharyngitis: a clinical entity? J Gen Intern Med. 1993;8:667-73.
12. **Bisno AL.** Group A streptococcal infections and acute rheumatic fever. N Engl J Med. 1991; 325:783-93.
13. **Centor RM, Witherspoon JM, Dalton HP.** Non-group A streptococci are associated with clinically significant sore throats. Clin Res. 1981;29:255.

14. **Petersen KM, Inglefinger JA, Komaroff AL, Aronson MD.** Non-group A streptococci in adults with pharyngitis. Clin Res. 1984;32:695A.

15. **Turner JC, Hayden GF, Kiselica D, et al.** Association of group C beta-hemolytic streptococci with endemic pharyngitis among college students. JAMA. 1990;264:2644-7.

16. **Meier FA, Centor RM, Graham L Jr, Dalton HP.** Clinical and microbiological evidence for endemic pharyngitis among adults due to group C streptococci. Arch Intern Med. 1990;150:825-9.

17. **Grayston JT.** Infections caused by *Chlamydia pneumoniae* strain *TWAR*. Clin Infect Dis. 1992;15:757-63.

18. **Hammerschlag MR, Chirgwin K, Roblin PM, et al.** Persistent infection with *Chlamydia pneumoniae* following acute respiratory illness. Clin Infect Dis. 1992;14:178-82.

19. **Komaroff AL, Aronson MD, Pass TM, Ervin CT.** The etiology of sore throat in adults. Clin Res. 1980;28:227.

20. **Bro-Jorgensen A, Jensen T.** Gonococcal pharyngeal infections: report of 110 cases. Br J Vener Dis. 1973;49:491 9.

21. **Granato PA, Schneible-Smith C, Weiner LB.** Use of New York City medium for improved recovery of *Neisseria gonorrhoeae* from clinical specimens. J Clin Microbiol. 1981;13:963-8.

22. **Pether JVS, Scott RJD, Hancock P.** Do meningococci cause sore throats? Lancet. 1994;344:1636.

23. **Tacket CO, Davis BR, Carter GP, et al.** *Yersinia enterocolitica* pharyngitis. Ann Intern Med. 1983;99:40-2.

24. **Miller RA, Brancato F, Holmes KK.** *Corynebacterium hemolyticum* as a cause of pharyngitis and scarlatiniform rash in young adults. Ann Intern Med. 1986;105:867-72.

25. **McCloskey RV, Eller JJ, Green M, et al.** The 1970 epidemic of diphtheria in San Antonio. Ann Intern Med. 1971;75:495-503.

26. **Frantz TD, Rasgon BM, Quesenberry CP Jr.** Acute epiglottitis in adults: analysis of 129 cases. JAMA. 1994;272:1358-60.

27. **Tynell E, Aurelius E, Brandell A, et al.** Acyclovir and prednisolone treatment for acute infectious mononucleosis: a multicenter, double-blind, placebo-controlled study. J Infect Dis. 1996;174:324-31.

28. **Steeper TA, Horwitz CA, Ablashi DV, et al.** The spectrum of clinical and laboratory findings due to human herpesvirus-6 (HHV-6) in patients with mononucleosis-like illnesses not due to EBV or CMV. Am J Clin Pathol. 1990;93:776-83.

29. **Bertram G, Dreiner N, Krueger GRF, et al.** Frequent double infection with Epstein-Barr virus and human herpesvirus-6 in patients with acute infectious mononucleosis. In Vivo. 1991;5:271-80.

30. **Akashi K, Eizuru Y, Sumiyoshi Y, et al.** Brief report: severe infectious mononucleosis-like syndrome and primary human herpesvirus 6 infection in an adult. N Engl J Med. 1993;329:168-71.

31. **Aronson MD, Komaroff AL, Pass TM, et al.** Heterophil antibody in adults with sore throat: frequency and clinical presentation. Ann Intern Med. 1982;96:505-8.

32. **Kaplan EL.** Unsolved problems in diagnosis and epidemiology of streptococcal infection. In: Wannamaker LW, Matsen IM, eds. Streptococci and Streptococcal Disease. New York: Academic Press; 1972:4-65.

33. **Halfon S, Davies AM, Kaplan O, et al.** Primary prevention of rheumatic fever in Jerusalem school children. Isr J Med Sci. 1968;4:809-14.

34. **Kaplan EL, Top FH, Dudding BA.** Diagnosis of streptococcal pharyngitis: differentiation of active infection from the carrier state in the symptomatic child. J Infect Dis. 1971; 123:490-501.

35. **Centor RM, Meier FA, Dalton HP.** Throat cultures and rapid tests for diagnosis of group A streptococcal pharyngitis. Ann Intern Med. 1986;105:892-9.

36. **Wegner DL, Witte DL, Schrantz RD.** Insensitivity of rapid antigen detection methods and single blood agar plate culture for diagnosing streptococcal pharyngitis. JAMA. 1992;267:695-7.

37. **Reed BD, Huck W, French T.** Diagnosis of group A beta-hemolytic streptococcus using clinical scoring criteria, Directigen 1-2-3 Group A streptococcal test, and culture. Arch Intern Med. 1990;150:1727-32.

38. **Evans AS, Niederman JC, Cenabre LC, et al.** A prospective evaluation of heterophil and Epstein-Barr virus specific IgM antibody tests in clinical and subclinical infectious mononucleosis: specificity and sensitivity of the tests and persistence of antibody. J Infect Dis. 1975;132:546-54.

39. **Petersen K, Phillips RS, Soukup J, et al.** The effect of erythromycin on resolution of symptoms among adults with pharyngitis not caused by group A streptococcus: a randomized controlled trial. J Gen Intern Med. 1997;12:95-101.

Acute Dysuria in Adult Women

21

Anthony L. Komaroff, MD

> **KEY POINTS**
>
> **Pretest Probabilities**
>
> - In nonpregnant adult women, any of at least seven different conditions may cause acute dysuria.
>
> - About two thirds of women with dysuria have lower urinary tract infections. These patients generally do not have symptoms of vaginitis or risk factors for subclinical pyelonephritis or infectious urethritis from sexually transmitted organisms.
>
> **Diagnostic Strategies**
>
> - Women with acute dysuria and pyuria are highly likely to have a treatable infection, although distinguishing the type of infection and the proper therapy requires additional data.
>
> - Urinalysis has a more important role and urine culture a less important role in the evaluation of dysuria than was previously believed.

BACKGROUND

In women who present with symptoms of acute dysuria, urinary frequency, or urinary urgency, clinicians may consider the diagnosis of urinary tract infection. When symptoms or signs suggesting acute pyelonephritis are present, the patient may need to be hospitalized. However, it is much more typical in office practice that women with urinary symptoms do not have findings suggesting acute pyelonephritis. For 30 years, the conventional view has been that 1) such patients have infection limited to the bladder; 2) the responsible micro-organisms are almost always the gram-negative coliforms; 3) the most valuable test is a urine culture: 4) the presence of greater than 100,000 bacteria/mL indicates a positive culture and proof of a urinary infection; and 5) patients with "positive" cultures should receive antibacterial treatment for 7 to 14 days.

Recent evidence seriously challenges each of these assumptions (1–4), as discussed in this chapter. We emphasize that this discussion pertains only to nonpregnant adult women without clinical evidence of acute pyelonephritis. Our comments are not applicable to pregnant women, girls, or males.

Urinary tract infections are often recurrent. Much has been learned about the biology of recurrent infection: Women born with a predisposition to recurrent infection often have a genetically determined increase in uroepithelial cell receptors that increase the adherence for *Escherichia coli* (5,6), or they may have a genetically determined reduction in certain blood group antigens on the uroepithelial cell surface that, when present, protect against the adherence of *E. coli* (7). When recurrent infection occurs with the same organism within 14 days of completing treatment, the recurrent infection is called a *relapse* and is indicative of upper tract infection that has not been eradicated. Recurrent infection with the same organisms after 14 days is sometimes called *persistent* infection and may also be indicative of upper tract infection. Recurrent infection with a different organism is called a *reinfection,* is indicative of lower tract infection, and is by far the most common cause of recurrent infections.

ESTIMATING PRETEST PROBABILITY

Acute Pyelonephritis

Acute pyelonephritis is a clinical entity suggested by dysuria, frequency, and urgency (although these symptoms sometimes may be absent) in association with fever, flank pain, nausea and vomiting, rigors, and costovertebral angle tenderness. Urinalysis almost always reveals marked pyuria and bacteriuria, and the urine culture colony count is almost always greater than 100,000 organisms per milliliter of urine (8). Hematuria and proteinuria also may be present during the height of the inflammation. Depending on how sick and frail the patient is, acute pyelonephritis can be managed by outpatient treatment with an oral antibacterial regimen or with hospitalization for parenteral therapy.

Subclinical Pyelonephritis

A surprising number of patients—as many as 30% in most primary care settings and 80% in emergency rooms serving indigent populations (9)—have what is called *subclinical pyelonephritis* (1,2). Although these patients appear clinically to have lower urinary tract infection, they actually have upper tract infection, as demonstrated by bilateral ureteral catheterization (10), the bladder wash-out technique (11,12), and the antibody-coated bacteria assay (13–15). These patients often have minimal symptoms that smolder for long periods, making infection difficult to eradicate. Many patients are likely to require prolonged therapy (e.g., 6 weeks of full-dose treatment) to eradicate a renal focus of infection. The optimal therapeutic regimen is unknown. At the initial visit, the urinalysis typically displays pyuria and bacteriuria; hematuria and proteinuria may also be transiently present. Urine culture almost always reveals more than 100,000 organisms/mL of urine (16).

Lower Urinary Tract Bacterial Infection
In most office practices, the most common cause of dysuria (in at least 60%–70% of patients) is lower urinary tract bacterial infection. Traditionally, such infections were categorized as either "cystitis" (i.e., inflammation of entire bladder but not of the upper tract) or "acute urethral syndrome" (i.e., inflammation of just the urethral mucosa). The former was supposedly characterized by colony counts of greater than 100,000 bacteria/mL of urine, and the latter by lower colony counts. Over the past 15 years, it has become apparent that many women with symptoms of lower urinary tract infection do indeed have colony counts of less than 100,000 bacteria/mL of urine (17–19), but the anatomic distinction between "cystitis" and "acute urethral syndrome" is probably invalid. Indeed, the traditional criterion of a "positive" culture—the presence of greater than 100,000 bacteria per milliliter—is not useful in symptomatic women (1,2,20). Instead, the work of Stamm and colleagues (21) indicates that the symptomatic woman with pyuria as shown by urinalysis and a colony count of greater than only 100 bacteria per milliliter of urine should be regarded as having lower urinary tract bacterial infection. This has been most solidly established for *E. coli* and for *Staphylococcus saprophyticus* infections. Treatment of lower tract bacterial infections with low colony counts (100–100,000 bacteria/mL urine) is demonstrably effective (22).

Chlamydial and Gonococcal Urethritis
Urethral infection with *Chlamydia trachomatis* accounts for a small fraction of cases of acute dysuria in women (16). Urinalysis typically reveals pyuria but not bacteriuria; hematuria is highly unusual, as is proteinuria. Urine culture typically is sterile, because the chlamydiae do not grow on the media used for urine bacterial cultures. Likewise, gonococcal infections of the urethra are the cause of dysuria in some women.

Other Types of Infectious Urethritis
Occasionally, urethritis may be caused by *Trichomonas vaginalis, Candida albicans*, or *Herpes simplex*. All of these forms of urethritis except candi-

dal urethritis typically produce pyuria (23). Urine cultures on conventional media are sterile.

Dysuria with No Recognized Pathogen

Some women with dysuria have no recognized pathogen. They also do not have pyuria and do not respond to antimicrobial treatment (16,22). The cause of the dysuria may be a urethral inflammation from trauma; desiccating agents, including estrogen deficiency in postmenopausal women; or other noninfectious factors.

Vaginitis

Patients with vaginitis may present with a chief symptom of dysuria and not of vaginal discharge or irritation, although these latter symptoms, even if not volunteered, almost always can be elicited (19,23,24). In some settings, vaginal infections actually are more frequent causes of the dysuria than are urinary infections (19). Typically, except when a trichomonal infection involves the urethra as well as the vagina, pyuria is absent (19,23). Evaluation of patients with vaginitis is discussed in Chapter 22.

There are insufficient data to estimate precisely the pretest probability of each of the preceding seven entities using history and physical examination data. More important, the literature suggests that the probability of each entity may differ strikingly from one practice setting to the next. For example, subclinical pyelonephritis and gonococcal urethritis have a greater probability in settings serving indigent inner-city women (9,25).

DIAGNOSTIC TESTS

Urinalysis

The urinalysis is valuable in the evaluation of patients with dysuria and in the diagnosis of urinary tract infection in the otherwise healthy adult woman, for several reasons. First and foremost, determining the presence or absence of pyuria is of great importance (1,16,26). Second, the presence of hematuria tends to rule out chlamydial and other forms of urethritis, as well as vaginitis; probably the same is true of proteinuria. When seen, leukocyte casts clearly indicate upper tract infection. Urine glucose may suggest previously unrecognized diabetes mellitus, which in turn raises the probability of papillary necrosis. Finally, patients with acute pyelonephritis have an impairment in the ability to concentrate urine, as reflected in the specific gravity.

The assessment of pyuria is imperfect. There is variability in the amount of supernatant in which the sediment pellet is resuspended and in the volume of urine placed under the cover-slip (27). A leukocyte counting chamber controls some of these variables (28–33) but has not been used widely in primary care settings. The value of pyuria has been established primarily by the work of Stamm and colleagues (16), who defined pyuria (using a counting chamber) as being eight or more leukocytes per cubic centimeter in uncentrifuged urine; this corresponds to approximately two leukocytes per high-power field in centrifuged urine sediment (34).

Leukocyte Esterase Test

Neutrophils contain several unique esterases not present in normal serum, urine, or kidney tissue. The leukocyte esterase test is a rapid method for detecting this esterase activity in urine (35). This test appears to be a highly specific measure of pyuria (specificity, 94%–98%) but is relatively less sensitive (sensitivity, 74%–96%) (35–37). Moreover, test sensitivity is lower in patients for whom the the pretest probabilities of urinary tract infection are lower, an example of spectrum bias (38). In one large study, the standard urinalysis proved more accurate than the leukocyte esterase test (39).

It is possible that the substitution of this rapid assay for microscopic examination may be cost-effective. However, further studies of its accuracy, as well as of the utility of other findings that can be obtained only by microscopic examination, such as casts, hematuria, and bacteriuria, must be performed before the potential role of this technique can be established.

Urine Culture

As is apparent from preceding comments, the urine culture as a first-line test is less valuable in women with acute dysuria than is the urinalysis. Its most important role may be in the follow-up of patients with recurrent infections rather than as part of an initial diagnostic test battery.

The following organisms are established urinary pathogens: *E. coli* (by far the most common pathogen), enterococcus, gram-negative coliforms other than *E. coli*, *S. saprophyticus* (40), and Group B streptococci (particularly in girls).

The urine culture is essential in identifying relapsing infections that are caused by the same organism. One practical difficulty arises in determining if recurrent infection with *E. coli* is the same organism or a different *E. coli*, because there are many strains of *E. coli* and because formal typing of isolates is not routinely performed. In general, when the antibiogram (pattern of antibacterial sensitivities) or the API number (a six-digit code used by laboratories to record the results of fermentations used to characterize bacteria) are the same as for the previous infection, then the organisms isolated are the same (i.e., the patient has relapsing or persistent infection).

Microscopic Examination of Vaginal Discharge

In patients with dysuria who also have symptoms of vaginal discharge or irritation, a speculum examination should be done. Any abnormal discharge (unusually copious, opaque, yellow or green colored, or foul smelling) should be examined microscopically. Patients who specifically deny having symptoms of vaginitis probably should not be subjected to a pelvic examination as part of the evaluation of acute dysuria (19).

Rapid Chlamydia and Gonococcus Tests

New polymerase chain reaction (PCR) and ligase chain reaction (LCR) tests for rapidly detecting chlamydial nucleic acids have been developed, with an estimated sensitivity of greater than 95% and an estimated specificity of greater than 97% in detecting cervical infection (41,42). Indeed, the PCR tests appear to be much more sensitive than conventional culture, and now constitute the "gold standard" for diagnosing *C. trachomatis* infection. The tests can be done using endocervical, urethral, or first-voided urine specimens; the latter may be the most sensitive. Because isolation of chlamydial organisms requires cell culture, which is an expensive and protracted test that is performed reliably in only a few laboratories and that may be relatively insensitive, the PCR test for chlamydia is likely to replace culture techniques. It has not been clearly established that it is superior to rapid chlamydial antigen detection techniques.

Likewise, tests for detecting gonococcal nucleic acids appear to have high sensitivity and specificity (43,44). Specimens for both tests can now be obtained with the same swab (44). The accuracy of the PCR tests in detecting a urethral infection with either chlamydial or gonococcal organisms as compared with detecting a cervical or pelvic infection has not been established as solidly.

DIAGNOSTIC STRATEGIES

The Single Episode of Dysuria

In women with dysuria, the presence of pyuria strongly suggests any of several treatable entities: acute pyelonephritis, subclinical pyelonephritis, lower urinary tract bacterial infection, chlamydial urethritis, and other urethritis. Conversely, pyuria is almost never present in patients in whom no recognized pathogen can be found; these patients also do not respond to antibacterial treatment (16). In addition, pyuria is usually absent in patients with vaginal infection. Patients with acute dysuria and pyuria (the "dysuria–pyuria syndrome") (26) therefore almost always benefit from immediate antibacterial treatment, and patients without pyuria do not. However, the finding of pyuria does not itself indicate what the treatment should be; that judgment is made on the basis of other data. Thus, the finding of pyuria on urinalysis appears to be only a predictor of the presence of a treatable infection. This finding also seems to be a better predictor than the presence of bacteria from a urine culture.

In the evaluation of a patient with dysuria, the patient first should always be asked about symptoms of vaginal discharge and irritation. If the patient has these symptoms, a pelvic examination and evaluation for vaginitis should be completed (see Chapter 22). Urinalysis and urine culture probably are unnecessary, although urinary and vaginal infections occasionally can co-exist (19,23).

Between 60% and 70% of women presenting with dysuria have lower urinary tract bacterial infections. In general, these patients do not have symptoms of vaginal discharge or irritation and do not have a history of risk factors for subclinical pyelonephritis or chlamydial or other forms of infectious urethritis (16) as described later in this chapter. In such patients, a urinalysis should be done, and those patients who have pyuria should receive treatment with a 3-day regimen of antibiotics such as trimethoprim-sulfamethoxazole or amoxicillin. In these patients, a urine culture at the initial visit is not necessary except in those patients who have had one or two previous symptomatic urinary infections during the past year. Patients with lower urinary tract bacterial infection and a urine culture colony count of greater than 100,000 bacteria/mL are treated with short-course (3-day) therapy just as successfully as patients with lower colony counts (45).

The possibility of subclinical pyelonephritis should be assessed by determining the presence of risk factors for this syndrome. These include 1) known underlying urinary tract disease; 2) diabetes mellitus or other conditions or therapies that produce an immunocompromised state; 3) urinary infections in childhood; 4) documented relapsing infection in the past; 5) symptoms for 7 to 10 days before seeking care (this also suggests chlamydial urethritis); 6) three or more previous urinary infections; or 7) acute pyelonephritis during the past year. Subclinical pyelonephritis also may be more likely in indigent, inner-city residents (14).

Although there are few data to support this policy, we recommend that patients with any one of these risk factors be managed as follows: A urinalysis and urine culture should be performed. For those patients with pyuria or leukocyte casts, immediate treatment with one of the standard antimicrobial agents is warranted. Many of these patients are likely to require prolonged therapy (e.g., 6 weeks of full-dose therapy) for the infection to be adequately treated. Every effort should be made to obtain a follow-up culture 2 to 4 days after therapy has been completed to be sure infection has been eradicated. In patients who have relapsing infection after a course of therapy (46), tests such as intravenous pyelography (IVP) or renal ultrasonongraphy are indicated.

Chlamydial urethritis is suggested if the patient has a sexual partner with recent urethritis, a new recent sexual partner, the stuttering (rather than abrupt) onset of symptoms over a period of days, and the absence of hematuria (15). A mucopurulent discharge from the cervical or urethral os that demonstrates leukocytes but no organisms is characteristic of chlamydial infection and is sufficient grounds for immediate treatment of this condition (47), even before the results of PCR testing return. Indeed, such classic findings probably should lead to immediate treatment with azithromycin; a single dose of 1 g orally that can be administered before the patient leaves the doctor's office is highly effective (48) and cost effective (49).

Gonococcal urethritis is more likely to occur in patients whose recent sexual partners have urethral discharge or in patients with a previous history of gonorrhea. It also is more likely in indigent inner-city women. We believe that patients with any of these risk factors for chlamydial or gonococcal urethritis should have a pelvic examination and urinalysis. Purulent discharge from the urethral or cervical os always should be Gram stained. A positive Gram stain is a sufficiently reliable indicator of gonorrhea (50,51) to lead to immediate treatment. In the patient with a high pretest probability of gonococcal urethritis based on clinical findings for whom the results of Gram stain are negative, culture or nucleic acid probe testing for gonorrhea or both are probably warranted.

Recurrent Dysuria

In women with a single episode of relapsing infection (as previously defined) or who have had three or more infections in the past year with the same organism (i.e., persistent infection) IVP or renal ultrasonography should be done; cystoscopic examination can be reserved for women with further recurrent infections or episodes of sterile dysuria in whom IVP or ultrasonography has not been revealing. In patients with recurrent infections that were not characterized as reinfections or relapses but that were probably mostly reinfections, IVP revealed a surgically correctable lesion in fewer than 1% of patients (52–54), and cystoscopy revealed a correctable lesion (e.g., urethral diverticulum) in as many as 4% (53,54). The yield of ultrasonography in such cases has not been carefully studied but is probably comparable to that of IVP (55).

CLINICAL PROBLEMS

Clinical Problem 1

A woman presents with dysuria without findings suggesting vaginitis, acute pyelonephritis, subclinical pyelonephritis, or urethritis.

Testing Strategy and Rationale

A urinalysis should be performed, and patients with pyuria should be treated with a 3-day antibiotic regimen (trimethoprim-sulfamethoxazole is preferred in patients who are not allergic to this agent). Urine culture is unnecessary unless there has been a symptomatic urinary infection within the past year.

Approximately two thirds of patients with acute dysuria fall into this category, in which an isolated lower tract bacterial infection is highly likely. The urinalysis finding of pyuria is both fairly sensitive and specific for bacterial infection in these patients. If the patient does not have pyuria, no treatment is given.

Clinical Example

A 28-year-old married woman presents with a 2-day history of dysuria. She has no other medical problems and no risk factors for sexually transmitted diseases. The urinalysis demonstrates 50 leukocytes and 5 erythrocytes per high-powered field. A moderate number of rodlike bacteria are also seen. She is given therapy with trimethoprim-sulfamethoxazole. No urine culture is obtained.

Clinical Problem 2

A woman with dysuria also has had acute pyelonephritis in the past year, a probable risk factor for subclinical pyelonephritis.

Testing Strategy and Rationale

If there are no symptoms of vaginitis, a urinalysis should be performed and a urine culture obtained. The patient should be treated promptly for possible subclinical pyelonephritis if pyuria or leukocyte casts are found. In all patients for whom the results of culture are positive, an additional culture should be obtained after treatment has been completed.

Clinical Example

A 30-year-old woman presents with a 10-day history of dysuria without symptoms of acute pyelonephritis or vaginitis. She reports having had an episode of acute pyelonephritis 6 months earlier. She has not had other previous problems with urinary infection. Because she has risk factors for subclinical pyelonephritis (previous acute pyelonephritis and a protracted period of symptoms before seeking care), both a urinalysis and a urine culture are obtained. Examination of the centrifuged sediment shows 20 leukocytes per high-power field, and antibiotic therapy is begun. The patient experiences prompt symptomatic improvement. The urine culture shows 100,000 *E. coli* bacteria per milliliter of urine, sensitive to all antibacterials tested. A follow-up urine culture is obtained after treatment to search for evidence of a relapse.

REFERENCES

1. **Komaroff AL.** Acute dysuria in women. N Engl J Med. 1984;310:368-75.

2. **Komaroff AL.** Urinalysis and urine culture in women with dysuria. Ann Intern Med. 1986; 104:212-8.

3. **Johnson JR, Stamm WE.** Urinary tract infections in women: diagnosis and treatment. Ann Intern Med. 1989;111:906-17.

4. **Stamm WE, Hooton TM.** Management of urinary tract infections in adults. N Engl J Med. 1993;329:1328-34.

5. **O'Hanley P, Low D, Romero I, et al.** Gal-Gal binding and hemolysin phenotypes and genotypes associated with uropathogenic *Escherichia coli*. N Engl J Med. 1985;313:414-20.

6. **Schaeffer AJ, Jones JM, Dunn JK.** Association of in vitro *Escherichia coli* adherence to vaginal and buccal epithelial cells with susceptibility of women to recurrent urinary tract infections. N Engl J Med. 1981;304:1062-6.

7. **Sheinfeld J, Schaeffer AJ, Cordon-Cardo C, et al.** Association of the Lewis blood-group phenotype with recurrent urinary tract infections in women. N Engl J Med. 1989;320:773-7.

8. **Kass EH.** Asymptomatic infections of the urinary tract. Trans Assoc Am Physicians. 1956;69:56-63.

9. **Savard-Fenton M, Fenton BW, Reller LB, et al.** Single-dose amoxicillin therapy with follow-up urine culture. Am J Med. 1982;73:808-13.

10. **Stamey TA, Govan DE, Palmer JM.** The localization and treatment of urinary tract infections: the role of bactericidal urine levels as opposed to serum levels. Medicine 1965;44:1-36.

11. **Fairley KF, Bond AG, Brown RB, Habersberger P.** Simple test to determine the site of urinary-tract infection. Lancet. 1967;2:427-8.

12. **Ronald AR, Boutros P, Mourtada H.** Bacteriuria localization and response to single-dose therapy in women. JAMA. 1976;235:1854-6.

13. **Fang LST, Tolkoff-Rubin NE, Rubin RH.** Efficacy of single-dose and conventional amoxicillin therapy in urinary-tract infection localized by the antibody-coated bacteria technic. N Engl J Med. 1978;298:413-6.

14. **Rubin RH, Fang LST, Jones SR, et al.** Single-dose amoxicillin therapy for urinary tract infection. JAMA. 1980;244:561-4.

15. **Buckwold FJ, Ludwig P, Harding GKM, et al.** Therapy for acute cystitis in adult women: Randomized comparison of single-dose sulfisoxazole vs. trimethoprim-sulfamethoxazole. JAMA. 1982;247:1839-42.

16. **Stamm WE, Wagner KF, Amsel R, et al.** Causes of the acute urethral syndrome in women. N Engl J Med. 1980;303:409-15.

17. **Gallagher DJA, Montgomerie JZ, North JDK.** Acute infections in the urinary tract and the urethral syndrome in general practice. Br Med J. 1965;1:622-6.

18. **Fairley KF, Carson NE, Gutch RC, et al.** Site of infection in acute urinary-tract infection in general practice. Lancet. 1971;2:615-8.

19. **Komaroff AL, Pass TM, McCue JD, et al.** Management strategies for urinary and vaginal infections. Arch Intern Med. 1978;138:1069-73.

20. **Kunin CM, White LV, Hua TH.** A reassessment of the importance of "low-count" bacteriuria in young women with acute urinary symptoms. Ann Intern Med. 1993;119:454-60.

21. **Stamm WE, Counts GW, Running KR, et al.** Diagnosis of coliform infection in acutely dysuric women. N Engl J Med. 1982;307:463-8.

22. **Stamm WE, Running K, McKevitt M, et al.** Treatment of the acute urethral syndrome. N Engl J Med. 1981;304:956-8.

23. **Demetriou E, Emans SJ, Masland RP.** Dysuria in adolescent girls: urinary tract infection or vaginitis? Pediatrics. 1982;70:299-301.

24. **Dans PE, Klaus B.** Dysuria in women. Johns Hopkins Med J. 1976;138:13-8.

25. **Curran JW.** Gonorrhea and the urethral syndrome. Sex Transm Dis. 1977;4:119-121.

26. **Komaroff AL, Friedland G.** The dysuria-pyuria syndrome. N Engl J Med. 1980;303:452-4.

27. **Gadeholt H.** Quantitative estimation of urinary sediment, with special regard to sources of error. Br Med J. 1964;1:1547-9.

28. **Little PJ.** A comparison of the urinary white cell concentration with the white cell excretion rate. Br J Urol. 1964;36:360-3.

29. **Mabeck CE.** Studies in urinary tract infections. IV. Urinary leucocyte excretion in bacteriuria. Acta Med Scand. 1969;186:193-8.

30. **Gadeholt H.** Quantitative estimation of cells in urine. An evaluation of the Addis count. Acta Med Scand. 1968;183:369 74

31. **Brumfitt W.** Urinary cell counts and their value. J Clin Pathol. 1965;18:550-5.

32. **Musher DM, Thorsteinsson SB, Airola VM.** Quantitative urinalysis: diagnosing urinary tract infection in men. JAMA. 1976;236:2069-72.

33. **Fairley K, Barraclough M.** Leucocyte-excretion rate as a screening test for bacteriuria. Lancet. 1967;1:420-1.

34. **Stansfeld JM.** The measurement and meaning of pyuria. Arch Dis Child. 1962;37:257-62.

35. **Kusumi RK, Grover PJ, Kunin CM.** Rapid detection of pyuria by leukocyte esterase activity. JAMA. 1981; 245:1653-5.

36. **Perry JL, Matthews JS, Weesner DE.** Evaluation of leukocyte esterase activity as a rapid screening technique for bacteriuria. J Clin Microbiol. 1982;15:852-4.

37. **Gelbart SM, Chen WT, Reid R.** Clinical trial of leukocyte test strips in routine use. Clin Chem. 1983;29:997-9.

38. **Lachs MS, Nachamkin I, Edelstein PH, et al.** Spectrum bias in the evaluation of diagnostic tests: lessons from the rapid dipstick test for urinary tract infection. Ann Intern Med. 1992;117:135-40.

39. **Blum RN, Wright RA.** Detection of pyuria and bacteriuria in symptomatic ambulatory women. J Gen Intern Med. 1992;7:140-4.

40. **Latham RH, Running K, Stamm WE.** Urinary tract infections in young adult women caused by *Staphylococcus saprophyticus*. JAMA. 1983;250:3063-6.

41. **LeBar WD.** Keeping up with new technology: new approaches to diagnosis of *Chlamydia* infection. Clin Chem. 1996;42:809-12.

42. **de Barbeyrac B, Rodriguez P, Dutilh B, et al.** Detection of *Chlamydia trachomatis* by ligase chain reaction compared with polymerase chain reaction and cell culture in urogenital specimens. Genitourin Med. 1995;71:382-6.

43. **Ho BS, Feng WG, Wong BK, Egglestone SI.** Polymerase chain reaction for the detection of *Neisseria gonorrhoeae* in clinical samples. J Clin Pathol. 1992;45:439-42.

44. **Wong KC, Ho BS, Egglestone SI, Lewis WH.** Duplex PCR system for simultaneous detection of *Neisseria gonorrhoeae* and *Chlamydia trachomatis* in clinical specimens. J Clin Pathol. 1995;48:101-4.

45. **Arav-Boger R, Leibovici L, Danon YL.** Urinary tract infections with low and high colony counts in young women. Arch Intern Med. 1994;154:300-4.

46. **Turck M, Anderson KN, Petersdorf RG.** Relapse and reinfection in chronic bacteriuria. N Engl J Med. 1966;275:70-3.

47. **Brunham RC, Paavonen J, Stevens CE, et al.** Mucopurulent cervicitis: the ignored counterpart in women of urethritis in men. N Engl J Med. 1984;311:1-6.

48. **Martin DH, Mroczkowski TF, Dalu ZA, et al, and the Azithromycin for Chlamydial Infections Study Group.** A controlled trial of a single dose of azithromycin for the treatment of chlamydial urethritis and cervicitis. N Engl J Med. 1992;327:921-5.

49. **Magid D, Douglas JM Jr, Schwartz JS.** Doxycycline compared with azithromycin for treating women with genital *Chlamydia trachomatis* infections: an incremental cost-effectiveness analysis. Ann Intern Med. 1996;124:389-99.

50. **Rothenberg RB, Simon R, Chipperfield E, Catterall RD.** Efficacy of selected diagnostic tests for sexually transmitted diseases. JAMA. 1976;235:49-51.

51. **Eschenbach DA, Buchanan TM, Pollock HM, et al.** Polymicrobial etiology of acute pelvic inflammatory disease. N Engl J Med. 1975;293:166-71.

52. **Fair WR, McClennan BL, Jost RG.** Are excretory urograms necessary in evaluating women with urinary tract infection. J Urol. 1979;121:313-5.

53. **Engel G, Schaeffer AJ, Grayhack JT, Wendel EF.** The role of excretory urography and cystoscopy in the evaluation and management of women with recurrent urinary tract infection. J Urol. 1979;123:190-1.

54. **Fowler JE, Pulaski ET.** Excretory urography, cystography, and cystoscopy in the evaluation of women with urinary-tract infection: a prospective study. N Engl J Med. 1981;304:462-5.

55. **Spencer J, Lindsell D, Mastorakou I.** Ultrasonography compared with intravenous urography in investigation of urinary tract infection in adults. Br Med J. 1990;301:221-4.

Acute Vaginitis

22

Lynn S. Bickley, MD

KEY POINTS

Pretest Probabilities

- Pretest probabilities for the different causes of acute vaginitis vary according to the clinical setting; the patient risk factors for sexually transmitted disease; and the origin of the discharge (vaginal as opposed to cervical).
- Discharges of vaginal origin may be caused by bacterial vaginosis, *Candida* species, or *Trichomonas vaginalis*.
- Discharges of cervical origin may be caused by *Neisseria gonorrhoeae*, *Chlamydia trachomatis*, or herpes simplex virus.

Diagnostic Strategies

- In cases of suspected vaginitis, initial diagnostic tests include the saline and potassium hydroxide (KOH) wet-mount preparations and the vaginal pH.
- For cases of suspected cervicitis, a cervical Gram stain and *N. gonorrhoeae* culture are warranted. The DNA probe test for *N. gonorrhoeae* is an alternative to culture. In patients at lower risk for *N. gonorrhoeae* and in those without evidence of *N. gonorrhoeae* on Gram stain, testing for chlamydia with one of the rapid diagnostic tests or culture may be indicated.
- In patients with complex or recurrent infections, cultures are warranted for definitive diagnosis.

BACKGROUND

Vaginal infection is one of the most common infections in women of reproductive age, accounting for 5 to 10 million health care visits per year. In general practices, as many as 8% of nonpregnant women report vaginal symptoms (1). The distribution of diagnosed vaginal, cervical, and urinary tract infection and absence of infection in a family practice residency clinic was 45%, 5%, 16%, and 40%, respectively (2). Infections of vaginal origin include bacterial vaginosis (BV); infection with *Candida* species, or vaginal candiasis (CSp); and *Trichomonas vaginitis*. The distribution of vaginal infections in office practices ranges from 20% to 50% for BV, 20% to 30% for CSp, and 5% to 10% for *T. vaginalis* (3).

Because as many as 25% of women who report having vaginal discharge have cervical infections (4), it is essential to distinguish cervical from vaginal discharges during the evaluations. The three principal causes of cervical discharge are *Chlamydia trachomatis*, *Neisseria gonorrhoeae*, and herpes simplex virus (HSV). Infection with *C. trachomatis* and *N. gonorrhoeae* carry risks of pelvic inflammatory disease (PID) and infertility in the range of 11% after a single episode of salpingitis, 23% after two episodes, and 54% after three or more episodes (5). The detection of vaginal and cervical infections has assumed new importance owing to recently documented risks for complications in pregnancy, especially for BV and *T. vaginalis* (1,6–8). Frequent vaginal and cervical infections also herald increased risk of infection from human papilloma virus, now linked to cervical dysplasia and carcinoma, and from human immmunodeficiency virus (HIV).

Vaginal and cervical infections arise from different types of epithelium. *Trichomonas vaginalis* and CSp infect the squamous epithelium, forming a continuous lining over the ectocervix and vagina. In contrast, BV disrupts the vaginal flora but does not produce an inflammatory response that attracts polymorphonuclear leukocytes (PMNs), giving rise to the term bacterial *vaginosis*. *Chlamydia trachomatis* and *N. gonorrhoeae* infect the thin vascular glandular columnar epithelium of the endocervix, commonly resulting in a mucopurulent discharge at the cervical os. Herpes simplex virus infects both zones of epithelium.

ESTIMATING PRETEST PROBABILITY

Bacterial Vaginosis

Bacterial vaginosis, the most common cause of increased vaginal discharge in symptomatic women, produces characteristic changes in the vaginal flora (Table 22-1). Because no single causative organism has been identified, diagnosis continues to be based on a combination of clinical criteria and the results of vaginal fluid microscopy. Widely used clinical criteria require three of four of the following findings for diagnosis: 1) thin homogeneous discharge; 2) vaginal pH of 4.5 or more; 3) clue cells on wet mount; and 4) a positive "whiff test," the release of a fishy aminelike odor when potassium hydroxide (KOH) is added to vaginal secretions. Because there is no counterpart in men, BV is not considered a sexually transmitted disease (STD).

Table 22-1. The Vaginal Ecosystem: Changes in the Vaginal Flora in Bacterial Vaginosis

	Normal Flora	Flora in Bacterial Vaginosis	Gram Stain Morphologic Features
Lactobaccilli	++++	+	Large gram-positive rods
Clue cells	+	++++	Epithelial cells with stippled borders (from adherent bacteria)
Anaerobes			
Gardnerella vaginalis	++	++++	Small gram-variable rods
Bacteroides	+	+++	Small gram-negative rods
Mobiluncas	+	+++	Curved gram-variable rods

Note: For micro-organisms, + = <1 organism per oil-immersion field; ++ = 1 to 5; +++ = 6 to 30; ++++ = >30. For clue cells, + implies absent or scant cells; ++++ implies multiple or many cells.

Vaginal Candidiasis

Vaginal candidiasis (CSp) affects 75% of women at least once in their lifetime, often occurring in conditions that disrupt the vaginal ecosystem. These include high estrogen states (menses and pregnancy), use of antibiotics, poorly controlled diabetes mellitus, and immunosuppression. The hallmark presenting symptom is vulvovaginal itching; the classic "cottage cheese" discharge is thick, white, and curdy. Twenty-five percent of affected women have no symptoms (9).

Trichomonas

Trichomonas vaginitis is caused by a flagellated protozoan, *T. vaginalis*, easily transmitted by sexual contact. Seventy percent of men and 85% of women contract the disease after a single sexual exposure (6). The characteristic discharge is thin, yellow or green, and frothy. Punctate hemorrhages may appear on the endocervix ("strawberry cervix") and vaginal walls. Common symptoms are vulvovaginal irritation, dysuria, and dyspareunia. Fifty percent of infected women and men may be asymptomatic (6).

Chlamydia trachomatis

Chlamydia trachomatis is the most common cause of cervical infection. It is detected in 4% to 13% of symptomatic women in office practices and in 20% to 30% of women in STD clinics. As many as 50% of women with mucopurulent cervicitis have chlamydia. The discharge is usually yellow or green. Cervical mucosa is often friable and bleeds easily.

Symptoms include increased discharge, dysuria, and vulvovaginal irritation. Only 60% of infected women are symptomatic, and only 50% have evidence of cervical infection on examination (10,11).

Neisseria gonorrhoeae
Gonococcal infections are seen in as many as 3% of women in office practices and as many as 17% in STD clinics. Symptoms occur 24 hours to 2 weeks after exposure to infection, and mucopurulent cervical discharge is noted in only 35% to 50%. At least 15% of women with endocervical gonococcal infection develop upper tract infection, and *N. gonorrhoeae* is recovered from peritoneal or tubal cultures in one half to two thirds of women with PID (12).

Herpes Simplex Virus
Herpes simplex virus is seen in approximately 1% to 3% of lower genital tract infections in office practices and the prevalence is as high as 48% in some STD clinics (13). Serologic studies suggest higher prevalence rates of HSV owing to the high percentage of women with latent infection and asymptomatic viral shedding or failure to culture atypical vulvar lesions such as fissures or furuncles (13). Herpes simplex virus produces characteristic painful vesicular lesions with associated dysuria, vaginal discharge, and tender inguinal adenopathy within 6 days of sexual contact with an infected partner. Approximately 70% of women report systemic symptoms such as fever and malaise. In primary HSV cervicitis, the cervix shows erythema, ulcerations, and mucopurulent discharge, with positive culture results occurring in 80% of women. In recurrent genital herpes, vulvar lesions are more common, and only 10% to 20% of women shed virus from the cervix.

Co-infections
In general office studies, more than 10% of women have more than one infection (14). For example, as many as 60% of women with *T. vaginalis* may have bacterial vaginosis (7). Approximately 13% of women with chlamydia have concurrent infection with *N. gonorrhoeae*, and approximately 30% of women with gonococcal infection have chlamydia (15).

Given the varied causes for acute vaginitis, estimating the pretest probability of specific vaginal or cervical infections is difficult. Symptoms and findings such as discharge characteristics often have poor predictive value (2–4,14,16,17). In addition, the prevalence of vaginal and cervical disease varies widely depending on the population studied, risk of STD, and assessment for coinfections or urinary tract infections (Table 22-2). In a carefully studied office population, approximately 35% of symptomatic patients had no infection; 32% of asymptomatic patients did have infection; and approximately 15% of infected patients had pelvic examinations with normal results (2). In

Table 22-2. Prevalence of Vaginal and Cervical Infection in Office Practices and STD Clinics

Type of Infection	Office/Clinic	STD Clinic
	← % →	
Vaginal infection		
Bacterial vaginosis	12–25	35–64
Trichomonas vaginalis	13–23	20–50
Candidiasis	20–25	25
Cervical infection		
Neisseria gonorrhoeae	3	17
Chlamydia trachomatis	4–13	15–30
Herpes simplex virus	1–3	1–48

STD – sexually transmitted disease.

some studies, the proportion of symptomatic women without documented infection increases to 50% (14).

To improve estimates of pretest probability, the clinical evaluation should include review of risk factors for STDs and HIV, use of proper technique to distinguish the origin of the discharge, and careful collection of specimens for microscopy and culture. Risk factors for STDs and HIV include age, number of sexual partners in the past month, sexual contact with an infected partner, history of previous STDs, and patient concern about HIV infections. To distinguish vaginal from cervical discharge, the cervix should be wiped clean with a large cotton-tipped swab; then, if no discharge from the cervical os is found or if the discharge from the os is clear, the discharge is more likely vaginal in origin. To minimize false-negative results, specimens for microscopy should be read promptly and swabs for culture should be plated with minimum delay.

DIAGNOSTIC TESTS

Evaluating diagnostic tests in acute vaginitis is problematic. Culture is the gold standard for diagnosis of most vaginal and cervical infections, but used alone, this test can delay treatment for 24 to 48 hours. Criteria for diagnosing BV and *Candida* on culture are not standardized, resulting in a wide variation in disease prevalence across studies (17–24). Although microscopy of vaginal and cervical specimens has been the cornerstone of office diagnosis, results depend on clinician skills at reading smears. Reports on newer tests for rapid diagnosis often fail to use culture to confirm the presence or absence of either the targeted disease or coinfections. A summary of the characteristics of common office and laboratory tests in the diagnosis of vaginal and cervical infections is discussed in this section and is summarized in Table 22-3.

Vaginal Infections

Because BV appears to result from an overgrowth of several colonizing anaerobic organisms, diagnosis has been hampered by lack of a simple, reliable office-based test or "gold-standard" culture. Although the composite clinical criteria noted previously are still widely used to identify study populations with BV, individual criteria lack sensitivity and specificity, especially in the presence of other infections. Currently, the most objective test for diagnosis is direct Gram stain of vaginal fluids (see Table 22-1) using a quantitative scoring system for three bacterial morphotypes: lactobacilli, *Gardnerella*, and "other" (predominantly anaerobes) (19–21). To achieve interobserver reliability, most studies have used trained microscopists to examine up to 20 fields at high powers of magnification (21–23). Clinicians, however, frequently lack the time or skill for reading such Gram stains, even with simplified scoring criteria (21,22).

The saline wet mount and the pH of vaginal secretions are useful office-based techniques for diagnosing suspected BV. The presence of clue cells on wet mount has a sensitivity of 98% and a specificity of approximately 90% (22). Using Gram stain, the sensitivity and specificity of clue cells for diagnosis is reported to be 80% and 91%, respectively (4). Scanning the wet mount for predominance of nonlactobacilli morphotypes also assists in confirming the diagnosis (23). Finding a normal vaginal pH (pH ≤ 4.4) and a predominance of lactobacilli make the diagnosis of BV much less likely (22,24).

An array of other tests for rapid office diagnosis of BV show promise but have not been widely studied or standardized. These include the amine test (adding KOH directly to the vaginal swab or secretions and sniffing for the fishy, aminelike odor); a colorimetric diamine oxidase test; tests for proline aminopeptidase and sialidases, which are enzymes released by anaerobes; and DNA probes for *Gardnerella vaginalis* (1,3,20,25). A definitive test for volatile organic acids released by anaerobes in vaginal wash specimens has high sensitivity (see Table 22-3) but relies on gas chromatography, which is not widely available.

In the diagnosis of *Candida* vaginitis, a positive KOH wet mount of vaginal secretions requires identification of budding yeast or branching mycelia. The sensitivity and specificity of this test compared with those of culture vary according to reader experience. Sensitivity averages about 60% but ranges from 34% to 84% (4,14,18,26,27), and specificity is 77% to 99% (26). Because 10% to 25% of asymptomatic women harbor

Table 22-3. Operating Characteristics of Common Diagnostic Tests for Vaginal and Cervical Infection

Diagnostic Test	Sensitivity	Specificity	Likelihood Ratio	
			Positive Result	Negative Result
	← % →			
Vaginal infection				
Bacterial vaginosis				
Gram stain of vaginal wash	97–100	99	97–100	0–0.03
"Whiff" test	38–92	93	5.4–13	0.09–0.67
Thin homogeneous discharge	42–80	88	3.5–6.7	0.23–0.66
Vaginal pH (pH ≥4.5)	52–97	94	8.7–16	0.03–0.51
Clue cells	80–98	90	8.0–9.8	0.02–0.22
Abnormal amines by chromatography	98	—	—	—
Vaginal candidiasis				
Potassium hydroxide preparation	~60 (range, 34–84)	77–99	2.6–60	0.40–0.52
Trichomonas vaginalis				
Saline wet mount	50–80	70–98	1.7–40	0.20–0.71
Direct fluorescent antibody	80–90	98	40–50	0.10–0.20
Pap smear	35–85	78–85	1.6–5.7	0.18–0.83
Culture	95	100	∞	0.05
Cervical infection				
Neisseria gonorrhoeae				
Cervix Gram stain	50–79	>90	5–7.9	0.23–0.56
N. gonorrhoeae culture— single cervical swab	85–90	98	43–45	0.10–0.15
DNA probe	~90	~96	~23	~0.10
Chlamydia trachomatis				
Cell culture—single cervical swab	70–80	98	35–40	0.2–0.31
Amplified DNA probes, ligase and polymerase chain reactions	>95	>99	95	0.05
Direct fluorescent antibody	70–87	97–99	23–87	0.13–0.31
Enzyme immunoassay	80–85	98	40–43	0.15–0.2
Herpes simplex virus				
Tzanck smear: vesicular/ pustular/crusted	67/54/17	85	4.3/3.6/1.1	0.41/0.54/0.98
Herpes simplex virus culture: vesicular/pustular/crusted	70/67/17	100	∞/∞/∞	0.30/0.33/0.83

CSp due to low-grade colonization, a "gold standard" of positive KOH or more than 2+ growth on culture or both has been recommended for definitive diagnosis of *Candida* vaginitis (27,28). In one study, saline wet mount had the same test parameters as the KOH mount, potentially saving an office procedure, but both were less accurate than Gram stain of vaginal secretions (sensitivity 65%, specificity 100%) (27).

The saline wet mount is a useful but imperfect test for in the diagnosis of trichomonas vaginalis. Although highly specific (70% to 98%), its sensitivity ranges from 50% to 80% (6,17,28,29). Loss of motility owing to cooling, low inoculum size, over-rapid scanning, and reader inexperience all reduce sensitivity. Direct fluorescent antibody (DFA) for *T. vaginalis* has shown promise, with a sensitivity of 80% to 86%, increasing to 90% when no other pathogens are present, and with a specificity of 98% (28). Diamond media for culture remains the gold standard, with a sensitivity of 95% (some strains of *T. vaginalis* do not grow in this medium); culture plus wet mount increase sensitivity to approximately 100% (6). Using Pap smear in the diagnosis of *T. vaginalis* is limited by variable and often low sensitivity as well as by only moderate specificity (28,30). The ratio of PMNs to clue cells on saline wet mounts can also be helpful; a ratio of greater than 1 was seen in 90% of patients with *T. vaginalis* and a ratio of less than 1 was noted in 75% of patients with BV (6).

Cervical Infections

The endocervical Gram stain is key to the evaluation of patients with mucopurulent cervical discharge. Presence of increased PMNs and gram-negative intracellular diplococci (GNID) confirms the diagnosis of gonococcal infection. Sensitivity of the cervical Gram stain compared with that of culture is 50% to 79%, with errors caused by the presence of background vaginal flora and reader inexperience; specificity is variable, but usually more than 90% (31,32). Increased PMNs in the absence of GNID on Gram stain raises suspicion of chlamydia (33).

Cervical cultures also have a role in the diagnostic evaluation. For *N. gonorrhoeae*, culture is 90% sensitive with the use of a single endocervical swab, increasing to 100% with the use of a second swab, usually from the rectum (34). Tissue culture is needed for isolating *C. trachomatis*. However, this technique is not widely available, and results may not be available for 4 to 7 days. Test characteristics are not as good as culture for *N. gonorrhoeae*, and sensitivity and specificity are 70% to 80% and 98%, respectively (10).

The most promising rapid diagnostic tests for chlamydia are amplified DNA probes using ligase and polymerase chain reactions, with sensitivity and specificity of approximately 95% and approximately 99%, respectively (35,36). A DFA test and an enzyme immunoassay have also been developed for use in the diagnosis of infection with *C.*

trachomatis. With experienced readers and use of the first cervical swab for the DFA specimen (and the second for culture), sensitivity and specificity for CT-DFA are 70% to 87% and 97% to 99%, respectively (11,37,38). The sensitivity decreases if readers are less experienced or if the first swab is not used for DFA testing. The enzyme immunoassay test has a sensitivity of 80% to 85% and a specificity of 98% (39). DNA probes for *N. gonorrhoeae* are being used increasingly. Sensitivity (approximately 90%) and specificity (approximately 96%) of this test are similar to those of culture (40,41). Although this technique is more expensive than culture, many logistical problems related to handing samples for culture are eliminated.

Vulvovaginal lesions suspicious for HSV, especially in women with a previous history of genital herpes, should be evaluated by Tzanck smear or viral culture or both. Tzanck smears are underused in the office diagnosis of genital HSV. After unroofing a vesicle or pustule, a sample is scraped from the base of the lesion and applied to a glass slide, stained with Toluidine blue, and examined under high-dry (40×) or oil-immersion (100×) lens for presence of multinucleated giant cells. Sensitivity and specificity are 65% and 85%, respectively (42). Sensitivity is highest for vesicular lesions (see Table 22-3). Cell culture is the gold standard, although sensitivity varies with the appearance of the lesion. Viral isolation rates are approximately 70% from vesicular and pustular lesions, decreasing to 20% if lesions are ulcerated or crusted (43). Virus is recovered more frequently from lesions that are primary or cutaneous than from lesions that are recurrent or of genital origin. Cell culture is cumbersome and may take as many as 7 days to yield positive results. In women with a first HSV infection, culture from multiple sites into one vial is recommended to improve diagnosis. Serologic assay for antibody to HSV-2 is advised for confirming recurrent genital herpes and identifying subclinical infection in sexually active women (13,44). Although in general DFA and enzyme immunoassay tests have not proved to be highly accurate (43,45,46), a rapid enzyme immunoassay test using mouse monoclonal antibody has recently shown high sensitivity for both early and late lesions (47).

DIAGNOSTIC STRATEGIES

Diagnosis of acute vaginitis requires characterization of the vaginal discharge and skill in interpreting simple office tests. Evaluation should target symptomatic women, because antimicrobial therapy is generally used only in symptomatic women with positive diagnostic test results and is used in asymptomatic women only if they report contact with an infected sexual partner.

Clinicians should assess risk factors for STDs and HIV in each patient, and be knowledgeable about the prevalence of the common causes of vaginal and cervical infection in their practice sites. The source of the discharge should be carefully ascertained during the pelvic examination. If the discharge appears vaginal in origin, then assessing the character of the discharge along with the vaginal pH, saline wet mount, and KOH wet mount should help to distinguish between bacterial vaginosis, candidal infection, and *T. vaginalis*. If BV is suspected, Gram stain of vaginal secretions can enhance diagnostic accuracy. If the results of these tests are inconclusive, several options are possible: empiric treatment for the most likely cause; further testing with a culture or rapid diagnostic test, such as DFA; or observation if the discharge appears physiologic. Urinalysis may also be helpful in some patients, as described in Chapter 21.

If cervicitis is present, cervical Gram stain should be obtained to look for GNID. If risk factors for STDs are present, culture for *N. gonorrhoeae* is also needed; however, testing for *N. gonorrhoeae* by DNA probe assay can be used instead of culture. If the cervical Gram stain is negative, then a decision needs to be made about whether to start empiric therapy or to wait for culture or DNA probe test results. This decision is influenced by the pretest probability, and therapy may be indicated when the pretest probability of gonococcal infection is high. In patients with negative Gram stains in which the probability of chlamydia is high, rapid diagnostic tests or culture for *C. trachomatis* may be helpful. If suspicious lesions are found, tests for HSV are warranted.

The studies of Komaroff (48) and Berg (2) show that the combination of symptoms and simple laboratory tests clearly enhance the posttest probability of cervical and vaginal infection but result in underdiagnosis of infections with *Candida*, *T. vaginalis*, and *C. trachomatis*. In patients not responding to treatment based on initial assessment, culture for yeast and trichomonas may be obtained on subsequent visits.

CLINICAL PROBLEMS

Clinical Problem 1
A young healthy woman is noted to have a scant white vaginal discharge on routine pelvic examination.

Testing Strategy and Rationale
No tests are indicated. In this clinical situation, the probability of an infection requiring diagnosis or specific treatment in a woman with no symptoms and a physiologic vaginal discharge is very low.

Clinical Example
A 40-year-old woman is seen for a routine gynecologic examination. She has no history of STD and reports that she has had no

recent sexual contacts. She is noted to have a scant white vaginal discharge. The patient has no symptoms of vaginal discharge or irritation. No further evaluation is needed at this time.

Clinical Problem 2
A young woman who reports multiple recent sexual partners reports symptoms of lower abdominal pain, dysuria, and yellow vaginal discharge.

Testing Strategy and Rationale
The patient should be asked about additional risk factors for STD and HIV, including infection with STDs in the past and contact with partners who may currently have STDs or HIV. The patient's menstrual, contraceptive, and pregnancy history must be obtained. The skin should be examined for rash, and a careful abdominal and pelvic examination should be performed.

In a young, sexually active woman, a purulent endocervical discharge with cervical or adnexal tenderness on bimanual examination is highly suggestive of PID. The probability of gonococcal infection and/or chlamydia cervicitis or salpingitis is more than 50%. Gram stain of the cervical discharge should be obtained. If the results are positive for *N. gonorrhoeae,* the diagnosis is relatively certain and treatment should be started; if the results are negative, then empiric therapy is often warranted. The patient should be treated for both gonococcal and chlamydial infection according to the Centers for Disease Control recommendations, and chlamydia culture is unnecessary. However, if the evaluation does not indicate *N. gonorrhoeae,* then further evaluation for *C. trachomatis* is indicated.

Clinical Example
A 28-year-old woman presents to the emergency department with symptoms of lower abdominal pain and vaginal discharge. Her examination reveals a low-grade fever, cervical motion tenderness, and cervicitis with cervical discharge. She has a history of previous STDs. Gram stain of the cervical discharge shows many white cells and gram-negative intracellular diplococci. An endocervical culture for *N. gonorrhoeae* is done, and treatment for gonococcal and *C. trachomatis* infection is initiated. Discussion about HIV status and HIV testing should also be undertaken.

REFERENCES

1. **O'Dowd TC, West RR, Winterburn PJ, et al.** Evaluation of a rapid diagnostic test for bacterial vaginosis. Br J Obstet Gynecol. 1996;103:366-70.

2. **Berg AO, Heidrich FE, Fihn SD, et al.** Establishing the cause of genitourinary symptoms in women in a family practice. JAMA 1984;251:620-5.

3. **Ferris DG, Hendrich J, Payne PM, et al.** Office laboratory diagnosis of vaginitis: clinician-performed tests compared with a rapid nucleic acid hybridization test. J Fam Pract. 1995;41:575-81.

4. **Eschenbach DA.** Vaginal infection. Clin Obstet Gynecol 1983;26:186-202.

5. **Ingalls RA, Rice PA.** Sexually transmitted disease. In: Noble J, Greene HL, Levinson W, et al, eds. Primary Care Medicine. St. Louis: Mosby–Year Book; 1996:855-85.

6. **Heine P, McGregor JA.** *Trichomonas vaginalis*: a reemerging pathogen. Clin Obstet Gynecol 1993;36(1):137-44.

7. **Soper DE.** Genitourinary infections and sexually transmitted diseases. In: Berek J S, Adashi E Y, Hillard PA, eds. Novak's Gynecology. 12th ed. Baltimore: Williams and Wilkins; 1996:429-45.

8. **Briselden AM, Hillier SL.** Evaluation of affirm VP microbial identification test for *Gardnerella vaginalis* and *Trichomonas vaginalis*. J Clin Microbiol. 1994;32(1):148-52.

9. **Freeman SB.** Common genitourinary infections. J Obstet Gynecol Neonatal Nurs. 1995;24:735-42.

10. **Stamm WE, Holmes KK.** *Chlamydia trachomatis* infections of the adult. In: Holmes KK, Mardh PA, Sparting PF, Weisner PJ, eds. Sexually Transmitted Diseases. New York: McGraw Hill; 1984:258-70.

11. **Livengood CH, Schmitt JW, Addison WA, et al.** Direct fluorescent antibody testing for endocervical chlamydia trachomatis: factors affecting accuracy. Obstet Gynecol. 1988;72:803-9.

12. **Sherrard J.** Modern diagnosis and management of gonorrhoea. Br J Hosp Med 1996;55:394-8.

13. **Koutsky LA, Stevens CE, Holmes K K, et al.** Underdiagnosis of genital herpes by current clinical and viral-isolation procedures. N Engl J Med. 1992;326:1533-9.

14. **Schaaf M, Perez-Stable E J, Borchardt K.** The limited value of symptoms and signs in the diagnosis of vaginal infections. Arch Intern Med 1990;150:1929-33.

15. **Braunstein H.** Gonorrhea as a marker for chlamydial infection [Letter]. JAMA 1987;:1330-1.

16. **Reed BD, Huck W, Zazove P.** Differentiation of *Gardnerella vaginalis, Candida albicans,* and *Trichomonas vaginalis* infections of the vagina. J Fam Pract 1989;28:673-80.

17. **Lossick TG.** Sexually transmitted vaginitis. Urol Clin North Am. 1984;11:141-53.

18. **Hill LVH, Embil JA.** Vaginitis: current microbiologic and clinical concepts. Can Med Assoc J. 1986;134:321-31.

19. **Spiegel CA, Amsel R, Holmes KK.** Diagnosis of bacterial vaginosis by direct Gram stain of vaginal fluid. J Clin Microb 1983;18:170-7.

20. **Hillier SL.** Diagnostic microbiology of bacterial vaginosis. Am J Obstet Gynecol. 1993;169(2 Pt 2):455-9.

21. **Nugent RP, Krohn MA, Hillier SL.** Reliability of diagnosing bacterial vaginosis is improved by a standardized method of Gram stain interpretation. J Clin Microb. 1991;29:297-301.

22. **Thomason JL, Gelbart SM, Anderson RJ, et al.** Statistical evaluation of diagnostic criteria for bacterial vaginosis. Am J Obstet Gynecol. 1990;162: 155-60.

23. **Thomason JL, Anderson RJ, Gelbart SM, et al.** Simplified Gram stain interpretive method for diagnosis of bacterial vaginosis. Am J Obstet Gynecol 1992;167:16-9.

24. **Eschenbach DA, Hillier S, Crichtlow C, et al.** Diagnosis and clinical manifestations of bacterial vaginosis. Am J Obstet Gynecol. 1988;158:819-28.

25. **Sonnex C.** The amine test: a simple, rapid, inexpensive method for diagnosing bacterial vaginosis. Br J Obstet Gynecol. 1995;102:160-1.

26. **Rothenberg RB, Simon R, Chipperfield E, Cutterall RD.** Efficacy of selected diagnostic tests for sexually transmitted diseases. JAMA 1976;235:49-51.

27. **Abbott J.** Clinical and microscopic diagnosis of vaginal yeast infection: a prospective analysis. Ann Emerg Med 1995;25:587-91.

28. **Bickley LS, Krisher K, Punsalang A Jr, et al.** Comparison of direct fluorescent antibody, acridine orange, wet mount and culture for detection of trichomonas vaginalis in women attending a public sexually transmitted diseases clinic. Sex Transm Dis. 1988;16:1024-8.

29. **Andrews H, Acheson N, Huengsberg M, et al.** The role of microscopy in the diagnosis of sexually transmitted infections in women. Genitourin Med. 1994;70:118-20.

30. **Kreiger JN, Tam MR, Stevens CE, et al.** Diagnosis of trichomoniasis: comparison of conventional wet mount examination with cytological studies, cultures, and monoclonal antibody staining of direct specimens. JAMA 1988;259:1223-7.

31. **Lossick JG, Smeltzer MP, Curran JW.** The value of cervical Gram stain in the diagnosis and treatment of gonorrhea in women in a venereal disease clinic. Sex Transm Dis. 1982;9:124-7.

32. **Goodhard ME, Ogden J, Zaidi AA, Kraus SJ.** Factors affecting the performance of smear and culture tests for the detection of *Neisseria gonorrhoeae*. Sex Transm Dis. 1981;9:63-9.

33. **Phillips RS, Hanff PA, Wertheimer A, et al.** Gonorrhea in women seen for routine gynecologic care: criteria for testing. Am J Med. 1988;85:177-82.

34. **Handsfield HH.** Gonorrhea and uncomplicated gonococcal infection. In: Holmes KK, Mardh PA, Sparting PF, Weisner PJ, eds. Sexually transmitted diseases. New York: McGraw Hill; 1984:205-20.

35. **Robinson AJ, Ridgway GL.** Modern diagnosis and management of genital *Chlamydia trachomatis* infection. Br J Hosp Med. 1996;55:388-93.

36. **Weinstock H, Dean D, Bolan G.** *Chlamydia trachomatis* infections. Infect Dis Clin North Am. 1994;8:797-819.

37. **Stamm WE, Harrison R, Alexander E R, et al.** Diagnosis of *Chlamydia trachomatis* infections by direct immunoflourescence staining of genital secretions. Ann Intern Med. 1984;101:638-44.

38. **Skolnik NS.** Screening for *Chlamydia trachomatis* infection. Am Fam Phys 1995;51:821-6.

39. **Jones MF, Smith TF, Houghm AJ, Herman JE.** Detection of *Chlamydia trachomatis* in genital specimens by the chlamydiazyme test. J Clin Microb 1984;20:465-7.

40. **Mahony JB, Luinstra KE, Tyndall M, et al.** Multiplex PCR for detection of *Chlamydia trachomatis* and *Neisseria gonorrhoeae* in genitourinary specimens. J Clin Microb 1995;33:3049-53.

41. **Schwebke JR, Zajackowski ME.** Comparison of DNA probe (Gen-probe) with culture for the detection of *Neisseria gonorrhea* in an urban STD programme. Genitourin Med. 1996;72:108-10.

42. **Solomon AR, Rasmussen JE, Varani T, Pierson CL.** The Tzanck smear in the diagnosis of cutaneous herpes simplex. JAMA 1984;251:633-5.

43. **Lafferty WE, Kroft S, Remington R, et al.** Diagnosis of herpes simplex virus by direct immunofluorescence and viral isolation from samples of external genital lesions in a high prevalence population. J Clin Microb. 1987;25:323-6.

44. **Corey L.** Genital herpes. In: Holmes KK, Mardh PA, Sparting PF, Weisner PJ, eds. Sexually Transmitted Diseases. New York: McGraw Hill; 1984: 449-74.

45. **Baker DA, Gonik B, Milch P, et al.** Clinical evaluation of a new herpes simplex virus ELISA: a rapid diagnostic test for herpes simplex virus. Obstet Gynecol. 1989;73:322-5.

46. **Warford AL, Levy RA, Rekrut K.** Evaluation of a commercial enzyme-linked immunoabsorbent assay for detection of herpes simplex virus antigen. J Clin Microb 1984;20:490-3.

47. **Cone RW, Swenson PD, Hobson AC, et al.** Herpes simplex virus detection from genital lesions: a comparative study using antigen detection (HerpChek) and culture. J Clin Microb. 1993;31:1774-6.

48. **Komaroff AL, Pass TM, McCue JD, et al.** Management strategies for urinary and vaginal infectious. Arch Intern Med. 1978;138:1068-73.

Human Immunodeficiency Virus Infection

23

Marguerite A. Urban, MD, and Richard C. Reichman, MD

KEY POINTS

Pretest Probabilities

- Estimating the probability of human immunodeficiency virus (HIV) infection is dependent on eliciting a careful history of previous risk-conferring behaviors or events.
- The most important risk histories include receptive anal intercourse among homosexual men, intravenous drug abuse with needle sharing, and vaginal or anal intercourse with HIV infected or potentially infected persons.

Diagnostic Strategies

- When initial enzyme immunoassay (EIA) serologic tests are repeatedly reactive, more specific confirmatory tests, such as the Western blot assay, should be performed.
- When the pretest probability of infection is low, suspicious or positive results should be repeated on a separate sample to exclude laboratory or human error.
- When the pretest probability of infection is high and EIA tests are repeatedly reactive, negative, or indeterminate, confirmatory tests should be repeated.
- When acute HIV infection is suspected, a negative EIA test result does not rule out infection. Alternative diagnostic testing, such as nucleic acid testing or viral culture, should be done, or repeat serologic testing should be pursued within 30 days if such alternative testing is not available.

BACKGROUND

Infection with the human immunodeficiency virus (HIV) has become an epidemic of staggering proportions. The Centers for Disease Control and Prevention (CDC) have classified HIV infection into three broad clinical categories: Category A—primary and asymptomatic HIV infection, which includes those cases with generalized lymphadenopathy; Category B—symptomatic HIV infection, but without opportunistic infections; and Category C—CDC–defined opportunistic infection or neoplasm or both (1). Persons with acquired immune deficiency syndrome (AIDS) are those persons with HIV infection in Category C and those in Categories A or B who also have a CD4 cell count of less than 200/mm^3. Worldwide, the World Health Organization (WHO) estimates that more than 22.6 million adults and children have been infected with HIV, resulting in more than 8.4 million AIDS cases (2).

HIV is transmitted through sexual contact, exposure to infected blood products via shared needles or transfusion, or from mother to infant either transplacentally at birth or through breast feeding. Within 2 to 6 weeks of initial infection, most persons develop a nonspecific mononucleosis-like syndrome manifested by fever, lymphadenopathy, rash, and occasionally, aseptic meningitis (3). These symptoms resolve spontaneously, and most infected persons then remain asymptomatic for several years. AIDS develops when immune function decline is significant, generally measured by a CD4 cell count of less than 200 cells/mm^3, or if a CDC–defined opportunistic infection or tumor is diagnosed (1). During initial infection, which is often referred to as seroconversion, acute infection, or primary infection, a burst of virus replication occurs that produces high levels of plasma viremia. Concomitantly, humoral and cellular immune responses to HIV antigens develop. During the asymptomatic or "clinically latent" phase, virus replication continues and produces detectable levels of circulating virus in most infected persons. Human immunodeficiency virus may be transmitted during all stages of infection.

Recent years have seen numerous advances in the understanding of HIV pathogenesis and improved methods of prophylaxis and diagnosis. However, despite this progress, most persons infected with HIV remain undiagnosed and thus are unable to benefit from these advances. The past 5 years have also been a time of intense study of new antiretroviral drugs. In general, the benefits of combination antiretroviral regimens have been most dramatic when administered to patients early in the course of the disease. This makes diagnosing HIV infection promptly even more urgent.

The diagnosis of HIV infection is dependent either on the identification of the virus or portions of the virus in the infected person or on the identification of an antigen-specific humoral immune response. To date, antibody testing has been the mainstay of laboratory diagnosis. Antibody tests are available for testing of blood, saliva, or urine. Identification of the virus may be accomplished by culture, identification of viral antigens, or identification of HIV DNA or RNA. These tests are not generally available for screening purposes but rather are used in research or specialized settings such as the screening of newborns or the screening of blood products. An exception is HIV RNA, which is currently widely available for monitoring response to therapy.

ESTIMATING PRETEST PROBABILITY

The pretest probability of HIV infection may be estimated based on a history of recognized risk behaviors or events that are associated with a high likelihood of infection. These include percutaneous exposure to potentially infected blood, either caused by sharing needles during intravenous drug use or from occupational exposure; a history of sexual risk behaviors such as male-to-male sex, multiple sexual partners, or sexual contact with a commercial sex worker; or a history of receiving blood products before 1985. Persons with a history of sexually transmitted diseases or with a sexual partner who engaged in any of the risk behaviors just mentioned is also at increased risk (3,4). The social stigma associated with many of these behaviors makes obtaining an accurate history a challenge for health care providers.

Numerous other variables increase the risk of contracting HIV, such as the prevalence of infection in the community where the risk behavior or event occurs, the presence or absence of other sexually transmitted diseases, related behaviors such as use of safer-sex practices, and possibly the viral burden of the HIV-source person. Finally, other individual characteristics may affect the pretest probability of infection. Some of these characteristics are apparent to the diagnostician, such as evidence of immune suppression on physical examination (e.g., oral thrush). Others are largely unknown, such as the presence or absence of genetic factors that have recently been found to be of importance in determining susceptibility to HIV infection (5).

Despite the numerous variables that may affect the ability to make an accurate assessment of pretest probability, some clear risk behaviors have been studied and some degrees of risk have been quantified, as shown in Figure 23-1 (4). These are helpful in viewing a population and in counseling persons about the risks of certain behaviors. The difficulties in obtaining accurate histories of socially sensitive study participants and the increasing benefit of early diagnosis and treatment supports the practice of "overtesting" in some situations in which one might expect a low pretest probability of infection.

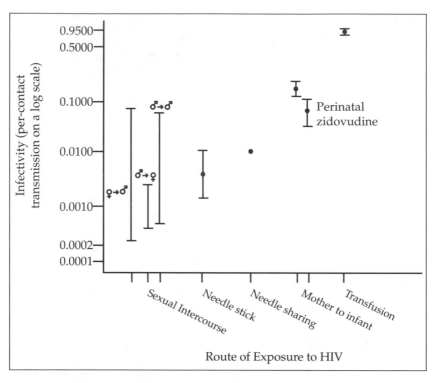

Figure 23-1. Per-contact probability of HIV transmission. The infectivity ranges for sexual contact were derived from a review of the literature; estimates for other routes of infection originated from a representative study. Note: ♀ → ♂ indicates female-to-male transmission; ♂ → ♀ indicates male-to-female transmission; and ♂ → ♂ indicates male-to-male transmission. Republished with permission from Royce RA, Sena A, Cates W Jr, Cohen MS. Sexual transmission of HIV. N Engl J Med. 1997;336:1072-8 [corrected figure in N Engl J Med. 1997;337:799].

DIAGNOSTIC TESTS

Serologic Testing

Enzyme Immunoassays
Enzyme immunoassays for HIV antibody testing were first introduced for blood bank screening in 1985 and are still the standard assay for initial HIV testing. These assays are inexpensive and practical for screening large numbers of samples. Briefly, serum from the patient is incubated with HIV viral proteins that are bound to a solid phase, such as a microtiter plate well. Human immunodeficiency–specific antibodies present in the serum bind to the HIV antigen on the plate, and the

remaining serum is washed away. Enzymatically labeled antibodies specific for human IgG are added to the wells, making a sandwich with the HIV antigen, the HIV-specific antibody from the patient, and the labeled IgG-specific antibody. A color reaction detects the entire complex and the amount of color reaction is recorded as an optical density. An optical density greater than a predetermined cutoff is reported as positive.

Enzyme immunoassay (EIA) tests have undergone several changes since the "first-generation" tests were released in 1985. The current "third-generation" assays use recombinant proteins as HIV antigens rather than use HIV antigens derived from lysates of whole virus cultured in human T lymphocytes. This change has been associated with improved sensitivity and specificity compared with the first-generation tests. In addition, third-generation assays use an enzyme-labeled antigen rather than antibody as the detection tool. This antigen detects IgM as well as IgG, leading to positive EIA test results earlier in the course of infection and to increased sensitivity of the assay (6).

As with most tests, false-positive and false-negative test results may occur. False-positive reactions have been reported to occur in patients who have had recent immune globulin administration and recent influenza vaccination and in the presence of antibodies to some HLA antigens, some autoantibodies, liver disease, and malignancies. False-negative EIA results have been reported in patients with hypogamma-globulinemia, variant strains of HIV, and most frequently, testing before seroconversion (3,7). Occasionally, patients with advanced AIDS have been reported to have a false-negative EIA test result, presumably owing to a loss of ability to make antibody. There have been rare reports of delayed seroconversion resulting in a negative EIA test result for an extended time after the initial infection (8).

The currently licensed EIA tests have been reported to have sensitivities ranging from 99.0% to 99.9% and specificities greater than 98.5%.

Western Blot

Western blot testing is generally reserved for confirmation of tests that are repeatedly positive by EIA. Western blot is more labor intensive and has an unacceptably high rate of "indeterminate" results. This test uses a membrane containing bands of individual HIV proteins or antigens that is incubated with patient serum. The membrane is then washed and any patient antibody specific for individual HIV antigens remains. This antigen antibody complex is detected by either an enzyme reaction or autoradiography. Positive results are visualized as bands at each reactive complex and show the presence of antibody in the patient's serum directed against a variety of HIV antigens.

Interpretation of Western blot results is dependent on the number and combination of bands present. Test results are reported as positive, negative, or indeterminate using established criteria. Current CDC criteria require the presence of any two of the following three bands for a test result to be considered positive: anti-p24, anti-gp41, or anti-gp120/160 bands. With negative test results, no bands correspond to viral antigens, and with indeterminate test results, there are some bands but not enough to meet the definition of a positive test result (9).

The sensitivity of Western blot has been reported to be greater than 96%, and the specificity has been reported to be between 99.4% and 99.9% (Table 23-1).

Immunofluoresence Antibody Testing

Immunofluoresence antibody testing (IFA) has been used as an alternative to Western blot for confirmatory testing. This test involves fixing HIV-infected cells to a slide and incubating the slide with patient serum. Patient antibodies that adhere to the HIV-infected cells are detected by fluorescein-labeled anti-human IgG antibodies. The slide is viewed with a fluorescence microscope and compared with positive and negative controls. Although IFA has been less well studied than Western blot, it has been reported to have similar sensitivity and specificity (10).

Urine and Saliva Serologic Testing

Human immunodeficiency virus testing using fluids other than blood has been proposed because it may have several benefits, including

Table 23-1. Operating Characteristics of Diagnostic Tests in the Evaluation of Human Immunodeficiency Virus Infections

Diagnostic Test	Sensitivity	Specificity	Likelihood Ratio	
			Positive Result	Negative Result
	← % →			
Enzyme immunoassay				
Blood	99.0–99.9	98.5	~66	~0.005
Urine	98.4–99.9	94.2–100	~33	~0.01
Saliva	98.6–99.1	~98.5	~66	~0.01
Western blot				
Blood	>96	99.4–99.9	~240	~0.04
Saliva	97.5–99.5	99.5	~197	~0.015
HIV Culture	40–97	100	⬅	0.03–0.6

EIA = enzyme immunoassay; HIV = human immunodeficiency virus.

improved acceptance of testing, ease of collection, and decreased risk of occupational needle-stick injuries.

An EIA test performed on urine was licensed by the Food and Drug Administration (FDA) in 1996. It detects IgG to HIV protein gp160. Sensitivity has been reported to range from 98.4% to 99.9%, and specificity has been reported to range from 94.2% to 100% (11). Currently, positive test results require a confirmatory blood test, although confirmatory Western blot testing using urine may be available in the near future.

In 1994, the FDA licensed a "saliva"-based EIA and confirmatory Western blot test kit. The patient applies a treated pad between the teeth and gums that collects mucosal transudate. The sensitivity of EIA has been reported to range from 98.6% to 99.1%, and the sensitivity of the Western blot portion of the oral test has been reported as 97.5% to 99.5%. The specificity of both EIA and Western blot testing is described as equivalent to that of serum testing (12).

Rapid Enzyme Immunoassay Testing

Several rapid screening EIA tests have been developed that yield results in several minutes. The one currently commercially available in the United States uses a mixture of latex beads coated with HIV antigen. The patient's serum is added, and a negative result is available in 10 minutes. Positive results need confirmation with traditional Western blot testing. Sensitivity and specificity have both been reported to be greater than 99% (13).

Home Testing

Companies have marketed FDA-approved blood serologic test kits that can be performed at home. The tests use a fingerstick method to obtain blood that is then sent to the company for EIA and Western blot testing, if necessary.

Virus Detection

Human Immunodeficiency Virus Culture

Viral culture is highly specific (100%), but its sensitivity ranges from 40% to 97% in persons known to be infected with HIV (10). This variability is most likely related to technical considerations and variable amounts of viremia during the course of HIV infection. Owing to the variable sensitivity and the labor-intensive nature of HIV culture techniques, viral culture is not frequently used to diagnose HIV infection.

Human Immunodeficiency Virus Antigen Detection

Detection of p24 antigen, an HIV core protein, can be accomplished using an enzyme immunoassay and serum from infected patients.

However, because the results of this test may be negative in as many as 50% of asymptomatic infected persons, its utility is limited.

Human Immunodeficiency Virus Nucleic Acid Tests

Human immunodeficiency virus nucleic acid tests are presently used to monitor disease progression and response to therapy. However, it is likely that these techniques will also be used for diagnostic purposes in the near future. Currently available tests, including polymerase chain reaction tests, nucleic acid sequence based amplification, and branched-chain DNA tests, detect very small quantities of HIV nucleic acids. Thus, the sensitivity of these tests is similar to and occasionally greater than that of HIV culture in some clinical settings. Other advantages of these tests over virus culture include a potential for rapid turnaround time, the possibility of laboratory automation, and the decreased risk of occupational exposure of laboratory workers to HIV in culture. The major disadvantage is the rate of false-positive results, generally arising from cross-contamination of the specimen or the laboratory with minute quantities of HIV nucleic acids, which are then detected by these highly sensitive assays (14).

DIAGNOSTIC STRATEGIES

In most situations, the usual approach to the diagnosis of HIV infection is to perform an initial screening EIA followed by a confirmatory Western blot for repeatedly positive EIA results. There are only a few situations in which this strategy may be misleading. When using a third-generation EIA assay, false-negative results can be anticipated during recently acquired infection—that is, infection contracted less than 30 days before testing. As discussed earlier in this chapter, false-negative test results may occur for other reasons, but this is rare. In those settings in which recent infection seems possible, such as a recent high-risk behavior or event or an illness consistent with seroconversion, a negative EIA result should be followed with either an alternative testing method such as virus culture, p24 antigen testing, or HIV nucleic acid detection, or the patient should be receive repeat testing within 15 to 30 days. Most experts would perform HIV nucleic acid testing or HIV culture or both. Results of nucleic acid testing are usually available before culture results, and nucleic acid testing is more widely available. Prompt diagnosis may become critically important if ongoing study results confirm benefits of antiretroviral therapy prescribed at the time of seroconversion.

The results of EIA must be interpreted in the context of pretest probability. Despite the impressive specificity of this test, the post-test probability of a repeatedly reactive EIA may be as low as 27% when the prevalence of disease is very low (15). For this reason, it is necessary to confirm positive EIA results with a highly specific confirmatory test such as the Western blot. When the results of both tests are positive, the diagnosis is confirmed. However, when the pretest probability is low, repeat testing is warranted to exclude the possibility of human error, such as mislabeling of specimens. Repeatedly positive EIA test results with negative confirmatory test results should be presumed to be negative when the pretest probability is low.

Repeatedly reactive EIA tests with indeterminate Western blot test results can be difficult to interpret. When the pretest probability of disease is high, a positive EIA test result followed by an indeterminate Western blot result may represent early infection or a false-negative Western blot result. Repeat testing withing 1 to 3 months should be considered; or, if available, alternative diagnostic testing such as virus culture or viral nucleic acid detection should be considered. When the pretest probability is low, the same scenario may or may not represent true infection. Options for repeat testing are the same. Patients at low risk for the disease with repeatedly indeterminate Western blot results are unlikely to be infected with HIV (16).

Diagnostic strategies may vary depending on the clinical scenario. Specialized settings such as blood banks and newborn HIV clinics have established protocols that are reviewed and altered as diagnostic technology changes. Recommendations by agencies such as the CDC and WHO about testing in these specialized situations are updated regularly.

CLINICAL PROBLEMS

Clinical Problem 1

A patient with multiple risk factors for HIV infection presents with an acute mononucleosis-like syndrome.

Testing Strategy and Rationale

In addition to the usual diagnostic workup for these symptoms, testing for HIV should be performed, because these symptoms of "mononucleosis" may represent acute HIV infection. Enzyme immunoassay should be performed, and if the results are positive, needs to be followed by confirmatory tests such as the Western blot. If the results of EIA are negative, acute infection remains a possibility, and additional testing should therefore be considered.

Clinical Example

A 24-year-old man reports symptoms of sore throat, fever, headache, and macular rash. The patient also reports that he is homosexual and has had two lifetime sexual partners. He had HIV serologic testing

Continued

done 6 months ago; the results were negative. He is currently in a monogamous relationship and does not use condoms.

In addition to the usual evaluation for these symptoms, repeat HIV testing is recommended. Results of the workup are unrevealing except in showing that the patient is mildly pancytopenic. The results of EIA are negative. Because this result may be a false-negative caused by acute infection, the patient is advised that HIV infection has not been excluded, and further diagnostic evaluation with repeat HIV serologic testing in 30 days is recommended. If available, HIV nucleic acid testing or culture may also be considered at this point.

Clinical Problem 2
A patient at low risk for HIV infection requests HIV testing.

Testing Strategy and Rationale
The potential risks and benefits of testing should be discussed with the patient, and if a decision is made to perform testing, EIA testing should be done first. The risks and benefits of such testing in patient at low risk for HIV infection should be discussed: The patient should be advised that a false-positive result could occur that may cause the patient considerable distress; that if the patient is infected with HIV, early diagnosis and treatment have been shown to be beneficial; and that a positive EIA test result would need to be followed by additional testing to distinguish true infection from a false-positive result.

Clinical Example
A 39-year-old mother of three requests HIV testing after reading a newspaper article about transfusion-related AIDS. She is concerned that she may have been infected during a blood transfusion received after the birth of one of her children, 2 years ago. She reports a history of three lifetime sexual partners and denies a history of sexually transmitted diseases, intravenous drug use, or receipt of other blood products. She believes her sexual partners would have been "low risk." The pretest probability of infection appears to be low. Although no sexual risk is identified, because the sexual histories of the partners are unknown, this could still be a potential route of exposure. Because blood supplies undergo routine screening, the risk of HIV infection from a blood transfusion is small. However, transfusion-associated HIV infection has occurred rarely in the past 10 years, most often associated with donation by persons with acute infections. The patient is advised that her risk of infection is very low, and she is counseled about the risks and benefits of testing. She decides to proceed with testing, and an EIA is ordered.

REFERENCES

1. Centers for Disease Control and Prevention. 1993 revised classification system for HIV infection and expanded surveillance case definition for AIDS among adolescents and adults. MMWR Morb Mortal Wkly Rep. 1992;41(No. RR-17):1-19.

2. World Health Organization. AIDS: the current global situation of the HIV pandemic. Weekly Epidemiologic Record. 1996;71(48):363-4.

3. **Chamberland ME, Ward JW, Curran JW.** Epidemiology and prevention of AIDS and HIV infection. In: Mandell GL, Bennett JE, Dolin R, eds. Principles and Practices of Infectious Diseases. 4th ed. New York: Churchill Livingstone; 1995:1174-203.

4. **Royce RA, Seña A, Cates Jr W, Cohen MS.** Sexual transmission of HIV. N Engl J Med. 1997;336:1072-8.

5. **Dean M, Carrington M, Winkler C, et al.** Genetic restriction of HIV-1 infection and progression to AIDS by a deletion allele of the CKR5 structural gene. Science. 1996;273:1856-62.

6. **Zaaijer HL, Exel-Oehlers PV, Kraaijeveld T, et al.** Early detection of antibodies to HIV-1 by third generation assays. Lancet. 1992;340:770-2.

7. **Hansen KN.** HIV testing. Emerg Med Clin North Am. 1995;13: 43-59.

8. Centers for Disease Control and Prevention. Persistent lack of detectable antibody in a person with HIV infection—Utah, 1995. MMWR Morb Mortal Wkly Rep. 1996;45:181-5.

9. Centers for Disease Control. Interpretation and use of the Western blot assay for serodiagnosis of human immunodeficiency virus type 1 infection. MMWR Morb Mortal Wkly Rep. 1989;38(Suppl 7):1-7.

10. Anonymous. Diagnostic tests for HIV: medical letter on drugs and therapeutics. 1997;39:81-3.

11. **Berrios DC, Avins AL, Haynes-Sanstad K, et al.** Screening for human immunodeficiency virus antibody in urine. Arch Pathol Lab Med. 1995;119:139-41.

12. **Gallo D, George JR, Fitchen JH, et al.** Evaluation of a system using oral mucosal transudate for HIV-1 antibody screening and confirmatory testing. OraSure HIV Clinical Trials Group. JAMA. 1997;277:254-8.

13. **Kassler WJ, Haley C, Jones WK, et al.** Performance of a rapid on-site human immunodeficiency virus antibody assay in a public health setting. J Clin Microb. 1995;33:2899-902.

14. **Owens DK, Holodniy M, Garber AM, et al.** Polymerase chain reaction for the diagnosis of HIV infection in adults: a meta-analysis with recommendations for clinical practice and study design. Ann Intern Med. 1996;124:803-15.

15. **Schwartz JS, Dans PE, Kinosian BP, et al.** Human immunodeficiency virus test evaluation, performance, and use: proposals to make good tests better. JAMA. 1988;259:2574-2579.

16. **Jackson JB, MacDonald KL, Cadwell J, et al.** Absence of HIV infection in blood donors with indeterminate western blot tests for antibody to HIV-1. N Engl J Med. 1990;322:217-22.

Infective Endocarditis

24

Diego G. Cahn-Hidalgo, MD, and Joseph D. Cappuccio, MD

KEY POINTS

Pretest Probabilities

- Making the diagnosis of infective endocarditis on the basis of clinical findings can be difficult because the signs and symptoms of this disease are neither sensitive nor specific. A high index of suspicion is required to identify the disease in patients with atypical presentations.

- Pretest probabilities for infective endocarditis are inexact. In patients with several specific findings, such as immunologic phenomena (Osler nodes, Roth spots), vascular phenomena (Janeway lesions, multiple arterial emboli), and new or changing heart murmur, the pretest probability is 80% to 90%. In patients with one or two sensitive but nonspecific findings, such as fever or unchanged heart murmur, the pretest probability is low.

Diagnostic Strategies

- The hallmark of the diagnosis of infective endocarditis is positive blood cultures. The persistence and nature of the organism are also important features of the disease. When the pretest probability is high, endocarditis can be diagnosed by positive blood cultures alone.

- Making the diagnosis of infective endocarditis is most confusing when one or more blood cultures yield unexpected results. Echocardiography may provide diagnostic information in such cases.

- The finding of vegetation(s) by echocardiography tends to confirm the diagnosis of infective endocarditis. However, because transthoracic echocardiography is not highly sensitive, a negative test does not exclude the disease. Transesophageal echocardiography is more sensitive and thus more helpful in excluding the diagnosis.

- The precise role of echocardiography in determining the prognosis for patients with infective endocarditis is uncertain.

BACKGROUND

The diagnosis and treatment of infective endocarditis, microbial infection of the heart, has changed dramatically from the preantibiotic era to the current era of antimicrobial drug therapy, echocardiography, and valvular heart surgery. Yet despite these diagnostic and therapeutic advances, the case fatality rate remains approximately 20% to 40%. This is mainly due to valve destruction with subsequent heart failure or overwhelming infection (1). Prosthetic valve endocarditis is associated with an even higher mortality rate of 40% to 80% (2).

A variety of infecting organisms, potential infective sources, and patient characteristics create heterogeneous clinical presentations of endocarditis. Although many patients have a typical presentation, a significant proportion have an atypical course. The clinician needs to maintain a high degree of suspicion with this latter group to avoid delays in diagnosis and possible complications of untreated infection. This chapter focuses on the role of primary clinical information, microbiological data, echocardiography, and laboratory studies in the evaluation of patients in whom infective endocarditis is suspected.

ESTIMATING PRETEST PROBABILITY

Determining the pretest probability of infective endocarditis requires the clinician to integrate data on the overall incidence of the disease, the presence of predisposing heart conditions or previous endocarditis, history of intravenous drug use, exposure to procedures causing bacteremia, and the clinical features seen at presentation (3–6).

The reported incidence of infective endocarditis in the general population varies between 1.7 and 3.8 cases per 100,000 persons per year (7,8). The incidence of infective endocarditis has remained fairly steady over recent decades: in Olmstead County, Minnesota, incidence rates were 4.3, 3.3, and 3.9 per 100,000 person-years, respectively, in each decade from 1950 through 1980 (9). Men are affected slightly more often than women. The incidence of infective endocarditis increases with age; many cases occur in those older than 50 years.

A predisposing cardiac lesion occurs in 60% to 80% of patients with native valve infective endocarditis (2). The spectrum of underlying cardiac lesions found in these patients has changed owing to the decline in the incidence of rheumatic heart disease, recognition of mitral valve prolapse, and increased use of intravenous drugs. The frequency of cardiac lesions in studies varies widely: mitral valve prolapse, 10% to 33%; degenerative heart disease, 1% to 32%; congenital heart disease, 10% to 20%; rheumatic heart disease, ~30%; and no underlying disease, 20% to 40%. Studies from the preantibiotic era include more rheumatic heart disease, whereas recent studies demonstrate higher occurrence rates of mitral valve prolapse, degenerative changes, and no underlying disease (2,10).

The source of the infecting organism remains undetermined in as many as 55% of reported cases. Intravenous drug abuse accounts for as many as 20% of cases, and dental procedures and disease are responsible for 11% to 25% (5,7,8,10–12).

Major infecting organisms are different for native valve endocarditis than for prosthetic valve infections. In native valves of patients who do not use intravenous drugs, 50% of patients have *Streptococcus viridans* as the infective agent, followed by *Staphylococcus aureus* in 20%; enterococci and other streptococci are the responsible organisms in 5% of patients each (13). In intravenous drug users, the major infecting organisms are quite different: *Staphylococcus aureus* is responsible for 57% of cases of infective endocarditis, *Streptococcus viridans* for 10%, enterococci for 8%, and gram-negative bacilli and fungi for 5% each. The organisms that cause prosthetic valve endocarditis include *Staphylococcus epidermis* in 33% of patients, gram-negative bacteria in 17%, *Staphylococcus aureus* in 15%, fungi in 10%, and *Streptococcus viridans* in 8%.

A spectrum of disease exists for those with endocarditis. Extremely virulent organisms such as *Staphylococcus aureus*, group A streptococci, or *Streptococcus pneumoniae* produce a rapid course with marked systemic signs, cardiac valve damage, and frequent metastatic infectious foci. At the other end of the spectrum, less virulent organisms, such as *S. viridans* and fastidious gram-negative organisms, produce milder forms of endocarditis with reduced systemic toxicity (13–15).

Clinical features of infective endocarditis are diverse and arise by one of four mechanisms: 1) systemic and local effects of the infection itself; 2) metastatic foci of infection; 3) systemic emboli; and 4) production of immunoglobulins or immune complexes with deposition in various tissues. The frequency with which various clinical manifestations occur has been documented in several series; the sensitivity of signs and symptoms can be estimated based on this (Table 24-1). However, specificity is not easily determined for most signs and symptoms. Fever of variable extent occurs in nearly 100% of patients sometime during the illness. A heart murmur is commonly found but may not be present at the initial presentation. More importantly, the classic "changing murmur" is truly uncommon, occurring in fewer than 20% of all cases. Musculoskeletal symptoms occur in as many as 50% of patients but are also found in many other conditions (16). Petechiae, once the most common cutaneous manifestation of infective endocarditis, are now much less prevalent (they occur in 12%–40% of cases) and are nonspecific. "Splinter" hemorrhages are also less common now than they were in the preantibiotic era and may be caused by trauma. Osler nodes are highly specific but are found in well under 50% of recent cases (17). Data from the preantibiotic era indicate a higher incidence of Osler nodes, attributable to more frequent infection by less virulent organisms. Reports of splenomegaly are variable. Retinal lesions, including Roth spots, occur in fewer than 10% of patients.

Table 24-1. Sensitivity of Signs and Symptoms in the Diagnosis of Infective Endocarditis

Clinical Finding	Sensitivity (%)
Symptoms	
Fever	84–100
Malaise	79
Weight loss	33–49
Dyspnea	28–42
Night sweats and chills	26–75
Musculoskeletal symptoms	10–53
Findings	
Any cardiac murmur	67–90
Changing cardiac murmur	7–16
Petechiae	12–40
Osler or Janeway lesion	10–50
Neurologic (focal or seizure)	10–20
Splenomegaly	9–75
Ocular emboli	3–8
Splinter hemorrhage	2–26

Because most of the signs and symptoms of infective endocarditis are either infrequent or nonspecific, the clinical diagnosis is difficult to make. Fever and a cardiac murmur, the most common signs in infective endocarditis, are frequently observed in other conditions. Clinical findings with greater specificity are observed less commonly. However, the clinician can assign high, intermediate, or low probability of infective endocarditis to patients, based on a combination of history and clinical findings. A patient with several specific clinical features of infective endocarditis such as Osler nodes or Roth spots has a high probability (perhaps 80%–90%) of infective endocarditis. Conversely, a patient with fever and a cardiac murmur alone has a low probability of infective endocarditis. Many patients in whom infective endocarditis is suspected have other combinations of clinical features and predisposing factors that give them intermediate pretest probabilities. Although such clinical estimates may be imprecise, they form the foundation for interpretation of the laboratory tests used to investigate suspected infective endocarditis.

DIAGNOSTIC TESTS

Blood Cultures

Positive blood culture results remain the mainstay of the laboratory diagnosis of infective endocarditis; expert clinicians often confirm the diagnosis of endocarditis on the basis of blood culture information alone (18). Culture data are important for confirming the diagnosis and choosing proper antibiotics. Documentable bacteremia, defined as one or more positive culture results, occurs in 77% to 90% of patients with infective endocarditis (19). In a study of 206 cases of culture-positive endocarditis, the first blood culture results were positive in 95% of patients, and one of the first two cultures drawn yielded positive results in 98% of cases (20). All cultures yielded positive results in 91% of cases. Hence, three sets of blood cultures are adequate in patients in whom infective endocarditis is suspected and who are at low risk for culture-negative disease.

Infective endocarditis with negative blood culture results accounts for 15% to 20% of cases. Reasons for the inability to isolate an organism include previous antibiotic treatment (as many as 60% of these cases), fungal disease, fastidious bacterial infections with nutritionally deficient streptococci, or atypical organisms such as *Chlamydia psittaci*, the HACEK organisms (*Haemophilus aphrophilus, Actinobacillus acetomycetemcomitans, Cardiobacterium hominis, Eikenella corrodens*, and *Kingella kingae*), *Brucella, Legionella, Neisseria*, or *Coxiella burnetti* (2,11).

The results of blood cultures among all patients with suspected bacteremia suggest that the specificity of a single positive blood culture result is between 75% and 95% (21,22). Thus, blood culture results are negative in as many as 95% of patients in whom infective endocarditis is suspected but who do not have the disease. If multiple positive culture results are required to support the diagnosis of infective endocarditis and if the offending organism is one that is known to produce endocarditis commonly, the specificity increases and approaches 100%, but sensitivity declines.

In the evaluation of patients with suspected endocarditis, attention should be given to the organism and pattern of positive blood culture results encountered. Sustained bacteremia (defined as multiple positive culture results over time with the same organism) is more likely to represent an endothelial infection characterized by constant seeding of the circulation than are sporadically positive blood culture results. Certain organisms are more likely to cause infective endocarditis. Bacteria such as *S. viridans*, coagulase-negative staphylococci, and enterococci cause sustained bacteremia almost exclusively in infective endocarditis. In some reports, more than 50% of patients with sustained coagulase-positive staphylococcal bacteremia have had infective endocarditis (23). Because inadequately treated staphylococcal endocarditis has a poor prognosis, most authorities recommend treatment regardless of whether other features of infective endocarditis are present (24). *Salmonella, Brucella*, and meningococci often cause bacteremia that lasts for days, but these organisms are rarely implicated as causative agents in infective endocarditis.

Thus, the sensitivity and specificity of bacteriologic data depends on the persistence of positive culture results as well as on the organism involved. The ranges for the operating characteristics of blood cultures are listed in Table 24-2.

Echocardiography

The reported sensitivity of transthoracic echocardiography (TTE) in detecting native valve vegetations ranges from 50% to 70%, whereas for transesophageal echocardiography (TEE) the sensitivity is between 90% and 100% (25–27). In prosthetic valve infections, the sensitivity of TTE is reported to be as low as 20%; TEE, on the other hand, has a sensitivity of 83% to 90% (28).

Echocardiographic criteria for infective endocarditis include an oscillating intracardiac mass on a valve, supporting structure, iatrogenic device, or a downstream regurgitant-jet site; an abscess; or new, partial dehiscence of prosthetic valve (3,4,25,26). The presence of valve thickening or nodules is not considered to be evidence of infective endocarditis (25).

Table 24-2. Operating Characteristics of Laboratory Tests in the Diagnosis of Infective Endocarditis*

Laboratory Finding	Sensitivity	Specificity
	←——————— % ———————→	
Blood cultures	77–96	75–95
Echocardiography		
Native valve: TTE	50–70	80–97
Native valve: TEE	90–100	~95
Prosthetic valve: TTE	~20	Uncertain
Prosthetic valve: TEE	83–90	Uncertain
Elevated erythrocyte		
Sedimentation rate	67–96	Poor
Circulating immune complex	80–100	Uncertain
C-reactive protein	~99	Uncertain
Rheumatoid factor	24–50	Uncertain
Anemia	50–80	Poor
Increased leukocyte count	~50	Uncertain
Microhematuria	25–50	Uncertain
Pyuria	~50	Uncertain
Teichoic acid antibody (staphylococcal bacteremia only)	67–90	70–90

TTE = transthoracic echocardiography; TEE = transesophageal echocardiography.
*Likelihood ratios not reported owing to the uncertainty of sensitivity and specificity.

As noted later in this chapter in the "Diagnostic Strategies" section, a positive TTE result makes it unnecessary to perform TEE; however, owing to the the low sensitivity of the study, a negative TTE result does not exclude the diagnosis of infective endocarditis (28). The positioning of the probe during TEE facilitates observation of the heart, thus enhancing the visualization of small vegetations sometimes not detected by TTE (27). Owing to the differences in sensitivity between TTE and TEE, use of TEE seems particularly important in those patients with suspected prosthetic valve infections. Finding dehiscence or a peri-prosthetic ring leak in such patients may indicate the need for urgent surgical intervention (25,29). Another role for TEE is to assess for abscess formation in patients with known infective endocarditis whose cardiac function is deteriorating (25,29).

The frequency of positive echocardiography results in patients who do not have infective endocarditis is between 3% and 20% (30,31). Differential diagnostic considerations include myxomatous valvular degeneration (mitral valve prolapse), tumors (myxomas), previous episodes of endocarditis, and ruptured chordae tendineae (32,33). Specificity is reported to decrease when the echocardiographer knows that infective endocarditis is under consideration (30).

Differences in the sensitivity of TTE compared with TEE may be more marked in older patients. In one study, the sensitivity of TTE decreased with the age of the patient, whereas the sensitivity of TEE was the same in all age groups (29). Because elderly patients with infective endocarditis may show fewer of the classic clinical and laboratory changes and also may have smaller vegetations than younger patients, TEE can result in more immediate diagnosis and treatment and in reduced mortality in these patients (29,34).

Echocardiography has also been used in determining the risk of embolization from an existing vegetation; however, this application remains controversial. In one study, when TTE was used to assess vegetation shape, attachment, mobility, and site, the procedure was not able to predict accurately the risk of embolization (35). The size of the vegetation did have some predictive value; vegetations larger than 1 cm were associated with a 50% risk of embolization, whereas the risk was 42% in patients with vegetations smaller than 1 cm.

Other Laboratory Findings

A variety of other laboratory abnormalities reported in patients with infective endocarditis are listed in Table 24-2. A normal or low erythrocyte sedimentation rate helps to exclude the diagnosis of infective endocarditis. Circulating immune complexes and C-reactive protein are fairly sensitive and, if the test results are negative, may exclude the diagnosis, although the duration of infective endocarditis may affect the sensitivity of these tests. None of the other single laboratory findings is sensitive or specific enough to be of help in confirming or excluding the disease.

In staphylococcal bacteremia, teichoic acid antibodies may help in predicting the severity of the illness and duration of the therapy. In more than 95% of patients with staphylococcal bacteremia, the test results are positive when undiluted serum is used. However, antibody titers of greater than 1:4 suggest serious infections such as endocarditis, osteomyelitis, or multiple metastatic abscesses. When used to separate patients with endocarditis from those with the limited bacteremia, the sensitivity ranges from 67% to 90%, and the specificity from 70% to 90% (36,37).

Immunoblotting can be used to determine the causative organism in some cases of culture-negative endocarditis (38). The use of antibody response to specific antigens can help to make a specific diagnosis; in one study, the test had a sensitivity of 85% for detecting streptococcal and enterococcal infections in patients with culture-negative endocarditis (39).

DIAGNOSTIC STRATEGIES

Serial blood cultures positive for organisms likely to cause endocarditis are important in the diagnosis of infective endocarditis. Table 24-3 shows the inferences that can be drawn from the results of blood cultures according to various pretest (clinical) estimates of the probability of infective endocarditis when it is assumed that the sensitivity and specificity of blood cultures are both 90%. It is apparent from this table that when the clinical suspicion is low, several negative culture results essentially exclude the diagnosis. Results that cause the greatest confusion are the unexpectedly positive results at low pretest probabilities and unexpectedly negative results when the clinical suspicion is high. The negative culture results in the context of high suspicion may represent specific situations such as antibiotic therapy within the past 7 days, fungal endocarditis, or true culture-negative disease.

In situations with unexpected culture results, the physician needs to pursue additional diagnostic studies to strengthen the case for or against endocarditis. As also shown in Table 24-3, a positive echocardiogram (assuming sensitivity and specificity of 60% and 95%, respectively, for TTE; and 95% and 95%, respectively, for TEE) is extremely helpful in strengthening the case for endocarditis when several blood culture results are unexpectedly positive with an organism known to cause infective endocarditis. The combination of both positive cultures and echocardiogram can increase the probability of infective endocarditis from 20% to greater than 95%, depending on the number of positive culture results and the organism identified. In this situation, a TTE with normal or negative findings is not particularly helpful,

Table 24-3. Post-test Probabilities for Blood Cultures and Echocardiography in the Diagnosis of Native Valve Infective Endocarditis

Diagnostic Test	Pretest Probabilities					
	20%		50%		80%	
	Positive Result	Negative Result	Positive Result	Negative Result	Positive Result	Negative Result
	←――――――――――――― % ―――――――――――――→					
Blood cultures	69	3	90	10	97	31
TTE and positive blood culture results	96	48	99	79	99	93
TTE and negative blood culture results	25	1	57	4	84	16
TEE and positive blood culture results	98	10	99	32	99	63
TEE and negative blood culture results	35	<1	68	1	90	2

TTE = transthoracic echocardiography; TEE = transesophageal echocardiography.

because the post-test probability of infective endocarditis may still be sufficiently high to warrant extended treatment with antibiotics; however, a TEE with negative findings is more reassuring. When the clinical suspicion of endocarditis is high, with a pretest probability of 80% but with negative blood culture results, a positive echocardiogram increases the post-test likelihood of disease back to more than 80%.

Echocardiography is helpful in strengthening a case for endocarditis in patients with unexpected negative blood culture results. However, TTE has limited utility in ruling out endocarditis because of its low sensitivity. The information in Table 24-3 suggests that TEE is more effective in reducing the probability of endocarditis.

In patients with prosthetic valves, prompt diagnosis and assessment of possible sequelae such as valve dehiscence or abscess formation are needed. The diagnostic approach can be further confused if the patient has received recent antibiotic therapy, which reduces the sensitivity of blood cultures. When the suspicion of endocarditis arises in patients with prosthetic valves, TEE is clearly useful, particularly in determining valve integrity.

The diagnostic approach just described is similar to that suggested by the "Duke criteria" for infective endocarditis. These criteria, developed in 1994, have emerged as a guide to the clinical diagnosis of infective endocarditis. The diagnosis is considered "definite" if two major criteria, one major and three minor criteria, or five minor criteria are met. The major criteria are 1) positive blood culture results with a typical organism from two separate blood cultures or persistent positive blood cultures drawn at at least 12-hour intervals or more than three positive blood cultures drawn over at least 1 hour and 2) evidence of definite echocardiographic abnormalities as discussed in the section on echocardiography earlier in this chapter. The six minor criteria are 1) predisposing heart condition or intravenous drug use; 2) fever (temperature >38 °C); 3) vascular phenomena; 4) immunologic phenomena; 5) echocardiogram consistent with but not meeting major criteria; and 6) positive blood culture results not meeting major criteria or serologic evidence of infection with an organism consistent with infective endocarditis (3,4). In their initial study, the "definite" endocarditis crtieria had a sensitivity of 80% in 69 confirmed cases (3).

In contrast, patients with a firm alternate diagnosis for the symptoms of endocarditis or who have had resolution of the concerning symptoms within less than 4 days of antibiotic treatment are classified as "rejected" for infective endocarditis. Finally, the remainder of the patients in whom infective endocarditis is suspected who do not meet either the "definite" or "rejected" category criteria fall into a "possible" category (3,4). For these patients, additional testing may be indicated, but the likelihood of infective endocarditis may still be relatively high. In such cases, the relative risks and benefits of empiric treatment compared with those of observation must be weighed carefully.

CLINICAL PROBLEMS

Clinical Problem 1
A patient presents with multiple clinical features suggesting endocarditis.

Testing Strategy and Rationale
In patients with many of the characteristics of infective endocarditis, the pretest probability is high. Three sets of blood cultures should be obtained at separate times. If the results are positive, they confirm the diagnosis (Table 24-3), and no further confirmatory testing is required. Echocardiogram should be performed if further assessment of cardiac complications is needed or if blood culture results are unexpectedly negative.

Clinical Example
A patient who uses intravenous drugs presents with a 1-week history of fever, chills, nocturnal sweats, and aching of multiple joints.

Continued

On examination, he appears extremely ill and fatigued. There are obvious stigmata of intravenous drug use, fever, and tachycardia. Several splinter hemorrhages are noted in addition to a single subconjunctival hemorrhage. The results of a lung examination are normal. The precordium is highly active, and a grade 2/6 holosystolic murmur is noted at the lower sternal border that increases with respiration. The results of the joint examination are normal. Blood cultures are obtained and should confirm the strong clinical suspicion of infective endocarditis.

Clinical Problem 2

A patient who presents with a clinical picture suggesting infection that requires immediate antibiotic therapy also has an intermediate probability of infective endocarditis.

Testing Strategy and Rationale

When infective endocarditis is being considered but pretest probability is intermediate, multiple positive or negative culture results cause the post-test probabilities to be very high or very low, respectively. Therefore, when the need for treatment is urgent but diagnostic uncertainty would be great with inadequate blood culture data, the clinician should rapidly obtain multiple cultures—ideally three—at intervals over a short period before initiating empiric treatment. Routine echocardiographic examination is not generally needed.

Clinical Example

A patient presents with fever of short duration (1–2 days), heart murmur, and microscopic pyuria. Only one blood culture and a urine culture are obtained, and antibiotic therapy for an urinary tract infection is started. Although the blood culture returns positive for alpha-streptococci, the patient becomes afebrile and the urine culture results are negative. Transthoracic echocardiography is performed and shows no vegetations.

This situation illustrates the dilemma that arises when the clinical picture is compatible with infective endocarditis but inadequate blood cultures are obtained. Does the patient have a persistent bacteremia with an organism likely to cause infective endocarditis, or does the patient have sporadic bacteremia caused by isolated infection, such as perinephric abscess? This demonstrates the rationale for obtaining multiple cultures. Depending on the pretest probability, the negative TTE may not reduce the probability of disease enough to exclude the diagnosis of infective endocarditis. Depending on the clinical situation, the patient's clinical course could be followed closely without further evaluation or treatment, or a TEE could be obtained.

REFERENCES

1. **King, JW, Shehane, RR, Lierl, J.** Infectious endocarditis at three hospitals in the same city: two study periods a decade apart. South Med J. 1986;79: 151-8.
2. **Kaye D.** Infective endocarditis. In: Fauci AS et al, eds. Harrison's Priniciples of Internal Medicine. 13th ed., New York: McGraw-Hill; 1994:520.
3. **Durack DT, Lukes AS, Bright DK.** New criteria for diagnosis of infective endocarditis: utilization of specific echocardiographic findings. Am J Med. 1994;96:200-9.
4. **Bayer AS, Ward JI, Ginzton LE, Shapiro SM.** Evaluation of new clinical criteria for the diagnosis of infective endocarditis. Am J Med. 1994;96:211-9.
5. **Mathew J, Addai T, Anand A, et al.** Clinical features, site of involvement, bacteriologic findings, and outcome of infective endocarditis in intravenous drug users. Arch Intern Med. 1995;155:1641-8.
6. **Shively BK.** Infective endocarditis. In: Crawford MH, ed. Diagnosis and Treatment in Cardiology. Norwalk, Appleton & Lange; 1995:370.
7. **King JW, Nguyen VQ, Conrad SA.** Results of a prospective statewide reporting system for infective endocarditis. Am J Med Sci. 1988;295:517-27.
8. **Skehan JD, Murray M, Mills PG.** Infective endocarditis. incidence and mortality in the North East Thames Region. Br Heart J. 1988;59:62-8.
9. **Griffin MR, Wilson WR, Edwards WD, et al.** Infective endocarditis; Olmsted County, Minnesota, 1950 through 1981. JAMA. 1985;254:1199-202.
10. **McKinsey DS, Ratts TE, Bisno AL.** Underlying cardiac lesions in adults with infective endocarditis; the changing spectrum. Am J Med. 1987;82: 681-8.
11. **Cunha BA, Gill V, Lazar JM.** Acute infective endocarditis. Infect Dis Clin North Am. 1996;10:811-34.
12. **Terpenning MS, Buggy BP, Kauffman CA.** Infective endocardidtis: clinical features in young and elderly patients. Am J Med. 1987;83:624-34.
13. **Bansal RC.** Infective endocarditis. Med Clin North Am. 1995;79(5):1205-40.
14. **Sandre RM, Shafran SD.** Infective endocarditis: review of 135 cases over 9 years. Clin Infect Dis. 1996;22:276-86.
15. **Berbari EF, Cockerill FR, Steckelberg JM.** Infective endocarditis due to unusual or fastidoious microorganisms. Mayo Clin Proc. 1997;72:532-42.
16. **Churchill MA, Geraci JE, Hunder GG.** Musculoskeletal manifestations of bacterial endocarditis. Ann Intern Med. 1977;87:754-9.
17. **Yee J, McAllister K.** Osler's nodes and the recognition of infective endocarditis: a lession of diagnostic importance. South Med J. 1987;80:753-8.
18. **Berlin JA, Abrutyn E, Strom Bl, et al.** Assessing diagnostic criteria for active infective endocarditis. Am J Cardiol. 1994;73:887-91.
19. **Weinstein L, Rubin RH.** Infective endocarditis—1973. Prog Cardiovasc Dis. 1973;16:239-74.
20. **Werner WS, Cobbs CG, Kaye D, Hook EW.** Studies on the bacteremia of bacterial endocarditis. JAMA. 1967;202:127-31.
21. **MacGregor RR, Beaty HN.** Evaluation of positive blood cultures: guidelines for early differentiation of contaminated from valid positive cultures. Arch Intern Med. 1972;130:84-7.

22. **Eisenberg JM, Rose JD, Weinstein AJ.** Routine blood cultures febrile outpatients. JAMA. 1976;236:2863-5.

23. **Wilson R, Hamburger M.** Fifteen years' experience with staphylococcal septicemia in a large city hospital: analysis of 55 cases in the Cincinnati General Hospital, 1940-1959. Am J Med. 1957;22:437-47.

24. **Watanakunakorn C, Tan JS, Phair JP.** Some salient features of *Staphylococcus aureus* endocarditis. Am J Med. 1973;54:473-81.

25. **Shapiro SM, Young E, De Guzman S, Ward J, et al.** Transesophageal echocardiography in diagnosis of infective endocarditis. Chest. 1994;105(2):377-82.

26. **Essop R.** Tranesophageal echocardiography in infective endocarditis: the standard for the 1990s? Am Heart J. 1995;130(2):402-4.

27. **Job FP, Franke S, Lethen H, et al.** Incremental value of biplane and multiplane tranesophageal echocardiography for the asessment of active infective endocarditis. Am J Cardiol. 1995;75:1033-7.

28. **Lowry RW, Zognbi WA, Baker WB, et al.** Clinical impact of transesophageal echocardiography in the diagnosis and management of infective endocarditis. Am J Cardiol. 1994;73:1089-91.

29. **Werner GS, Schulz R, Fuchs JB, et al.** Infective endocarditis in the elderly in the era of transesophageal echocardiography: clinical features and prognosis compared with younger patients. Am J Med. 1996;100(1):90-7.

30. **Tape TG, Panzer RJ.** Echocardiography, endocarditis, and clinical information bias. J Gen Intern Med. 1986;1:300-4.

31. **Stratton JR, Werner JA, Pearlman AS, et al.** Bacteremia and the heart: serial echocardiographic findings in 80 patients with documented or suspected bacteremia. Am J Med. 1982;73:851-8.

32. **Chandraratna PAN, Langevin E.** Limitations of the echocardiogram in diagnosing valvular vegetations in patients with mitral valve prolapse. Circulation. 1977;56:436-8.

33. **Markiewicz W, Peled B, Alroy G, et al.** Endocardiography in infective endocarditis: lack of specificity in patients with valvular pathology. Eur J Cardiol. 1979;10:247-57.

34. **Slama MA, Novara A, Van de Putte P, et al.** Diagnostic and therapeutic implications of transesophageal echocardiography in medical ICU patients with unexplained shock, hypoxemia, or suspected endocarditis. Intens Care Med. 1996;22:916-22.

35. **Heinle S, et al.** Value of transthoracic echocardiography in predicting embolic events in active infective endocarditis. Am J Cardiol. 1994;74:799-801.

36. **Wheat J, Kohler RB, Garten M, White A.** Commercialy available (endostaph) assay for teichoic acid antibodies. Arch Intern Med. 1984;144:261-4.

37. **Tuazon CU, Sheagren JN.** Teichoic acid antibodies in the diagnosis of serious infections with *Staphylococcus aureus*. Ann Intern Med. 1976;84:543-6.

38. **Clark I, Burnie JP.** Immunoblotting and culture positive endocarditis. J Clin Pathol. 1991;44:152-6.

39. **Burnie JP, Clark I.** Immunoblotting in the diagnosis of culture negative endocarditis caused by streptococci and enterococci. J Clin Pathol. 1995;48:1130-6.

Acute Sinusitis

25

Joshua Chodosh, MD

KEY POINTS

Pretest Probabilities

- Predisposing factors for sinusitis include upper respiratory infections, dental abscesses, and long-term use of over-the-counter vasoconstrictor nasal sprays. The role of allergic rhinitis is controversial.
- Independent clinical predictors of sinusitis include a history of poor response to nasal decongestants, a colored nasal discharge, maxillary toothache, purulent secretion, and abnormal transillumination. Patients with four or five of these findings have a high probability of sinusitis, whereas those without any findings have a low probability.

Diagnostic Strategies

- The "gold standard" for the diagnosis of sinusitis is the presence of infected secretions demonstrated by sinus puncture and lavage. However, this procedure is performed infrequently.
- The diagnosis of sinusitis and decisions about therapy can often be made on the basis of clinical information alone.
- The sensitivity of plain radiographs in detecting maxillary sinusitis is at least 70%, and the specificity approaches 100%. When maxillary sinus infection is suspected, a single Water's view is nearly as reliable as a complete series.
  - *Sen/Spec 70/100*
- Sinus computed tomography is the noninvasive "gold standard" for sinusitis and the test of choice when surgical treatment is considered. However, the specificity of computed tomography may be as low as 65%.
  - *Sen/Spec 100/65*

BACKGROUND

Diagnosing acute sinusitis can be challenging. Predisposing factors, such as upper respiratory infections, dental abscesses, and long-term use of over-the-counter vasoconstrictor nasal sprays may be confused with sinusitis. In addition, the role of allergic rhinitis is controversial (1–3).

There is consensus that antibiotics are required for the rapid resolution of bacterial sinusitis (4,5). Chronic or recurrent symptoms of asthma and obstructive pulmonary disease may be more difficult to control in patients who have sinusitis (6,7). Accurate identification and treatment of bacterial sinusitis is also important because of the risk of serious complications that may occur, including orbital cellulitis, osteomyelitis, meningitis, and cavernous sinus thrombosis (8,9). However, these factors must be weighed against the risks of inappropriate use of antibiotics in patients who do not have acute sinusitis.

The most rigorous clinical studies of patients with acute sinusitis, although few in number, are summarized in this chapter. Such studies have attempted to define the signs and symptoms that provide the greatest predictive power for diagnosing sinusitis (10–13). However, although the "gold standard" for sinusitis has been the finding of infected secretions demonstrated by sinus puncture and lavage from the ostial area (14), this procedure is performed infrequently and is usually done only by otolaryngologists. In addition, studies often did not use the same "gold standard," making it difficult to compare results.

ESTIMATING PRETEST PROBABILITY

National surveys and other reports provide some information on the prevalence of sinusitis, but findings may be inflated owing to the frequency of other common conditions with similar presentations and the infrequent use of the "gold standard." It is well known that "sinusitis" is often diagnosed and is the fifth most common diagnosis for which antibiotics are prescribed (15). In addition, of those surveyed about recent health problems, 14% of the United States population report having "sinusitis" (16).

Several predisposing factors, when present, should increase the clinician's suspicion for sinusitis. These include a history of a previous upper respiratory infection, the presence of an upper molar dental abscess, long-term use of over-the-counter vasoconstrictor nasal sprays, and (according to some studies) a history of allergic rhinitis.

Several important clinical findings have been generated by Williams and colleagues (10) in a prospective evaluation of 247 consecutive men presenting to a university-affiliated Veterans Affairs medical center with symptoms of nasal discharge, facial pain, or self-suspected "sinusitis." This study evaluated the operating characteristics of historical and physical examination findings for sinusitis, using a set of four-view sinus radiographs as the criterion standard. The prevalence of sinusitis in this study was 38%. Those features having the best independent performance in the diagnosis of sinusitis were the historical findings of no improvement with the use of nasal decongestants, a colored nasal discharge, and maxillary toothache and the physical findings of purulent nasal secretion and abnormal transillumination (Table 25-1). Predicted probability increased with each additional independent predictor; in patients with all five clinical predictors, the probability of sinusitis was 92%, whereas in patients with none of these predictors, the probability was 9% (Table 25-2). Thus, these results could be used as a "scoring system" to help estimate the probability of acute sinusitis. Of interest in this study is the finding that the clinician's "overall" impression, although not necessarily one that can be applied universally, was also an important clinical predictor with a likelihood ratio of 4.7 for "high probability" assessments and 0.4 for "low probability" assessments. The clinician's impression of high probability for sinus disease had an accuracy of 74% in this study (10).

Clinical predictors of sinusitis reported in a recent Norwegian study (11) are also presented in Table 25-1. A history of previous upper

Table 25-1. Operating Characteristics of Clinical Signs and Symptoms in the Diagnosis of Acute Sinusitis

Clinical Finding	Likelihood Ratio (95% CI)	
	Positive Result	**Negative Result**
Criterion standard: Four-view sinus radiography*		
No improvement with decongestants	2.1 (1.4–3.1)	0.7 (0.6–0.9)
Colored nasal discharge	1.5 (1.2–1.9)	0.5 (0.4–0.8)
Purulent nasal secretion on examination	2.1 (1.5–3.0)	0.7 (0.5 0.8)
Abnormal transillumination	1.6 (1.3–2.0)	0.5 (0.4–0.7)
Maxillary toothache	2.5 (1.2–5.0)	0.9 (0.8–1.0)
Criterion standard: Computed tomography†		
Purulent secretion in nasal cavity‡	5.5	0.5
Double sickening‡	2.1	0.4
Purulent rhinorrhea‡	1.5	0.3
Unilateral facial pain	1.7	0.7
Nasality	1.4	0.4
Hyposmia/anosmia	1.4	0.5

*Adapted from Williams JW, Simel DL, Roberts L, Samsa GP. Clinical evaluation for sinusitis: making the diagnosis by history and physical examination. Ann Intern Med. 1992; 117:705-10.
†Adapted from Lindboek M, Hjortdahl P, Johnsen UL. Use of symptoms, signs, and blood tests to diagnose acute sinus infections in primary care: comparison with computed tomography. Fam Med. 1996;28:183-8.
‡Independently associated with computed tomography.

Table 25-2. Probability of Sinusitis Based on Clinical Predictor Variables*

Numbers of Factors Present	Predicted Probability of Sinusitis (%)	Likelihood Ratio
0	9	0.1
1	21	0.5
2	40	1.1
3	63	2.6
4	81	6.4
5	92	6.4

*Overall prevelance of sinusitis in this study was 38%.

Adapted with permission from Williams JW, Simel DL, Roberts L, Samsa GP. Clinical evalution for sinusitis: making the diagnosis by history and physical examination. Ann Intern Med. 1992; 117:705-10.

respiratory infection, referred to as "double sickening," was found to have an independent likelihood ratio of 2.1 using computed tomography (CT) as the criterion standard. (This finding was not supported in the study by Williams [10], but it was dropped from data collection after just one third of that study group had been evaluated.) Purulent secretion above the inferior turbinate was 100% specific in this study, but evaluations used an ENT microscope that is not routinely used in primary care settings. In addition, this finding was noted in only 6 of 127 CT-positive cases. The diagnostic value of finding purulent material draining in the posterior pharynx has not been evaluated in published studies.

DIAGNOSTIC TESTS

The use of diagnostic tests beyond the history and examination is largely determined by the need for a more immediate and definitive diagnosis. The gold standard for maxillary sinusitis, the area most frequently involved in acute sinusitis (17–19) has been sinus puncture, lavage, and aspiration of secretions from the antrum. Studies of diagnostic tests including radiography, CT, magnetic resonance imaging, and ultrasonography have generated some controversy.

Transillumination

The utility of transillumination in the diagnosis of sinusitis has been questioned, in part because it is "operator-dependent." Its potential diagnostic value is in detecting abnormal findings of the maxillary sinuses. Transillumination of frontal sinuses is problematic owing to their often asymmetric and unreliable development (18). The best known method for transillumination is performed in a fully darkened room with the light source placed over the infraorbital rim while it is shielded from the examiner's eyes and the degree of light transmission is compared through both sides of the hard palate. Time is needed for visual adaptation to darkness. Of three studies with otolaryngologists, this technique was found to be clinically useful in two (20) but not in the third (21). Williams (10) reported a likelihood ratio of 1.6 for unilateral opaqueness or dullness and 0.5 for bilateral normal transillumination. Agreement among inexperienced examiners is poor (10).

Radiography

Several studies have demonstrated good correlation between plain radiographs, involving four-view radiographs, and antral puncture, although sample sizes have been small (18,20,22,23). This correlation has benefited from the frequency of maxillary sinus involvement in acute sinusitis as well as from the differential degree of radiographic resolution favoring the maxillary over ethmoid or sphenoid areas (17–19). Plain radiographs have a sensitivity of approximately 70% for sinusitis, with CT as the criterion standard (Table 25-3). The low sensitivity is caused in part by ethmoid and sphenoid anatomy limiting radiographic resolution. Individual ethmoid air cells may be opacified but radiographically obscured by the air density of surrounding normal cells (24). Because the sphenoid sinuses are anatomically deep with multiple overlying structures, the accuracy of the radiographic images is compromised (18). Thus, air-fluid levels or opacification, two of the radiographic findings of sinusitis, may be missed on plain radiography (25). Although CT affords greater resolution of the ethmoid and sphenoid areas, concerns about its specificity may falsely lower the sensitivity of plain radiographs when CT is used as the criterion standard.

The high frequency of maxillary sinusitis, 88% in one study (25), has led to the suggestion of obtaining a single Water's view radiograph, which images the maxillary sinus quite well, instead of the standard four-view series. Excellent agreement between these two methods has been demonstrated (25,26).

Computed Tomography

Computed tomography is considered by many to be the radiographic criterion standard for sinusitis and is the study required for surgical guidance in refractory or complicated cases. However, we found no studies that compared the results of CT directly with those of sinus aspiration.

Table 25-3. Operating Characteristics of Diagnostic Tests for Acute Sinusitis

Diagnostic Test	Definition of Positive Result	Sensitivity	Specificity	Likelihood Ratio	
				Positive Result	Negative Result
		← ─── % ─── →			
Transillumination (maxillary with mini-mag lite)	Normal, dull, or opaque (reduced or no light transmission)	73	54	1.6	0.5
Four-view radiography (CT as criterion standard)	Mucosal thickening ≥3 mm; air-fluid level; complete opacification	70	88	5.8	0.3
Single Water's view radiograph (four-view radiograph as criterion standard) for maxillary sinus	Mucosal thickening ≥6 mm; air-fluid level; complete opacification	82	86	5.9	0.2
Computed tomography	Mucosal thickening; air-fluid level; complete opacification	100	65	2.9	0.0

CT = computed tomography.

Although CT is highly sensitive and a normal scan virtually rules out sinus disease, the specificity of sinus CT has been questioned (27,28). In a prospective study of 666 asymptomatic patients (those suspected of having sinus disease were excluded) having cranial CT scans for reasons other than acute sinusitis, an abnormality in one or more paranasal sinuses indicative of sinus disease was noted in 43% (28). The most frequent finding in that study was mucosal thickening of the ethmoid sinus. Another study of 100 asymptomatic patients demonstrated that 39% had paranasal clouding, with isolated ethmoid cells as the most common abnormality (29). Twenty-one of these 39 patients had involvement of at least two sinuses, but chart review for most showed a history of sinus infection in just one patient. In a third study, abnormalities of one or more sinuses were noted on CT scans in 22 of 31 patients who reported nasal or head congestion associated with common colds (27). Another study with more rigorous exclusion criteria nevertheless demonstrated finding 16% positive CT scans in asymptomatic patients (30). These findings underscore the need for careful patient selection and test interpretation when CT is being considered or is used in patients with possible sinusitis.

Other Modalities

Ultrasonography had shown initial promise as a noninvasive diagnostic test, but studies have not supported its use (31). Magnetic resonance imaging may demonstrate greater definition in certain instances, particularly with regard to infectious complications and neoplasms, but should be used only rarely owing to its poor resolution of bone and thus its generally poor clinical utility for the endoscopic surgeon (32).

DIAGNOSTIC STRATEGIES

For most cases of suspected sinusitis, obtaining specific data from the history and physical examination provides important diagnostic information. The clinical history should include inquiry about the presence or absence of colored nasal discharge, maxillary toothache, poor response to decongestants, unilateral facial pain, and previous upper respiratory infection. Physical examination should include nasal inspection for purulent secretions and palpation for sinus tenderness. If performed routinely, transillumination may also be helpful. The initial evaluation should also include an assessment for the complications of acute sinusitis discussed earlier in this chapter.

The use of diagnostic tests beyond the history and examination is largely determined by the need for a more definitive answer, but in general should not be routinely used in the initial evaluation for sinusitis. The diagnosis of sinusitis can often be made or excluded, and decisions about antibiotic therapy may often be made, on the basis of clinical information alone (14).

Radiographic evaluation should be reserved for refractory or complicated presentations that increase the likelihood of other serious diseases or complications or for patients in whom the probability of sinusitis, based on the information from the history and physical examination, is neither high enough to justify antibiotic treatment nor low enough to warrant only symptomatic therapy. One example is patients with multiple antibiotic allergies for whom antibiotic therapy has additional risks. Although treatment failures may be due to inappropriate antibiotic selection or duration of therapy, treatment failures when broad-spectrum agents are used warrant the use of imaging studies.

If symptoms suggest maxillary sinus disease, a single Water's view radiograph should be considered. Patients with a high post-test probability of sinusitis despite a negative plain radiograph or those with a complicated presentation should be evaluated with a sinus CT. Computed tomography is more likely to be helpful in patients with a severe presentation or a history suggestive of chronic disease, either of which may necessitate endoscopic evaluation and surgery (33).

CLINICAL PROBLEMS

Clinical Problem 1
A patient presents with symptoms highly suggestive of acute sinusitis.

Testing Strategy and Rationale
A careful history and targeted physical examination should be performed that specifically evaluate for symptoms and findings of sinusitis (see Table 25-1). The clinician should inquire about previous upper respiratory infection, decongestant use, colored nasal discharge, and maxillary toothache, and the examination should include nasal inspection and possibly transillumination. In patients who have multiple factors associated with sinusitis, radiography is often not necessary.

Clinical Example
A 25-year-old man presents with a history of a painful pressure over the left cheek for the past 10 days which has not responded to decongestants. He has also noted yellow-colored nasal discharge. Physical examination reveals purulent nasal secretion, and the results of transillumination are abnormal. The probability of acute sinusitis is believed to be high for this patient, because he has four of the five clinical predictors for sinusitis (10), and treatment is begun without performing additional studies.

Clinical Problem 2
A patient with multiple antibiotic allergies requests evaluation because of "sinus trouble."

Testing Strategy and Rationale
A careful history should be done specifically inquiring about decongestant use, colored nasal discharge, maxillary toothache, and previous upper respiratory infection. Physical examination should include nasal inspection and transillumination (provided that the clinician is experienced in this method). Imaging studies should be used only if the probability of disease is neither high nor low enough to guide decisions concerning therapy.

Clinical Example
A 40-year-old man who has had multiple adverse antibiotic reactions associated with many previous treatments for "sinusitis" presents for evaluation. He cannot relate specific details about previous episodes. He has noted nasal congestion and colored nasal discharge for the past 5 days. He has had some improvement with

intermittent use of decongestants. He has not had a toothache. His examination shows boggy, erythematous nasal mucosa but no purulent discharge. The results of transillumination are normal.

Based on the clinical presentation, the probability of sinusitis is estimated to be no more than 20% (see Tables 25-1 and 25-2), and it is decided that decongestant therapy without antibiotics should be the initial treatment. However, the patient is convinced that he has sinusitis and requests antibiotics. A single Water's view radiograph is obtained and is normal. This result reduces the probability of sinusitis to approximately 5%, and symptomatic treatment alone is given.

REFERENCES

1. **Willet LR, Carson JL, Williams JW.** Current diagnosis and management of sinusitis. J Gen Intern Med. 1994;9:38-45.

2. **Kennedy DW, Gwaltney JM Jr, Jones JG.** Medical management of sinusitis: educational goals and management guidelines. Ann Otol Rhinol Laryngol. 1995;176:22-30.

3. **Zinreich J.** Imaging of inflammatory sinus disease. Otolaryngol Clin North Am. 1993;26:535-47.

4. **Evans FO, Syndor JB, Moore WE, et al.** Sinusitis of the maxillary antrum. N Engl J Med. 1975;293:735-9.

5. **Axelsson A, Chidekel N, Grebelius N, Jensen C.** Treatment of acute maxillary sinusitis: a comparison of four different methods. Acta Otolaryngol (Stockh). 1970;70:71-6.

6. **Slavin RG.** Relationship of nasal disease and sinusitis to bronchial asthma. Ann Allergy. 1982;49:76-80.

7. **Friedman WH, Katsantonis GP, Slavin RG, et al.** Sphenoidectomy: its role in the asthmatic patient. Otolaryngol Head Neck Surg. 1982;90:171-7.

8. **Ramsey PG, Weymuller EA.** Complications of bacterial infection of the ears, paranasal sinuses, and oropharynx in adults. Emerg Med Clin North Am. 1985;3:143-60.

9. **Meyers BR.** Bacterial sinusitis. J Fam Pract. 1984;18:117-8, 123-7.

10. **Williams JW, Simel DL, Roberts L, Samsa GP.** Clinical evaluation for sinusitis: making the diagnosis by history and physical examination. Ann Intern Med. 1992;117:705-10.

11. **Lindboek M, Hjortdahl P, Johnsen UL.** Use of symptoms, signs, and blood tests to diagnose acute sinus infections in primary care: comparison with computed tomography. Fam Med. 1996;28:183-8.

12. **Berg O, Carenfelt C.** Analysis of symptoms and clinical signs in the maxillary sinus empyema. Acta Otolaryngol (Stockh). 1998;105:343-9.

13. **van Duijn NP, Brouwer HJ, Lamberts H.** Use of symptoms and signs to diagnose maxillary sinusitis in general practice: comparison with ultrasonography. BMJ. 1992;305:684-7.

14. **Williams JW, Simel DL.** Does this patient have sinusitis? Diagnosing acute sinusitis by history and physical examination. JAMA. 1993;270:1242-6.

15. **Williams JW Jr.** Sinusitis: beginning a new age of enlightenment. West J Med. 1995;163:80-2.

16. Prevalence of selected chronic conditions. Vital Health Stat 10. 1986; Jul (155):1-66.

17. **Williams JW, Roberts L Jr, Distell B, Simel DL.** Diagnosing sinusitis by x-ray: is a single Water's view adequate? J Gen Intern Med. 1992;7:481-5.

18. **MacLeod B.** Paranasal sinus radiography. Emerg Med Clin North Am. 1991;9:743-55.

19. **Axelsson A, Jensen C.** The roentgenologic demonstration of sinusitis. Am J Roentgenol. 1974;122:621-7.

20. **Evans FO, Syndor JB, Moore WE, et al.** Sinusitis of the maxillary antrum. N Engl J Med. 1975;293:735-9.

21. **Spector SL, Lotan A, English G, Philpot I.** Comparison between transillumination and the roentgenogram in diagnosing paranasal sinus disease. J Allergy Clin Immunol. 1981;67:22-6.

22. **Axelsson A, Grebelius N, Chidekel N, Jensen C.** The correlation between the radiological examination and the irrigation findings in maxillary sinusitis. Acta Otolaryngol. 1970;69:302-6.

23. **Wilson NW, Jalowayski AA, Hamburger RN.** A comparison of nasal cytology with sinus x-rays for the diagnosis of sinusitis. Am J Rhinol. 1988;2:55-9.

24. **Som PM, Lawson W, Biller HF, Lanzieri CF.** Ethmoid sinus disease: CT evaluation in 400 cases. Radiology. 1986;159:591-7.

25. **Burke TF, Guertler AT, Timmons JH.** Comparison of sinus x-rays with computed tomography scans in acute sinusitis. Acad Emerg Med. 1994;1:235-9.

26. **Hayward MW, Lyons K, Ennis WP, Rees J.** Radiography of the paranasal sinuses: one or three views? Clin Radiol. 1990;41:163-4.

27. **Gwaltney JM Jr, Phillips CD, Miller RD, Riker DK.** Computed tomographic study of the common cold. N Engl J Med. 1994;330:25-30.

28. **Havas TE, Motbey JA, Gullane PJ.** Prevalence of incidental abnormalities on computed tomographic scans of the paranasal sinuses. Arch Otolaryngol Head Neck Surg. 1998;114:856-9.

29. **Lloyd GAS.** CT of the paranasal sinuses: study of a control series in relation to endoscopic surgery. J Laryngol Otol. 1990;104:477-81.

30. **Calhoun KH, Waggenspack GA, Simpson CB, et al.** CT evaluation of the paranasal sinuses in symptomatic and asymptomatic populations. Otolaryngol Head Neck Surg. 1991;104:480-3.

31. **Pfister R, Lutolf M, Schapowal A, et al.** Screening for sinus disease in patients with asthma: a computed tomography-controlled comparison of A-mode ultrasonography and standard radiosurgery. J Allergy Clin Immunol. 1994;94:804-9.

32. **Zinreich SJ.** Imaging of chronic sinusitis in adults: x-ray, computed tomography, and magnetic resonance imaging. J Allergy Clin Immunol. 1992;90:445-51.

33. **Slavin RG.** Sinusitis: present state of the art. Allergy Proc. 1991;12:163-5.

Osteomyelitis

26

David R. Lambert, MD

KEY POINTS

Pretest Probabilities

- Osteomyelitis is relatively uncommon in adults except those with predisposing conditions such as a history of diabetic foot ulcers, trauma, and orthopedic surgery.
- The pretest probability is increased in patients older than 50 years of age who have fever and localized long bone or back pain.
- Approximately 50% of patients with diabetes and foot ulcers who are referred for testing are found to have osteomyelitis.

Diagnostic Strategies

- Although radiography is a useful first step in the diagnostic approach and is helpful in excluding other diagnoses, this test has low sensitivity in patients with early osteomyelitis and its results may be difficult to interpret in patients with vascular insufficiency.
- In patients with osteomyelitis who have fever and bone pain, the results of blood cultures are positive in no more than 40% to 60% of patients. When the results are positive, the test identifies the causative organism.
- In patients in whom the probability of osteomyelitis is intermediate or high after results of radiography are found to be normal, magnetic resonance imaging or fine-needle bone biopsy should be performed because of the high specificity of these tests.
- In patients in whom the probability of disease is relatively low after results of radiography are found to be normal, a technetium 99m bone scan, if interpreted to maximize sensitivity, is indicated. A negative result should rule out the diagnosis.
- Bone biopsy is the gold standard for diagnosis.

BACKGROUND

Osteomyelitis generally develops by one of the following mechanisms: 1) hematogenous seeding from bacteremia; 2) spread from a contiguous focus of infection, often associated with injury or a surgical procedure; and 3) in association with vascular insufficiency. In one study of adults with osteomyelitis, 19% of cases were caused by hematogenous spread, 47% were caused by contiguous infection, and 34% were related to vascular insufficiency (1). Hematogenous spread is the most common mechanism for patients between 1 and 20 years of age.

Although many patients present with fever and localized bone pain, others report only limb pain with nonspecific symptoms. A high index of suspicion is often required to identify the disease. Although generally not fatal, complications of osteomyelitis include paralysis from vertebral osteomyelitis, the need for limb amputations, and chronic osteomyelitis with draining fistula. This chapter focuses on the evaluation of adult patients with suspected osteomyelitis.

ESTIMATING PRETEST PROBABILITY

To estimate the pretest probability of osteomyelitis, clinicians need to integrate information regarding the prevalence of the disease in various age groups, the presence or absence of predisposing conditions (e.g., sickle cell disease, hemodialysis, and intravenous drug use), and the clinical presentation. Osteomyelitis is relatively uncommon: A 7-year study in England found a case rate for hematogenous osteomyelitis of seven cases/one million adults/year (2). The incidence is higher in men, growing children, elderly persons, and immunocompromised patients. Environmental, social, and geographic factors have also been reported to be important in outbreak rates (3).

The different mechanisms for osteomyelitis are associated with different risk factors and clinical presentations. In adults, hematogenous seeding is most often found in patients older than 50 years of age and usually involves the vertebrae (60%) or long bones (30%) (1,2,4). The lumbar vertebrae are the most frequently affected sites in the spine (2,5). Patients with long-bone involvement usually present with 7 to 10 days of fever and localized bone pain. The results of blood cultures are positive in approximately 50% of patients and nearly always show *Staphylococcus aureus* (3,6).

Vertebral osteomyelitis has a much more indolent and subtle presentation. Patients are more often men (2:1) and are likely to present with neck or back pain and stiffness. Many present with dull, constant pain of many weeks' duration, and some patients have atypical presenting symptoms such as occipital, chest, or abdominal pain (4,5). Only 50% are febrile on presentation (4). Less than one fourth of patients present with a positive straight-leg raising test or with neurologic deficits (6). A clinical sign believed to be useful (although its sensitivity is not known) is marked tenderness when the involved vertebrae is pressed or percussed. Although the genitourinary tract, skin, and respiratory tract are the most frequent sources of primary infection, in one third of patients there is no obvious source. Thus, one should have a high suspicion of vertebral osteomyelitis in adults presenting with fever, back pain, and stiffness.

Contiguous osteomyelitis usually affects the femur or tibia of older adults who have a history of trauma or orthopedic surgery (2). In one study, 86% of patients with contiguous osteomyelitis had open reduction of fractures and were usually diagnosed within 1 month of the predisposing event; however, the diagnosis was delayed somewhat in patients who had had surgery (7). Fever, swelling, and erythema are present in about half the patients. Pain is a variable finding and can be difficult to rely on, because many patients have recently undergone surgery. However, unexpectedly severe pain with or without purulent drainage should raise the suspicion for osteomyelitis.

Nearly all patients with osteomyelitis in association with vascular insufficiency have diabetes. The foot is most commonly involved. The classic presentation is a nonhealing foot ulcer without systemic manifestations (4,8). Associated fluctuance or erythema further increases suspicion for bone infection. Insertion of a sterile probe into a diabetic foot ulcer with palpation of bone has a sensitivity of 66% and a specificity of 85% for the diagnosis of osteomyelitis (9).

DIAGNOSTIC TESTS
Information presented in this section and in Table 26-1 is severely limited in terms of providing detailed information on test sensitivity and specificity. This is a result of studies that suffer from several methodologic problems, including lack of a consistently applied gold standard, referral bias, incorporation bias, and lack of blinded test interpretation.

Cultures
Blood cultures often identify the causative organism in patients with osteomyelitis, particularly in those with acute presentations. They have been reported to be positive in 40% to 60% of patients with hematogenous osteomyelitis (1,5). Recovery of an organism appears to occur less frequently in patients with vertebral involvement (5). Data on rates of positive blood culture results in patients with other forms of osteomyelitis are lacking. Because hematogenous osteomyelitis tends to be monomicrobial and originates from bacteremia, the rate of positive blood culture results with this cause is probably higher than with other causes. Osteomyelitis in the presence of vascular insufficiency is

Table 26-1. Estimates of the Operating Characteristics of Diagnostic Tests for Osteomyelitis

Type of Osteomyelitis	Diagnostic Test	Sensitivity	Specificity
		←———— % ————→	
Hematogenous, nonvertebral	Radiography	"Low"	"Moderate to high"
	Bone scan	72	50
	MRI	67–95	88
Hematogenous, vertebral	Radiography	48	?
	Bone scan	71	?
	CT	65	?
	MRI	100	?
Contiguous	Radiography	"Low"	?
	Bone scan	67–100	"Low"
	MRI	75	"Moderate to high"
Vascular insufficiency	Radiography	22–60	81–94
	Bone scan	50–100	25–70
	MRI	60–99	80–100

MRI = magnetic resonance imaging; CT = computed tomography.
Adapted from references 1,2,4,5,10–24.

usually caused by a local polymicrobial infection without bacteremia. Nonetheless, a blood culture that is positive for an organism known to cause osteomyelitis in a patient in whom the disease is suspected substantially increases the probability of osteomyelitis.

Much attention has been given to wound cultures in patients with contiguous osteomyelitis and in patients with diabetes and foot ulcers in an effort to determine the causative organism. The degree of concordance between wound cultures and deep, surgical bone cultures has varied from less than 50% to 70%. One prospective study that demonstrated a higher concordance involved cleansing the area before a deep wound culture was obtained from nonpedal wounds (25). Although there is little evidence to support obtaining cultures from foot lesions of patients with diabetes, some argue that cultures can be helpful in determining the presence of methicillin-resistant S. aureus. Bone aspiration culture has a reported yield of 60% when done before the administration of antibiotics (10).

Other Laboratory Tests: Erythrocyte Sedimentation Rate and C-Reactive Protein
The erythrocyte sedimentation rate (ESR) is a nonspecific measure of inflammation that can sometimes be helpful in the diagnosis of

osteomyelitis. In a study of adults with hematogenous osteomyelitis, the ESR was more than 30 mm/h in 95% of cases (2). Another report showed that the ESR was more than 50 mm/h in 76% of patients with hematogenous osteomyelitis of the spine (11). In patients with contiguous osteomyelitis, the ESR may be normal, and postoperative patients without osteomyelitis may have an elevated ESR caused by the surgical procedure. Elderly patients tend to have a higher ESR at baseline and a more prolonged increase in the ESR with surgery. An elevated ESR is not helpful in detecting osteomyelitis in those with vascular insufficiency, because these patients frequently have comorbid conditions that can also lead to an increased value (8).

The C-reactive protein (CRP) functions much the same way as the ESR. Although CRP is believed to be more sensitive for inflammation with a more rapid change than the ESR, in patients with localized bone infection the ESR may be elevated and the CRP may be normal (12). Thus, CRP adds little if any incremental benefit to the ESR in the diagnosis of osteomyelitis.

The serum leukocyte count is a poor indicator of osteomyelitis because it is neither sensitive nor specific (1,12). Other laboratory tests such as measurement of calcium, phosphorus, and alkaline phosphatase are of no value in the diagnosis of osteomyelitis (1).

Radiography

Plain bone radiographs are the least sensitive of all radiologic tests for osteomyelitis, but they are relatively specific. The earliest change associated with osteomyelitis is the subtle finding of soft tissue swelling, but this is not specific (26). Radiographic changes caused by osteomyelitis take at least 10 to 14 days to occur and in most cases are not seen before 3 or 4 weeks. Radiographic changes caused by vertebral osteomyelitis may not be evident for several months (6). Early radiographs can, however, exclude other diseases such as tumors or occult fractures.

Radionuclide Scanning

The most commonly used radionuclide scan uses technetium-99m pyrophosphate (^{99}Tc). In osteomyelitis, uptake, caused by hyperemia of soft tissue, can occur 10 to 14 days before changes on plain radiographs are present. Although the test is highly sensitive for various types of osteomyelitis, it is not specific (see Table 26-1). In particular, specificity declines when other bone disease is present (27). False-negative scans have been reported and may occur in as many as 8% of patients with diabetes who have foot ulcers in whom osteomyelitis has been shown by biopsy (28,29).

Bone scans may be problematic in patients with diabetes and vascular insufficiency. A meta-analysis of ^{99}Tc bone scans (most of which used triple-phase scans) for foot osteomyelitis in patients with diabetes or other vascular conditions concluded that the test performed poorly; using receiver operating characteristic analysis, at a sensitivity of 90%, the test's specificity was approximately 46% (30). (Of note, in the studies reviewed for this meta-analysis, between 40% and 60% of patients evaluated for possible osteomyelitis were actually found to have the disease.)

Studies using indium leukocyte scanning to diagnose osteomyelitis found it to be more specific than the bone scan but less sensitive, especially in indolent infections. Some suggest using it in conjunction with the ^{99}Tc bone scan. Although gallium scans are reported to be more specific than bone scans, they are not as sensitive because large amounts of purulent material with "active" leukocytes must be present for osteomyelitis to be detected (13,31). Antigranulocyte antibody scans have been used mostly in research settings, are not readily available, and appear to add little to the other radionuclide scans.

Computed Tomography and Magnetic Resonance Imaging

Computed tomography (CT) has been used in the diagnosis of osteomyelitis. Although CT can visualize surrounding soft tissues, it is prone to some image degradation owing to artifacts caused by bone or metal (32).

Magnetic resonance imaging (MRI) has largely replaced CT in the evaluation of osteomyelitis. Magnetic resonance imaging allows for early diagnosis by detecting early marrow changes caused by inflammatory cells. Although relatively expensive, MRI can delineate the extent of osteomyelitis and guide surgical resection, improving its cost-effectiveness. This study also performs well in difficult clinical situations such as foot infections in patients with diabetes. In such a case, the sensitivity is increased by obtaining multiplanar images, using a surface coil, accurately positioning the patient, and using contrast agents (14,15). It is considered the best diagnostic test for vertebral infections (13).

Bone Biopsy

Surgical bone biopsy to find histologic changes remains the gold standard for diagnosing osteomyelitis. Fine-needle bone biopsy was noted to be 87% sensitive and 93% specific when compared with surgical biopsy (10).

DIAGNOSTIC STRATEGIES

In approaching patients with possible osteomyelitis, the diagnostic strategy may vary somewhat depending on the site and possible cause of the disease. In addition, it is difficult to recommend a specific strategy because of the limited information concerning test characteristics.

In most cases, the initial study should be radiography to look for changes caused by osteomyelitis and to exclude other processes. Plain radiographs are more likely to be positive in patients who have had symptoms for at least 2 to 3 weeks. If radiographic changes are present, further studies are aimed at identification of the organism through blood cultures, bone aspiration, or bone biopsy.

When radiography yields negative results, what the next steps should be becomes less clear. Obtaining an ESR can help in some cases; because it is generally elevated in those with osteomyelitis caused by hematogenous spread or vascular insufficiency, a normal test result reduces the likelihood of disease. Also, detecting a palpable bone using a sterile probe in patients with diabetes who have foot ulcers increases the odds of osteomyelitis fourfold.

If the probability of osteomyelitis is intermediate or high, the next test should be one with high specificity, such as MRI or fine-needle biopsy. Positive MRI or fine-needle biopsy results confirm the diagnosis. Depending on the test used and clinical picture, negative results could necessitate additional testing.

When the results of radiography are negative and the probability of disease is relatively low, a ^{99}Tc bone scan is a reasonable test, assuming it is read with a goal of obtaining maximum sensitivity. Although follow-up testing is needed when the result is positive, a negative result should adequately rule out the diagnosis.

When the probability of disease remains high despite normal results with tests such as MRI or fine-needle biopsy, options include open biopsy, empiric treatment, and clinical observation.

In patients with a suspected contiguous focus of infection, plain radiographs are often difficult to interpret when the patient has had previous surgery or trauma. Although MRI may be helpful, surgical exploration and biopsy are often needed to confirm the diagnosis.

CLINICAL PROBLEMS

Clinical Problem 1
A patient with vascular insufficiency has a foot ulcer and a clinical presentation highly suspicious for osteomyelitis.

Testing Strategy and Rationale
Radiography should be performed. If the results are positive, the clinician should attempt to identify the causative organism and begin treatment. If the results are negative, either MRI or fine-needle bone biopsy should be performed, owing to the high clinical suspicion in this case. A positive result with either test confirms the diagnosis. Given its low specificity, nuclear scanning would be less helpful.

Continued

Clinical Example

A 55-year-old man with diabetes, neuropathy, and vascular disease presents with an ulcer he noticed 1 week ago (he does not perform regular foot examinations). Associated erythema is noted. He has a low-grade fever. The ulcer is fairly deep, and bone is palpable using a sterile probe.

The clinical assessment is that the probability of osteomyelitis is high in this patient. Magnetic resonance imaging is performed; the results are positive and the diagnosis is confirmed.

Clinical Problem 2

A patient has bony pain and fever, but the clinical suspicion of osteomyelitis is low.

Testing Strategy and Rationale

In this case, initial radiography is a good choice to look for changes associated with osteomyelitis and also to exclude other disease processes. If the results are negative, bone scanning should be done if suspicion remains high. A normal ESR may also be helpful in showing a reduced probability of disease.

Clinical Example

A 70-year-old man presents with 2 days of increasing pain in his right lower tibia. He fell 2 days ago but sustained minimal injury. About 2 weeks ago he was hospitalized for a severe urinary tract infection. He has not noted any fever or chills in the past week. Physical examination reveals a tender leg with minimal ecchymosis but no erythema, warmth, or open skin areas. ESR is elevated at 45 mm/h.

Although this clinical presentation likely represents only trauma, the possibility of hematogenously spread osteomyelitis causes concern because the patient's symptoms seem out of proportion to the injury. The elevated ESR could be the result of osteomyelitis, the patient's advanced age, or recent infection. Radiography is done, and the results are normal. Bone scanning is performed, and the results of this also are negative. The patient is given symptomatic treatment.

REFERENCES

1. **Waldvogel FA, Medoff G, Swartz MN.** Osteomyelitis: a review of clinical features, therapeutic considerations and unusual aspects (Part I). N Engl J Med. 1970;282:198-206.
2. **Markus HS.** Haematogenous osteomyelitis in the adult: a clinical and epidemiologic study. Q J Med. 1989;266:521-7.

3. **Gillespie WJ.** Epidemiology in bone and joint infection. Infect Dis Clin North Am. 1990;4:361-76.

4. **Waldvogel FA, Medoff G, Swarta MN.** Osteomyelitis: a review of clinical features, therapeutic considerations and unusual aspects (Part III). N Engl J Med. 1970;282:316-21.

5. **Sapico FL, Montgomerie JZ.** Vertebral osteomyelitis. Infect Dis Clin North Am. 1990;4:539-50.

6. **Waldvogel FA, Vasey H.** Osteomyelitis: the past decade. N Engl J Med. 1980;303:360-70.

7. **Waldvogel FA, Medoff G, Swarta MN.** Osteomyelitis: a review of clinical features, therapeutic considerations and unusual aspects (Part II). N Engl J Med. 1970;282:260-6.

8. **Armstrong DG, Lavery LA, Sariaya M, Ashry H.** Leukocytosis is a poor indicator of acute osteomyelitis of the foot in diabetes mellitus. J Foot Ankle Surg. 1996;35:280-3.

9. **Grayson ML, Gibbons GW, Balough K, et al.** Probing to bone in infected pedal ulcers: a clinical sign of underlying osteomyelitis in diabetic patients. JAMA. 1995;273:721-3.

10. **Howard CB, Einhorn M, Dagan R, et al.** Fine-needle bone biopsy to diagnose osteomyelitis. J Bone Joint Surg. 1994;76-B:311-4.

11. **Schulak DJ, Rayhack JM, Lippert FG, Convery FR.** The erythrocyte sedimentation rate in orthopaedic patients. Clin Orthop.1982;167:197-202.

12. **Unkila-Kallio L, Kallio M, Eskola J, Peltola H.** Serum C-reactive protein, erythrocyte sedimentation rate, and white blood cell count in acute hematogenous osteomyelitis of children. Pediatrics. 1994;93:59-62.

13. **Haas DW, McAndrew MP.** Bacterial osteomyelitis in adults: evolving considerations in diagnosis and treatment. Am J Med. 1996;101:550-61.

14. **Wang A, Weinstein D, Greenfield L, et al.** MRI and diabetic foot infections. Magn Reson Imaging. 1990;8:805-9.

15. **Morrison WB, Schweitzer ME, Wapner KL, et al.** Osteomyelitis in feet of diabetics: clinical accuracy, surgical utility, and cost-effectiveness of MR imaging. Radiology. 1995;196:557-64.

16. **Croll SD, Nicholas GG, Osborn MA, et al.** Role of magnetic resonance imaging in the diagnosis of osteomyelitis in diabetic foot infections. J Vasc Surg. 1996;24:266-70.

17. **Levine SE, Neagle CE, Esterhai JL, et al.** Magnetic resonance imaging for the diagnosis of osteomyelitis in the diabetic patient with a foot ulcer. Foot Ankle Int. 1994;15:151-6.

18. **Lee SM, Lee RG, Wilinsky J, et al.** Magnification radiology in osteomyelitis. Skeletal Radiol. 1986;15:625-7.

19. **Scheidler J, Leinsinger G, Pfahler M, Kirsch CM.** Diagnosis of osteomyelitis: accuracy and limitations of antigranulocyte antibody imaging compared to three-phase bone scan. Clin Nucl Med. 1994;19:731-7.

20. **Ritter M, Richter W, Leinsinger G, et al.** Granulocytes and three-phase bone scintigraph for differentiation of diabetic gangrene with and without osteomyelitis. Diabetes Care. 1992;15:1014-9.

21. **Newman L, Waller J, Palesro C, et al.** Leukocyte scanning with ^{111}In is superior to magnetic resonance imaging in diagnosis of clinically unsuspected osteomyelitis in diabetic foot ulcers. Diabetes Care. 1992;15:1527-30.

22. **Ivancevic V, Dodig D, Livakovic M, et al.** Comparison of three-phase bone scan, three-phase 99m-Tc-HM-PAO leukocyte scan and 67-gallium scan in chronic bone infection. Prog Clin Biol Res. 1990;355:189-98.

23. **Williamson M, Quenzer R, Rosenberg R, et al.** Osteomyelitis: sensitivity of 0.0064 T MRI, three-phase bone scanning and indium scanning with biopsy proof. Magn Reson Imaging. 1991;9:945-8.

24. **Myers SP, Wiener SN.** Diagnosis of hematogenous pyogenic vertebral osteomyelitis by magnetic resonance imaging. Arch Intern Med. 1991;151: 683-7.

25. **Perry CR, Pearson RL, Miller GA.** Accuracy of cultures of material from swabbing of the superficial aspect of the wound and needle biopsy in the preoperative assessment of osteomyelitis. J Bone Joint Surg. 1991;73-A: 745-9.

26. **Bravo AA, Bruskoff BL, Perner R.** A review of osteomyelitis with case presentation. J Am Podiatr Med Assoc. 1985;75:83-9.

27. **Schauwecker DS.** The scintigraphic diagnosis of osteomyelitis. AJR Am J Roentgenol.1992;158:9-18.

28. **Burdge DR, Gribble MJ.** Histologically proven pressure sore–related osteomyelitis in the setting of negative technetium bone scans. Am J Phys Med Rehab. 1993;72:386-9.

29. **Park NM, Wheat LJ, Siddiqui AR, et al.** Scintigraphic evaluation of diabetic osteomyelitis. J Nucl Med. 1982;23:569-73.

30. **Littenberg B, Mushlin AI.** Technetium bone scanning in the diagnosis of osteomyelitis: a meta-analysis of test performance. J Gen Intern Med. 1992;7:158-63.

31. **Gentry LO.** Osteomyelitis: options for diagnosis and management. J Antimicrob Chemother. 1988;21(Suppl C):115-28.

32. **Lew DP, Waldvogel FA.** Osteomyelitis. N Engl J Med. 1997;336:999-1007.

Syphilis and Neurosyphilis   **27**

Mark A. Shelly, MD

KEY POINTS

Pretest Probabilities

- A history of sexual contact and the clinical appearance of skin lesions can give a high pretest probability of primary or secondary syphilis.
- It is uncommon for neurosyphilis to present in its classic form. Most patients are asymptomatic or have nonspecific symptoms and signs.

Diagnostic Strategies

- When early syphilis is suspected, nontreponemal tests (the rapid plasma reagin [RPR] or Venereal Disease Research Laboratory test [VDRL]) effectively confirm or screen for the disease.
- Treponemal tests, such as the fluorescent treponemal antibody absorption test (FTA-Abs), provide increased specificity for confirming nontreponemal tests and added sensitivity in detecting past infection.
- A negative serum FTA-Abs test result excludes the diagnosis of neurosyphilis.
- Lumbar puncture is indicated in patients with late syphilis and in certain patients at high risk for treatment failure.
- Infection with human immunodeficiency virus (HIV) alters the response to treatment of syphilis; thus, the possibility of HIV infection should be considered in the diagnostic approach to patients with syphilis.

BACKGROUND

The diagnostic approach to syphilis varies with the clinical stage and duration of the disease. Syphilis results from infection with the spirochete *Treponema pallidum*, usually by direct contact with infectious lesions during sexual intercourse.

Early syphilis includes primary, secondary, and early latent syphilis. Primary syphilis occurs approximately 3 weeks after exposure and manifests as a painless, indurated genital ulcer (chancre) at the inoculation site. The absence of a recognized ulcer is common, especially in reinfection. Secondary syphilis is a systemic illness with a prominent rash, frequently involving the palms and soles, beginning 6 weeks to several months after exposure. Secondary syphilis may relapse, usually within 1 year after infection. Syphilis is infectious during primary and secondary stages. Public health officials define early syphilis as the first year after infection, when transmission is most likely to occur.

Latent syphilis is the asymptomatic period between primary–secondary and tertiary syphilis. During the latent period, cerebrospinal fluid (CSF) abnormalities represent an asymptomatic form of neurosyphilis (1). Approximately one third of patients who do not receive treatment develop tertiary syphilis, which appears years after initial infection. Among those persons initially infected, tertiary syphilis manifests as benign late syphilis (skin gumma) in 16% of patients, with symptomatic cardiovascular or neurologic syndromes in 10% and 6.5%, respectively (2).

ESTIMATING PRETEST PROBABILITY

The prevalence of syphilis declined dramatically with the use of penicillin in the 1940s. Routine serologic tests have yielded positive results in 6% to 17% of university hospital inpatients, 1% to 2% of community hospital outpatients, and 5% to 6% of elderly patients with dementia (3). The incidence of early syphilis varies geographically and among different populations in the United States, with most cases occurring in cities. In 1995, the incidence of early and late syphilis was 6 and 20 cases, respectively, per 100,000 persons (4).

The prevalence of syphilis in the general population has dropped to the point that routine screening is no longer recommended, except in patients at risk for sexually transmitted disease (STD) and in pregnancy, to prevent congenital syphilis. A history of any STD increases the chance of past syphilis exposure. Only half of the patients seropositive for syphilis, however, give a history of previous STD (5).

A history of sexual contact or the clinical appearance of skin lesions is highly suggestive of primary or secondary syphilis. Thirty percent of persons who do not receive treatment after having sexual contact with persons with infectious syphilis develop syphilis (6); consequently, patients with exposure to known infectious syphilis should receive empiric therapy.

The manifestations of neurosyphilis are protean. Infrequently, neurosyphilis presents in its classic form, with tabes dorsalis, lancinating pains, loss of proprioception, and wide-based ataxia. Signs such as cognitive decline, reflex changes, pupillary abnormalities, visual loss, deafness, and cranial nerve palsies are nonspecific. Even the often emphasized Argyll Robertson pupil is nonspecific, caused more frequently by diabetes mellitus than neurosyphilis. Neurosyphilis may resemble stroke, dementia, psychosis, chronic headaches, new onset seizures, and myelitis. A significant subset (as many as 30%) of patients with neurosyphilis are asymptomatic and can be diagnosed only by lumbar puncture (7). Based on synthesis of data from several studies, the pretest probability of neurosyphilis for a patient with serologic late latent syphilis is 6% to 7% (8–14).

DIAGNOSTIC TESTS

Treponema pallidum cannot be cultured by routine methods; culturing the organism by animal inoculation is confined to research use. Without specific microbiologic or microscopic identification available in most cases, the diagnosis relies heavily on serologic evidence of infection.

Dark-field Examination

When skin lesions are evident, dark-field examination of fresh exudate from these lesions can provide a definitive diagnosis. Unfortunately, a dark-field microscope and experienced personnel are not usually available. Some laboratories use a direct fluorescent antibody test (DFA-TP) to examine a dry slide of exudate to help provide microscopic identification. The DFA-TP results can confirm the presence of *T. pallidum* infection, even in locations such as the mouth where saprophytic treponemes make dark-field examination uninterpretable, and the procedure does not need to be performed on the same day as the dark-field examination (15).

Nontreponemal Serologic Tests

The nontreponemal serologic tests for syphilis detect a heterogeneous group of antibodies, called reagins, that bind a cardiolipin-lecithin complex in vitro. Laboratories use several similar tests, including the rapid plasma reagin (RPR), Veneral Disease Research Laboratory (VDRL), and toluidine red unheated serum test (TRUST). The sensitivity and specificity of the modern nontreponemal tests are similar. Because of their low cost and ease of use, the nontreponemal tests are recommended over the treponemal tests for screening patients at risk for the disease. (For simplicity, the RPR represents nontreponemal tests in this chapter.)

The RPR varies with the stage and course of illness. In initial infection, the chancre develops before the antibodies: In approximately one in four patients, the results of the RPR are negative during primary syphilis. As the duration of the disease after exposure increases, the RPR titer increases and remains elevated through the secondary stage of syphilis. In almost 100% of patients with secondary syphilis and early latent syphilis, the results of the RPR are positive at a titer of 1:8 or higher. When the titer is very high, it may test falsely negative unless done on diluted serum (a prozone phenomenon) (16). After this point, the RPR wanes through late latent syphilis to a sensitivity of 73% (Table 27-1).

The specificity of the nontreponemal tests, such as the RPR, varies among populations. A false-positive RPR can result from acute or chronic infections, autoimmune diseases (e.g., systemic lupus erythematosus), chronic diseases such as malignancy, and aging. In the general population, specificity of the tests approaches 97%; but in a population with a low prevalence of syphilis infection, the occurrence of biologic false-positives can account for more than 25% of the positive findings (3). False-positive results are often transient and rarely reach a titer greater than 1:8 (16,17).

Because the nontreponemal tests are reported as titers correlating with disease activity, they help monitor response to antibiotic therapy. With adequate penicillin treatment, the RPR should decline by at least a factor of four over the course of 6 months for primary syphilis and over the course of 12 months for secondary syphilis. The RPR usually declines further, becoming nonreactive in a time course roughly correlating with the duration of untreated infection (17). As many as 20% of treated cases of secondary or later syphilis remain in a stable, "serofast" state in which the RPR remains positive at a low titer indefinitely.

Table 27-1. Operating Characteristics of Serologic Tests in the Stages of Syphilis

Stage of Syphilis	Sensitivity		Specificity	
	RPR	FTA-Abs	VDRL	FTA-Abs
	←		%	→
Primary	72	91	*	98–99
Secondary	100	100	*	98–99
Latent	73	100	*	98–99
Tertiary	77	100	*	98–99
Screening	86	99	97	98–99

RPR = rapid plasma reagin; FTA-Abs = fluorescent treponemal antibody absorbed; VDRL = Venereal Disease Research Laboratory.

*VDRL specificity variable by stage and proportion of population tested that has autoimmune or other chronic disease

Because titers vary between alternative nontreponemal tests, the same technique should be used to follow titers.

Treponemal Tests

The treponemal tests show specific antibodies against *T. pallidum*. The most commonly available test in the United States is the fluorescent treponemal antibody absorption test (FTA-Abs) test. After absorbing non-specific antibody against nonpathogenic treponemes, the patient's serum is applied to a slide coated with spirochetes; a fluorescent anti-immunoglobulin is applied; the resulting fluorescence is rated on a scale of zero to 4+. Borderline and 1+ reactions should be repeated because they are nonspecific; persistently borderline reactions are considered negative results (15).

Other specific treponemal tests are available. Hemagglutination assays, such as the *T. pallidum* hemagglutination assay or the micro-hemagglutination assay for *T. pallidum*, show agglutination of sensitized sheep erythrocytes if the specific antibody is present. Hemagglutination assays can quantitate specific antibodies, but these titers do not reliably correlate with disease activity or with response to therapy (15). In the *T. pallidum* immobilization test, specific antibodies in the patient's serum immobilize the spirochetes. Once the standard for specificity, this test is now available in only a few research laboratories.

The sensitivity of the FTA-Abs test exceeds that of the nontreponemal tests even in early syphilis. The higher specificity of the assay, approximately 98%, makes the FTA-Abs test useful in identifying biologic false-positive results among patients with positive nontreponemal tests. Rare false-positive FTA-Abs test results have been reported with other spirochetal infections, such as Lyme disease, and in some cases of lepromatous leprosy and lupus erythematosus (18). The hemagglutination tests may have a slightly higher specificity for syphilis, but sensitivity is comparable to that of the FTA-Abs test.

Unlike the nontreponemal tests, the FTA-Abs persists indefinitely, even after adequate treatment of the infection, and does not correlate with disease activity. This test cannot distinguish previous infection from reinfection.

Lumbar Puncture

Infection of the central nervous system is one of the most serious consequences of syphilis. The lumbar puncture is frequently used in this evaluation. Tests on CSF differ in their ability to indicate neurosyphilis, and test evaluation is made problematic by the lack of a gold standard definition or diagnostic test for neurosyphilis.

The CSF cell count and protein are often elevated in neurosyphilis but are of uncertain and probably low specificity in patients with neurologic symptoms or signs. The leukocyte count correlates better with disease activity and with treatment. Based on combined results from several series (5,19–24), leukocyte pleocytosis (>5 cells/mm³) occurs in approximately 63% of cases (Table 27-2). The sensitivity of a combined abnormal CSF leukocyte count or elevated CSF protein level is approximately 80% to 90% or higher, because some patients without pleocytosis have an abnormal protein (25–27).

The CSF-VDRL is an important serologic marker for neurologic involvement, with almost 100% specificity for neurosyphilis (17). Rare false-positive results can occur when the CSF sample has been visibly contaminated with blood in a patient for whom the serum VDRL test result is positive. The sensitivity of the CSF-VDRL is debated, with estimates ranging from 27% to 79%. Recent reports give a combined sensitivity of 52% (see Table 27-2) (5,19–24), a low estimate because some studies used CSF treponemal tests (such as the CSF-FTA) to diagnose neurosyphilis. Unlike the serum nontreponemal tests, the CSF-VDRL does not reliably change with treatment.

Treponemal tests of the CSF (CSF-FTA) lack specificity for neurosyphilis. The results of CSF-FTA are frequently positive in patients with syphilis (17), but they may also be positive in as many as 4.5% of patients with a negative peripheral FTA-Abs test result (26). A small amount of blood contamination may be enough to cause a false-positive result (28). The results of CSF-FTA-Abs are not positive as often as they are with CSF-FTA, but they remain of uncertain significance (29). Although a negative CSF-FTA test result is strong evidence against neurosyphilis, a positive test result is of little diagnostic value. The Centers for Disease Control and Prevention (CDC) recommends that FTA testing no longer be done routinely on CSF samples.

Various other tests have been used to evaluate for neurosyphilis. Inflammation in the central nervous system may be associated with local immunoglobulin production (e.g., oligoclonal bands or elevated IgG index). Because the hemagglutination assay can be titered, an index of treponemal antibody production in the CSF can measure local

Table 27-2. Operating Characteristics of Cerebrospinal Fluid Abnormalities in the Diagnosis of Neurosyphilis

CSF Abnormalities	Sensitivity	Specificity
	%	%
CSF-VDRL (positive result)	52 (27–79)	100
Elevated CSF leukocytes	63 (31–82)	Uncertain
Elevated CSF protein	48 (23–100)	Uncertain

CSF = cerebrospinal fluid; VDRL = Venereal Disease Research Laboratory.

antibody production (1). These tests have yet to receive widespread clinical use (7).

DIAGNOSTIC STRATEGIES

The laboratory approach to the diagnosis of syphilis varies with the clinical stage suggested by the patient's history and examination. The decision to do a lumbar puncture to evaluate for neurosyphilis also varies with the stage of the disease. The impact of HIV infection is discussed separately.

In the case of primary syphilis, the patient should receive treatment on the basis of a typical clinical presentation, before any serologic test result is known. The diagnosis may be confirmed with dark-field microscopy or DFA-TP examination of the chancre. An RPR should be done to follow disease activity and to confirm an effective cure, bearing in mind that the RPR test result is negative at presentation in one fourth or more of these patients. Although there are fewer false-negative results with the FTA-Abs, this test does not distinguish reinfection from previous infection and therefore is less useful during the early stage of the disease.

Suspected secondary syphilis can be evaluated with the RPR; the FTA-Abs offers little advantage of RPR in terms of sensitivity, although because of its higher specificity, the FTA-Abs can be used to distinguish syphilitic infection from other diseases known to cause positive reagin test results. In secondary syphilis, the RPR titer is rarely less than 1:8.

The RPR remains sensitive during early latent syphilis. An inexpensive and reliable test, it is well suited for screening asymptomatic patients at risk for the disease. Some cases of tertiary syphilis may lose reactivity on RPR testing. In elderly persons with neurologic symptoms but for whom the pretest probability of infection is low, some experts prefer the FTA-Abs for case finding, owing to the difference in sensitivity between the VDRL and FTA-Abs and the lower specificity of the VDRL (15). However, it is unlikely this will identify any persons who will benefit from treatment, because those with negative RPR test results in this setting are unlikely to have ongoing inflammation (7).

A positive serologic test result for syphilis raises the question of neurosyphilis and the need for a lumbar puncture. The purpose of examining CSF is to identify those patients with neurosyphilis or those at risk for developing neurosyphilis (asymptomatic neurosyphilis).

Lumbar puncture is of little diagnostic value during early syphilis. In untreated primary and secondary syphilis, abnormal findings in the CSF are seen in 13% and 25% to 40% of patients, respectively; neurosyphilis develops in only 6.5% of patients, even if syphilis is left untreated. The specificity of the lumbar puncture for predicting subsequent neurosyphilis is low during early syphilis, and neurosyphilis rarely occurs after treatment of early syphilis with the recommended therapies.

Lumbar puncture has greater diagnostic potential during late syphilis. Cerebrospinal fluid abnormalities in asymptomatic patients peak at 12 to 18 months after exposure, decreasing to 20% at 3 years, 12.9% at 10 years, and 6.3% at 20 years (7). In late syphilis, the prevalence of elevated protein, positive CSF-VDRL results, and pleocytosis in the CSF decreases, although it may remain as high as 30% (13).

The decision to perform lumbar puncture in patients with asymptomatic late syphilis is still controversial. It is recommended by some experts (17), whereas others argue that the number of improved outcomes from treating abnormal lumbar punctures may be less than the complication rate (27). Central to this argument are several issues: the efficacy of current recommended treatments for late syphilis (30); the prevalence of neurosyphilis in the untreated, asymptomatic patient for whom the RPR or FTA-Abs yields positive test results; and the diagnostic characteristics of lumbar puncture.

It is generally agreed that patients with neurologic symptoms and evidence of untreated syphilis (by history or positive serologic test) should have a lumbar puncture to assess for neurosyphilis. Even with the possibility of false-positive results, a positive CSF-VDRL result in this setting would be compelling evidence for a trial of antibiotic therapy owing to the high specificity of the test. Findings in the CSF limited to pleocytosis or elevated CSF protein would not be specific enough to exclude other causes of the patient's symptoms. Progression from asymptomatic to symptomatic neurosyphilis usually occurs during the first 30 years after infection: If infection occurred more than 30 years before evaluation and the patient is not yet symptomatic, a lumbar puncture may be unnecessary (31).

Centers for Disease Control and Prevention guidelines (32) suggest six settings in late syphilis in which a lumbar puncture should be done: 1) in patients with neurologic signs or symptoms; 2) in patients with serologic evidence of a treatment failure (the RPR increases fourfold or fails to decrease to less than 1:32); 3) the serum nontreponemal titer is 1:32 or greater; 4) in patients with other evidence of active syphilis (e.g., aortitis, gumma, iritis); 5) in patients for whom nonpenicillin therapy is planned; and 6) in patients in whom an HIV antibody test result is positive.

Infection with the Human Immunodeficiency Virus

With the emergence of acquired immunodeficiency syndrome (AIDS), the standard recommendations for the diagnosis and management of syphilis have been challenged. There are case reports of early and severe neurosyphilis in patients with concurrent HIV infection. According to many reports, atypical presentations may be more common in HIV but are certainly not out of the range of the protean manifestations of syphilis recorded in the past (33). Incomplete information precludes adjustment of the pretest probability of neurosyphilis on the basis of HIV status alone (8). A growing body of literature suggests that the HIV-positive patient may be at increased risk for treatment failure using standard recommended guidelines.

Syphilis serologic results may be altered by HIV infection. A case has been reported of an initially negative RPR test result in a patient with AIDS and secondary syphilis (34), but most often the nontreponemal titers have been normal or high (32).

Although HIV infection may affect decisions about treatment of early syphilis, the value of lumbar puncture in predicting patients at risk for later neurosyphilis remains low. Abnormalities found in CSF correlate with the isolation of *T. pallidum*, although test sensitivity is unchanged, and the specificity remains low.

Lumbar puncture in asymptomatic patients with late latent syphilis is likely to be valuable because these patients are at higher risk for treatment failure. The CDC recommends a lumbar puncture in patients with late syphilis with concurrent HIV but does not currently advise a lumbar puncture in early syphilis. Follow-up in these patients should be frequent to watch for treatment failures (32).

CLINICAL PROBLEMS

Clinical Problem 1
A patient with a history of treated syphilis presents with signs and symptoms of primary syphilis.

Testing Strategy and Rationale
If available, dark-field microscopy or DFA-TP should be done on fluid from the base of a chancre. The appropriate serologic test is the RPR. The results of FTA-Abs would be positive from previous exposure. Treatment for early syphilis should be initiated, regardless of serologic test results. Follow-up serologic testing should be done to confirm successful therapy.

Clinical Example
A 27-year-old man with a history of treated syphilis presents with a chancre 3 weeks after a sexual encounter with a new partner. Given the sexual encounter, appropriate incubation period, and a painless genital ulcer, the pretest suspicion for syphilis is high. A negative RPR result would not be uncommon. Treatment should result in healing of the chancre; an RPR titer at 6 months after treatment should be negative (or should be at least one fourth of the initial titer).

Continued

Clinical Problem 2

A patient has nonspecific neurologic signs and a history suggesting a risk of previous syphilis.

Testing Strategy and Rationale

When one is considering neurosyphilis, the RPR remains a reasonable test for case finding. To rule out infection in the distant past, the FTA-Abs adds sensitivity. The pretest probability of syphilis is increased by any history of sexually transmitted diseases. If the results of the serum FTA-Abs are positive, the test should be followed up with lumbar puncture.

Clinical Example

A 60-year-old woman is admitted to a nursing home for progressive dementia. Although not currently sexually active, she was treated for gonorrhea on several occasions as recently as 15 years ago. The test results of an RPR are positive. If the FTA-Abs is also positive, lumbar puncture should be done to evaluate for neurosyphilis. A positive CSF-VDRL would prove neurosyphilis, and the patient should be treated. However, this test alone would have a low sensitivity. Cerebrospinal fluid pleocytosis or elevated protein would be suggestive of neurosyphilis even in the absence of a reactive CSF-VDRL, raising the probability sufficiently to justify treatment.

REFERENCES

1. **Tramont EC.** *Treponema pallidum* (syphilis). In: Mandell GL, Bennet JE, Dolin R, eds. Principles and Practice of Infectious Diseases. New York: Churchill Livingstone; 1996:2117-33.
2. **Clark EG, Danbolt N.** The Oslo study of the natural history of untreated syphilis: an epidemiologic investigation based on a re-study of the Boeck-Bruusgaard material: a review and appraisal. J Chron Dis. 1955;2:311-4.
3. **Ho P, Pein F, Pruett K.** Routine serologic testing for syphilis in a community medical practice. West. J Med. 1980;132:485-7.
4. Centers for Disease Control and Prevention. Summary of notifiable diseases, United States, 1995. MMWR Morb Mortal Wkly Rep. 1995;44:73.
5. **Hooshmand H, Escobar MR, Kopf SW.** Neurosyphilis: a study of 241 patients. JAMA. 1972;219:726-9.
6. **Sparling PF.** Natural history of syphilis. In: Holmes KK, Mardh PA, Sparling PF, et al, eds. Sexually Transmitted Diseases. New York: McGraw-Hill; 1991:213-9.
7. **Swartz MN.** Neurosyphilis. In: Holmes KK, Mardh PA, Sparling PF, et al, eds. Sexually Transmitted Diseases. New York: McGraw-Hill; 1991:231-46.

8. Lukehart SA, Hook EWd, Baker-Zander SA, et al. Invasion of the central nervous system by *Treponema pallidum*: implications for diagnosis and treatment. Ann Intern Med. 1988;109:855-62.

9. Dans PE, Cafferty L, Otter SE, Johnson RJ. Inappropriate use of the cerebrospinal fluid Venereal Disease Research Laboratory (VDRL) test to exclude neurosyphilis. Ann Intern Med. 1986;104:86-9.

10. Traviesa DC, Prystowsky SD, Nelson BJ, Johnson KP. Cerebrospinal fluid findings in asymptomatic patients with reactive serum fluorescent treponemal antibody absorption tests. Ann Neurol. 1978;4:524-30.

11. Ducas J, Robson HG. Cerebrospinal fluid penicillin levels during therapy for latent syphilis. JAMA. 1981;246:2583-4.

12. Dijkstra JW. Asymptomatic neurosyphilis. Int J Dermatol. 1983;22:581-9.

13. Graman PS, Trupei MA, Reichman RC. Evaluation of cerebrospinal fluid in asymptomatic late syphilis. Sex Transm Dis. 1987;14:205-8.

14. Kelley RE, Bell L, Kelley SE, Lee SC. Syphilis detection in cerebrovascular disease. Stroke. 1989;20:230-4.

15. Larsen SA, Steiner BM, Rudolph AH. Laboratory diagnosis and interpretation of tests for syphilis. Clin Microb Rev. 1995;8:1-21.

16. Jurado RL, Campbell J, Martin PD. Prozone phenomenon in secondary syphilis. Has its time arrived? [See comments]. Arch Intern Med. 1993; 153:2496-8.

17. Larsen SA, Hunter EF, Creighton ET. Syphilis. In: Holmes KK, Mardh PA, Sparling PF, et al, eds. Sexually Transmitted Diseases. New York: McGraw-Hill; 1990:927-34.

18. Jaffe HW, Musher DM. Management of reactive syphilis serology. In: Holmes KK, Mardh PA, Sparling PF, et al, eds. Sexually Transmitted Diseases. New York: McGraw-Hill; 1990:935-9.

19. Luger A, Schmidt BL, Steyrer K, Schonwald E. Diagnosis of neurosyphilis by examination of the cerebrospinal fluid. Br J Vener Dis. 1981;57:232-7.

20. Lee JB, Kim SC, Lee S, et al. Symptomatic neurosyphilis. Int J Dermatol. 1983;22:577-80.

21. Burke JM, Schaberg DR. Neurosyphilis in the antibiotic era. Neurology. 1985;35:1368-71.

22. Wolters EC. Neurosyphilis: a changing diagnostic problem? Eurn Neurol. 1987;26:23-8.

23. Smikle MF, James OB, Prabhakar P. Diagnosis of neurosyphilis: a critical assessment of current methods. South Med J. 1988;81:452-4.

24. Davis LE, Schmitt JW. Clinical significance of cerebrospinal fluid tests for neurosyphilis. Ann Neurol. 1989;25:50-5.

25. Zenker PN, Rolfs RT. Treatment of syphilis, 1989. Rev Infect Dis. 1990;12: S590-609.

26. Simon RP. Neurosyphilis. Arch Neurol. 1985;42:606-13.

27. Wiesel J, Rose DN, Silver AL, et al. Lumbar puncture in asymptomatic late syphilis: an analysis of the benefits and risks. Arch Intern Med. 1985;145 465-8.

28. **Davis LE, Sperry S.** The CSF-FTA test and the significance of blood contamination. Ann Neurol. 1979;6:68-9.

29. **Bracero L, Wormser GP, Bottone EJ.** Serologic tests for syphilis: a guide to interpreting in various stages of disease. Mt Sinai J Med. 1979;46:289-92.

30. **Greene BM, Miller NR, Bynum TE.** Failure of penicillin G benzathine in the treatment of neurosyphilis. Arch Intern Med. 1980;140:1117-8.

31. **Jaffe HW, Kabins SA.** Examination of the cerebrospinal fluid in patients with syphilis. Rev Infect Dis. 1982;45:842-7.

32. **Centers for Disease Control and Prevention.** 1993 Sexually transmitted diseases treatment guidelines. MMWR Morb Mortal Wkly Rep. 1993;42 1-102.

33. **Hook EWI.** Syphilis and HIV infection. J Infect Dis. 1989;160:530-4.

34. **Hicks CB, Benson PM, Lupton GP, Tramont EC.** Seronegative secondary syphilis in a patient infected with the human immunodeficiency virus (HIV) with Kaposi sarcoma. Ann Intern Med. 1987;107:492-5.

Respiratory Problems

Pulmonary Embolism   28

Eric J. Anish, MD, and Raymond J. Mayewski, MD

KEY POINTS

Pretest Probabilities

- Among patients presenting with possible pulmonary embolism (PE), between 20% and 30% actually have an embolism. Although information from the history, physical examination, chest radiography, electrocardiography, and arterial blood gas analysis can help revise the pretest probability of PE, further testing is usually needed to establish the diagnosis.

- A normal partial pressure of oxygen in arterial blood (Pao_2 ≥80 mm Hg) or a normal alveolar-arterial oxygen gradient does not exclude the diagnosis of pulmonary embolism.

- Patients with suspected PE should be evaluated for conditions that could place them at risk for thromboembolic disease.

Diagnostic Strategies

- With rare exceptions, a normal perfusion scan excludes a diagnosis of pulmonary embolism.

- The combination of high-probability ventilation–perfusion (V/Q) scan and either intermediate or high clinical suspicion of pulmonary embolism generally allows one to make a diagnosis of PE.

- The combination of low-probability V/Q scan and low clinical suspicion of pulmonary embolism allows one reliably to exclude a diagnosis of PE.

- The remaining patients with V/Q scans that demonstrate abnormalities generally require further diagnostic testing, which should begin with an evaluation of the lower extremities for venous thrombosis.

- When noninvasive studies do not adequately rule in or rule out a diagnosis of PE, pulmonary angiography remains an extremely valuable diagnostic test.

BACKGROUND

The diagnosis of pulmonary embolism (PE) is frequently considered in the evaluation of patients with acute, otherwise unexplained respiratory symptoms such as dyspnea or pleuritic chest pain. It is estimated that each year PE develops in more than 600,000 patients, resulting in as many as 60,000 deaths (1). Thus, venous thromboembolism is the third most common acute cardiovascular disease, exceeded only by cardiac ischemia and stroke (2). Unfortunately, PE is underdiagnosed; it has been estimated that no more than one third of emboli detected at autopsy were diagnosed antemortem. Consequently, the mortality from thromboembolic disease has remained virtually unchanged over the past several decades (3).

Because untreated PE results in substantial morbidity and mortality and invasive angiographic procedures may not be readily available, clinicians must often make treatment decisions when a definitive diagnosis is still somewhat uncertain. However, the proper use of clinical information and the noninvasive tests permit a diagnosis of thromboembolic disease or safely exclude this diagnosis in most patients being evaluated for possible PE, without the need for pulmonary angiography.

ESTIMATING PRETEST PROBABILITY

The clinical presentation of pulmonary embolism is highly variable and is determined by the severity of vascular obstruction; the size, number, and distribution of the emboli; the patient's age; and the presence of underlying cardiopulmonary disorders (4). Unfortunately, presenting symptoms are nonspecific; the signs and symptoms so commonly seen in patients with PE are also found in the conditions that mimic PE (Table 28-1). Although dyspnea or tachypnea or pleuritic chest pain is seen in more than 95% of patients with PE, none of these findings is very specific. The classic presentation of acute onset dyspnea, pleuritic chest pain, and hemoptysis is seen in only a small percentage of patients with confirmed PE (5).

Several investigators have studied the utility of arterial blood gas analysis in evaluating patients for possible PE. Although in patients with confirmed PE, a reduced partial pressure of oxygen in arterial blood (PaO_2) (<80 mm Hg) or an increased alveolar-arterial oxygen gradient (A-aO_2) (>20 mm Hg) is found in <u>most</u> patients, it is certainly not uncommon to find a normal PaO_2 or A-aO_2, particularly in patients with minimal pulmonary vascular obstruction (5,6). In the Prospective Investigation of Pulmonary Embolism Diagnosis (PIOPED) study, among patients without pre-existing cardiopulmonary disease there was no difference in room air PaO_2 or in the A-aO_2 gradient between those persons who had PE at angiography and those who did not (6).

Table 28-1. Operating Characteristics of Symptoms, Signs, and Laboratory Tests in the Diagnosis of Pulmonary Embolism in Patients Without Pre-existing Cardiac or Pulmonary Disease

Symptom, Sign, and Laboratory Test	Sensitivity	Specificity	Likelihood Ratio	
			Positive Result	Negative Result
	← % →			
Symptom				
Dyspnea	73	28	1.0	0.96
Pleuritic pain	66	41	1.1	0.83
Immobilization	56	67	1.7	0.66
Recent surgery	54	69	1.7	0.67
Cough	37	64	1.0	0.98
Leg swelling	28	78	1.3	0.92
Leg pain	26	76	1.1	0.97
Hemoptysis	13	92	1.6	0.95
Palpitations	10	82	0.6	1.1
Wheezing	9	89	0.8	1.0
Sign				
Tachypnea (>20 breaths/min)	70	32	1.0	0.94
Crackles	51	60	1.3	0.82
Tachycardia (>100 beats/min)	30	76	1.3	0.92
S_4	24	86	1.7	0.88
Increased P_2	23	87	1.8	0.89
Deep venous thrombosis	11	89	1.0	1.0
Temperature >38.5 °C	7	88	0.6	1.1
Pleural friction rub	3	98	1.5	0.99
Cyanosis	1	98	0.5	1.0
Laboratory				
Chest radiography any abnormality	84	34	1.3	0.47
Chest radiography pleural effusion	48	69	1.5	0.75
Pao_2 <80 mm Hg	74	30	1.1	0.87

Adapted from Stein PD, Terrin ML, Hale CA, et al. Clinical, laboratory, roentgenographic, and electrocardiographic findings in patients with acute pulmonary embolism and no pre-existing cardiac or pulmonary disease. Chest. 1991;100:598-603.

Certainly, the presence of a low Pao_2 and increased A-aO_2-gradient may increase a clinical suspicion of PE; however, normal values do not exclude the diagnosis. (Unfortunately, if patients who have marked hypoxia are excluded from analyses in which Pao_2 is measured because they are "too sick" to have had blood gases measured on room air, the sensitivity for the finding of hypoxia is decreased.)

Chest radiography and electrocardiography (ECG) are often performed in the evaluation of patients with suspected PE. Although studies may reveal abnormalities, again, the findings are often nonspecific. For example, data from PIOPED revealed that the most common abnormality found on chest radiography was atelectasis or a pulmonary parenchymal abnormality, which was seen in 68% of patients with PE and in 48% of patients without PE (5). Small pleural effusions were noted in about half of the patients with PE. Classic findings such as a wedge-shaped infarct (Hampton's hump) or a prominent central pulmonary artery and decreased pulmonary vascularity (Westermark's sign) are not commonly seen (5,7). Approximately 70% of patients with PE have some ECG abnormality. The most common abnormalities are nonspecific ST segment or T-wave changes, which are seen in approximately 50% of patients with PE (5). The classic right ventricular ECG strain pattern of $S_1Q_3T_3$ is not commonly seen; and when it is seen, it is usually in the setting of massive PE (7). Although ECG is never diagnostic for PE, it can be very helpful in identifying other conditions in which the clinical presentations may be similar to those of PE, such as myocardial ischemia or pericarditis.

In estimating the likelihood of PE, it is imperative to consider risk factors for the development of venous thromboembolism. As noted in Table 28-1, a history of immobilization or recent surgery has predictive value. One must also be concerned about PE in patients with primary or acquired (secondary) hypercoagulable states (8–10). Some investigators have reported that as many as 95% of patients with confirmed PE have a predisposing medical condition (5).

In estimating the pretest probability of PE, information from the PIOPED study is helpful. In that study, approximately 30% of those suspected of having PE were found to actually have a PE (5). In another study, Hull and colleagues (11) reported that among 21% of patients who presented to an emergency department for evaluation of pleuritic chest pain, PE was a cause of the pain. These baseline prevalences can be modified based on findings from the initial evaluation. For example, a previously healthy patient with recent immobilization, leg swelling, hemoptysis, and a small pleural effusion on chest radiography has a pretest probability for PE of approximately 60%.

DIAGNOSTIC TESTS

Ventilation–Perfusion Lung Scanning

Of all of the noninvasive tests available for the evaluation of a suspected PE, ventilation–perfusion (V/Q) scanning remains one of the most useful. As described below, certain scan patterns are highly specific for

PE, and normal findings on perfusion scintigraphy virtually exclude the diagnosis of clinically significant embolism (12).

Perfusion studies are performed by injecting isotopically labeled macroaggregates of albumin intravenously, and the ventilation studies are performed by inhalation of radioactive aerosols (1). The distribution of the radioactive materials within the lung is recorded, and each is compared to a standard chest radiograph. Abnormalities found on perfusion scan alone are nonspecific and can be seen in several other cardiopulmonary diseases. However, when perfusion and ventilation scans are combined, certain patterns occur that can be used to estimate the likelihood of PE. Pulmonary embolism often results in areas of increased V/Q ratio—that is, areas of normal ventilation with decreased to absent blood flow. In contrast, pulmonary parenchymal disorders that result in defects in perfusion are usually associated with diminished or absent ventilation. The ventilation–perfusion abnormality resulting from PE is termed V/Q "mismatch," whereas that seen with parenchymal disease has been labeled a "matched" defect (13). Based on the size of the defect and the degree of V/Q "mismatch," an abnormality found on V/Q scan can be classified as high probability, intermediate or indeterminate probability, or low probability for PE (Table 28-2) (13,14). Likelihood ratios for various patterns derived from PIOPED data are presented in Table 28-2; a high-probability scan has a likelihood ratio of 7.3, whereas a low-probability scan has a ratio of 0.14 (14).

Although there has been some reluctance to pursue V/Q scans in patients with underlying cardiopulmonary disease, studies have shown that the presence of such conditions or an abnormal baseline chest radiograph does not eliminate the diagnostic utility of V/Q scanning in patients with acute PE (15). Although the presence of underlying cardiopulmonary disease may increase the likelihood that the scan will not be diagnostic, this study remains a valuable tool in the initial evaluation of PE in these patients.

Studies of Peripheral Veins
When the combined results of V/Q scanning and pretest probability leave the diagnosis uncertain, many would argue that a noninvasive study of the lower extremities for venous thrombosis is a reasonable step (16). A detailed discussion of the diagnostic approach to suspected deep venous thrombosis is presented in Chapter 9.

The search for venous thrombosis is considered useful because such thrombi occur in approximately 70% of patients with angiographically proven PE (1). If a study of the lower extremities yields positive results, a diagnosis of venous thromboembolism can be made. This approach eliminates the need for diagnostic tests that are costly

Table 28-2. Likelihood Ratios for Results of Ventilation–Perfusion Scans in the Diagnosis of Pulmonary Embolism

Scan Pattern	Patients with PE (*n*)	Patients without PE (*n*)	Likelihood Ratio for Result
High probability (e.g., multiple segmental or larger defects with mismatch or perfusion defect much larger than matching ventilation or chest radiograph defect)	102	14	7.3
Intermediate (indeterminate) probability (e.g., indeterminate with chest radiograph defect similar in size to V/Q mismatch)	105	217	0.48
Low probability (e.g., single moderate mismatch or perfusion defect much smaller than matching ventilation or chest radiograph defect)	39	273	0.14
Near normal/normal	5	126	0.04
Normal	0	21	0

33%

Data from The PIOPED Investigators. Value of the ventilation/perfusion scan in acute pulmonary embolism: results of the Prospective Investigation of Pulmonary Embolism Diagnosis (PIOPED). JAMA. 1990;263:2753.

or invasive or both (e.g., pulmonary angiography). Although a positive lower extremity study is extremely helpful; a negative test result cannot usually be used to exclude a diagnosis of PE, because in almost 30% of patients with established PE, thrombus is not detected on lower extremity studies (1).

Pulmonary Angiography

Pulmonary angiography remains the "gold standard" for the diagnosis of PE. This study is extremely sensitive for detecting clinically significant PE and can detect clots as small as 0.5 mm. With rare exceptions, a normal angiogram excludes the diagnosis of emboli in all but the smallest pulmonary vessels (7).

Despite its diagnostic value, pulmonary angiography is an invasive study that necessitates right-heart catheterization and intravenous contrast material, both of which carry some associated risk. However, when the study is performed by experienced angiographers, the morbidity and mortality are low. Among the 1111 patients who underwent pulmonary angiography in the PIOPED study, there were 9 (1%) major nonfatal complications and 5 (0.5%) deaths. However, not all of the deaths were necessarily related to the procedure itself (17). Additional studies have found even lower complication rates: one large retrospective analysis of 1434 patients found a 2% incidence of immediate nonfatal complications and only 2 deaths (0.1%) (18). Pulmonary angiography therefore remains an extremely valuable diagnostic test for PE; nevertheless, it must be used judiciously.

Computed Tomography

Because of the limitations of V/Q scanning and the invasiveness of conventional pulmonary angiography, there has been a growing interest in additional noninvasive tests for evaluating patients with suspected PE. Recent technical developments in computed tomography (CT), namely helical (spiral) CT and electron-beam CT, have substantially improved visualization of the pulmonary vasculature (19). Several recent studies have reported on the accuracy of these new modalities in the detection of acute pulmonary artery clot. Sensitivity and specificity of these tests in the detection of central clots have been reported to be between 95% and 100%. Currently, the accuracy of CT in detecting of smaller peripheral clots in vessels distal to the segmental branches appears to be lower than that of conventional pulmonary angiography. However, the clinical significance of this is unclear (19–21).

Computed tomography does offer the potential benefit of assessing conditions other than PE, such as abnormalities of the lung parenchyma, mediastinum, hilum, pericardium, and chest wall, which may be causing the patient's symptoms. However, well-designed, large, prospective clinical trials to assess patient outcomes are required before CT can routinely replace conventional testing in the evaluation of patients suspected of having PE.

Magnetic Resonance Imaging

Magnetic resonance imaging (MRI) is also evolving as a noninvasive means of visualizing clots in the pulmonary arteries, and technical advances in this method continue to be made. It also has the advantage of not requiring iodinated contrast material. Studies have indicated that the sensitivity of MRI in detecting emboli varies with clot size and vessel location. As with CT scans, the ability of MRI to detect small clots in vessels at and beyond segmental branches is limited. Furthermore, the detection of clots in vessels with "in-plane" orientation is also limited (19).

Studies have found overall sensitivities between 90% and 100% and specificities of 60% to 80% for the detection of PE (19,22). An additional consideration is the potential to combine pulmonary magnetic resonance angiography with magnetic resonance venography of the peripheral vascular system, thus providing a thorough evaluation for thromboembolic disease (19). However, at present, more clinical experience is needed with pulmonary magnetic resonance angiography before it can be routinely used in the evaluation of patients with possible PE.

Plasma D-Dimer Levels

In addition to imaging studies, investigators are evaluating certain laboratory tests in patients with suspected PE. It is well accepted that tests such as leukocyte count and a variety of serum chemistries have little diagnostic value. However, the plasma D-dimer level has been receiving attention recently. D-dimer is released into the circulation when a cross-linked fibrin clot undergoes fibrinolysis (23). In theory, one should see increased levels of plasma D-dimer in patients with PE.

Some investigators have reported that a low concentration of plasma D-dimer (usually <500 ng/mL) measured by the enzyme-linked immunosorbent assay (ELISA) technique may be used to rule out acute PE, because it has been reported to have sensitivity of between 90% and 100% (23–26). Of note, use of the latex agglutination assay has not been shown to be as reliable (25). Although low D-dimer levels may be helpful in excluding a diagnosis of PE, an elevated value is quite nonspecific. False-positive test results are seen in many conditions; for example, they may be seen in surgical and trauma patients and in those with renal disease. Specificity values in the 25% to 45% range have been reported (23–26). Although these are promising results, at present the data are insufficient to allow reliance on this test. Improvements in the standardization and calibration of the various assays must be achieved and larger clinical trials must be completed before the D-dimer test can play a larger role in the routine evaluation of patients in whom PE is suspected.

DIAGNOSTIC STRATEGIES

Most patients who have symptoms of dyspnea or chest pain have a condition other than PE. Initial evaluation of such patients should therefore be directed toward the elucidation of these more commonly encountered problems such as musculoskeletal pain, respiratory tract infection, or myocardial ischemia. Frequently, a careful history and physical examination, together with chest radiography and ECG, allow one to make a diagnosis with confidence and eliminate PE from further consideration. However, in patients for whom PE remains a concern, information from the history, physical examination, chest radiography and blood gas analysis is neither sufficiently sensitive nor specific to exclude or confirm the diagnosis of PE. Therefore, additional diagnostic testing must be pursued.

In most such patients, V/Q scanning is the next step. A normal perfusion scan essentially excludes a diagnosis of PE. However, in nearly 90% of patients referred for V/Q scanning, some abnormality is found. The perfusion and ventilation defects must then be compared to determine the diagnostic impact of the scan (see Table 28-2). If the pretest probability of PE is intermediate or high and the V/Q scan reveals a "high-probability" pattern of defects, the patient should be considered to have PE (Table 28-3). No further diagnostic testing is usually required, unless thrombolytic therapy is being considered—in which case, according to some, pulmonary angiography should be performed. If the pretest probability of PE is low, a low-probability V/Q scan should lead one confidently to rule out PE (see Table 28-3). Patients with any other combination of clinical probability and V/Q scan result generally require further diagnostic investigation; patients with indeterminate V/Q scans make up most of this group.

Further diagnostic testing should continue with an evaluation of the lower extremities for clots. The choice of procedure depends on test availability and local expertise. If the clinical suspicion for PE is high, the lung scan is not "high-probability," and lower extremity studies are negative, many authorities recommend proceeding with pulmonary angiography (16). In other patients with indeterminate V/Q scans and a single negative lower extremity test, many believe that serial noninvasive leg tests are an appropriate approach, provided that these patients have good cardiopulmonary reserve (e.g., no evidence of right-heart failure, Pao_2 >50 mm Hg while breathing room air, and hemodynamic stability); if there does not appear to be adequate reserve, pulmonary angiography should be pursued (16). This approach has been validated by studies showing good outcomes without anticoagulant therapy in such patients in whom the results of serial testing remain negative (27,28).

Table 28-3. Post-test Probabilities of Pulmonary Embolism Based on Ventilation/Perfusion Scanning

Scan Pattern	Pretest Probabilities		
	20%	50%	80%
	←	%	→
High probability	65	88	97
Intermediate/indeterminate probability	11	32	66
Low probability	4	12	36
Near normal/normal	1	4	14
Normal	0	0	0

*See Table 28-2 for definitions of scan patterns.

The exact role of newer diagnostic modalities such as CT, magnetic resonance angiography, and plasma D-dimer in the evaluation of patients with suspected PE continues to be investigated.

CLINICAL PROBLEMS

Clinical Problem 1

A previously healthy young patient has findings occasionally associated with PE, such as pleuritic chest pain and fever, but no predisposing factors for thromboembolic disease.

Testing Strategy and Rationale

A history should be obtained, and a physical examination and chest radiography should be performed. The lack of predisposing risk factors makes a diagnosis of PE rather unlikely. A pulmonary infection is the most likely cause of this patient's symptoms.

Clinical Example

A 25-year-old woman presents with an acute onset of pleuritic pain, fever, and nonproductive cough. She has no previous history of thromboembolic disease and no other predisposing risk factors such as recent immobilization. On physical examination, her temperature is 38.5 °C, she is not tachypneic or tachycardic, and lung examination reveals scattered rales at the right base. Oxygen saturation obtained by pulse oximetry is 98% on room air. Because the history and examination are not suggestive of pericarditis or myocardial ischemia, ECG is not performed. Owing to the focal findings on lung examination, chest radiography is performed and reveals a small infiltrate in the right lower lobe. Based on this information, the likelihood that this patient has had a PE is quite low and further evaluation for PE is not indicated.

Clinical Problem 2

An elderly, hospitalized patient recovering from a myocardial infarction complicated by congestive heart failure experiences an abrupt onset of dyspnea and hypoxia.

Testing Strategy and Rationale

After the history and physical examination, ECG should be performed immediately to evaluate this patient for possible myocardial ischemia. This patient's advanced age, his history of congestive heart failure, and his prolonged bed rest all place him at significant risk for PE. If the ECG is not diagnostic, chest radiography, blood gas analysis, and V/Q scanning should be done. The clinical suspicion of PE is at least intermediate, if not high. Therefore, a "high-probability" V/Q scan determines a sufficiently high post-test probability of PE such that appropriate therapy can be initiated without additional testing. Otherwise, only a normal V/Q scan is likely to obviate the need for further diagnostic evaluation.

Clinical Example

An 80-year-old man has been recently admitted for an acute myocardial infarction complicated by congestive heart failure. On the sixth day of his convalescence, he suddenly develops dyspnea and hypoxemia (PaO_2 = 48 mm Hg on room air) without any significant changes on ECG and no appreciable findings of congestive heart failure on examination. Chest radiography shows only mild heart failure.

V/Q scanning is done. It is read as "high probability," and treatment for PE is started. However, if it had been "low probability," additional testing beginning with lower extremity studies for thrombus would have been indicated owing to the intermediate to high pretest probability.

REFERENCES

1. **Hirsh J, Hoak J.** Management of deep vein thrombosis and pulmonary embolism: a statement for healthcare professionals. Circulation. 1996;93:2212-45.

2. **Giuntini C, Di Ricco G, Marini C, et al.** Epidemiology. Chest. 1995;107:3S-9S.

3. **Palla A, Petruzzelli S, Donnamaria V, et al.** The role of suspicion in the diagnosis of pulmonary embolism. Chest. 1995;107:21S-24S.

4. **Manganelli D, Palla A, Donnamaria V, et al.** Clinical features of pulmonary embolism: doubts and uncertainties. Chest. 1995;107:25S-32S.

5. **Stein PD, Terrin ML, Hales CA, et al.** Clinical, laboratory, roentgenographic, and electrocardiographic findings in patients with acute pulmonary embolism and no pre-existing cardiac or pulmonary disease. Chest. 1991;100:598-603.

6. **Stein PD, Goldhaber SZ, Henry JW.** Alveolar-arterial oxygen gradient in the assessment of acute pulmonary embolism. Chest. 1995;107:139-43.

7. **Palevsky HI, Kelley MA, Fishman AP.** Pulmonary thromboembolic disease. In: Fishman AP, Elias JA, Fishman JA, et al, eds. Fishman's Pulmonary Diseases and Disorders. New York: McGraw-Hill; 1998:1297-329.

8. **Bauer KA.** The hypercoagulable state. In: Beutler E, Lichtman MA, Coller BS, et al, eds. Williams Hematology. New York: McGraw-Hill; 1995:1531-50.

9. **Anderson AA, Wheeler HB.** Venous thromboembolism: risk factors and prophylaxis. Clin Chest Med. 1995;16:235-51.

10. **Goldhaber SZ, Morpurgo M.** Diagnosis, treatment, and prevention of pulmonary embolism: report for the WHO/International Society and Federation of Cardiology Task Force. JAMA. 1992;268:1727-33.

11. **Hull RD, Raskob GE, Carter CJ, et al.** Pulmonary embolism in outpatients with pleuritic chest pain. Arch Intern Med. 1988;148:838-44.

12. **Hull RD, Raskob GE, Coates G, et al.** Clinical validity of a normal perfusion lung scan in patients with suspected pulmonary embolism. Chest. 1990;97:23-6.

13. **Arroliga AC, Matthay MA, Matthay RA.** Pulmonary thromboembolism and other pulmonary vascular diseases. In: George RB, Light RW, Matthay MA, et al, eds. Chest Medicine: Essentials of Pulmonary and Critical Care Medicine. Baltimore: Williams & Wilkins; 1995:271-302.

14. The PIOPED Investigators. Value of the ventilation/perfusion scan in acute pulmonary embolism: results of the Prospective Investigation of Pulmonary Embolism Diagnosis (PIOPED). JAMA. 1990;263:2753-9.

15. **Stein PD, Coleman RE, Gottschalk A, et al.** Diagnostic utility of ventilation/perfusion lung scans in acute pulmonary embolism is not diminished by pre-existing cardiac or pulmonary disease. Chest. 1991;100:604-6.

16. ACCP Consensus Committee on Pulmonary Embolism. Opinions regarding the diagnosis and management of venous thromboembolic disease. Chest. 1996;109:233-7.

17. **Stein PD, Athanasoulis C, Alavi A, et al.** Complications and validity of pulmonary angiography in acute pulmonary embolism. Circulation. 1992;85:462-8.

18. **Perlmut LM, Braun SD, Newman GE, et al.** Pulmonary arteriography in the high-risk patient. Radiology. 1987;162:187-9.

19. **Gefter WB, Hatabu H, Holland GA, et al.** Pulmonary thromboembolism: recent developments in diagnosis with CT and MR imaging. Radiology. 1995;197:561-74.

20. **Van Rossum AB, Pattynama PM, Tjin ER, et al.** Pulmonary embolism: validation of spiral CT angiography in 149 patients. Radiology. 1996;201:467-70.

21. **Bluemke DA, Chambers TP.** Spiral CT angiography: an alternative to conventional angiography. Radiology. 1995;195:317-9.

22. **Matsumoto AH, Tegtmeyer CJ.** Contemporary diagnostic approaches to acute pulmonary emboli. Radiol Clin North Am. 1995;33:167-83.

23. **Bounameaux H, de Moerloose P, Perrier A, et al.** Plasma measurement of D-dimer as diagnostic aid in suspected venous thromboembolism: an overview. Thromb Haemost. 1994;71:1-6.

24. **Bounameaux H, Cirafici P, de Moerloose P, et al.** Measurement of D-dimer in plasma as diagnostic aid in suspected pulmonary embolism. Lancet. 1991;337:196-200.

25. **Ginsberg JS, Brill-Edwards PA, Demers C, et al.** D-dimer in patients with clinically suspected pulmonary embolism. Chest. 1993;104:1679-84.

26. **Goldhaber SZ, Simons GR, Elliot CG, et al.** Quantitative plasma D-dimer levels among patients undergoing pulmonary angiography for suspected pulmonary embolism. JAMA. 1993;270:2819-22.

27. **Stein PD, Hull RD, Pineo G.** Strategy that includes serial noninvasive leg tests for diagnosis of thromboembolic disease in patients with suspected acute pulmonary embolism based on data from PIOPED. Arch Intern Med. 1995;155:2101-4.

28. **Hull RD, Raskob GE, Ginsberg JS, et al.** A noninvasive strategy for the treatment of patients with suspected pulmonary embolism. Arch Intern Med. 1994;154:289-97.

Solitary Pulmonary Nodule   **29**

Thomas G. Tape, MD

KEY POINTS

Pretest Probabilities

- Forty to fifty percent of solitary pulmonary nodules discovered in the course of regular medical care are malignant. Solitary nodules discovered during mass-screening chest radiography have no more than a 10% risk of being malignant.

- Granulomas, caused by diseases such as tuberculosis, histoplasmosis, and coccidioidomycosis, are the most frequent causes of benign solitary nodules.

- The risk of malignancy depends on the patient's age and smoking history and on the size and appearance of the lesion.

- Lesions that have certain patterns of calcification on chest radiography or that have been stable in size for more than 2 years are nearly always benign.

Diagnostic Strategies

- Computed tomography helps further define the lesion and any associated disease. Occasionally it can confirm the benign nature of a lesion.

- Transthoracic needle aspiration biopsy may be helpful in confirming malignancy when surgery would not be indicated for subsequent therapy. The low frequency of obtaining adequate material for a specific diagnosis of benign lesions limits its utility.

- Lung biopsy, either by thoracotomy or by the less invasive videothoracoscopy, is the definitive diagnostic procedure in the evaluation of solitary pulmonary nodules.

BACKGROUND

Finding a solitary pulmonary nodule on routine chest radiography is a common and often frustrating problem. We define a solitary pulmonary nodule as a discrete pulmonary density of 6 cm or less without symptoms referable to the nodule. (Although the criteria for defining a solitary nodule vary among studies, with some studies using a size as low as 2 to 3 cm for the purpose of definition, most of the studies reviewed for this chapter were based on the 6-cm cutoff.) The differential diagnosis is extensive, but primary lung carcinoma and infectious granulomas account for most of the lesions. The likelihood of malignancy is usually high enough to warrant a definitive diagnosis. Although surgery is often the treatment of choice for localized malignancies, it is not appropriate for metastatic disease and is usually not needed for benign lesions (1–3). Thus, the goal of the evaluation of a solitary pulmonary nodule is to differentiate malignancies requiring surgical intervention from benign lesions that can be safely observed.

ESTIMATING PRETEST PROBABILITY

Approximately 40% of solitary pulmonary nodules reported in older series proved to be malignant (2–4). Recent reports found a 50% prevalence of malignant nodules (5,6). The nodules reported in these studies were discovered on chest radiographs obtained in the course of general medical care. When chest radiography was performed in the general public for mass screening purposes, the prevalence of solitary pulmonary nodules was about 1 per 1000 persons and the likelihood that a solitary nodule was malignant was in the range of 4% to 10% (7,8).

The risk of malignancy is strongly related to several clinical features (4,9). The effects of patient age, the size of the lesion, the appearance of the lesion, and the patient's smoking history on the pretest probability are shown in Table 29-1. In one study, radiologists who explicitly incorporated the likelihood ratios for patients' clinical characteristics made more accurate estimates of malignant risk than unaided expert readers (10). The presence of calcium in the nodule seen on plain chest radiography is an important predictor of benign disease. A nodule with central, laminated, diffuse, or popcorn calcification is highly unlikely to be malignant (8,11–14). Eccentric or stippled calcification patterns, however, may be seen in malignant lesions (12,14).

If previous chest radiographs are available, any changes noted in the lesion are helpful in assessing its malignant potential. Although benign lesions may grow at rates identical to those of malignant neoplasms, a nodule that is stable in size over a period of at least 2 years is virtually never malignant (12).

Consideration should also be given to where the patient resides and to travel history. Histoplasmomas are common causes of solitary pulmonary nodules in the Midwest (12), and coccidioidomas are common in the Southwest (13).

Table 29-1. Likelihood Ratios for Malignancy in Patients with Solitary Pulmonary Nodules

Finding	Likelihood Ratio
Patient's age, y	
20–29	0.05
30–39	0.24
40–49	0.94
50–59	1.90
60–69	2.64
>69	4.16
Smoking history	
Never smoked	0.19
Current cigarette smoker	2.27
Pipe or cigar smoker	1.00
Ex-cigarette smoker	0.92
Ex-pipe or cigar smoker	0.55
Hemoptysis	5.08
Previous malignancy	4.95
Size of lesion	
0–1.0 cm	0.52
1.1–2.0 cm	0.74
2.1–3.0 cm	3.67
>3.0 cm	5.23
Edge characteristics (chest radiography)	
Ill defined	2.51
Well defined, lobular	1.27
Well defined, smooth	0.36
Edge characteristics (computed tomography)	
Smooth	0.30
Lobulated	0.74
Irregular or spicular	5.54
Location	
Upper or middle lobe	1.22
Lower lobe	0.66

Adapted from Gurney JW. Determining the likelihood of malignancy in solitary pulmonary nodules with Bayesian analysis: part I. Theory. Radiology. 1993;186:405-13.

DIAGNOSTIC TESTS

Computed Tomography

Although computed tomography (CT) rarely provides further information about the location and size of the nodule, it may disclose associated disease such as hilar adenopathy or other pulmonary nodules that are missed on plain radiography. Computed tomography can identify a subset of patients with benign lesions based on high CT density numbers (15,16). Although its sensitivity is 99.5% (Table 29-2), the specificity (proportion of benign nodules diagnosed as benign) is only 17% (16). Combining contrast enhancement with thin-section CT (17, 18) shows promise in differentiating benign from malignant lesions but has not yet been systematically studied.

Magnetic Resonance Imaging

The role of magnetic resonance imaging (MRI) in evaluating pulmonary nodules has not been determined. Compared with CT, it has better contrast resolution but inferior spatial resolution. It may be more sensitive than CT for identifying nodules adjacent to blood vessels (19). At present, there are no reports using MRI criteria to separate benign

Table 29-2. Operating Characteristics of Diagnostic Tests for Solitary Pulmonary Nodule

Test	Sensitivity	Specificity	Likelihood Ratio	
			Positive Result	Negative Result
	←——— % ———→			
Standardized CT scan density				
<165 Hounsfield units	99	17	1.2	0.06
Transbronchial bmiopsy				
<2.0 cm nodule	25	*		
2.0–2.9 cm nodule	40	*		
3.0–4.0 cm nodule	56	*		
Transthoracic needle biopsy	94	94	16	0.06
Malignant result			48	
Indeterminate result			0.66	
Negative result			0.03	

CT = computed tomography.
*Although the false-positive rate is less than 1%, as many as 85% of benign nodules have inadequate material for specific diagnosis.

from malignant nodules. Therefore, MRI cannot yet be recommended in the workup of a solitary pulmonary nodule.

Positron Emission Tomography

Compared with normal tissue, lung tumors have increased uptake of 2-[^{18}F]-fluoro-2-deoxy-D-glucose (FDG) that can be demonstrated with positron emission tomography (PET) imaging. Preliminary studies report near perfect sensitivity in detecting malignancy, with specificity in the 80% to 90% range (20,21). However, this promising technology is not yet widely available.

Flexible Fiberoptic Bronchoscopy

Flexible fiberoptic bronchoscopy allows direct visualization of the central airways, with provision for bronchial brushing and washing and fluoroscopically guided transbronchial biopsy of pulmonary nodules. In experienced hands, the rate of serious complications for transbronchial biopsy is remarkably low: 0.2% death rate, 5.5% pneumothorax rate, and 1% to 4% hemorrhage of more than 50 mL (22,23). The diagnostic accuracy of transbronchial biopsy is primarily determined by whether adequate tissue from the nodule has actually been obtained. The rate of definitive diagnoses, both benign and malignant, ranges from 36% to 77% in various studies (24). The sensitivity for diagnosing malignant nodules is highly dependent on nodule size: 25% for nodules less than 2 cm, 40% for nodules 2 to 2.9 cm, and 56% for nodules 3 to 4 cm (25). Although false-positive diagnoses of malignancy are only rarely reported, the specificity of the test is limited by the large number of inadequate or nonspecific specimens. In one series, only 15% of benign lesions were definitively diagnosed; the other biopsies were indeterminant (24). In practice, surgery is often needed, regardless of the results of the bronchoscopy (26,27). Fiberoptic bronchoscopy should not be a routine part of the solitary pulmonary nodule workup.

Transthoracic Needle Biopsy

Transthoracic needle aspiration is performed by placing a needle directly into the nodule under fluoroscopic guidance and making repeated passes while aspirating tissue. The tissue fragments that are obtained are sent for histologic examination, and the remainder of the aspirate is sent for cytologic examination. The procedure is relatively safe when done by experienced personnel. However, in 11% to 24% of patients, a pneumothorax develops, with 5% to 14% of patients requiring insertion of a chest tube (28,29). Minor hemoptysis is reported in about 10% of biopsies (30).

The diagnostic accuracy of the transthoracic biopsy is generally higher than that of transbronchial biopsy, with sensitivity for malignancy ranging from 86% to 98% and specificity ranging from 71% to 99% (28–34). These operating characteristics were calculated assuming that indeterminant results were incorrect diagnoses. The sensitivity is again dependent on the size of the lesion (25) as well as on the location (35). The sensitivity can be increased by repeating inadequate or indeterminant biopsies (29,36) and by using specialized biopsy needles that obtain more tissue (30,33). Data from several of the larger series (28–30,32) yield the following estimates of likelihood ratios: 48 for a malignant biopsy, 0.66 for an indeterminant biopsy, and 0.03 for a negative biopsy. The finding of a specific benign histology is infrequently obtained in practice because benign neoplasms are difficult to penetrate with the needle (28,37).

Sputum Cytology

Although noninvasive and relatively cheap, cytologic examination of the sputum rarely results in a definitive diagnosis. In a study of 101 consecutive cases of solitary pulmonary nodules, cytologic examination of the sputum yielded a definitive diagnosis in only one patient (23). The sensitivity of this test is in the range of 10% to 20% and varies with cell type and location of the tumor (28,38). Nevertheless, a positive result is specific for malignancy and may obviate the need for more invasive workup.

Lung Biopsy

Lung biopsy is the gold standard for establishing specific diagnoses in patients with a solitary pulmonary nodule and will generally be needed when the benign nature of the lesion cannot be determined by less invasive means. Until recently, lung biopsy required open thoracotomy. With the advent of videothoracoscopy, lung biopsy and resection can now be performed with much less pain and a shorter hospital stay (39,40). In some cases, lung biopsy can be done without general anesthesia (41).

DIAGNOSTIC STRATEGIES

The first step in the diagnostic evaluation is to analyze the plain chest radiograph for evidence of benign calcification patterns and to compare the nodule with earlier radiographs for stability over time. If either criterion is met, the lesion can be considered benign and observation is appropriate. Otherwise, an estimate of the risk of malignancy should be made, taking into account the size of the nodule and the patient's age and smoking history.

The next step is controversial. Cummings and colleagues performed a decision analysis of patients with solitary pulmonary nodules of malignant potential based on their chest radiographic appearance (42). The strategies were 1) observation with serial chest radiography; 2) biopsy (transbronchial or transthoracic) with observation for indeterminant results; 3) biopsy with thoracotomy for indeterminant results; and 4) immediate thoracotomy. The observation strategy was slightly preferred when the pretest probability of malignancy was less than 3%; the biopsy/observation strategy was preferred when the probability of malignancy was between 3% and 48%; the biopsy/surgery strategy was preferred when the probability of malignancy was between 48% and 68%; and the immediate surgery strategy was preferred when the pretest probabilities were greater than 68%. However, because the differences in calculated life expectancies were so small (i.e., a "close call"), other factors not included in the model should be considered when deciding how to care for an individual patient. Such factors include the results of CT, the local expertise in performing invasive tests, regional differences in the prevalence of histoplasmosis and coccidioidomycosis, and the patient's preferences. If PET scanning is available, it can be performed after CT to further evaluate patients at low risk for malignancy. In addition, this analysis did not consider thoracoscopy as an option. Its lesser morbidity compared with that of thoracotomy makes immediate lung biopsy a more attractive option in some cases.

If the decision is made to perform a needle biopsy, transthoracic fine needle aspiration biopsy is usually preferred to fiberoptic bronchoscopy. Table 29-3 shows the effect of pretest probability of malignancy on post-test probabilities for various fine needle aspiration biopsy results. The finding of a malignant aspirate generally requires no further diagnostic investigation unless the cell type is in doubt. The finding of a specific benign histology effectively rules out malignancy except at very high pretest probabilities. Indeterminant or nonspecific benign results should, in general, be evaluated further.

Table 29-3. Post-test Probability of Malignancy Based on Transthoracic Needle Biopsy Results

Biopsy Results	Pretest Probability		
	20%	50%	80%
	←	%	→
Malignant	92	98	99
Indeterminate or inadequate	14	40	73
Negative	0.8	3	11

CLINICAL PROBLEMS

Clinical Problem 1
A small, uncalcified peripheral nodule that was not seen on previous chest radiographs is detected. The patient is a nonsmoker.

Clinical Strategy and Rationale
Computed tomography should be performed to search for benign calcification patterns and to rule out associated disease. Clinically, the probability that this lesion is malignant is low because it is small and the patient is a nonsmoker. If the CT scan shows a benign calcification pattern or high CT density, it can be safely assumed that the lesion is benign and the patient may be followed with periodic chest films to assure stability. Otherwise, PET should be done next, if available. If it is not available, consider a transthoracic needle aspiration biopsy.

Clinical Example
A 50-year-old patient with asthma is noted to have a 2-cm nodule located peripherally in the right upper lobe. The lesion was not seen on chest radiography done 3 years earlier. A CT scan shows a popcorn pattern of calcification. The most likely diagnosis is hamartoma. Follow-up chest radiographs are scheduled to assure stability of the nodule.

Clinical Problem 2
A large pulmonary nodule is incidentally discovered in a patient who smokes.

Testing Strategy and Rationale
The large nodule size and smoking history increase the probability of malignancy to greater than 50%. A CT scan should be done to search for lymph node involvement and for other lung nodules. If there is evidence of metastasis, a transthoracic needle aspiration biopsy would be the least invasive way to make the diagnosis. If there is no evidence of metastatic disease, the patient should proceed directly to lung biopsy and subsequent resection by videothoracoscopy and/or thoracotomy.

Clinical Example
A 55-year-old woman injured in a motor vehicle accident is discovered to have a 4-cm mass with an irregular border located in the left lower lobe. She has a 30-pack-year history of smoking. Computed tomography confirms the mass along with multiple small nodules in the right lung and multiple enlarged left hilar

Continued

lymph nodes. There is also a 3-cm lesion in the right lobe of the liver. Because the clinical picture suggests metastatic lung cancer, surgery is not indicated as a treatment option. Transthoracic needle aspiration biopsy shows squamous cell carcinoma.

REFERENCES

1. **Nandi PL, Tang SC, Mok CK, et al.** Pulmonary coin lesions: a ten-year review of 239 cases. Aust N Z J Surg. 1981;51:56-8.

2. **Seybold WD.** Solitary or "coin" lesions of the lung: analysis of 2,258 recorded cases. Postgrad Med. 1964;424-30.

3. **Steele JD.** The solitary pulmonary nodule: report of a cooperative study of resected asymptomatic solitary pulmonary nodules in males. J Thorac Cardiovasc Surg.1963;46:21-39.

4. **Cummings SR, Lillington GA, Richard RJ.** Estimating the probability of malignancy in solitary pulmonary nodules: a Bayesian approach. Am Rev Repir Dis. 1986;134:449-52.

5. **Libby DM, Henschke CI, Yankelevitz DF.** The solitary pulmonary nodule: update 1995. Am J Med. 1995;99:491-6.

6. **Lovich SF, Samples TL, Ostrow LB, Kline AL.** The solitary pulmonary nodule: a recent military experience. Mil Med. 1990;155:266-8.

7. **McClure CD, Boucot KR, Shipman GA, et al.** The solitary pulmonary nodule and primary lung malignancy. Arch Environ Health. 1961;3:127-39.

8. **Holin SM, Dwork RE, Glaser S, et al.** Solitary pulmonary nodules found in a community-wide chest roentgenographic survey: a five-year follow-up study. Am Rev Tuberc. 1959;79:427-39.

9. **Gurney JW.** Determining the likelihood of malignancy in solitary pulmonary nodules with Bayesian analysis: part I. Theory. Radiology. 1993;186:405-13.

10. **Gurney JW.** Determining the likelihood of malignancy in solitary pulmonary nodules with Bayesian analysis: part II. Application. Radiology. 1993;186:415-22.

11. **Neff TA.** The science and humanity of the solitary pulmonary nodule. Am Rev Respir Dis. 1986;134:433-4.

12. **Godwin JD.** The solitary pulmonary nodule. Radiol Clin North Am. 1983;21:709-21.

13. **Winn RE.** Solitary pulmonary nodule in the southwest: coccidioidoma or carcinoma? Arch Intern Med. 1986;146:250-1.

14. **Lillington GA.** Management of the solitary pulmonary nodule. Hosp Pract. 1993;28:41-8.

15. **Siegelman SS, Zerhouni EA, Leo FP, et al.** CT of the solitary pulmonary nodule. AJR Am J Roentgenol. 1980;135:1-13.

16. **Zerhouni EA, Stitik FP, Siegelman SS, et al.** CT of the pulmonary nodule: a cooperative study. Radiology. 1986;160:319-27.

17. **Yamashita K, Matsonobe S, Tsuda T, et al.** Solitary pulmonary nodule: preliminary study of evaluation with incremental dynamic CT. Radiology. 1995;194:399-405.

18. **Swensen SJ, Brown LR, Colby TV, Weaver AL.** Pulmonary nodules: CT evaluation of enhancement with iodinated contrast material. Radiology. 1995:194:393-8.

19. **Müller NL, Gamsu G, Webb WR.** Pulmonary nodules: detection using magnetic resonance and computed tomography. Radiology. 1985;155:687-90.

20. **Dewan NA, Gupta NC, Redepenning LS, et al.** Diagnostic efficacy of PET-FDG imaging in solitary pulmonary nodules: potential role in evaluation and management. Chest. 1993;104:997-1002.

21. **Patz EF, Goodman PC.** Positron emission tomography imaging of the thorax. Adv Chest Radiol. 1994;32:811-23.

22. **Sheldon RL.** Flexible fiberoptic bronchoscopy. Prim Care. 1985;12:299-315.

23. **Fulkerson WJ.** Fiberoptic bronchoscopy. N Engl J Med. 1984;311:511-5.

24. **Fletcher EC, Levin DC.** Flexible fiberoptic bronchoscopy and fluoroscopically guided transbronchial biopsy in the management of solitary pulmonary nodules. West J Med. 1982;136:477-83.

25. **Wallace JM, Deutsch AL.** Flexible fiberoptic bronchoscopy and percutaneous needle lung aspiration for evaluating the solitary pulmonary nodule. Chest. 1982;81:665-71.

26. **Torrington KG, Kern JD.** The utility of fiberoptic bronchoscopy in the evaluation of the solitary pulmonary nodule. Chest. 1993;104:1021-4.

27. **Goldberg SK, Walkenstein MD, Steinbach A, Aranson R.** The role of staging bronchoscopy in the preoperative assessment of a solitary pulmonary nodule. Chest. 1993;104:94-7.

28. **Khouri NF, Meziane MA, Zerhouni EA, et al.** The solitary pulmonary nodule: assessment, diagnosis, and management. Chest. 1987;91:128-33.

29. **Sagel SS, Ferguson TB, Forrest JV, et al.** Percutaneous transthoracic aspiration needle biopsy. Ann Thorac Surg. 1978;26:399-404.

30. **Wescott JL.** Direct percutaneous needle aspiration of localized pulmonary lesions: results in 422 patients. Radiology. 1980;137:31-5.

31. **Poe RH, Tobin RE.** Sensitivity and specificity of needle biopsy in lung malignancy. Am Rev Respir Dis. 1980;122:725-9.

32. **Young GP, Young I, Cowan DF, Blei RL.** The reliability of fine-needle aspiration biopsy in the diagnosis of deep lesions of the lung and mediastinum: experience with 250 cases using a modified technique. Diagn Cytopathol. 1987;3:1-7.

33. **Böcking A, Klose KC, Kyll HJ, Hauptmann S.** Cytologic versus histologic evaluation of needle biopsy of the lung, hilum and mediastinum: sensitivity, specificity, and typing accuracy. Acta Cytol. 1995;39:463-71.

34. **Mitruka S, Landreneau RJ, Mack MJ, et al.** Diagnosing the indeterminate pulmonary nodule: percutaneous biopsy versus thorascopy. Surgery. 1995;118-676-84.

35. **Berquist TH, Bailey RB, Cortese DA, Miller WE.** Transthoracic needle biopsy: accuracy and complications in relation to location and type of lesion. Mayo Clin Proc. 1980;55:475-81.

36. **Gobien RP, Valicenti JF, Paris BS, Daniell C.** Thin-needle aspiration biopsy: methods of increasing the accuracy of a negative prediction. Radiology. 1982;145:603-5.

37. **Sinner WN.** Fine-needle biopsy of hamartomas of the lung. Am J Rev 1982;138:65-9.
38. **Midthun DE, Swensen SJ, Jett JR.** Clinical strategies for solitary pulmonary nodule. Annu Rev Med. 1992;43:195-208.
39. **Santambrogio L, Nosotti M, Bellaviti N, Mezzetti M.** Videothoracoscopy versus thoracotomy for the diagnosis of the indeterminate solitary pulmonary nodule. Ann Thorac Surg. 1995;59-868-71.
40. **Mack MJ, Hazelrigg SR, Landreneau RJ, Acuff TE.** Thoracoscopy for the diagnosis of the indeterminate solitary pulmonary nodule. Ann Thorac Surg. 1993;56:825-32.
41. **Landreneau RJ, Mack MJ, Hazelrigg SR, et al.** The role of thoracoscopy in the management of intrathoracic neoplastic processes. Semin Thorac Cardiovasc Surg. 1993;5:219-28.
42. **Cummings SR, Lillington GA, Richard RJ.** Managing solitary pulmonary nodules: the choice of a strategy is a "close call." Am Rev Respir Dis. 1986; 134:453-60.

Pleural Effusions

30

Gary W. Wahl, MD, and William J. Hall, MD

KEY POINTS

Pretest Probabilities

- Congestive heart failure, infection, and malignancy are the most common causes of pleural effusions.
- The principal disease processes to be excluded in the presence of a nonpurulent pleural exudate are malignancy and tuberculosis.
- In patients with pleural exudates for whom no specific diagnosis is evident after testing, the probability of developing a malignancy at a later date is at least 30%.

Diagnostic Strategies

- The most critical determination in diagnosing pleural effusions is distinguishing between transudates and exudates by proper interpretation of pleural fluid protein and lactic dehydrogenase levels.
- When a transudative effusion is found, more extensive testing of pleural fluid or a pleural biopsy is generally not needed.
- When the fluid is an exudate, pleural fluid cytologic testing and closed pleural biopsy are usually the most useful tests unless the cause of the effusion is obvious, such as a pneumonia.
- In certain clinical settings (e.g., parapneumonic effusions), selective or serial testing of pleural fluid may have important prognostic value.

BACKGROUND

Pleural effusions occur in the course of many diseases. The initial and most important step in evaluating pleural effusions is to differentiate between the two fundamental pathophysiologic mechanisms of fluid accumulation in the pleural space (1,2). Pleural fluid accumulates as a *transudate* when the usual balance of osmotic and hydrostatic forces controlling fluid movement is altered and a low-protein ultrafiltrate of plasma develops. This occurs in congestive heart failure, cirrhosis, and hypoproteinemic states. An *exudative* effusion forms when breakdown of vascular integrity or inhibition of lymphatic drainage occurs, as with infection, inflammatory response, or malignancy. From a diagnostic standpoint, verification of a transudative process directs the subsequent workup away from the pleural space toward a consideration of systemic disease. An exudative process requires a more extensive diagnostic approach to the pleural space and warrants a search for more serious disease, especially occult malignancy.

Evaluation of a pleural effusion that develops in the course of a bacterial pneumonia is especially problematic. When bacteria and abundant leukocytes are present (i.e., an empyema), tube thoracostomy and prolonged hospitalization may be required. Failure to recognize this complication could be life threatening. However, most parapneumonic effusions are sterile, and 90% of these resolve with antibiotic therapy alone. The term "complicated parapneumonic effusion," which is discussed further in the "Diagnostic Tests" section later in this chapter, describes a sterile exudative effusion associated with bacterial pneumonia that requires tube thoracostomy for adequate control (3).

ESTIMATING PRETEST PROBABILITY

Pleural effusions develop in a wide variety of local and systemic disease processes (4–20). Estimates of the frequency of the most common causes of pleural effusions are summarized in Table 30-1 (1,17–19). The cause can often be deduced from attendant clinical circumstances (e.g., congestive heart failure, pneumonia, or known malignancy). When pleural effusions occur that have no obvious cause, an appropriate

Table 30-1. Causes of Pleural Effusions

Cause	%
Congestive heart failure	11–47
Parapneumonic	15–33
Malignancy	15–27
Lung cancer	5–13
Breast cancer	1–5
Lymphoma	0–3
Other malignancy	4–7
Pulmonary embolism	0–11
Tuberculosis	0–33
Other	1–23

Data from references 1, 17, 18, and 19.

diagnostic evaluation should be done because the effusion may be the harbinger of serious disease.

Pain associated with pleural effusion usually indicates an exudative process (1). Other common symptoms, such as cough, shortness of breath, or chest pressure do not distinguish between exudative and transudative processes. Exudates unrelated to pneumonia most often result from malignancy, such as lung cancer, breast cancer, and lymphoma, or from tuberculosis. Ninety percent of transudates are related to congestive heart failure, and these are frequently bilateral (20). Pleural effusions occur in 20% to 50% of patients with documented pulmonary emboli (21). These effusions are often small, may be either exudates or transudates, and have no distinctive features (4,21–23). A hemorrhagic pleural effusion is neither commonly associated with pulmonary embolism nor specific for the diagnosis (24).

In those with past exposure to asbestos, benign asbestos effusion is a common cause of exudative effusion. As with other forms of asbestos-related lung disease, there may be a latent period of 10 to 40 years between exposure and illness. The effusions may be unilateral but can be sequentially bilateral (25). Patients are frequently asymptomatic.

DIAGNOSTIC TESTS

The first step in the diagnostic evaluation is usually a thoracentesis. The pleural fluid is then analyzed using a variety of biochemical tests and cytologic examinations. The proper selection and sequencing of these tests requires an understanding of their operating characteristics as well as an estimate of the probability of various causes of the disease.

Biochemical and Hematologic Evaluation of Pleural Fluid

Protein and lactic dehydrogenase (LDH) levels are the best markers of an exudative process (Table 30-2). Elevated LDH and protein concentrations are both indicative of an exudate (26). Slightly improved operating characteristics are achieved by comparing the ratio of pleural fluid to blood concentrations. Based on a retrospective study, Light (26) proposed criteria for identifying exudates; these criteria are now the "gold standard." An exudate is diagnosed when at least one of three criteria are met: 1) a ratio of pleural fluid to blood protein greater than 0.5; 2) a ratio of pleural fluid to blood LDH greater than 0.6; and 3) pleural fluid LDH more than two thirds the upper limit of normal for blood LDH. Subsequent studies in unselected populations have confirmed the validity of these criteria in diagnosing exudates (27). However, when these criteria are used, 10% to 20% of transudates are misdiagnosed as exudates, most commonly when congestive heart failure has been treated with diuretics. In these patients, a fluid cholesterol level of less than 55 mg/dL or a fluid to plasma cholesterol ratio of less than 0.3 suggests a transudate (17,18).

Table 30-2. Operating Characteristics of Diagnostic Tests Used to Confirm the Presence of an Exudative Pleural Effusion

Diagnostic Test	Definition of Positive Result	Sensitivity	Specificity	Likelihood Ratio	
				Positive Result	Negative Result
		← % →			
Lactic dehydrogenase	>200 U/L	70	100	∞	0.30
Lactic dehydrogenase ratio	>0.6	86	98	43	0.14
Protein	>3g/dL	89	91	10	0.12
Protein ratio	>0.5	90	98	45	0.10
Triad*		99	98	50	0.01

*Triad: at least one of these three criteria present—1) lactic dehydrogenase >200 U/L; 2) lactic dehydrogenase ratio >0.6; or 3) protein ratio >0.5.

An increased number of leukocytes or erythrocytes is of little value in the initial characterization of pleural fluid. Although relatively specific for an exudate, a high leukocyte count (>10,000/mm^3) is found infrequently (28). One milliliter of blood in 500 mL of pleural fluid causes a red tinge to the fluid, and therefore many "bloody" pleural effusions result from extravasation of small amounts of blood into the pleural space during thoracentesis (1). Leukocyte counts are highly variable in effusions associated with tuberculosis (29).

Glucose levels are not specific for any particular disease process, although effusions caused by rheumatoid arthritis (30,31) can cause extremely low levels of pleural fluid glucose. Low complement levels have been reported to differentiate effusions caused by rheumatic diseases, chiefly rheumatoid arthritis and lupus, from those due to other causes (Table 30-3) (32). Acute inflammation of the pancreas may be associated with pleural effusions, and pleural fluid amylase levels are elevated in approximately 90% of these cases (6). Adenosine deaminase levels of more than 70 U/L are seen only in effusions caused by tuberculosis, rheumatoid disease, or empyema (33).

Various criteria for prospectively identifying "complicated parapneumonic effusions" are listed in Table 30-3. Although the presence of frank pus is always an indication for tube thoracostomy, leukocyte pleocytosis alone is not a reliable predictor of the need for drainage (28). However, low pleural fluid pH and glucose and high LDH are indicators of severe disease that is unlikely to resolve without drainage. A pH below 7.0, glucose level less than 40 mg/dL, or LDH level greater than 1000 U/L are all highly predictive of a complicated parapneumonic effusion (3,5,34,35).

Table 30-3. Operating Characteristics of Noncytologic Tests for Establishing the Specific Causes of Pleural Effusions

Diagnostic Test	Defintion of Positive Result	Sensitivity	Specificity	Likelihood Ratio	
				Positive Result	Negative Result
	←————%————→				
Complicated parapneumonic effusion/empyema					
pH	<7.0	70	100	∞	0.30
	<7.2	90	87	6.9	0.12
Lactic dehydrogenase	>1000 U/L	100	80	4.9	0
Glucose	<40 mg/dL	78	100	∞	0.22
Leukocyte count	>10,000/mm³	50	60	1.3	0.83
Rheumatoid arthritis					
Complement (CH50)	<10 U/mL	83	87	6.4	0.19
Chylous effusion					
Apperance	Turbid	47	98	25	0.53
Triglyceride	>110 mg/dL	73	100	∞	0.26
	>50 mg/dL	100	75	4.4	0
Pancreatitis					
Amylase	>5000 U/L	90	—	—	—

Pleural Fluid Culture

The yield of pleural fluid culture in tuberculosis is variable and generally unacceptably low (29,36), with a reported sensitivity of 24%, although specificity approaches 100%.

Pleural Fluid Cytologic Examination

Both cytologic examination of fluid and histologic evaluation of biopsy specimens are reasonably sensitive tests (Table 30-4), and when positive for malignancy, also often help delineate cell type and the primary site of tumor (37–39).

Pleural Biopsy

When cytologic and microbiologic studies of exudative fluid are not diagnostic, most recommend that closed pleural biopsy be performed (40). The sensitivity of combined cytologic examination and pleural biopsy for malignancy when an exudative effu-

Table 30-4. Operating Characteristics of Cytologic Examination or Pleural Biopsy or Both in Establishing the Cause of an Exudative Pleural Effusion

Diagnostic Test	Sensitivity	Specificity	Likelihood Ratio	
			Positive Result	Negative Result
	←———%———→			
All diagnoses				
Cytologic examination	63	100	∞	0.37
Cytologic examination and pleural biopsy	68	99	68	0.32
Malignancy		m		
Cytologic examination and pleural biopsy	65	100	∞	0.35
Tuberculosis				
Culture	24	100	∞	0.76
Culture and pleural biopsy	90	100	∞	0.10

sion is present is 65%, and the specificity of the combined tests is reported to be 100% (37–39) (see Table 30-4). The operating characteristics for tuberculosis are a sensitivity of 90% and a specificity of 100% (37,41).

Although pleural biopsy evaluation is highly specific for either malignancy or tuberculosis, a common histologic finding on pleural biopsy is nonspecific inflammatory response, occurring in 50% to 70% of reported cases (37,42,43). In approximately 60% to 65% of these patients, the effusion gradually resolves with no further sequelae, whereas malignancy develops in approximately 30% to 35%, often within 2 years (37,44). Tuberculosis is a very uncommon cause of "nonspecific inflammation" (37,39). Video-assisted thoracoscopy (VATS) can detect malignancy in these patients, but many feel early diagnosis is unimportant, because therapeutic options for pleural malignancy are limited (1). Fiberoptic bronchoscopy may be useful if the patient has a history of hemoptysis or if chest radiography shows a mass, infiltrate, or atelectasis (45).

Chylous Effusions

The presence of chyle in pleural fluid indicates either interruption of the thoracic duct, as may occur in trauma, or inhibition of lymphatic drainage, often suggesting malignancy. Gross appearance of the fluid is not a sensitive indicator of the presence or absence of chyle, but simple measurement of triglyceride levels usually identifies chylous effusions (46) (see Table 30-3).

DIAGNOSTIC STRATEGIES

Many pleural effusions occur in clinical settings that make the diagnosis readily deducible—for example, congestive heart failure or pneumonia. The more perplexing cases generally involve a unilateral effusion. In this setting, the possibility of malignancy is often the major diagnostic consideration. Effusions caused by tuberculosis, pulmonary embolism, collagen vascular disease, and asbestos exposure are less common.

The diagnostic process begins with a careful history and physical examination to guide the subsequent testing. Particular attention should be paid to tobacco use and occupational exposures. Physical examination should be directed toward the most common malignancies associated with pleural effusions: primary carcinoma of the lung and metastatic carcinoma of the breast.

A diagnostic thoracentesis should be the next step. Ideally, fluid should be analyzed initially for protein and LDH to determine if the effusion is an exudate or transudate. If local laboratory facilities offer rapid service, these determinations should be done before any other testing. If the fluid proves to be a transudate, no further invasive studies are necessary. If the effusion is found to be an exudate, a 100 to 200 mL sample of fluid should be sent for additional tests appropriate to the clinical situation. Commonly ordered tests include measurements of pH and glucose, cell count, cytologic examination, and culture for bacteria or acid fast bacilli or both.

If the cause of a pleural exudate cannot be determined by pleural fluid analysis, a closed pleural biopsy usually should be done. If the results are nondiagnostic, the subsequent course of action is determined by the individual clinical setting. Serial observation, repeat closed pleural biopsy, fiberoptic bronchoscopy, or VATS are all considerations.

Because the characteristics of pleural effusions related to pulmonary embolism are nonspecific, the workup of patients with suspected pulmonary embolism should focus on diagnostic tests such as ventilation–perfusion scans (see Chapter 28), rather than on evaluating the pleural fluid. The diagnosis of benign asbestos pleural effusion is based on a history of asbestos exposure and the exclusion of other probable causes of the effusion. The fluid is usually straw colored, but can be bloody, and the chemical and cellular analyses are nonspecific. The presence of other asbestos-related changes on radiography are substantially more likely in patients with benign asbestos pleural effusion than in those with idiopathic effusions (47).

CLINICAL PROBLEMS

Clinical Problem 1

A patient develops a pleural effusion during the course of a bacterial pneumonia.

Testing Strategy and Rationale

The pH of the pleural fluid should be measured and a bacterial culture obtained. Pleural effusions are a relatively common complication of bacterial pneumonia, occurring in 30% to 50% of cases. A small proportion are "complicated parapneumonic effusions." Although thick pus and bacteria are not present, without drainage these effusions can produce persistent fever and pain and may lead to the formation of a restrictive rind.

Determination of pH is the best marker of a complicated effusion and facilitates selection of the appropriate therapeutic strategy. Measurements of pleural fluid glucose and LDH levels may also be helpful in such cases.

Clinical Example

A 78-year-old woman who resides in a nursing home is hospitalized with a right lower lobe pneumonia caused by *Klebsiella pneumoniae*. Despite appropriate antibacterial therapy, a right-sided pleural effusion develops on the fourth day of therapy. She remains febrile. Based on clinical judgment, the probability that this is a "complicated effusion" that will require a chest tube for resolution is estimated to be approximately 50%. Analysis of fluid obtained at thoracentesis shows a leukocyte count of more than 10,000/mm³, an absence of bacteria, and a pH of 7.1. Using likelihood ratios for these tests (see Table 30-3), the presence of leukocytes yields a revised post-test probability of 55% and is therefore of marginal benefit. However, the pH less than 7.2 is diagnostically useful, and causes the revised probability of a complicated effusion to be 87%. Most would proceed with chest tube drainage. Conversely, had the pH determination been greater than 7.2, the post-test probability of a "complicated effusion" would be only 10%.

Clinical Problem 2

A unilateral pleural effusion is discovered in an asymptomatic, middle-aged patient who smokes.

Testing Strategy and Rationale

Thoracentesis should be performed to determine if the effusion is an exudate and, if so, cytologic examination of the fluid needs to be done. If measurement of protein and LDH levels indicate that the effusion is a transudate, the diagnostic approach should focus on systemic disease such as congestive heart failure or cirrhosis. An exudative pleural effusion in a patient in this age range who smokes strongly suggests malignancy. If fluid cytologic examination is not diagnostic, a pleural biopsy should be done. If a tuberculin skin test is done, a positive result may only indicate previous infection.

Clinical Example
A 60-year-old man presents with a unilateral effusion. A tuberculin skin test is positive, and he has a history of moderate tobacco use. Analysis of pleural fluid shows an exudate, and cytologic examination demonstrates no malignant cells. A closed pleural biopsy shows only "nonspecific inflammation" and no evidence of granulomas or abnormal cells.

Using the operating characteristics from Table 30-4, post-test probabilities can be calculated. If the pretest probability of malignancy is 75% and of tuberculosis is 25%, a nonspecific, negative finding causes the post-test probability of malignancy to be approximately 50%, whereas the probability of tuberculosis decreases to less than 5%. Because the likelihood of malignancy is still relatively high, subsequent steps such as serial observation or repeat biopsy are discussed with the patient.

REFERENCES

1. **Light RW.** Pleural Disease. 3rd ed. Philadelphia: Lea & Febiger; 1995.
2. **Wang N.** Anatomy and physiology of the pleural space. Clin Chest Med. 1985;6:3-16.
3. **Light RW.** Management of parapneumonic effusions. Arch Intern Med. 1981;141:1339-41.
4. **Dalen JE.** Pulmonary embolism, pulmonary hemorrhage, and pulmonary infarction. N Engl J Med. 1977;296:1431-5.
5. **Light RW, Girard WM, Jenkinson SG, George RB.** Parapneumonic effusions. Am J Med. 1980;69:507-9.
6. **Kaye MD.** Pleuropulmonary complications of pancreatitis. Thorax. 1968;23:297-306.
7. **Logue RB, Rogers JV, Gay BB.** Subtle roentgenographic signs of left heart failure. Am Heart J. 1963;65:464-73.
8. **Plum GE, Bruwer AJ, Clagett OT.** Chronic constrictive pericarditis: roentgenographic findings in 35 surgically proved cases. Proc Mayo Clin. 1957;32:555-6.
9. **Liberman FL, Hidemure R, Peters RL, Reynolds RB.** Pathogenesis and treatment of hydrothorax complicating cirrhosis with ascites. Ann Intern Med. 1966;64:341-51.

10. **Dressler W.** The post-myocardial infarction syndrome. Arch Intern Med. 1959;103:28-42.

11. **Cohen S, Hossain S.** Primary carcinoma of lung: a review of 417 histologically proved cases. Dis Chest. 1966;49:67-73.

12. **Goldsmith HS, Bailey HD, Callahan EL, Beattie EJ.** Pulmonary lymphagitic metastases from breast carcinoma. Arch Surg. 1967;94:483-8.

13. **Vieta JO, Craver LF.** Intrathoracic manifestations of the lymphomatoid diseases. Radiology. 1941;37:138-58.

14. **Fine NL, Smith LR, Sheedy PF.** Frequency of pleural effusions in mycoplasma and viral pneumonias. N Engl J Med. 1970;283:790-3.

15. **Bynum LJ, Wilson JE.** Radiographic features of pleural effusions in pulmonary embolism. Am Rev Respir Dis. 1978;117:829-34.

16. **Walker WC, Wright L.** Rheumatoid pleuritis. Ann Rheum Dis. 1967;26:467-74.

17. **Valdes L, Pose A, Suarez J.** Cholesterol: a useful parameter for distinguishing between pleural exudates and transudates. Chest. 1991;99:1097-102.

18. **Suay VG, Moragon EM, Viedma EC.** Pleural cholesterol in differentiating transudates and exudates. Respiration. 1995;62:57-63.

19. **Marel M, Miroslava Z, Stasny B, Light RW.** The incidence of pleural effusion in a well-defined region. Chest 1993;104:1486-9.

20. **Kinasewitz G, Fishman A.** Pleural dynamics and effusions. In: Fishman A, ed. Pulmonary Diseases and Disorders. New York: McGraw-Hill; 1988;2117-38.

21. **Bynum LJ, Wilson JE III.** Characteristics of pleural effusions associated with pulmonary embolism. Arch Intern Med. 1976;136:159-62.

22. **Talbot S, Worthington BS, Roebuck EJ.** Radiographic signs of pulmonary embolism and pulmonary infarction. Thorax. 1973;28:198-203.

23. **Hefner J.** Pleural effusions from pulmonary thromboembolism. Semin Respir. Med. 1987;9:59-64.

24. **Griner PF.** Pleural fluid following pulmonary infarction. JAMA. 1967;202:947-9.

25. **Britton MG.** Asbestos pleural disease. Br J Dis Chest. 1982;76: 1-10.

26. **Light RW, MacGregor MI, Luchsinger PC, Ball WC.** Pleural effusions: the diagnostic separation of transudates from exudates. Ann Intern Med. 1972;77:507-13.

27. **Peterman TA, Speicher CE.** Evaluating pleural effusions. A two-stage laboratory approach. JAMA. 1984;252:1051-3.

28. **Light RW, Erazon YC, Ball WC.** Cells in pleural fluid: their value in differential diagnosis. Arch Intern Med. 1973;132:854-60.

29. **Berger HW, Mejia EM.** Tuberculous pleurisy. Chest. 1973;63:88-92.

30. **Light RW, Ball WC.** Glucose and amylase in pleural effusions. JAMA. 1973;225:257-60.

31. **Lillington GA, Carr DT, Mayne JG.** Rheumatoid pleurisy with effusion. Arch Intern Med. 1971;128:764-8.

32. **Halla JT, Schroehenloher RE, Volanakis JE.** Immune complexes and other laboratory features of pleural effusions: a comparative study of rheumatoid

arthritis, systemic lupus erythematosus, and other diseases. Ann Intern Med. 1980;92:748-52.

33. **Ocana IM, Martinez JM, Seguna RM, et al.** Adenosine deaminase in pleural fluids. Chest. 1983;84:51-3.

34. **Light RW, MacGregor MI, Ball WC, Luchsinger PC.** Diagnostic significance of pleural fluid pH and pCO_2. Chest. 1973;64:591-6.

35. **Potts DE, Levin DC, Sahn SA.** Pleural fluid pH in parapneumonic effusions. Chest. 1976;70:328-30.

36. **Levine H, Metzger W, Lacua D.** Diagnosis of tuberculous pleurisy by culture of pleural biopsy specimen. Arch Intern Med. 1970;126:269-73.

37. **Poe RE, Israel RH, Utell MJ, et al.** Sensitivity, specificity, and predictive values of closed pleural biopsy. Arch Intern Med. 1984;144:325-8.

38. **Niden AH, Burrows B, Kasik JE.** Percutaneous pleural biopsy with a curetting needle. Am Rev Respir Dis. 1961;84:37-41.

39. **Hampson F, Karlish AJ.** Needle biopsy of the pleura in the diagnosis of pleural effusion. Lancet. 1958;2:1349-53.

40. **Mstitz P, Purves M, Pollard A.** Pleural biopsy in diagnosis of pleural effusions. Mayo Clin Proc. 1980;55:700-6.

41. **Scharer L, McClement JH.** Isolation of tubercle bacilli from needle biopsy specimens of parietal pleura. Am Rev Respir Dis. 1968;97:466-8.

42. **VanHoff DD, Livolsi V.** Diagnostic reliability of needle biopsy of the parietal pleura. Am Rev Respir Dis. 1967;97:466-9.

43. **Scerbo J, Keltz H, Stine DJ.** A prospective study of closed pleural biopsy. JAMA. 1971; 218:377-80.

44. **Ryan CJ, Rodgers RF, Vani KK, Hepper NG.** The outcome of patients with pleural effusion of indeterminate cause at thoracotomy. Mayo Clin Proc. 1981;56:145-9.

45. **Poe RH, Levy PC, Israel RH, et al.** Use of fiberoptic bronchoscopy in the diagnosis of bronchogenic carcinoma. Chest 1994;105:1663-7.

46. **Staate BA, Ellefson RD, Budahn LL, et al.** The lipoprotein profile of chylous and non-chylous pleural effusion. Mayo Clin Proc. 1980;55:700-4.

47. **Martensson G, Hagberg S, Pettersson K, Thiringer G.** Asbestos pleural effusion: a clinical entity. Thorax. 1987;42:646-51.

Chronic Obstructive Lung Disease

31

Catherine Chiu Tan, MD, and Raymond J. Mayewski, MD

KEY POINTS

Pretest Probabilities

- Between 10% and 20% of smokers eventually develop severe chronic obstructive lung disease (COLD).

- Chronic respiratory symptoms, such as cough and sputum production, are neither highly sensitive nor specific when considering the diagnosis of early or mild COLD.

- A history of smoking more than 70 pack-years and a finding of diminished breath sounds on physical examination greatly increase the probability that a patient has moderate or severe COLD.

Diagnostic Strategies

- Because of their low sensitivity, conventional spirometric tests do not appear to be useful in screening for early COLD.

- Among patients with more severe symptoms, spirometric tests are helpful to confirm the presence of COLD, to exclude other diseases that may produce similar symptoms, and to monitor the severity of disease and the impact of therapy. Many of these tests can be performed simply and inexpensively using office spirometry.

BACKGROUND

Approximately 30% of adults in the United States smoke cigarettes (1). Between 10% and 20% of these individuals will eventually develop disabling chronic obstructive lung disease (COLD) (2). This disorder is the fifth leading cause of death and second most common cause of Social Security–compensated disability (3). The estimated prevalence of chronic bronchitis is 30 per 1000, whereas that for emphysema is 10 per 1000 (4-6).

The hallmark of these disorders is airflow obstruction during expiration either through alteration of the bronchial tubes (bronchitis) or destruction of pulmonary parenchyma (emphysema). Investigations into the natural history of these disorders have established the central role of cigarette smoking in the development of COLD (2,7,8). Furthermore, a dose-dependent relationship has been demonstrated between cigarette smoking and the clinical and pathologic severity of COLD (2,7,9). The diagnosis of these disorders is often made either by history (i.e., symptoms of chronic cough, sputum production, wheezing, or shortness of breath); by findings on physical examination; or by the demonstration of airflow obstruction using pulmonary function tests.

Because early detection of COLD may provide an incentive for patients to avoid future disability through cessation of smoking, it is appropriate to compare the relative merits of the medical history and physical examination with those of pulmonary function tests for this purpose. In addition, an assessment of the value of pulmonary testing in differentiating COLD from other conditions that may cause similar symptoms is in order. Finally, the use of pulmonary function tests in monitoring patients with COLD will be reviewed.

ESTIMATING PRETEST PROBABILITY

The sensitivity and specificity of respiratory symptoms in the diagnosis of COLD is difficult to determine because the definition of chronic bronchitis in most epidemiologic surveys is based on the presence of symptoms. Not unexpectedly, respiratory symptoms are common in patients with emphysema (10). However, others report little correlation between symptoms and the presence of abnormalities of small airways (11), which are believed to be the earliest manifestations of COLD (12-14). Symptoms may strongly correlate with smoking history, but not with airflow obstruction (2). Large epidemiologic surveys have found chronic cough or persistent sputum production in 25% to 33% of male cigarette smokers (5,15-17). These data suggest that the medical history is neither very sensitive nor specific when considering the early diagnosis of COLD. The maximum sensitivity of noting chronic cough and/or sputum production in the young smoker is 30% to 40%.

However, as the smoking history progresses (i.e., a more than 20 pack-year history), aspects of the history and physical examination may aid in diagnosing COLD. Holleman and colleagues (18) demonstrated that the number of years of tobacco use and the history of patient-reported wheezing were independent predictors of airflow obstruction. The likelihood ratio for a positive result was 3.1 and for a negative result was 0.58. In addition, the presence of wheezing on physical examination was found to be a predictor of airflow obstruction. Likewise, in patients with moderate COLD, eliciting a history of more than 70 pack-years of tobacco use and a physical examination finding of diminished breath sounds had a sensitivity of 67% and specificity of 98% (positive likelihood ratio of 34 and negative likelihood ratio of 0.34) (19).

DIAGNOSTIC TESTS

Pulmonary Function Tests

In Early Detection of COLD

Conventional spirometric tests of airway obstruction are more often abnormal in the advanced stages of COLD than they are early in the disease (2,10,11,20–31). The sensitivity and specificity of these tests in the literature varies greatly, as shown in Table 31-1. This is due in part to variation both in the severity of disease in the sampled populations and in the definition of the normal value. (In most studies, abnormal has been defined as < 70% or 80% of predicted values in healthy, non-smoking, age-matched study participants.)

Table 31-1. Operating Characteristics for Conventional Spirometric Tests in Smokers*

Diagnostic Test[†]	Sensitivity	Specificity	Likelihood Ratio	
			Positive Result	Negative Result
	← % →			
In a young, minimally symptomatic, or <20 pack-year smoker				
FEV_1	5–15	95	1–3	~1
FEV_1/FVC	10–12	90	~1	~1
MMEFR	20	80	~1	~1
In a middle-aged, moderately symptomatic, or >20 pack-year smoker				
FEV_1	10–40	90	1–4	0.7–1
FEV_1/FVC	20–50	90	2–5	0.6–0.9
MMEFR	20–40	80	1–2	0.8–1

*FEV_1 = expiratory volume during first second of forced expiration; FEV_1/FVC = the ratio of FEV_1 to forced vital capacity; MMEFR = maximal mid-expiratory flow rate.

[†]Predicted normals are based on regression analysis of height, sex, and age. Abnormal results are defined as <80% of predicted.

Overall, it appears that in young smokers, conventional spirometric tests show abnormalities as often in those with as in those without COLD. The FEV_1 (expiratory volume during the first second of forced-expiration) is abnormal in approximately 10% of younger smokers, and the maximal midexpiratory flow rate (MMEFR) is abnormal in approximately 20%. In older or more symptomatic patients, these tests are abnormal in 30% to 40% of patients with COLD and in as many as 20% of those without COLD. The sensitivities of specialized tests of peripheral airway and parenchymal abnormalities, which are believed to represent the earliest pathologic manifestations of COLD, are also low and are not generally helpful in the detection and management of patients with COLD.

When faced with young patients with a history of smoking in whom the diagnosis of COLD is suspected, data suggest that a history of chronic cough, sputum production, wheezing, or shortness of breath on exertion is about as sensitive as the currently available spirometric pulmonary function tests. Unfortunately, neither the history nor pulmonary testing is sufficiently sensitive to facilitate the early diagnosis of COLD. Although specialized tests of small airway disease may be somewhat more sensitive, their specificity has not been established, and therefore they cannot be recommended for early disease detection.

When symptoms and signs of COLD are well established in severely diseased patients, all of the results of conventional spirometric and peripheral airway tests of pulmonary function are likely to be abnormal. Casanova and colleagues (32) demonstrated that there was generally no effect of pulmonary function test results in the management of patients with known obstructive lung disease. Therefore, their use in this circumstance seems only to confirm a presumptive diagnosis.

Differential Diagnosis

It is not uncommon for smokers to have severe respiratory symptoms on the basis of cardiovascular or nonobstructive pulmonary disease because the prevalence of these disorders is also high in such patients. The conventional spirometric pulmonary function tests (i.e., FEV_1 and ratio of FEV_1 to forced vital capacity [FVC]) are quite helpful in distinguishing COLD from other causes of severe respiratory symptoms. Because the sensitivity of these tests approaches 100% in patients with severe symptoms caused by COLD, this diagnosis can be excluded with a high degree of confidence (i.e., post-test probability approaches zero) when they are normal in a severely symptomatic patient. The specificity of these tests can be as high as 90% if a normal FEV_1 is defined as >80% of predicted mean values. This specificity results in a high post-test probability when COLD is suspected on clinical grounds. Spirometric tests are therefore valuable in determining the presence of COLD when severe symptoms are present, and the cause is not obvious.

Patient Management

Certain spirometric tests such as FEV_1 and MMEFR correlate well with advancing COLD (2,30). They are valuable in assessing both disease progression and the impact of therapeutic interventions in the patient with established and moderately advanced COLD. Redelmeier and colleagues (33) showed that a change in FEV_1 of more than 112 mL correlated with a noticeable difference in dyspnea in patients with known COLD. Other pulmonary function tests such as residual volume, total lung capacity, airway resistance/conductance, or chest radiography do not generally add to the information gained from FEV_1 or MMEFR in monitoring such patients (34).

DIAGNOSTIC STRATEGIES

Certain aspects of the medical history can be a sensitive "test" in the diagnosis of moderate or severe COLD. A productive cough in a cigarette smoker that occurs at least three months per year for two consecutive years is considered very suggestive for COLD. Many patients overlook certain coughing patterns, such as the morning "cigarette cough" or the cough of "lingering colds," and the physician must pursue such symptoms when considering the possibility of COLD.

When the cigarette-smoking patient is asymptomatic, the results of neither conventional spirometric nor specialized tests for small airways disease are likely to be abnormal. Therefore, the use of these tests is not recommended and may actually be used by some patients as "evidence" that smoking has not been detrimental to their health.

Pulmonary function testing can be used to confirm the presence of COLD in the symptomatic smoking patient because the specificities of these conventional spirometric tests are high (about 90%) and, if positive, usually establishes the diagnosis. Although a dozen or more standard pulmonary function tests are available for use, three spirometric tests are routinely used to establish the diagnosis of COLD: FEV1, FVC, and FEV1/FVC. These three tests can be easily and economically performed in the office using a portable spirometer. Maximal midexpiratory flow rate can also be measured, but although it has greater sensitivity, it is less specific and therefore has likelihood ratios similar to the other measures. These same tests are also the most sensitive in following the course of COLD or the response to conventional therapy with bronchodilators.

The use of more specialized pulmonary function tests that are usually performed in a pulmonary laboratory should be reserved for those patients who require provocation testing. These include those who are methylcholine challenged, those whose preoperative assessment indicates the testing, or those in whom other respiratory illnesses are strongly suspected (e.g., interstitial, restrictive, or oxygen-diffusion diseases).

Chest radiography is of little value in the diagnosis of COLD in minimally or moderately symptomatic patients and has no value in the assessment of progressive disease severity. It is reasonable, however, to obtain a chest radiograph in patients (particularly those who smoke) with respiratory symptoms to exclude the possibilities of infection, malignancy, or bullous disease that may mimic the signs and symptoms of COLD. Repeat screening chest radiographs, however, are not recommended owing to their lack of sensitivity for COLD and the lack of evidence that screening radiographs improve the overall survival of those who smoke.

CLINICAL PROBLEMS

Clinical Problem 1

A middle-aged patient with a long history of smoking has a productive cough and exertional dyspnea.

Testing Strategy and Rationale

A careful history of cough frequency and duration should be obtained, and chest radiography should be performed. Office spirometry should be also be done. A careful history that identifies the presence of a productive cough for at least 3 months per year for 2 years is highly suggestive for COLD in a cigarette-smoking patient. Initial chest radiography would exclude the less likely possibility of malignancy, parenchymal infection, or other radiologically evident pulmonary disease. Simple office spirometry would include the FEV_1, and FEV_1/FVC ratio. These latter tests are highly specific for COLD (90%), and, if positive, they would virtually confirm the diagnosis in a patient with a suspected high probability of disease based on the history.

Clinical Example

A 55-year-old man reports a continuous productive cough over the past three winters (January through April). He has smoked two packs of cigarettes per day since the age of 22 years. A few expiratory wheezes during forced expiration are detected. The likelihood of COLD is estimated to be at least 80%, and testing is obtained using office spirometry. Should the office spirometry reveal a reduced FEV_1 or a reduced FEV_1/FVC ratio, then the post-test probability for COLD would be approximately 95%. If these same

Continued

tests were normal, the post-test probability for COLD would be reduced, but only to approximately 75%.

Clinical Problem 2

A routine examination is performed for a young asymptomatic patient who smokes.

Testing Strategy and Rationale

A history and a physical examination should be performed. No spirometry is needed. Conventional measures of lung function with either office or laboratory spirometry are usually normal in a young asymptomatic smoker. Such tests add virtually no useful information regarding the presence or absence of COLD. Furthermore, the more sensitive small airway function tests available do not identify the 10% or 20% of patients who will develop significant COLD in the future.

Clinical Example

A history and physical examination are performed on a 30-year-old woman who has smoked one pack of cigarettes per day since the age of 25 years. The history is negative for cough, and the results of the physical examination are normal. The probability of COLD in this patient is estimated to be low, but screening by the use of office spirometry is considered. The post-test probability for COLD for an abnormal FEV_1 or an FEV_1/FVC ratio would only be about 33%, if the pretest probability is as high as 20%. The post-test probability if these tests were negative would remain at about 20%. The use of these tests, therefore, in such patients would not be sufficient to either confirm or exclude early COLD with any degree of certainty. Therefore, pulmonary testing should not be ordered, but the patient should be counseled to stop smoking.

REFERENCES

1. **The Health Consequences of Smoking: Nicotine Addiction.** A Report of the Surgeon General, DHHS Publication Number (PHS) 89-8411, 1989.
2. **Fletcher C, Peto R, Tinker C, Speezer FE**: The Natural History of Chronic Bronchitis and Emphysema. Oxford University Press; 1976:1-104.
3. **Murray JF, Nadel JA.** Textbook of Respiratory Medicine. Philadelphia: WB Saunders; 1988:1001-3.
4. Smoking and Health, A Report of the Surgeon General, DHEW Publication No. (PHS) 79-50066, G-7 to G-52, 1979.
5. **LeBowitz MD, Knudson RJ, Burrows B.** Tuscon epidemiologic study of obstructive lung diseases. Am J Epidemiol. 1975;102:137-52.

6. Prevalence of Selected Chronic Respiratory Conditions, United States 1970, NCHS Vital and Health Statistics, Series 10, No. 84, DHEW Publication No. (HRA) 74-1511, 1973.

7. **Fletcher C.** Some recent advances in the prevention and treatment of chronic bronchitis and related disorders with special reference to the effects of cigarette smoking. Proc R Soc Med. 1965;58:918-32.

8. **Stuart-Harris CH.** The pathogenesis of chronic bronchitis and emphysema. Scot Med J. 1965;10:93-99.

9. **Auerbach O, Hammond EC, Garfinkel L, Benante C.** Relation of smoking and age to emphysema. Whole lung study. N Eng J Med. 1972;286:853-7.

10. **Buist AS, VanFleet DL, Ross BB.** A comparison of conventional spirometric tests and the test of closing volume in an emphysema screening center. Am Rev Respir Dis. 1973;107:735-43.

11. **Bosman J, Bodef, Ghezzo RH, Martin R, Macklem PT.** The relationship between symptoms and functional abnormalities in the clinically healthy cigarette smokers. Am Rev Respir Dis. 1976;114:297-304.

12. **Hogg JC, Macklem PJ, Thurlbeck WM.** Site and nature of airway obstruction in chronic obstructive lung disease. N Eng J Med. 1968;275:1355-60.

13. **Brown R, Woolcock AJ, Vincent NJ, Macklem PT.** Physiological effects of experimental airway obstruction with beads. J Appl Physiol. 1969;27: 328-35.

14. **Macklem PT, Mead J.** Resistance of central and peripheral airways measured by a retrograde catheter. J Appl Physiol. 1967;22:395-401.

15. **Sharp JT, Paul O, Lepper MH, et al.** Prevalence of chronic bronchitis in an American male urban industrial population. Am Rev Respir Dis. 1965;91: 510-20.

16. **Hepper NG, Hyatt RE, Fowler WS.** Detection of chronic obstructive lung disease. Arch Environ Health. 1969;19:806-13.

17. **Higgins ITT.** Tobacco smoking, respiratory symptoms, and ventilatory capacity: studies in random samples of the population. Br Med J. 1950; 2:325-9.

18. **Holleman DR, Simel DL, Goldberg JS.** Diagnosis of obstructive airways disease from the clinical examination. J Gen Intern Med 1993;8:63-8.

19. **Badgett RG, Tanaka DJ, Hunt DK, et al.** Can moderate chronic obstructive pulmonary disease be diagnosed by history and physical findings alone? Am J Med. 1993;94:188-96.

20. **Buist AS, Ross BB.** Quantitative analysis of the alveolar plateau in the diagnosis of early airway obstruction. Am Rev Respir Dis. 1973;108: 1078-87.

21. **Benson MK.** The closing volume as a screening test in smokers. Scand J Resp Dis. 1974;95(suppl):84-90.

22. **Dirkson H, Janzon L, Lindell SE.** Influence of smoking and cessation of smoking in lung function. A population study of closing volume and nitrogen washout. Scand J Respir Dis. 1974;85(Suppl):266-74.

23. **Marco M, Minette A.** Lung function changes in smokers with normal conventional spirometry. Am Rev Respir Dis. 1976;114:732-38.

24. **Armstrong JG, Woolcock AJ.** Lung function in asymptomatic cigarette smokers-the single breath N2 test. Aust N Zealand J Med. 1976;6:123-6.

25. **Knudson RJ, Lebowitz MD, Burton AP, Knudson DE.** The closing volume test. Evaluation of nitrogen and holus methods in a random population. Am Rev Respir Dis. 1977;115:423-4.

26. **Manfreda J, Nelson N, Chermiack RM.** Prevalence of respiratory abnormalities in a rural and urban community. Am Rev Respir Dis. 1978;117: 215-26.

27. **Niewoehner DE, Kleinderman J, Rice DB.** Pathologic changes in the peripheral airways of young cigarette smokers. N Engl J Mcd.1974;291: 755-8.

28. **Thurlbeck SM, Henderson JA, Fraser RG, Bates DV.** Chronic obstructive lung disease. Medicine 1970;49:81-145.

29. **Doll R, Peto R.** Mortality in relation to smoking: 20 years' observations on male British doctors. Br Med J. 1976;2:1525-36.

30. **Walter S, Naney NR, Collier CR.** Changes in forced expiratory spirogram in young male smokers. Am Rev Respir Dis. 1979;119:717-24.

31. **Knudson RJ, Burrows B, Lebowitz M.** The maximal expiratory flow-volume curve: its use in the detection of ventilatory abnormalities in a population study. Am Rev Respir Dis. 1976;114:871-9, 1976.

32. **Casanova JE, Kaufman J.** Utility of pulmonary function testing in the management of chronic obstructive pulmonary disease. J Gen Intern Med. 1993; 8:448-50.

33. **Redelmeier DA, Goldstein RS, Min ST, Hyland RH.** Spirometry and dyspnea in patients with chronic obstructive pulmonary disease. Chest. 1996; 109:1163-8.

34. **Bates DV.** The fate of the chronic chronic bronchitis: a report of the ten-year follow-up in the Canadian Department of Veteran's Affairs Coordinated Study of Chronic Bronchitis. Am Rev Respir Dis. 1973;108:1043-65.

Sarcoidosis

32

Robert H. Poe, MD

KEY POINTS

Pretest Probabilities

- Sarcoidosis most commonly affects young adults and frequently presents with bilateral hilar lymphadenopathy (BHA), either alone or associated with pulmonary infiltrates, skin, or eye lesions.

- The prevalence and severity of sarcoidosis vary among population groups from less than 1 to 64 per 100,000 persons. The peak incidence is in patients in the third decade of life.

- In more than 90% of patients, chest radiography reveals abnormalities, and yet as many as 30% of patients are totally asymptomatic.

Diagnostic Strategies

- In asymptomatic patients or in patients with uveitis or erythema nodosum as the sole clinical manifestation, the presence of BHA is highly specific for sarcoidosis. For patients in whom BHA is found, no further diagnostic evaluation is usually required, although basing the diagnosis on the presence of BHA carries a small risk of misdiagnosis.

- Flexible fiberoptic transbronchial lung biopsy and scalene node/mediastinal node biopsy are highly sensitive and specific for sarcoidosis. Node biopsy is more sensitive in patients with BHA who do not have parenchymal lung infiltration (stage I disease), whereas transbronchial lung biopsy is often the preferred test in patients with parenchymal lung infiltrates (stage II or III disease).

- The angiotensin-converting enzyme (ACE) level is not recommended for diagnosis in patients with suspected sarcoidosis owing to its variable and often low specificity.

- Clinical observation of patients with sarcoidosis is sensitive for the detection of changes in disease activity. In such patients, the ACE level does not offer any additional information and is not recommended.

BACKGROUND

A chest radiograph showing bilateral hilar adenopathy (BHA) or bilateral parenchymal disease or both in the minimally symptomatic or asymptomatic patient poses a difficult diagnostic problem. Three considerations are usually entertained in these situations: 1) sarcoidosis, 2) neoplasm, or 3) infection such as tuberculosis. Pneumonoconioses, hypersensitivity pneumonitis, and collagen vascular disease could cause a similar appearance on radiography, but such diseases are frequently apparent from the history or examination.

Because the more serious possible disorders, neoplasm and tuberculosis, generally require prompt treatment, the initial diagnostic strategy has frequently used highly invasive and highly specific procedures for disease identification. Alternatively, however, the confirmation of the least serious possibility, sarcoidosis, can eliminate the more serious diseases from further consideration. Moreover, the diagnostic procedures currently available for sarcoidosis are typically less invasive and in most patients with a benign, self-limiting disease could obviate the need for tests associated with greater morbidity.

Sarcoidosis is a multisystem granulomatous disorder of unknown cause, most commonly affecting young adults and presenting most frequently with BHA with and without pulmonary infiltrates (1). The diagnosis is made by demonstrating either the presence of noncaseating granulomas in multiple organs or on the basis of highly specific clinical findings as described below.

Sarcoidosis is classified into stages according to the abnormality found on chest radiography: Stage 0—normal chest radiograph; stage I—BHA (with or without paratracheal adenopathy); stage II—BHA and parenchymal lung infiltrates; stage III—parenchymal lung infiltrates without BHA; and stage IV—bullae, cysts, and emphysematous changes.

Numerous immunologic abnormalities occur in this disorder, including bronchoalveolar lymphocyte proliferation and activation, peripheral lymphopenia with hypergammaglobulinemia, and cutaneous anergy (2–5).

ESTIMATING PRETEST PROBABILITY

The prevalence and severity of sarcoidosis vary in different population groups. In the United States, the prevalence among whites is about 5 per 100,000 and 40 per 100,000 for blacks. Many patients are young (<40 years old), asymptomatic, and present with stage I disease (i.e., BHA) (6,7). No more than 10% of young patients with stage I disease have either uveitis or erythema nodosum at the time of presentation; however, either of these findings in patients with BHA has a specificity for sarcoidosis approaching 100% (6–9). Generally, younger asymptomatic patients with stage I disease have a benign self-limiting course that does not require treatment. Older patients are more often symptomatic, with nonrespiratory symptoms and stage II or stage III disease. These patients have a less favorable prognosis and often require treatment. Patients presenting with dyspnea and airway obstruction generally show progressive disease and respond poorly to treatment (10).

Many other clinical findings are seen in sarcoidosis patients, such as hepatosplenomegaly, cranial nerve palsy, and constitutional symptoms (6–8). These manifestations lack both sensitivity and specificity for sarcoidosis and are commonly observed in diseases that are included in the differential diagnosis (e.g., lymphoma and tuberculosis). Certain skin manifestations, such as malar nodules (lupus pernio) or large violaceous plaques, are highly specific for sarcoidosis but are found in only a minority of patients (6,7,11).

The initial clinical evaluation with chest radiography defines certain sensitive and specific clinical patterns that enable confident estimation of the probability of sarcoidosis. Chest radiography is the most important diagnostic test and often first raises the question of the disease, many times unexpectedly. In a study of nearly 100 patients with sarcoidosis and of more than 1900 patients with lymphoma and other neoplastic diseases, BHA with or without paratracheal adenopathy or parenchymal pulmonary infiltration (i.e., stage I and II patterns) was present in 74 of 99 patients with sarcoidosis (sensitivity = 75%) and in only 26 of 1913 patients with neoplasm (specificity = 99%) (12). Of 397 patients with tuberculosis or possible fungal disease, only 3 had BHA (specificity = 99%). Additionally, 39 of 74 patients with sarcoidosis and BHA were totally asymptomatic or had either uveitis or erythema nodosum (sensitivity = 53%); none of the patients with neoplastic illness and BHA had these clinical findings. Therefore, the presence of BHA alone in asymptomatic patients or in the patient with uveitis or erythema nodosum strongly suggests the diagnosis of sarcoidosis, possibly making further diagnostic testing unnecessary.

When the findings other than BHA are shown by radiography, such as pleural effusion or a mediastinal mass, or when the patient is symptomatic or older than 40 years of age, the probability of sarcoidosis decreases to approximately 50% to 75%. Although the likelihood of neoplasm in these particular patients with BHA is still low, the possibility of inflammatory or hypersensitivity lung disease cannot be as reliably excluded. Such patients usually require additional diagnostic evaluation.

DIAGNOSTIC TESTS

Kveim-Siltzbach Test

The Kveim-Siltzbach test has been historically a diagnostic marker of sarcoidosis. However, because of the difficulty in obtaining reliable antigen and the availability of more specific tests, the Kveim reaction is now rarely used.

Transbronchial Lung Biopsy

Flexible fiberoptic transbronchial lung biopsy is commonly used for the diagnosis of sarcoidosis. A biopsy that demonstrates multiple, non-caseating granulomas and that yields negative results for acid-fast organisms is considered pathognomonic for sarcoidosis (specificity = 100%). The procedure is easily performed by experienced physicians and is usually well tolerated. Positive results depend on the number of specimens obtained (13) and the radiographic stage of the disease. The sensitivity in stage 0 to stage I disease has been reported to average 66% and in stage II and stage III averages between 80% and 83% (Table 32-1) (13). Higher yields can be achieved by increasing the number of biopsies to 10 in stage I disease (5 may be adequate in stage II and stage III disease) and by directing the biopsy to the lobe with the most involvement.

Table 32-1. Operating Characteristics of Diagnostics Tests and Procedures for Sarcoidosis

Diagnostic Test	Definition of Positive Result	Disease Stage	Sensitivity	Specificity	Likelihood Ratio	
					Positive Result	Negative Result
			←———— % ————→			
Chest radiography						
BHA in asymptomatic patients	BHA	I/II	75	99	75	0.25
Transbronchial lung biopsy	Noncaseating granuloma	0/I	66	100	∞	0.34
		II/III	83	100	∞	0.17
Thoracic node biopsy	Noncaseating granuloma					
No scalene node palpable		All	70	100	∞	0.30
Scalene node palpable		All	85	100	∞	0.15
Mediastinoscopy		All	85	100	∞	0.15
ACE test	Assay dependent	I	61	95*	12	0.41
		II	77	95*	15	0.24
		III	93	95*	19	0.07

*Specificity highly variable (see text). ACE = angiotensin-converting enzyme; BHA = bilateral hilar adenopathy.

Scalene/ Mediastinal Node Biopsy

Before the use of flexible transbronchial lung biopsy, scalene node biopsy was the most frequently used invasive procedure in the diagnosis of sarcoidosis. The sensitivity of this procedure is 80% to 90% when the scalene nodes are palpable and 70% when nodes are not palpable (14). The yield also varies with the surgeon and the extent of scalene fat pad dissection performed; generally, a more extensive dissection leads to greater sensitivity.

Mediastinoscopy is an extension of the scalene node biopsy technique and has a sensitivity of 85% in patients with hilar or mediastinal adenopathy or both (15). When the biopsy demonstrates multiple, acid-fast negative, noncaseating granulomas, the specificity is virtually 100%. The procedure is generally well tolerated.

Serum Angiotensin-Converting Enzyme

Angiotensin-converting enzyme (ACE) is present in lung tissue, vascular endothelium, and noncaseating granulomas (16,17). The serum concentration of this enzyme is elevated in most patients with active, untreated sarcoidosis and in approximately 40% of patients with chronic, untreated disease (16–19).

The sensitivity of the ACE assay depends on the chemical method used and the stage of the disease. Both the older spectrophotometric assays and newer radioimmunoassays are reliable when performed by competent laboratories (20,21). ACE levels reflect the metabolic activity of the activated macrophage, and increased levels correlate with increased granulomatous activity. The enzyme level correlates better with pulmonary sarcoidosis than with disease elsewhere in the body (22). The sensitivity of the ACE level varies with the stage of sarcoidosis: stage I = 61%, stage II – 77%, stage III = 93%; however, the ACE level is reduced in many patients who receive corticosteroids (16,17,19).

Estimates for the specificity of the ACE level are controversial. Elevated levels have been reported in such common disorders as osteoarthritis, ethanol-related liver disease, hyperthyroidism, systemic fungal disease such as coccidioidomycosis, diabetes mellitus, and rarer disorders as Gaucher disease, leprosy, berylliosis, Lennert lymphoma, and lymphangiolmyomatosis (16,17,23). Because the ACE level can be elevated in patients with both common disorders and diseases likely to be considered in the differential diagnosis of sarcoidosis, it is not recommended for use in critical diagnostic situations.

Some suggest that the measurements of the ACE level can be used in patients with established sarcoidosis to detect a change in disease activity that requires treatment (20,21). However, changes in ACE levels correlate more with changes in corticosteroid dosage than with disease activity (22). Furthermore, serial measurements of ACE level have not yet been shown to be more sensitive than clinical observation in assessing disease activity (22).

Bronchoalveolar Lavage

Bronchoalveolar lavage (BAL) is a relatively simple procedure accomplished by positioning a flexible fiberoptic bronchoscope in a distal lung subsegment, instilling aliquots of physiologic saline, and removing the sample using low suction. The procedure, which is well tolerated and is associated with a low morbidity, allows rapid access to alveolar cells (2,24). Lavage fluid in patients with sarcoidosis shows an increase in both the absolute number of alveolar lymphocytes and the proportion of T lymphocytes (2,24). A decrease in T lymphocytes may occur when the disease becomes inactive and after corticosteroid therapy (25). The percent of T lymphocytes found by lavage may be able to characterize the degree of alveolitis present (2,25). Early reports suggested that BAL might be a valuable test for sarcoidosis (2). However, similar abnormalities are seen in patients with hypersensitivity pneumonitis, mycobacterial infections, methotrexate-induced lung disease, cytomegalovirus infection, *Pneumocystis carinii* pneumonia, talc pneumoconiosis, asbestosis, and berylliosis (26). The helper-suppressor ratio may be a better index, because the lymphocytes in nonsarcoid disease are generally both T and B lymphocytes with resultant low helper-suppressor cell ratios.

Although the BAL procedure appears promising, considerable variability exists in both the technique and methods used for cell analysis; hence, the precise sensitivity or specificity cannot be estimated. The utility of BAL in the diagnosis of sarcoidosis has yet to be established.

Lung and Tissue Biopsy

Open lung biopsy has a sensitivity and specificity for the diagnosis of sarcoidosis of nearly 100%. However, an open lung biopsy is rarely necessary, and this approach is gradually being replaced by thoracoscopy (27).

Many other organs can demonstrate noncaseating granulomas in patients with sarcoidosis. In patients with BHA but with no obvious extrathoracic abnormalities, 70% of percutaneous liver biopsies show noncaseating granulomas (28). However, the specificity of liver biopsy is controversial, because noncaseating hepatic granulomas can also be seen in patients with viral infection, inflammatory bowel disease, primary biliary cirrhosis, some lymphomas, and tuberculosis (although if the patient has tuberculosis, staining may demonstrate acid-fast bacilli). For this reason, we do not recommend the use of the liver biopsy in the diagnosis of sarcoidosis.

Biopsy of the minor salivary glands is a simple outpatient technique with a sensitivity approaching 60% (29). Sarcoid granulomas may also be obtained from obvious conjunctival follicles but blind biopsy of the conjunctiva is usually unrewarding; one series, however, reports a sensitivity of 47% (30).

Gallium 67 Lung Scan

Activated macrophages in sarcoid tissue accumulate gallium, which may therefore be used to detect active granulomas, and pulmonary inflammatory and immune effector cells constituting the alveolitis concentrate the isotope. However, uptake of gallium by the lung parenchyma is not diagnostic of sarcoidosis, because it occurs in most interstitial lung disorders with an active alveolitis as well as in neoplastic tissue. Increased uptake of gallium in the intrathoracic lymph nodes in sarcoidosis does not correlate with the alveolitis and has only a weak correlation with the clinical signs and symptoms and the radiographic stage and pattern of disease (31). In some cases, whole-body gallium imaging, including uptake in lacrimal and salivary glands, may improve the sensitivity of the test and reduce the need for invasive biopsy procedures in asymptomatic patients (32). Gallium uptake is suppressed by corticosteroids. Overall, owing to the limited value of the information to be gained in most patients, the expense of the test, and the inconvenience of the 48- to 72-hour delay necessary to complete the study, we do not recommend this study for routine use in the diagnostic evaluation of sarcoidosis.

Computed Tomography

Computed tomography, especially using the newer high-resolution technique, is sensitive in delineating the presence and extent of parenchymal abnormalities in sarcoidosis; it is more sensitive than standard chest radiography in demonstrating intrathoracic sarcoidosis (33). This may prove to be of benefit to the 5% of patients with extrathoracic sarcoidosis and for whom the results of chest radiography are normal, but it is not recommended for routine diagnostic use.

DIAGNOSTIC STRATEGIES

The history, physical examination, and chest radiography are the most important initial diagnostic procedures in patients in whom sarcoidosis is suspected. The presence of BHA with or without parenchymal disease in asymptomatic patients or in patients with uveitis or erythema nodosum strongly suggests the diagnosis, and often in such cases no further diagnostic testing is needed. Nearly half of all patients with sarcoidosis present with these findings and therefore can be spared further invasive diagnostic procedures.

Patients with similar findings on chest radiography but who are symptomatic or have other significant physical findings require investigation. We estimate that the probability of sarcoidosis in such patients may still be 50% to 75%. In such patients, biopsy of palpable adenopathy or skin lesions should be done, because the sensitivity and specificity of these procedures is high: 90% and 100%, respectively. A biopsy demonstrating noncaseating granulomas with negative acid-fast stains confirms the diagnosis of sarcoidosis. A negative biopsy result reduces the probability of sarcoidosis to approximately 10%; therefore, additional studies would probably be needed to evaluate for other disorders.

The choice of further diagnostic procedures in patients in whom sarcoidosis is suspected and who do not exhibit the features noted previously should be based on the morbidity associated with the procedure and the pattern present on the chest radiograph. Scalene or mediastinal node biopsy is recommended for patients with either stage 0 or stage I disease, because its sensitivity is slightly greater than that of transbronchial lung biopsy (70%–85%, compared with 66%). Transbronchial lung biopsy is recommended when chest radiography suggests stage II or stage III disease, because the sensitivity of this procedure approaches that of mediastinoscopy, which is associated with greater morbidity.

We do not recommend the serum ACE level to diagnose sarcoidosis because of its low sensitivity in stage I disease and its uncertain specificity. Liver biopsy is likewise not recommended because its

Table 32-2. Post-test Probability of Sarcoidosis Based on Results of Selected Diagnostic Procedures*

Diagnostic Test	Radio-graphic Stage	Pretest Probability					
		20%		50%		80%	
		Positive Result	Negative Result	Positive Result	Negative Result	Positive Result	Negative Result
		%					
Chest radiography							
BHA in asymptomatic patients	I/II	95	6	99	20	>99	50
Transbronchial lung biopsy	0/I	100	8	100	25	100	58
	II/III	100	4	100	15	100	40
Thoracic node biopsy							
Scalene (no scalene node palpable)	All	100	7	100	23	100	55
Mediastinoscopy	All	100	4	100	13	100	38

BHA = bilateral hilar adenopathy.

*Angiotensin-converting enzyme (ACE) test is not included owing to its variable specificity.

specificity is not known and because other procedures associated with less morbidity (i.e., scalene/mediastinal node and transbronchial lung biopsy) are at least as sensitive as this test and are highly specific. Bronchoalveolar lavage should be regarded as investigational at present and should not be performed for diagnostic purposes. Pulmonary function testing with measurement of lung volumes and diffusing capacity may also be a part of the evaluation, because patients may have abnormalities whether symptoms are present or not.

Table 32-2 summarizes the post-test probabilities for tests and procedures used routinely in the diagnosis of sarcoidosis.

CLINICAL PROBLEMS

Clinical Problem 1
Bilateral hilar lymphadenopathy is seen on chest radiography in a young, asymptomatic patient.

Testing Strategy and Rationale
A careful history should be obtained, and a physical examination should be performed. In asymptomatic patients, BHA is virtually pathognomonic for sarcoidosis, having a specificity of almost 100% in such patients, and therefore usually confirms the diagnosis of sarcoidosis. Approximately half of all patients with sarcoidosis present in this manner. Pulmonary function testing should be considered, but no further diagnostic testing is required. The physical examination of such patients may reveal minor abnormalities, but the absence of symptoms is the important factor that increases the specificity of BHA to almost 100%. The physical examination is important, however, to assess cardiac, neurologic, and pulmonary findings, which are frequently affected by sarcoidosis and may necessitate treatment or close follow-up. Generally, young, asymptomatic patients have a benign course without treatment. Repeat chest radiography within 12 to 18 months or at any time symptoms develop is recommended.

Clinical Example
A 25-year-old woman presents who was discovered to have BHA during a routine medical assessment at her place of employment. She is asymptomatic, and on careful examination no abnormalities are detected. The specificity of these findings is virtually 100% and therefore confirms the presence of sarcoidosis. No further diagnostic testing is usually required.

Continued

Clinical Problem 2

A patient with BHA found on chest radiography also has symptoms such as cough, fever, and malaise.

Testing Strategy and Rationale

A careful physical examination should be performed, and if no abnormalities are found, a scalene node biopsy or transbronchial biopsy should be done, depending on whether lung infiltrates are absent or present. The presence of BHA in symptomatic patients still favors the diagnosis of sarcoidosis. As many as 50% to 75% of such patients prove to have this disease. However, the likelihood of other potentially serious diseases (e.g., malignancy) remains, and further diagnostic testing is usually required.

Physical examination is extremely important, because most patients who have malignancy have either organomegaly or adenopathy. If adenopathy is discovered, a biopsy should be done immediately. If no adenopathy is found or if organ biopsy cannot safely be performed, scalene/mediastinal node biopsy is preferred in patients without infiltrates, because it is more sensitive in stage I sarcoidosis; whereas transbronchial lung biopsy is preferred in patients with infiltrates, because it is nearly as sensitive as mediastinoscopy in stage II or stage III disease but has lower morbidity (see Table 32-1).

Clinical Example

A 30-year-old man presents with night sweats, weight loss of 15 lb, and cough. Although the results of the physical examination are normal, chest radiography reveals BHA without infiltrates. The probability of sarcoidosis is therefore approximately 70%, and a mediastinal node biopsy is done to confirm the suspicion. If the results of the biopsy are negative (i.e., no noncaseating granulomas are found), the post-test probability of sarcoidosis is reduced to approximately 40% and further tests are needed; if the results of the biopsy are positive, the post-test probability of sarcoidosis is 100% and no further testing is required.

REFERENCES

1. **James DG, Turiaf J, Hosoda YY, et al.** Description of sarcoidosis: report of the subcommittee on clarification and definition. In: Siltzbach LE, ed. 7th International Conference on Sarcoidosis and Other Granulomatous Disease. New York: The New York Academy of Sciences; 1976:742.
2. **Crystal RB, Roberts WE, Hunninghake GW, et al.** Pulmonarysarcoidosis: a disease characterized and perpetuated by activated lung T-lymphocytes. Ann Intern Med. 1981;94:73-94.

3. **Daniele RP, Dauber JH, Rossman MD.** Immunologic abnormalities in sarcoidosis. Ann Intern Med. 1980;92:406-16.

4. **Hunninghake GW, Gadek JE, Young RC Jr, et al.** Maintenance of granuloma formation in pulmonary sarcoidosis by T-lymphocytes within the lung. N Engl J Med. 1980;302:594-8.

5. **Hunninghake GW, Fulmer JD, Young RC Jr, et al.** Localization of the immune response in sarcoidosis. Am Rev Respir Dis. 1979;120: 49-57.

6. **Siltzbach LE.** Sarcoidosis: clinical features and management. Med Clin North Am. 1967;51:483-502.

7. **Kirks DR, Greenspan RH.** Sarcoid Radiol Clin North Am. 1973;11:279-94.

8. **Kataria YP, Shaw RA, Campbell PB.** Sarcoidosis: an overview. Clin Notes Resp Dis. 1982;20:3-16.

9. **Neville E, Walker AN, Geraint James D.** Prognostic factors predicting the outcome of sarcoidosis: an analysis of 818 patients. Q J Med. 1983;208: 525-33.

10. **DeRemee RA, Anderson HA.** Sarcoidosis: a correlation of dyspnea and roentgenographic stage and pulmonary function changes. Mayo Clin Proc. 1974;49:742-5.

11. **Sharma OP.** Cutaneous sarcoidosis: clinical features and management. Chest. 1972;61:320-5.

12. **Winterbauer RH, Belic N, Moores KD.** A clinical interpretation of bilateral hilar adenopathy. Ann Intern Med. 1973;78:65-71.

13. **Rothe RA, Fuller PB, Byrd RB, et al.** Transbronchoscopic lung biopsy in sarcoidosis: optimum number and sites for diagnosis. Chest. 1980;77:400-2.

14. **Lillington GA, Jamplis RW.** Scalene node biopsy. Ann Intern Med. 1963; 59:101-10.

15. **Munkgaard S, Neukerch F.** Comparison of biopsy procedures in intrathoracic sarcoidosis. Acta Med Scand. 1979;205:179-82.

16. **Lewis RJ, Caccavale RJ, Sisler GE.** Imaged thoracoscopic lung biopsy. Chest. 1992;102:60-2.

17. **Studdy PR, Lapworth R, Bird R.** Angiotensin converting enzyme and its clinical significance: a review. J Clin Pathol. 1983;36:938-47.

18. **Studdy PR, Bird R, James DG.** Serum angiotensin converting enzyme in sarcoidosis and other granulomatous disorders. Lancet. 1978; 2:1131-4.

19. **Allen RK.** A review of angiotensin converting enzyme in health and disease. Sarcoidosis. 1991;8:95-100.

20. **Baughman RP, Ploysongsang Y, Roberts RD, et al.** Effects of sarcoid and steroids on angiotensin converting enzyme. Am Rev Respir Dis. 1983;128: 631-3.

21. **Cushman DW, Cheung HS.** Spectrophotometric assay and properties of the ACE of rabbit lung. Biochem Pharmacol. 1971;20:1637-48.

22. **Ryan JW, Chung A, Amuous C, et al.** A simple radioassay for ACE. Biochemistry. 1977;167:4-20.

23. **James DG, Williams WJ.** Immunology of sarcoidosis. Am J Med. 1982;72:5-8.

24. **Romer FK.** Angiotensin-converting enzyme activity in sarcoidosis and other disorders. Sarcoidosis. 1985;2:25-34.

25. **Rossman MD, Dauber JH, Cardello ME, et al.** Pulmonary sarcoidosis: correlation of serum angiotensin converting enzyme with blood and bronchoalveolar lymphocytes. Am Rev Respir Dis. 1982;125:366-8.

26. **Ceuppens JL, Lacquet LM, Mariën G, et al.** T-cell subsets in pulmonary sarcoidosis: correlation with disease activity and effect of steroid treatment. Am Rev Respir Dis. 1984;129:563-8.

27. **Daniele RP, Elias JA, Epstein PE, et al.** Bronchoalveolar lavage: role in the pathogenesis, diagnosis and management of interstitial lung disease. Ann Intern Med. 1985;102:93-108.

28. **Israel HL, Goldstein A.** Hepatic granulomatosis and sarcoidosis. Ann Intern Med. 1973;79:669-78.

29. **Nessan VJ, Jacoway JR.** Biopsy of minor salivary glands in the diagnosis of sarcoidosis. N Engl J Med. 1979;301:922-4.

30. **Karma A.** Ophthalmic changes in sarcoidosis. Acta Ophthalmologica. 1979;57:141.

31. **Line BR, Hunninghake GW, Keogh BA, et al.** Gallium-67 scanning to stage the alveolitis of sarcoidosis: correlation with clinical studies, pulmonary function studies and bronchoalveolar lavage. Am Rev Respir Dis. 1981;123:440-6.

32. **Israel HL, Albertine KH, Park CH, et al.** Whole-body gallium-67 scans: role in diagnosis of sarcoidosis. Am Rev Respir Dis. 1991;144:1182-6.

33. **Muller NL, Kullnig P, Miller RR.** The CT findings of pulmonary sarcoidosis. Analysis of 25 patients. AJR Am J Roentgenol. 1989;152:1179-85.

Mediastinal Mass   **33**

Thomas G. Tape, MD

KEY POINTS

Pretest Probabilities

- The differential diagnosis of a mediastinal mass is extensive. Common diagnoses include metastatic cancer, various primary neoplasms, lymphoma, vascular abnormalities, and inflammatory lesions.

- Many patients are asymptomatic when the mediastinal mass is discovered.

- Fewer than 50% of primary mediastinal tumors are malignant, but the presence of symptoms at the time of diagnosis increases the likelihood of malignancy.

Diagnostic Strategies

- Chest radiography and computed tomography (CT) are the most useful noninvasive tests to define the location and extent of a mediastinal mass. Magnetic resonance imaging (MRI) is better than CT for evaluating posterior mediastinal masses. Further diagnostic testing should be individualized.

- Most patients with lesions that could be neoplastic require tissue biopsy for definitive diagnosis.

- Fine-needle aspiration biopsy is the least morbid method of obtaining tissue for diagnosis. The test accurately identifies malignancy; however, nonmalignant aspirates usually require confirmation by actual tissue biopsy.

- Histologic examination of tissue obtained during videothoracoscopy or open thoracotomy is the gold standard for diagnosis of a mediastinal mass.

BACKGROUND

A wide variety of lesions may present as a mediastinal mass. The differential diagnosis includes various types of cysts, hernias, diverticula, vascular abnormalities, inflammatory processes, and primary and metastatic neoplasms.

The discovery of a mediastinal mass is usually made by chest radiography. In many cases, it is discovered incidentally on a chest radiograph that is being done for some other reason (1–3). Some patients may have various symptoms including cough, dyspnea, pain, hoarseness, and dysphagia.

The gold standard for diagnosis of a mediastinal mass is surgical biopsy. In cases of benign tumors or resectable malignancies, surgery is the treatment of choice as well. However, many mediastinal masses do not require surgical intervention. The goal of diagnostic testing is to obtain a definitive diagnosis by the least invasive means.

ESTIMATING PRETEST PROBABILITY

Primary mediastinal tumors are rare; the incidence has been estimated at 1 in 3400 admissions to a university hospital (1). Thymomas, lymphomas, germ-cell tumors, neurogenic tumors, and benign cysts each accounts for more than 10% of primary lesions (1–7). Other types of tumors occur less frequently, and less than 50% of all primary lesions are malignant. The presence of symptoms attributable to the mass correlates with malignancy. In one study, about 60% of symptomatic patients had malignant tumors, whereas over 80% of asymptomatic patients had a benign diagnosis (6).

Other causes of mediastinal masses are much more common than primary tumors, but the incidence of these other causes has not been well studied. One report by Lyons and colleagues (8) describes the frequency of specific causes of mediastinal masses (Table 33-1). Sixty percent of these masses were benign, mainly caused by an inflammatory diseases such as sarcoidosis. Lymphomas accounted for most of the malignant lesions. These data should be interpreted with caution because the increasing incidence of lung carcinoma and more frequent use of chest radiography have clearly changed the case mix of mediastinal masses.

Clinically useful estimates of pretest probability can be obtained from reports of fine needle aspiration biopsy of mediastinal masses. Patients in these studies had been previously evaluated with noninvasive diagnostic tests, thereby ruling out many of the diagnoses listed in Table 33-1. Pooling the data from three studies (9–11), carcinoma accounted for 51% of cases overall, lymphoma for 16%, various benign lesions for 10%, thymoma for 9%, neurogenic tumors for 3%, and teratoma for 3%. The balance were various rare malignant tumors. Therefore, most patients presenting for fine needle aspiration biopsy had a malignancy.

Because mediastinal masses are often discovered incidentally, the history and physical examination may be completely normal. Findings, when present, may include cough, dyspnea, pain, hoarseness, dysphagia, weight loss, fever, tracheal deviation, evidence of superior vena

Table 33-1. Frequency of Specific Causes of Mediastinal Masses

Type	Number of Cases	Percentage of Total
Cysts (thymic, pericardial, other)	22	2.8
Hernias, diverticula, achalasias	42	5.4
Vascular abnormalities		
Aneurysms of great vessels and heart	36	4.6
Vascular abnormalities	32	4.1
Cardiac metastasis and hemangiomas	15	1.9
Neoplams		
Malignant lymphomas	203	25.9
Hodgkin lymphoma	146	
Lymphosarcoma	40	
Other lymphomas	17	
Other neoplasms	123	15.7
Teratoma and dermoid	35	
Thymoma	26	
Metastatic growths	34	
Other neoplasms	28	
Inflammation	278	35.4
Sarcoid	160	
Histoplasmosis	53	
Tuberculoma	48	
Other	17	
Miscellaneous (includes goiter)	33	4.2
Total	784	100

Adapted from Lyons HA, Calvy GL, Sammons BP. The diagnosis and classification of mediastinal masses: a study of 782 cases. Ann Intern Med. 1959;51:897-929.

cava obstruction, and signs of myasthenia gravis (5,6). The location of the mass, as discussed in the next section, can help to narrow the differential diagnosis.

DIAGNOSTIC TESTS

Chest Radiography
The mediastinal mass is frequently discovered on chest radiography. The posterior/anterior and lateral chest radiographs are useful mainly

in localizing the mass, which may narrow the differential diagnosis. Thymoma, teratoma, substernal thyroid goiter, and lymphoma are common diagnoses in the anterior mediastinum. Metastatic disease, aortic aneurysms, and cysts are common lesions in the middle mediastinum. Neurogenic tumors and paravertebral abscesses are common masses of the posterior mediastinum (12,13).

Computed Tomography

The chest computed tomography (CT) scan gives further clarification of the location, size, and anatomic relationships of the mass (14). With the use of radiocontrast media, vascular abnormalities can be differentiated from tumors (15,16). However, CT is not reliable in differentiating cysts from solid tumors (17). In patients with myasthenia gravis, the CT scan is the most useful noninvasive test to identify thymoma. Its sensitivity approaches 100%, but it can not distinguish thymic hyperplasia from tumor (18). In general, the CT scan or an alternative imaging scan such as magnetic resonance imaging (MRI) or sonography will be needed to plan the approach if either surgery or fine-needle aspiration biopsy is being considered.

When imaged by CT, teratomas frequently have fat, fluid-containing cystic areas and calcifications. Although the exact specificity of these findings is not known, the infrequently observed finding of fat-fluid levels is reported to be highly specific (19).

Magnetic Resonance Imaging

Magnetic resonance imaging offers no advantage over CT in imaging the anterior and middle mediastinum except in cases where iodinated contrast media are contraindicated (20–27). Magnetic resonance imaging is more expensive than CT, it can not detect small calcifications within lymph nodes, and it has inferior spatial resolution. However, MRI is the best tool for evaluating posterior mediastinal masses, which are often of neurogenic origin (28). It can determine whether the tumor involves the spinal canal without the need for intrathecal contrast.

Ultrasonography

Parasternal and suprasternal sonography, transthoracic echocardiography, and transesophageal echocardiography have been reported to have diagnostic accuracy approaching that of CT in identifying and localizing selected mediastinal masses (29–33). Ultrasonography is best at evaluating tumors of the supra-aortic, pericardial, and paratracheal regions and can differentiate pericardial cysts from pericardial effusions (34). Ultrasound can also be used to guide fine-needle aspiration biopsy (35–37). At present however, the reported experience with mediastinal sonography is insufficient to recommend that it replace CT scanning.

Miscellaneous Tests

Other studies can be applied in some patients who may be suspected of having the potential for specific problems. Barium swallow is effective in identifying hernias and diverticula of the upper gastrointestinal tract. The radioiodine scan is useful in the workup of anterior mediastinal masses in which a substernal thyroid is a possibility, but a hypofunctioning goiter may result in a false-negative scan (38). If a vascular abnormality is suspected and the CT scan is nondiagnostic, angiography, either conventional or using MRI, is indicated. Superior venacavography achieved with nuclear-medicine techniques may be helpful in determining the site and extent of obstruction in patients having the superior vena cava syndrome (39). If a germ-cell tumor is a possibility, tumor markers such as alpha-fetoprotein and human chorionic gonadotropin should be assayed. Evaluation of a posterior mass with clinical suspicion of spinal cord compression may require myelography in cases where the MRI scan is nondiagnostic.

Invasive Diagnostic Tests

Fine-needle Aspiration Biopsy

Fine-needle aspiration biopsy is performed by placing a narrow-gauge needle into the mediastinal mass using fluoroscopy, CT, or ultrasonography for guidance, thereby obtaining material for cytopathologic examination. The procedure is remarkably free of major complications. From reports in the literature (9–11,40–46), the incidence of pneumothorax is 15% to 20%, but few cases required insertion of a chest tube. One series sampled five "masses" that were found to be aortic aneurysms without ensuing complications (10). Minor hemoptysis is also frequently reported. Fine-needle aspiration is quite accurate both in identifying malignant cells and in determining their specific histology (Table 33-2). Combining data from several studies (9–11,44), its sensitivity is 82% and its specificity is 100%. In deriving these operating characteristics, inadequate, indeterminant, and benign aspirates were all considered negative results (not diagnostic of malignancy). Likelihood ratios for the various test results are as follows: infinite for a malignant aspirate, 0.3 for an inadequate or indeterminant aspirate, and 0.1 for a benign aspirate. A study limited to anterior mediastinal masses reported a lower sensitivity (63%), which was mainly owing to the difficulty of identifying lymphoma (46).

Lymph-node Biopsy

Scalene lymph-node biopsy and/or mediastinoscopy for lymph-node biopsy are indicated if there is a suspicion of mediastinal lymphadenopathy, and the diagnosis has not been made by less invasive means. Scalene lymph node biopsy (whether or not there are palpable nodes) is most useful in diagnosing lymphoma and sarcoidosis; its sensitivity is 70% to 90% (12). The specimen should generally also be sent for culture.

Mediastinoscopy

Mediastinoscopy is used to obtain tissue from superior mediastinal masses and paratracheal lymph nodes. It is most helpful in the staging of bronchogenic cancer and lymphoma. When applied to the diagnosis of mediastinal masses in general, it has a rather low (32%) sensitivity for finding malignancy because of the limited area of the mediastinum accessible for biopsy (47). For lesions within the range of the mediastinoscope, the sensitivity is 93% (48). Thus, a negative mediastinoscopy does not rule out malignancy.

Surgical Biopsy

Surgical biopsy is the gold standard for establishing specific diagnoses in patients with mediastinal masses. Because mediastinal tumors have a pretest probability of malignancy of at least 20% and often much higher, surgery will generally be needed if a definitive diagnosis cannot be made by less invasive means. In a series of 129 patients requiring surgery for mediastinal mass, the diagnosis had not been established preoperatively in 32% (49). When the diagnosis is known, surgery may still be required for treatment.

The recent development of videothoracoscopy allows biopsy and removal of many mediastinal masses with much less morbidity than conventional thoracotomy (50,51). This endoscopic surgical technique can reach all the mediastinal compartments and is particularly well

Table 33-2. Operating Characteristics of Diagnostic Procedures in the Diagnosis of Mediastinal Masses

Diagnostic Test	Sensitivity	Specificity	Likelihood Ratio	
			Positive Result	Negative Result
	←——— % ———→			
Fine-needle aspiration biopsy	82	100	∞	0.18*
Scalene node biopsy	70–90	100	∞	0.10–0.30
Mediastinoscopy	32–93[†]	100	∞	0.07–0.68
Surgical biopsy	100	100	∞	0

*"Negative" fine-needle aspiration biopsy results include benign histologic findings (likelihood ratio = 0.1) and indeterminate and inadequate specimens (likelihood ratio = 0.3)

[†]The lower number is for all patients, the higher number is for patients who have lesions within reach of the mediastinoscope.

suited for evaluating anterior masses and lymph nodes in the aorticopulmonary and periazygous regions (50). If videothoracoscopy is unavailable, an open surgical approach should be used to obtain tissue for definitive diagnosis.

DIAGNOSTIC STRATEGIES

Chest radiography should be the first step in the diagnostic evaluation. Then, depending on the clinical setting and radiographic findings, including location, one or more tests may be indicated that, when positive, may be adequate to make a definitive diagnosis. These tests, which are not part of the evaluation of all patients, include barium swallow to evaluate suspected esophageal tumors, diverticula, or hernias; radioiodine scan to evaluate suspected substernal thyroid; and ultrasonography if a cystic lesion is a consideration. The remaining patients should have a CT or MRI scan to better define the location and extent of the mass. The major utility of these noninvasive tests is in defining the location of the mass and differentiating tumors from anatomic anomalies. Because of the wide variety of mediastinal tumors, many of which are malignant, subsequent tissue biopsy is often required.

If the diagnosis is still uncertain, a fine-needle aspiration biopsy is indicated when technically feasible. Table 33-3 shows the effect of pretest probability of malignancy on post-test probabilities for various fine-needle aspiration biopsy results. Because there are no false-positive diagnoses of malignancy, the finding of malignant cells requires no further diagnostic investigation unless the specific histology of the cells can not be determined. However, except for situations when the pretest probability of malignancy is very low, a benign, indeterminant, or inadequate specimen should generally be worked up further with a surgical biopsy because the post-test probability of malignancy in these situations is not negligible. When there is a suspicion that the mass represents lymph nodes, then a scalene lymph node biopsy or medi-

Table 33-3. Post-test Probabilities for Fine-needle Aspiration Biopsy in the Diagnosis of Mediastinal Masses

Biopsy Result	Pretest Probability		
	20%	50%	80%
	←————————— % —————————→		
Malignant cells	100	100	100
Indeterminate or inadequate specimen	7	23	55
Negative	2	9	29

astinoscopy should be considered because hilar nodes are difficult to sample by fine-needle aspiration. If these procedures are not indicated or nondiagnostic, then surgery, videothoracoscopy if available, may be needed for definitive diagnosis and, if appropriate, resection of the lesion.

CLINICAL PROBLEMS

Clinical Problem 1

An asymptomatic patient is noted to have unilateral hilar fullness suggesting lymphadenopathy.

Testing Strategy and Rationale

The suspicion of hilar lymphadenopathy should be confirmed by CT. Hilar lymph nodes are technically difficult to sample by fine-needle aspiration, and the specimen is often uninterpretable. Therefore, if tissue is required for histopathology, one should consider scalene lymph-node biopsy or mediastinoscopy. Otherwise videothoracoscopy or open thoracotomy should be performed for definitive diagnosis.

Clinical Example

A 45-year-old woman is discovered to have left hilar fullness on a chest radiograph taken after a fall from a ladder. The patient has no symptoms other than chest-wall tenderness. A CT scan suggests left hilar and paratracheal lymphadenopathy. The patient requires further evaluation with either scalene lymph-node biopsy, mediastinoscopy, or videothoracoscopy. Subsequent lymph-node histology shows non-Hodgkin lymphoma.

Clinical Problem 2

A patient has an anterior mediastinal mass.

Testing Strategy and Rationale

If the CT scan suggests the possibility of retrosternal thyroid, a radioiodine scan should be obtained. Otherwise tissue for histopathologic diagnosis should be obtained by fine-needle aspiration or surgical biopsy.

Clinical Example

A 25-year-old man complains of anorexia and fatigue. A chest radiograph shows an anterior mediastinal mass, which is confirmed by a CT scan. The mass appears distinct from the thyroid gland. Fine-needle aspiration biopsy shows a germ-cell tumor.

REFERENCES

1. **Silverman NA, Sabiston DC Jr.** Primary tumors and cysts of the mediastinum. Curr Probl Cancer. 1977;2:1-55.

2. **Fontenelle LJ, Armstrong RG, Stranford W, et al.** The asymptomatic mediastinal mass. Arch Surg. 1971;102:98-102.

3. **Benjamin SP, McCormack LJ, Effler DB, Groves LK.** Primary tumors of the mediastinum. Chest. 1972;62:297-303.

4. **Wychulis AR, Payne WS, Clagett OT, Woolner LB.** Surgical treatment of mediastinal tumors. J Thorac Cardiovasc Surg. 1971;62:379-92.

5. **Conkle DM, Adkins RB Jr.** Primary malignant tumors of the mediastinum. Ann Thorac Surg. 1972;14:553-67.

6. **Davis RD Jr, Oldham HN Jr, Sabiston DC Jr.** Primary cysts and neoplasms of the mediastinum: recent changes in clinical presentation, methods of diagnosis, management, and results. Ann Thorac Surg. 1987;44: 229-37.

7. **Mullen B, Richardson JD.** Primary anterior mediastinal tumors in children and adults. Ann Thorac Surg. 1986;42:338-45.

8. **Lyons HA, Calvy GL, Sammons BP.** The diagnosis and classification of mediastinal masses: a study of 782 cases. Ann Intern Med. 1959;51:897-929.

9. **Weisbrod GL, Lyons DJ, Tao LC, Chamberlain DW.** Percutaneous fine-needle aspiration biopsy of mediastinal lesions. AJR Am J Roentgenol. 1984;143:525-9.

10. **Westcott JL.** Percutaneous needle aspiration of hilar and mediastinal masses. Radiology. 1981;141:323-9.

11. **Adler OB, Rosenberger A, Peleg H.** Fine-needle aspiration biopsy of mediastinal masses: evaluation of 136 experiences. AJR Am J Roentgenol. 1983; 140:893-6.

12. **Lillington GA, Jamplis RW.** A Diagnostic Approach to Chest Diseases. Baltimore: Williams & Wilkins Co; 1977:436-61.

13. **Stark P.** Imaging mediastinal tumors. CA. 1987;37:211-24.

14. **Livesay JJ, Mink JH, Fee HJ, et al.** The use of computed tomography to evaluate suspected mediastinal tumors. Ann Thorac Surg. 1979;27:305-11.

15. **Crowe JK, Brown LR, Muhm JR.** Computed tomography of the mediastinum. Radiology. 1981;128:75-87.

16. **Godwin JD, Herfkens RL, Skiöldebrand CG, et al.** Evaluation of dissections and aneurysms of the thoracic aorta by conventional and dynamic CT scanning. Radiology. 1980;136:125-33.

17. **Marvasti MA, Mitchell GE, Burke WA, Meyer JA.** Misleading density of mediastinal cysts on computerized tomography. Ann Thorac Surg. 1981;31:167-70.

18. **Moore AV, Korobkin M, Powers B, et al.** Thymoma detection by mediastinal CT: patients with myasthenia gravis. AJR Am J Roentgenol. 1982;138: 217-22.

19. **Moeller KH, Rosado de Christenson ML, Templeton PA.** Mediastinal mature teratoma: imaging features. AJR Am J Roentgenol. 1997;169:985-90.

20. **Siegel JM, Nadel SN, Glazer HS, Sagel SS.** Mediastinal lesions in children: comparison of CT and MR. Radiology. 1986;160:241-4.

21. **Levitt RG, Glazer HS, Roper CL, et al.** Magnetic resonance imaging of mediastinal and hilar masses: comparison with CT. AJR Am J Roentgenol. 1985;145:9-14.

22. **Poon PY, Bronskill MJ, Menkelman MR, et al.** Magnetic resonance imaging of the mediastinum. J Can Assoc Radiol. 1986;37:173-81.

23. **Von Schulthess GK, McMurdo K, Tscholakoff D, et al.** Mediastinal masses: MR imaging. Radiology. 1986;158:289-96.

24. **Epstein DM, Kressel H, Gefter W, et al.** MR imaging of the mediastinum: a retrospective comparison with computed tomography. J Comput Assist Tomogr. 1984;8:670-6.

25. **Batra P, Brown K, Collins JD, et al.** Mediastinal masses: magnetic resonance imaging in comparison with computed tomography. J Natl Med Assoc. 1991;83:969-74.

26. **Ikezoe J, Takeuchi N, Tsuyoshi J.** MRI of anterior mediastinal tumors. Radiat Med. 1992;10:176-83.

27. **Rice TW.** Benign neoplasms and cysts of the mediastinum. Semin Thorac Cardiovasc Surg. 1992;4:25-33.

28. **Saenz NC, Schnitzer JJ, Eraklis AE, et al.** Posterior mediastinal masses. J Pediatr Surg. 1993;28:172-6.

29. **Wernecke K, Peters PE, Galanski M.** Mediastinal tumors: evaluation with suprasternal sonography. Radiology. 1986;159:405-9.

30. **Wernecke K, Potter R, Peters PE, Koch P.** Parasternal mediastinal sonography: sensitivity in the detection of anterior mediastinal and subcarinal tumors. AJR Am J Roentgenol. 1988;150:1021-6.

31. **Mancuso L, Pitrolo F, Bondi F, et al.** Echocardiographic recognition of mediastinal masses. Chest. 1988;93:144-8.

32. **Wernecke K, Vassallo P, Pötter R, et al.** Mediastinal tumors: sensitivity of detection with sonography compared with CT and radiography. Radiology. 1990;175:137-43.

33. **Leestuzzi C, Nicholosi GL, Mimo R, et al.** Usefulness of transesophageal echocardiography in evaluation of paracardia neoplastic masses. Am J Cardiol. 1992;70:247-51.

34. **Friday RO.** Paracardiac cyst: diagnosis by ultrasound and puncture. JAMA. 1973;226:82.

35. **Saito T, Kobayashi H, Sugama Y, et al.** Ultrasonically guided needle biopsy in the diagnosis of mediastinal masses. Am Rev Respir Dis. 1988;138:679-84.

36. **Samad SA, Sharifah NA, Zulfiqar MA, et al.** Ultrasound guided percutaneous biopsies of suspected mediastinal lesions. Med J Malaysia. 1993;48:421-6.

37. **Hsu WH, Chaing CD, Hsu JY, et al.** Ultrasonically guided needle biopsy of anterior mediastinal masses: comparison of carcinomatous and non-carcinomatous masses. J Clin Ultrasound. 1995;23:349-56.

38. **Bonte FJ, Curry TS.** Radionuclide scanning in the diagnosis of mediastinal masses. Semin Roentgenol. 1969;4:33-40.

39. **Miyame T.** Interpretation of ^{99m}Tc superior vena cavograms and results of studies in 92 patients. Radiology. 1973;108:339-52.

40. **Jareb M, Us-Krašovec M.** Transthoracic needle biopsy of mediastinal and hilar lesions. Cancer. 1977;40:1354-7.

41. **Gobien RP, Skucas J, Paris BS.** CT-assisted fluoroscopically guided aspiration biopsy of central hilar and mediastinal masses. Radiology. 1981; 141:443-7.

42. **Jereb M.** The usefulness of needle biopsy in chest lesions of different sizes and locations. Radiology. 1980;134:13-5.

43. **Sterrett G, Whitaker D, Shilkin KB, Walters M.** The fine needle aspiration cytology of mediastinal lesions. Cancer. 1983;51:127-35.

44. **Linder J, Olsen GA, Johnston WW.** Fine-needle aspiration biopsy of the mediastinum. Am J Med. 1986;81:1005-8.

45. **Böcking A, Klose KC, Kyll HJ, Hauptmann S.** Cytologic versus histologic evaluation of needle biopsy of the lung, hilum and mediastinum. Acta Cytol. 1995;39:463-71.

46. **Herman SJ, Holub RV, Weisbrod GL, Chamberlain DW.** Anterior mediastinal masses: utility of transthoracic needle biopsy. Radiology. 1991;108: 167-70.

47. **Schoolmeesters JEPV.** Experience with the Artronix Torso-Cat-Scanner in the examination of the thorax, particularly the mediastinum: comparison with mediastinoscopy and operation. Diagn Imag. 1983;52:93-100.

48. **Naylor AR, Elliott RC, Walker WS, et al.** Role of mediastinoscopy in the diagnosis of mediastinal masses. J R Coll Surg Edinb. 1990;35:98-100.

49. **Blegvad S, Lippert H, Simper LB, Dybdhal H.** Mediastinal tumours: a report of 129 cases. Scand J Thorac Cardiovasc. 1990;24:39-42.

50. **Landreneau RJ, Makc MJ, Hazelrigg SR, et al.** The role of thoracoscopy in the management of intrathoracic neoplastic processes. Semin Thorac Cardiovasc Surg. 1993;5:219-28.

51. **Yim APC.** Video-assisted thoracoscopic management of anterior mediastinal masses. Surg Endosc. 1995;9:1184-8.

Musculoskeletal and Immunologic Problems

Acute Monarticular Arthritis　34

N. Paul Hudson, MD

KEY POINTS

Pretest Probabilities

- In otherwise healthy adults, acute monarthritis is usually caused by gout or gonococcal arthritis.
- Gonococcal arthritis typically occurs in healthy young persons.
- Acute gouty arthritis is uncommon in premenopausal women.
- Co-occurrence of gout and rheumatoid disease is rare.
- Nongonococcal joint infection usually occurs in patients who are elderly or chronically ill.

Diagnostic Strategies

- Joint aspiration is the diagnostic standard for infectious and crystal-induced arthritis. Identification of synovial crystals is highly sensitive and 100% specific.
- Measurement of serum uric acid is a poor test for the presence or absence of gout.
- Gram stain of synovial fluid is fairly sensitive (~65%) for nongonococcal joint sepsis.
- Gonococcal arthropathy is rapidly responsive to antibiotic therapy; a therapeutic trial may be the only method to confirm the diagnosis.

BACKGROUND

The differential diagnosis of acute monarthritis is extensive; most rheumatic diseases can present in this way. The disorders that require prompt, specific treatment are infectious and crystal-induced arthritis, which are the focus of this chapter. Ideally, these diagnoses are made by synovial fluid analysis. Difficulties arise when synovial fluid is unavailable or when analysis is inconclusive. Crystal-induced disease is not destructive acutely, but the patient usually wants prompt relief. The outcome of joint sepsis varies depending on the organism and the timing of appropriate treatment. Thus, timely therapeutic choices must be made.

ESTIMATING PRETEST PROBABILITY

The approach to the patient with acute monarthritis varies depending on the patient's age, sex, and medical history. In healthy adult patients with acute monarthritis, the probability of nongonococcal joint sepsis is estimated to be less than 10%. Pyogenic joint infections in adults are seen primarily in ill and elderly persons, except in cases of trauma or parenteral drug abuse (1). Gonococcal arthropathy (GA) is a disease that occurs in sexually active adults; it is more common in women than in men, and in patients with complement deficiency (2). Gouty arthritis is a disease that occurs in adult men and elderly women (3). Thus, in adolescents, young adults, and premenopausal women, GA is more likely to occur, whereas in older men, gout is more likely to occur. In younger men, the likelihood of the two diseases may be similar.

Findings that suggest gonococcal arthropathy include prodromal myalgias, migratory arthralgias, fever, dermatitis, or tenosynovitis. These findings are seen in approximately 65% of patients (1). Diagnostic criteria for gouty arthritis have been formulated for research purposes (4). These criteria identify the most characteristic clinical findings (Table 34-1). When six or more are present, the sensitivity is 87% and the specificity is 96%. Acute gouty arthritis is typically an episodic monarthritis that develops rapidly with exquisite pain, heat, erythema, and swelling. First metatarsophalangeal arthritis (podagra) is common, and patients are not febrile

Table 34-1. Criteria for Diagnosis of Gouty Arthritis

More than one attack of acute arthritis

Development of maximal inflammation in 1 day

Monarthritis

Joint erythema

First metatarsophalangeal pain or swelling

Unilateral first metatarsophalangeal acute arthritis

Unilateral tarsal acute arthritis

Tophus (suspected or proven)

Asymmetric joint swelling (by radiography or examination)

Hyperuricemia

Bone cysts without erosions on radiography

Negative joint fluid culture

unless multiple joints are involved (5). A history of a similar disorder responsive to colchicine, renal colic (urate stone), or subcutaneous nodules (tophi) suggests gout. Pseudogout, which results from deposition of calcium pyrophosphate dihydrate crystals (CPPD), is so named because its clinical presentation is similar to gouty arthritis. It frequently affects the knee or wrist, attacks may be precipitated by trauma, and it also occurs more frequently in older patients.

In patients with monarthritis who are elderly or chronically ill, nongonococcal joint sepsis is more likely. In rheumatoid arthritis, the likelihood of acute gout is very small (6), so acute monarthritis should be assumed to be caused by a flare of disease or infection. Crystal-induced disease is typically recurrent and may cause a monarticular flare. Gonococcal arthropathy is also a possible diagnosis in these patients.

DIAGNOSTIC TESTS

Immunologic Tests
Immunologic tests have minimal value in the diagnosis of acute monarticular arthritis. Diagnosis of any connective tissue disease requires having a chronic polyarthritis for the rheumatoid factor or antinuclear antibody (ANA) to have meaning. The erythrocyte sedimentation rate and C-reactive protein only confirm the obvious inflammation. None of the diagnoses under consideration should be excluded using these studies.

Radiographs
Radiographs are useful only for detecting trauma, pathologic fracture, or acute calcific tendonitis (7). Thus, they are helpful only in cases of monarticular arthritis when there is concern that trauma or pathologic fracture may be producing local swelling and pain. Chondrocalcinosis, associated with pseudogout, may be seen on a radiograph, but its presence does not exclude a septic joint.

Serum Uric Acid
Measurement of the serum uric acid level has modest utility. Hyperuricemia is common and often asymptomatic. In the Framingham study, gout occurred in participants with normal uric acid levels (8). The sensitivity and specificity of an elevated serum urate level for gouty arthritis are about 90% and 54%, respectively (Table 34-2). Thus, an elevated level is not specific for gout and a normal level does not completely rule out the diagnosis.

Synovial Fluid Analysis
Synovial fluid analysis, based on cell counts, cell differential, Gram stain, and crystal examination, is the most useful study for acute

monarthritis. An leukoctye count of more than 3000/mm^3 with more than 70% polymorphonuclear leukocytes (PMNs) indicates inflammation. In infected joints, the leukocyte count is usually greater than 50,000, with more than 90% PMNs (9). A Gram stain of joint fluid is positive in 65% of patients with pyogenic infection, ranging from 75% with staphylococcal infection to 50% for gram-negative organisms to less than 25% for gonococcal disease (1).

Acute crystal-induced disease causes synovial leukocytosis with leukocyte and PMN counts comparable to those of joint sepsis. Microscopic examination for crystals of monosodium urate (gout) has a sensitivity of 85% and is nearly 100% specific (4). However, sepsis may coexist with crystal disease (10). The less obvious CPPD crystals are seen in only 60% to 70% of aspirates from those patients with pseudogout.

Crystal Examination of Tophi

Tophaceous deposits are present in no more than 30% of gout patients, but confirmation by crystal examination is 99% specific for gouty arthritis (4).

Table 34-2. Operating Characteristics of Diagnosis Tests for Monarticular Arthritis

Diagnostic Test	Sensitivity	Specificity	Likelihood Ratio	
			Positive Result	Negative Result
	←——— % ———→			
Gouty arthritis				
Criteria (6+)	87	96	22	0.13
Criteria (5+)	95	89	8.6	0.05
Serum urate level >7 mg/dL	90	54	1.9	0.19
Crystal examination	85	99	85	0.15
Tophus (proven)	30	99	30	0.71
Gonococcal septic arthritis				
Synovial culture	25	99	25	0.75
Gram stain	25	99	25	0.75
All other cultures	50	99	50	0.50
Nongonococcal septic arthritis				
Gram stain	65	99	65	0.35
Blood culture	50	95	10	0.52

DIAGNOSTIC STRATEGIES

In patients with acute monarthritis, joint aspiration and synovial fluid analysis are critical for definitive diagnosis. A clinical history of gout and identification of a tophus may provide near certainty without a joint aspiration (Table 34-3). A Gram stain and culture should be obtained in elderly or chronically ill patients, regardless of crystal examination results.

In a previously healthy young woman with monarthritis, gono-coccal disease is highly likely if gout cannot be crystal-proven. Although joint fluid Gram stain or cultures or both are positive in fewer than 25% of cases, the chance of a bacteriologic diagnosis is vastly improved by culturing the blood, cervix and urethra, and other possible sources of gonococcal bacteremia (1). A prompt response (48 to 72 hours) to appropriate antibiotics supports the diagnosis. A similar strategy applies to young men. In young adults, the possibility of reactive arthritis (arthritis occurring after an acute infection) presenting as monarthritis, instead of the usual polyarthritis, may also be considered.

Table 34-3. Post-test Probabilities of Monarticular Arthritis Based on Results of Diagnostic Tests

Diagnostic test	Pretest Probabilities					
	20%		50%		80%	
	Positive Result	Negative Result	Positive Result	Negative Result	Positive Result	Negative Result
	←			%		→
Gouty arthritis						
Criteria (6+)	85	3	95	12	99	34
Criteria (5+)	68	1	89	5	97	17
Serum urate level > 7 mg/dL	32	5	66	16	88	43
Crystal examination	95	4	99	14	99+	39
Tophus (proven)	88	15	96	41	99	74
Gonococcal septic arthritis						
Gram stain	86	16	96	43	99	75
Synovial culture	86	16	96	43	99	75
All other cultures	93	11	98	34	99+	67
Nongonococcal septic arthritis						
Gram stain	94	8	98	26	99+	58
Blood culture	71	12	91	35	98	68

In healthy older men and postmenopausal women, gout is more likely. When the diagnosis is not confirmed by microscopic examination for synovial crystals or by Gram stain of synovial fluid, five or more clinical criteria strongly suggest gout, especially if the patient does not have clinical features of disseminated gonococcal disease. In patients who do not have five or more criteria for gout, empiric treatment for gonococcal disease may be indicated as a therapeutic and diagnostic maneuver, depending on the clinical evaluation, anticipating prompt response to antibiotics or confirmation by culture results.

In elderly or chronically ill patients with acute monarthritis, joint sepsis should be suspected, even in patients who do not have fever or leukocytosis. Treatment for joint sepsis should be initiated unless crystals are identified and the Gram stain is negative. The presence of hyperuricemia, which may be caused by renal insufficiency, salicylates, or diuretics, is difficult to interpret in these patients and should not influence therapy.

In evaluating patients with acute monarthritis, clinicians need to remember that most rheumatic diseases can present as monarthritis. Thus, when the evaluation outlined above fails to confirm that either crystal-induced or infectious arthritis is likely, other rheumatic disorders must then be considered.

CLINICAL PROBLEMS

Clinical Problem 1
A healthy young adult has a first episode of monarthritis.

Testing Strategy and Rationale
The joint should be aspirated, and synovial fluid analysis should be performed. Immunologic studies and measurement of the serum uric acid level are not indicated, nor are radiographic studies unless trauma is suspected. The high probability of gonococcal arthritis can be offset only by the specificity of finding crystals on examination of the fluid.

Clinical Example
A 28-year-old sexually active woman presents with a first episode of right knee pain and swelling. She reports that she has not had previous myalgias and has no skin lesions. Aspirate of the knee yields cloudy fluid with a leukocyte count of 35,000/mm^3 and 85% PMNs. Unless monosodium urate crystals are seen, gonococcal arthritis is highly likely and treatment should be started.

Clinical Problem 2

A middle-aged patient with a history of several episodes of monarthritis presents with what he presumes is another episode of "gout".

Testing Strategy and Rationale

The joint should be aspirated and synovial fluid analysis should be performed. In a patient who has had multiple episodes of monarthritis, gout may or may not be the cause of the current episode. Unless he is chronically ill or immunosuppressed, nongonococcal joint sepsis is highly unlikely. A careful history, joint aspiration, and serum urate may all be useful in making a diagnosis. Immunologic studies and radiography are not indicated.

Clinical Example

A 45-year-old man presents with a 2-day history of wrist stiffness, a low-grade fever, and a "gouty flare" of the right knee. Although he has had similar attacks in the past, none have been crystal-proven and none have involved the knee. He denies dysuria or urethral discharge. He takes a diuretic for hypertension and has a serum urate level of 7.9 mg/dL. His clinical evaluation detects only three of the criteria for gouty arthritis. Aspirate of fluid from the knee shows a leukocyte count of 65,000/mm^3 with 92% PMNs, and examination for organisms and crystals yields negative results. Despite the patient's history of "gout," owing to the absence of crystals and because the patient has few clinical criteria for gouty arthritis, a presumptive diagnosis of gonococcal arthritis is made and treatment with antibiotics is begun.

REFERENCES

1. **Goldenberg DL, Reed JI.** Medical progress: bacterial arthritis. N Engl J Med. 1985;312:764-71.
2. **O'Brien JP, Goldenberg DL, Rice PA.** Disseminated gonococcal infection: a prospective analysis of 49 patients and a review of pathophysiology and immune mechanisms. Medicine. 1983;62:395-406.
3. **Levinson DJ.** Clinical gout and the pathogenesis of hyperuricemia. In: McCarty DJ, ed. Arthritis and Allied Conditions: A Textbook of Rheumatology. Philadelphia: Lea and Febiger; 1989:1645-76.
4. **Wallace SL, Robinson H, Masi AT, et al.** Preliminary criteria for the classification of the acute arthritis of primary gout. Arth Rheum. 1977; 20:895-900.
5. **Hadler NM, Franck WA, Bress NM, et al.** Acute polyarticular gout. Am J Med. 1974; 56:715-9.

6. **Rizzoli AJ, Trujeque L, Bankhurst AD.** The coexistence of gout and rheumatoid arthritis: case reports and review of the literature. J Rheumatol. 1980;7:316-24.

7. **Claudepierre P, Rahmouni A, Bergamasco P, et al.** Misleading clinical aspects of hydroxyapatite deposits: a series of 15 cases. J Rheumatol. 1997;24:531-5.

8. **Hall AP, Barry PE, Dawber TR, et al.** Epidemiology of gout and hyperuricemia: a long term population study. Am J Med. 1967;42:27-37.

9. **Krey PR, Bailen DA.** Synovial fluid leukocytosis. Am J Med. 1979;67:436-42.

10. **Lurie DP, Musil G.** Staphylococcal septic arthritis presenting as acute flare of pseudogout: clinical, pathological and arthroscopic findings with a review of the literature. J Rheumatol. 1983; 10:503-6.

Low Back Pain Syndromes   **35**

Daniel J. Mazanec, MD

KEY POINTS

Pretest Probabilities

- Low back pain is common, with a lifetime prevalence for adults of 60% to 90%. In as many as 80% of persons with acute low back pain, a precise anatomic cause cannot be identified. Nonmechanical causes of acute low back pain whose identification affects treatment, such as cancer, infection, and aortic aneurysm, are identified in fewer that 1% of unselected populations with low back pain.

- In patients older than 65 years, lumbar spinal stenosis is a common cause of low back pain.

- In patients with chronic low back pain for which the cause is unknown, a specific cause is eventually identified in as many as 15% of cases—most often malignancy, visceral causes (endometriosis, inflammatory bowel disease), or inflammatory spondyloarthropathy.

- In patients with chronic low back pain for which the cause is unknown, complicating psychosocial problems including anxiety, depression, litigation, compensation, and substance abuse are present in as many as 60% of cases.

Diagnostic Strategies

- Lumbar spine radiography is not indicated in the initial evaluation of most patients with acute low back pain.

- In selected patients with acute low back pain and in most patients with chronic low back pain (>6 weeks' duration) anteroposterior and lateral lumbar spine radiographs are appropriate.

- In patients in whom infectious or neoplastic causes of low back pain are suspected, bone scanning or magnetic resonance imaging should be performed.

Continued

- In patients with radicular symptoms unresponsive to conservative therapy, imaging studies, such as magnetic resonance imaging or computed tomography, should be performed at the time of surgical consultation.
- In patients in whom inflammatory spondyloarthropathy is suspected, a posteroanterior radiography of the pelvis is the initial test of choice.

BACKGROUND

Low back pain is an extremely common problem in adult patients, with an annual incidence of approximately 5% and a lifetime prevalence of 60% to 90% (1,2). Approximately 1% of patients with back pain describe true radicular symptoms, or sciatica, resulting from compression and/or inflammation of one or more lumbosacral nerve roots (1). Back symptoms may be acute (<6 weeks' duration) or chronic (>6 weeks' duration), mechanical or nonmechanical. Mechanical causes of low back pain or radicular symptoms result from structural spinal abnormalities. Nonmechanical causes include inflammatory and malignant spinal conditions as well as nonspinal sources—for example, hip osteoarthritis, diabetic neuropathy, aortic aneurysm. Table 35-1 lists the common causes of low back pain.

In as many as 85% of patients, the precise anatomic source of acute low back pain cannot be identified (1,2). For example, clinical features are not reliable in establishing whether the facet joint or the lumbar disk is the cause of pain in persons with acute low back pain (3,4). However, serious, nonmechanical causes of low back pain such as malignancy or infection are rare, occurring in fewer than 1% of patients with low back pain presenting to primary care physicians (5,6). Furthermore, the natural history of acute back pain is favorable—the median time to recovery is 14 days and most persons with this condition return to work within 1 month (7,8). In most patients with acute low back pain, if the initial careful history and physical examination fail to reveal "red flags" of serious underlying disease, further diagnostic testing is unnecessary. Patients who do not respond to conservative therapy and have persistent or worsening symptoms merit further evaluation.

The evaluation of patients with persistent chronic back pain should focus on identifying common mechanical causes of chronic back pain. Serious, nonmechanical causes such as malignancy or infection should be considered, the adequacy of previous treatment should be assessed, and the presence of complicating psychosocial problems that may be barriers to recovery should be sought.

Sciatica, radiating leg pain often extending below the knee, is noted in 1.5% of persons with back pain (9). In younger patients, true radicular pain is most often a result of lumbar nerve root compression or inflammation by a herniated lumbar disk or both. At least 70% of patients with disk herniation and sciatica improve substantially with

Table 35-1. Common Causes of Low Back Pain

Acute	Chronic
Mechanical	Mechanical
Fracture	Degenerative disk/joint disease
Disk herniation	Severe spondylolisthesis
Myofascial strain/sprain	Severe kyphoscoliosis
Facet syndrome	Nonmechanical
Nonmechanical	Disk space infection
Visceral	Osteomyelitis
Aneurysm	Malignancy
Endometriosis	Multiple myeloma
Inflammatory bowel disease	Metastatic
Renal colic	Spondyloarthropathy
Pancreatitis	Fibromyalgia
Penetrating ulcer	Paget disease
Prostatitis	
Pelvic inflammatory disease	

nonoperative, "conservative" therapy within 2 to 4 weeks (10). In persons older than 50 years of age, spinal stenosis is a frequent cause of radicular leg pain. The natural history of untreated spinal stenosis is not well studied but perhaps as many as two thirds of persons with symptomatic stenosis show no significant worsening when followed for as long as 4 years (11). Preliminary study suggests nonoperative treatment may be effective in as many as two thirds of persons with this condition (12). As with nonsciatic low back pain, further initial diagnostic evaluation beyond careful history and physical examination is not indicated unless cauda equina syndrome is suspected or rapidly progressive weakness is noted. Urgent surgical therapy may be required in these situations. In evaluating patients with sciatica, the possibility of "pseudosciatica" caused, for example, by hip disease, trochanteric bursitis, or meralgia paresthetica must also be considered.

This chapter focuses on the diagnostic evaluation of patients with acute and chronic back pain as well as with sciatica. In the evaluation of all these groups, the frequent low likelihood of finding a specific cause for the back pain and the response to nonoperative, nonpharmacologic therapy are important considerations when planning even noninvasive diagnostic studies. Identification of patients requiring urgent, specific therapy is emphasized in this chapter.

ESTIMATING PRETEST PROBABILITY

The prevalence of patients with nonmechanical back pain requiring specific therapy is estimated to be approximately 1%. In a large primary care series, the most common systemic disease resulting in back pain (i.e., malignancy) was found in 0.66% of all patients (5). The prevalence of ankylosing spondylitis in a general population is estimated to be 0.1% to 0.3% (13).

Infectious causes such as diskitis or osteomyelitis are found in fewer than 0.01% of patients in a primary care practice (6). Compression fractures (acute mechanical pain) are found in approximately 4% of patients with acute back pain in the primary care setting (9). Sacral insufficiency fractures were reported in 0.16% of patients admitted to a hospital from an internal medicine practice and may present as low back pain (14). Sets of clinical historical criteria useful in identifying patients with a higher probability of back pain resulting from malignancy (5), spondyloarthropathy (15,16), infection (17), and fracture (9,14) are detailed in Table 35-2.

Physical findings in patients with acute low back pain are frequently not helpful in identifying the cause of pain. Clinical tests to examine and stress sacroiliac joints are unreliable and do not appear to help distinguish between ankylosing spondylitis and noninflammatory back disorders (18,19). In patients suspected of having "discogenic" back pain, a controversial entity, no significant association was found between historical and examination findings and positive discography results (4). The lumbosacral facet joints may be a source of pain in some persons—that is, the lumbar facet syndrome. However, no set of clinical features has been found to correlate with relief of back pain produced by injection of the facet joint with a local anesthetic (3). Furthermore, no correlation between facet block results and the outcome of surgical or nonoperative treatment was demonstrated in a study of 126 patients undergoing diagnostic facet injection (20).

Chronic low back pain is often complicated by psychosocial problems such as compensation, litigation, psychiatric disorders, and substance abuse. Fifty-nine percent of 200 patients with chronic low back pain were found by structured psychiatric interview to have at least one current psychiatric diagnosis, most commonly major depression, substance abuse, or anxiety disorders (21). Assessment for evidence of psychological distress, such as vegetative signs of depression, should be considered in persons with chronic nonspecific low back pain. The "pain drawing" is a useful screening technique for nonorganic issues (22,23). In pain drawings, patients mark the nature and distribution of their pain on a standard silhouette of the human body; nonanatomic distribution of markings and markings outside the figure suggest a high likelihood of nonorganic pain. The Waddell tests, a set of five observations made during the physical examination, are also useful in identifying patients with psychosocial problems (24). The sensitivity of a high Waddell score (>3) for the presence of nonorganic problems is

Table 35-2. Identification of Patients with High Probability of Back Pain from Malignancy, Infection, Fracture, or Spondyloarthropathy

Clinical Criteria	Sensitivity	Specificity	Likelihood Ratio Positive Result	Likelihood Ratio Negative Result
	← % →			
For malignancy				
Age >50 y	77	71	2.7	0.32
Unexplained weight loss	85	94	14.0	0.16
History of cancer (except skin)	31	98	16.0	0.70
Visit within last month for problem not improving	31	91	3.1	0.77
Any of the above findings	100	37	1.6	0
For osteomyelitis				
Intravenous drug abuse, urinary tract infection, or skin infection	40	NA	—	—
For spondyloarthropathy				
Pain >3 months	71–86	9–54	0.8–1.9	0.3–3.2
Morning stiffness of the back	64–95	29–59	0.9–2.3	0.1–1.2
Onset of symptoms at age <35 y	90	30	1.3	0.33
Insidious onset of symptoms	53–88	51–76	1.1–3.7	0.2–0.9
Discomfort improves with exercise	69–75	45–90	1.3–7.5	0.3–0.7
Pain makes patient get out of bed at night	65	79	3.1	0.44
Any four of first five criteria	95	85	6.3	0.06
For fracture				
Age >50 y	84–100	28	~1.3	~0.11
Trauma	30–63	85	2–4	0.4–0.8
Corticosteroid use	6–13	99.5	~10	~0.9

approximately 80% (Table 35-3). False-positive results occur in approximately 20% of patients tested (23).

In a patient younger than 55 years of age, the presence of sciatica (i.e., leg pain radiating posterolaterally down the leg to below the knee)

Table 35-3. Identification of Patients with High Probability of Psychosocial Problems Complicating Back Pain

Clinical Criteria	Sensitivity	Specificity	Likelihood Ratio	
			Positive Result	Negative Result
	← % →			
Waddell test score >3	82	80–100	~8	~0.2
Pain drawing	93			

is strongly suggestive of disk herniation and radiculopathy. Leg pain is typically greater than back pain and may be associated with numbness or paresthesia. The suspicion of a disk herniation is further supported by the finding of a positive ipsilateral straight leg-raise test result (sensitivity, approximately 80%) defined by reproduction of radicular leg pain with elevation of the affected leg less than 60 degrees in the supine position (9). The contralateral straight leg-raise test with reproduction of sciatica on elevation of the contralateral limb further increases the probability of herniation (25). Other important findings (Table 35-4), identified in approximately 50% of patients with lower lumbar radiculopathy, include ankle reflex loss and weakness of the extensor hallucis longus (26).

Lumbar canal stenosis leads to decompressive spinal surgery in 0.1% of adults older than 65 years of age (27). Although the actual prevalence of symptomatic stenosis is unknown, it is probably much higher. Historical features most strongly associated with the diagnosis of lumbar canal stenosis include older age, severe lower extremity pain, pseudo-claudication, and absence of pain when seated (28). Strongly suggestive physical findings include wide-based gait, abnormal Romberg test result, and thigh pain after 30 seconds of lumbar extension.

DIAGNOSTIC TESTS

Plain Lumbosacral Radiography

The sensitivity of technically adequate lumbosacral radiographs for causes of back pain requiring specific or urgent therapy is depicted in Table 35-5. For infectious causes, sensitivity ranges from up to 90% for osteomyelitis to 25% for disk space infection (6). The sensitivity of plain lumbar radiographs for vertebral fracture approaches 99%, but radiography of the pelvis is relatively insensitive (31%) in identifying sacral insufficiency fractures (6,14). The sensitivity for malignancy is approximately 65% to 70%. These estimates are based on data obtained at the patient's first visit. Radiography is much less sensitive early in the course

Table 35-4. Identification of Patients with High Probability of Radiculopathy from Disk Herniation and Spinal Stenosis

Clinical Criteria	Sensitivity	Specificity	Likelihood Ratio	
			Positive Result	Negative Result
	←——— % ———→			
For herniated disk/radiculopathy				
Sciatica	95	—	—	—
Positive ipsilateral straight leg-raise test result	80	40	1.3	0.5
Crossed straight-leg raise test result	25	90	2.5	0.8
Great toe extensor weakness	50	70	1.7	0.7
Impaired ankle reflex	50	60	1.3	0.8
For lumbar canal stenosis				
Age >65 y	77	69	2.5	0.3
Severe lower extremity pain	65	67	2.0	0.5
No pain when seated	46	93	6.6	0.6
Wide-based gait	43	97	14	0.6
Abnormal Romberg test result	39	91	4.3	0.7
Thigh pain after 30 seconds of lumbar extension	51	69	1.6	0.7

of infection and malignancy (29). Reliable data regarding the specificity of plain radiographs for neoplastic or infectious causes of back pain are not available, but estimates range from 90% for osteomyelitis to 25% for epidural infection (30).

The addition of oblique and spot lateral views to the standard anteroposterior (AP) and lateral views of the lumbar spine adds additional information in only 2% of cases while significantly increasing radiation exposure (31). Follow-up or serial examinations are also of low yield. In a large hospital series, 64% of follow-up examinations demonstrated no interval change and 32% demonstrated only expected healing or progressive degenerative change (32). Although lateral lumbosacral spine radiographs obtained with spinal flexion and extension are sometimes used to demonstrate "instability" (excess or abnormal anterior or posterior movement of adjoining vertebral bodies with spinal movement), clinically signifi-

Table 35-5. Operating Characteristics of Diagnostic Tests in the Evaluation of Back Pain

Diagnostic Test	Sensitivity	Specificity	Likelihood Ratio	
			Positive Result	Negative Result
	←————%————→			
For malignancy				
Plain radiography	70	90	7.0	0.33
Bone scanning	~95	70	3.2	0.07
CT	95	80	4.8	0.06
MRI	~97	?	—	—
ESR (>20 mm/h)	78	67	24	0.33
For osteomyelitis				
Plain radiography	80–90	70–90	2.7–9.0	0.11–0.29
Bone scanning	95	70	3.2	0.07
CT	95	80	4.8	0.06
MRI	96	92	12	0.04
ESR (>20 mm/h)	71–94	?	—	—
For vertebral fracture				
Plain radiography	99	31	1.4	0.03
Bone scanning	92	?	—	—
For spondyloarthropathy				
PA pelvic radiograph	50	90	5.0	0.56
CT	80	70	2.7	0.29
B27 (white pts.)	92	92	12	0.09
B27 (black pts.)	50	98	25.0	0.51
For Lumbar disk disease				
CT	~85	~65	2.4	0.23
MRI	~85	~70	2.8	0.5
Myelography	~75	~70	2.5	0.36

CT = computed tomography; ESR = erythrocyte sedimentation rate; MRI = magnetic resonance imaging; PA = posteroanterior.

cant "instability" warranting consideration of surgical fusion is not consistently defined.

Several commonly reported radiographic findings are of questionable clinical significance. These include disk space narrowing, spondylosis, lumbarization, sacralization, Schmorl nodes, spina bifida occulta, and disk calcification (33). No significant correlation between disk space height narrowing and low back pain can be demonstrated (34). In addition to the doubtful clinical importance of these radiographic observations, marked variability of interpretation of plain lumbar radiographs by different observers has been noted (35).

A single posteroanterior (PA) radiograph of the pelvis can be unequivocally interpreted in 70% to 80% of patients with low back pain in whom spondylitis is a diagnostic consideration (36). A plain PA view of the pelvis showing inflammatory changes in the sacroiliac joints has a sensitivity of approximately 50% for spondylitis (37). The sensitivity may be higher in well-established disease. In circumstances when the PA view is equivocal for changes of spondylitis, a series of views (PA, obliques, angled PA) has increased sensitivity (approximately 80%) and typically resolves the ambiguity (36).

Plain radiography is not helpful in the diagnosis of lumbar disk herniation; however, preoperative standing lateral plain radiographs may disclose an unsuspected spondylolisthesis that may affect the surgical decision to perform a fusion procedure in addition to the laminectomy or discectomy. Plain radiographs do not provide direct evidence of lumbar canal stenosis, although they may reveal degenerative changes consistent with its pathogenesis.

Radionuclide Imaging (Bone Scanning)

Radionuclide imaging is an excellent technique for the early detection of bone abnormalities. In general, infectious, neoplastic, or inflammatory disease that disturbs normal bone metabolism and is associated with increased osteoblastic activity results in increased activity on bone scan. This abnormality is detected on bone scan before abnormalities are detected by radiography. For example, in osteomyelitis, bone scans may show abnormality within 1 day of onset, whereas radiography may not reveal abnormality for 2 weeks (38). The sensitivity of the bone scan in detecting osteomyelitis is approximately 95% (39). Radionuclide imaging has been reported to have a sensitivity as high as approximately 97% in detecting bony malignancy in patients with musculoskeletal symptoms without known previous cancer (40). Approximately 30% of lesions identified on bone scan are benign and do not affect treatment (40,41).

Single photon emission computed tomography (SPECT) has been evaluated in the detection of sacroiliitis in patients with clinical features suggestive of spondyloarthropathy but in whom no diagnostic changes on plain radiographs are seen (42). The sensitivity of SPECT in these patients was 38%, with a specificity of 100%.

Computed Tomography

The sensitivity of computed tomography (CT) is comparable to that of bone scintigraphy in the detection of infectious or malignant causes of back pain. Osteomyelitis typically produces an early increase in vascular congestion, which can be detected by CT long before changes are seen in plain radiographs. The specificity of CT for infectious or malignant disease of the spine is approximately 80%. Computed tomography is superior to magnetic resonance imaging (MRI) in the evaluation of bony disease (e.g., fracture) and is less costly (43).

Computed tomography is more sensitive (80%) than radiography in detecting sacroiliitis (37). The specificity of this study is approximately 70%.

Computed tomography compares favorably with myelography and MRI in the detection of lumbar disk herniation, with a sensitivity of 72% to 97% (43–45). Abnormalities are present in 35% of asymptomatic persons by lumbar CT scan, including disk herniation, facet degeneration, and spinal stenosis (46). The sensitivity of CT for lumbar canal stenosis is approximately 80% (47).

Myelography

Myelography is clearly a more invasive procedure than CT or MRI. Severe headache occurs after this procedure in 5% to 10% of patients (43). The sensitivity of myelography in identifying disk herniation is slightly less than that of CT and MRI—approximately 75%. (43–45) The specificity for symptomatic disk herniation is 63% to 76% (44,48). In comparison with routine CT, myelography does offer visualization of the thoracolumbar junction, affording the opportunity to diagnose clinically silent spinal tumors in this region (45). Intrathecal enhanced CT (CT-myelography) is not superior to CT alone in identifying disk herniation (sensitivity, 77%) (43).

Magnetic Resonance Imaging

In a comparative study of patients with a high likelihood of vertebral osteomyelitis, MRI has been shown to have a sensitivity of 96% and a specificity of 92%. In this study, bone scanning had a sensitivity of 90% but a specificity of only 78% (49). Magnetic resonance imaging is probably also more sensitive than bone scanning in the detection of malignant causes of back pain (50). Other advantages of MRI over bone scanning in the evaluation of infectious or malignant disease include a better assessment of paravertebral soft tissue as well as differentiation of degenerative change from infection. The bone scan, on the other hand, offers whole-body surveillance.

Magnetic resonance imaging is highly sensitive for disk herniation and spinal stenosis, approximately 85%, about the same as CT and superior to myelography (43). Gadolinium-enhanced MRI is useful in assessing postoperative patients in whom enhancing epidural scar can be distinguished from recurrent disk herniation. As with CT, abnormalities are frequently detected by MRI in asymptomatic persons. Disk bulge is found in more than 50% of asymptomatic persons and disk herniation in 28% to 36% (51,52). Nonintervertebral disk abnormalities, including Schmorl nodes, facet arthropathy, and spinal stenosis, are also common findings in asymptomatic patients.

Discography

Lumbar discography is a controversial procedure based on the concept that internal disk disruption is a potential cause of back pain (53). The test evaluates the qualitative pain response as well as quantitative anatomy by injection of contrast material into the disk. Reproduction of typical symptoms by injection of the suspected symptomatic disk coupled with minimal symptoms when a "control" disk is injected is interpreted as identifying the suspect disk as the cause of pain (43). The sensitivity and specificity of this test for this entity are not known.

Erythrocyte Sedimentation Rate

The erythrocyte sedimentation rate (ESR), although quite nonspecific, has a role in the diagnostic evaluation of low back pain in selected circumstances. Measurement of the ESR is the most sensitive serologic test for detecting malignant causes of back pain. An ESR greater than 20 mm/h has been found to have a sensitivity of 78% and a specificity of 67% for an underlying malignancy in patients with low back pain.

In patients in whom ankylosing spondylitis is suspected, elevation of the ESR is noted in approximately 55% of those with active disease (54). Estimates of the specificity of the ESR in this clinical situation are not available but would be expected to be relatively low. The sensitivity of an elevated ESR for infectious causes of back pain (e.g., osteomyelitis) ranges from 71% to 94% (6). Again, specificity data are not available but would be expected to be relatively low.

HLA-B27 Antigen

The histocompatibility antigen, HLA-B27, has been associated with inflammatory spondyloarthropathy, particularly ankylosing spondylitis. Ninety-two percent of white patients with ankylosing spondylitis are B27-positive; only 50% of black patients with ankylosing spondylitis test positive for the antigen. The specificity of B27 for ankylosing spondylitis is 92% in white persons and 98% in black persons (55).

DIAGNOSTIC STRATEGIES

Most patients with acute low back pain improve with simple treatment advice (i.e., to continue ordinary activities as much as they can be tolerated), and many have relief of pain within 2 weeks (56). Serious causes requiring urgent, specific treatment are identified in fewer than 1% of patients. Thus, in most patients with acute low back pain, no immediate diagnostic studies are indicated beyond a careful history and physical examination (57). In patients who have a higher probability of infectious or neoplastic causes of pain based on the clinical assessment, diagnostic tests are indicated. Table 35-6 provides post-test probabilities for the diagnostic studies at various pretest probabilities.

When the pain is confined to the low back and the pretest suspicion of malignancy or infection is high, bone scanning, MRI, or CT should be obtained, generally after initial radiography. Although MRI and CT have slightly better test characteristics (the decision to choose one over the other may depend on local expertise), bone scanning should be considered if the pain is more generalized or if surveillance of the entire skeleton is desired. If the bone scan identifies increased uptake in the lumbar spine suggestive of malignancy or infection, MRI or CT is often required to clearly delineate the lesion.

When back symptoms persist beyond 4 to 6 weeks, reassessment of the original diagnosis, screening for psychosocial barriers to re-

Table 35-6. Post-test Probabilities for Diagnostic Tests in the Evaluation of Back Pain

Diagnostic Test	Pretest Probability					
	20%		50%		80%	
	Positive Result	Negative Result	Positive Result	Negative Result	Positive Result	Negative Result
	←			%		→
For malignancy						
Plain radiography	64	8	88	25	97	56
Bone scanning	44	2	76	7	93	22
CT	55	1	83	6	95	20
ESR >20 mm/h	37	8	70	25	90	57
For osteomyelitis						
Plain radiography	60	5	86	17	96	44
Bone scanning	44	2	76	7	93	22
CT	55	1	83	6	95	19
MRI	75	1	92	4	98	14
For lumbar disk disease						
CT	38	5	71	19	91	48
MRI	41	5	74	18	92	46
Myelography	38	8	71	26	91	59

CT = computed tomography; ESR = erythrocyte sedimentation rate; MRI = magnetic resonance imaging.

covery, and re-evaluation of the prescribed therapy are required. Plain AP and lateral lumbosacral radiographs may now be indicated for most patients. The Waddell tests and pain drawings may be useful in assessing the presence of nonorganic problems that may delay recovery.

In patients presenting with probable sciatica, the initial history and physical examination should further refine the probability of radiculopathy secondary to lumbar disk herniation. Most patients with disk herniation and sciatica respond within 6 weeks to nonoperative treatment. Surgery is indicated in patients who do not respond to medical management or who are unwilling to wait 6 to 12 weeks for relief of symptoms (58). Urgent, immediate imaging and surgical consultation is indicated in the rare situation of cauda equina syndrome characterized by bowel or bladder dysfunction, leg weakness, and saddle anesthesia. Earlier imaging and surgical consideration may also be appropriate when progressive muscle weakness is noted in the distribution of the involved nerve root. With these uncommon exceptions, a trial of aggressive nonoperative care is appropriate in patients with sciatica and suspected disk herniation. Diagnostic studies are generally not required until surgical intervention is contemplated. As noted above, radiography is rarely of diagnostic value in the preoperative evaluation of sciatica. Magnetic resonance imaging and CT appear to have similar operating characteristics for the diagnosis of lumbar disk herniation, although one of these modalities may be favored based on local expertise. Myelography is slightly less sensitive, is more invasive, and more expensive.

Spinal stenosis is a clinical diagnosis that is confirmed radiographically. Table 35-4 lists the pretest clinical features helpful in recognizing this condition. The natural history of spinal stenosis is not well characterized. Some patients respond to nonoperative treatment. Diagnostic imaging is appropriate only in patients being referred for surgical consideration. Radiography may reveal degenerative changes consistent with spinal stenosis but is not diagnostic. Because stenosis is often a multilevel process, MRI and CT-myelography are techniques of choice, as they view more of the thoracolumbar spine than standard lumbar CT.

In patients in whom ankylosing spondylitis or other spondyloarthropathy is suspected based on clinical criteria, PA radiography of the pelvis is the initial diagnostic test of choice. In patients in whom the clinical history suggests a high pretest probability of spondylitis but in whom the single plain radiograph is nondiagnostic, HLA-B27 testing should be done. A positive test result increases the likelihood of spondylitis, whereas a negative test result in this situation virtually excludes the diagnosis in white patients. A series of plain radiographs (obliques, angled PA view) or CT may clarify equivocal situations.

CLINICAL PROBLEMS

Clinical Problem 1
A previously healthy patient presents with acute low back pain.

Testing Strategy and Rationale
In the absence of "red flags" for malignancy or infection, no diagnostic studies beyond the history and physical examination are required. In most cases of acute low back pain, a precise anatomic basis for the pain is not identified and the natural history is prompt, full recovery.

Clinical Example
A 42-year-old man presents with a 4-day history of waist-level lumbar pain that occurred after a weekend camping trip. The pain does not radiate and is relieved when he sits in his recliner or lies supine on the floor. He has continued to work but has curtailed his recreational jogging program. Careful review of systems and medical history are remarkable only for seasonal asthma. He takes no medications. Physical examination reveals limited lumbar flexion and extension but no other abnormalities.

This patient has nonspecific acute low back pain, commonly referred to as lumbar strain or mechanical low back pain. The prognosis for full functional recovery and resolution of symptoms without specific therapy within 2 weeks is excellent. No "red flags" for malignancy or infection are present. No diagnostic testing is indicated at this time. He should be advised to return within 3 to 4 weeks for re-evaluation if symptoms persist or worsen.

Clinical Problem 2
An elderly patient presents for evaluation of acute atraumatic low back pain.

Testing Strategy and Rationale
Anteroposterior and lateral radiography of the lumbar spine should be performed. In patients older than 50 years of age, the likelihood of neoplastic and infectious causes of back pain is higher. Spontaneous pelvic fractures occur almost exclusively in the elderly. Because the sensitivity of radiography for malignancy or infection is low, particularly early in the disease course, additional tests such as bone scanning, MRI, or CT should be performed in patients who are judged to be high risk by clinical evaluation. If a fracture is suspected but the results of radiography are normal, bone scanning or CT should be performed. Measurement of the

ESR can be useful in some cases to guide decisions about diagnostic studies.

Clinical Example

A 64-year-old woman presents with a 6-week history of progressively worsening lumbar pain. The pain is constant and frequently awakens her from sleep. She notes increased fatigue and has lost 10 pounds. Physical examination is unremarkable.

The likelihood that the cause of pain is malignant or infectious in this patient is greatly increased by her age, progressively worsening symptoms, nocturnal pain, and weight loss. Radiography and measurement of the ESR should be performed. Given the strongly suggestive clinical picture, if radiography is unrevealing or nonspecific, bone scanning or MRI should be done.

REFERENCES

1. **Frymoyer JW.** Back pain and sciatica. N Engl J Med. 1988;318:291-300.
2. **Deyo RA.** Early diagnostic evaluation of low back pain. J Gen Intern Med. 1986;1:328-38.
3. **Schwarzer AC, Aprill CN, Derby R, et al.** Clinical features of patients with pain stemming from the lumbar zygapophyseal joints: is the lumbar facet syndrome a clinical entity? Spine. 1994;19:1132-7.
4. **Schwarzer AC, Aprill CN, Derby R, et al.** The prevalence and clinical features of internal disc disruption in patients with chronic low back pain. Spine. 1995;20:1878-83.
5. **Deyo RA, Diehl AK.** Cancer as a cause of back pain: frequency, clinical presentation, and diagnostic strategies. J Gen Intern Med. 1988;3:230-8.
6. **Liang M, Komaroff AL.** Roentgenograms in primary care patients with acute low back pain: a cost-effectiveness analysis. Arch Intern Med. 1982;142:1108-12.
7. **Anderson GJB, Svensson HO, Oden A.** The intensity of work recovery in low back pain. Spine. 1983;8:880-4.
8. **Gilbert JR, Taylor DW, Hildebrand A, Evans C.** Clinical trial of common treatments for low back pain in family practice. BMJ. 1985;291:791-5.
9. **Deyo RA, Rainville J, Kent DL.** What can the history and physical examination tell us about low back pain. JAMA. 1992;268:760-5.
10. **Bell GR, Rothman RH.** The conservative treatment of sciatica. Spine. 1984;9:54-6.
11. **Johnsson K, Rosen I, Uden A.** The natural course of lumbar spinal stenosis. Acta Orthop Scand. 1990; 61(Suppl 237):24.
12. **Mazanec DJ, Segal AM, Drucker Y, et al.** Symptomatic lumbar canal stenosis (LCS): a nonoperative management trial. Arthritis Rheum. 1996; 39(Suppl):S133.

13. **Coughlan ES, McCarthy C.** Ankylosing spondylitis: a comparison of clinical and radiographic features in men and women. Irish Med J. 1993;86: 120-2.

14. **Grasland A, Pouchot J, Mathieu A, et al.** Sacral insufficiency fractures: an easily overlooked cause of back pain in elderly women. Arch Intern Med. 1996;156:668-74.

15. **Calin A, Porta J, Fries JF, et al.** Clinical history as a screening test for ankylosing spondylitis. JAMA. 1977;237:2613-4.

16. **Gran JT.** An epidemiological survey of the signs and symtoms of ankylosing spondylitis. Clin Rheumatol. 1985;4:161-9.

17. **Waldvogel FA, Vasey H.** Osteomyelitis: the past decade. New Engl J Med. 1980;303:360-70.

18. **Russell AS, Maksymowych W, LeClercq S.** Clinical examination of the sacroiliac joints: a prospective study. Arthritis Rheum. 1981;24:1575-8.

19. **Dreyfuss P, Dreyer S, Griffen J, et al.** Positive sacroiliac screening tests in asymtomatic adults. Spine. 1994;19:1138-43.

20. **Esses SI, Moro JK.** The value of facet joint blocks in patient selection for lumbar fusion. Spine. 1993;18:185-90.

21. **Polatin PB, Kinney RK, Gatchel RJ, et al.** Psychiatric illness and chronic low-back pain. The mind and the spine—which goes first? Spine. 1993;18:66-71.

22. **Mann NH, Brown MD, Hertz DB, et al.** Initial-impression diagnosis using low back pain patient pain drawings. Spine. 1993;18: 41-53.

23. **Chan CW, Goldman S, Illstrup DM, et al.** The pain drawing and Waddell's nonorganic physical signs in chronic low back pain. Spine. 1993; 18:1717-22.

24. **Waddell G, McCulloch JA, Kummel E, Venner RM.** Nonorganic physical signs in low-back pain. Spine. 1980;5:117-25.

25. **Schaum SM, Taylor TKF.** Tension signs in lumbar disc prolapse. Clin Orthop. 1971;75:195-204.

26. **Hakelius A, Hindmarsh J.** The comparative reliability of preoperative diagnostic methods in lumbar disc surgery. Acta Orthop Scand. 1972;43: 234-8.

27. **Katz JN, Dalgas M, Stucki G, Lipson SJ.** Diagnosis of lumbar spinal stenosis. Rheum Dis Clin North Am. 1994;20:471-83.

28. **Katz JN, Dalgas M, Stucki G, et al.** Degenerative lumbar spinal stenosis: diagnostic value of the history and physical examination. Arthritis Rheum. 1995;38:1236-41.

29. **Ardan GM.** Bone destruction not demonstrable by radiography. Br J Radiol. 1951;24:107.

30. **Deyo RA.** Plain roentgoenography for low back pain: finding needles in a haystack. Arch Intern Med. 1989;149:27-9.

31. **Rhea JT, DeLuca SA, Llewellyn HJ, et al.** The oblique view: an unnecessary component of the initial adult lumbar spine examination. Radiology. 1980;134:45-7.

32. **Scavone JG, Latshaw RF, Rohrer GV.** Use of lumbar spine films. JAMA. 1981;246:1105-8.

33. **Nachemson AL.** The lumbar spine: an orthopedic challenge. Spine. 1976;1:59-70.

34. **Dabbs VM, Dabbs LG.** Correlation between disc height narrowing and low back pain. Spine. 1990;15:1366-9.

35. **Coste J, Paollagi JB, Spira A.** Reliability of interpretation of plain lumbar spine radiographs in benign, mechanical low back pain. Spine. 1991;16: 426-8.

36. **Ryan LM, Carrera GF, Lightfoot RW, et al.** The radiographic diagnosis of sacroiliitis. Arthritis Rheum. 1983;26:760-3.

37. **Kozin F, Carrera GF, Ryan LM, et al.** Computed tomography in the diagnosis of sacroiliitis. Arthritis Rheum. 1981;24:1479-85.

38. **Handmaker H, Leonards R.** The bone scan in inflammatory ossous disease. Semin Nucl Med. 1976;6:95-105.

39. **Duszynski DO, Kuhn JP, Afshani E, Riddlesberger MM.** Early radionuclide detection of acute osteomyelitis. Radiology. 1975;117:337-40.

40. **Jacobson AF.** Musculoskeletal pain as an indicator of occult malignancy: yield of bone scintigraphy. Arch Intern Med. 1997;157:105-9.

41. **Kelen GD, Noji EK, Peter ED.** Guidelines for use of lumbar spine radiography. Ann Emerg Med. 1986;15:245-51.

42. **Hanly JG, Mitchell MJ, Barnes DC, MacMillan L.** Early recognition of sacroiliitis by magnetic resonance imaging and single photon emission computed tomography. J Rheumatol. 1994;21:2088-95.

43. **Luers PR.** Lumbosacral spine imaging: physioanatomic method. Curr Probl Diagn Radiol. 1992;(Sept/Oct):151-213.

44. **Haughton VM, Eldevik OP, Magnaes B, et al.** A prospective comparison of computed tomography and myelography in the diagnosis of herniated lumbar disks. Neuroradiology. 1982;142:103-10.

45. **Bell GR, Rothman RH, Booth RE, et al.** A study of computer-assisted tomography. II. Comparison of metrizamide myelography and computed tomography in the diagnosis of herniated lumbar disc and spinal stenosis. Spine. 1984;9:552-6.

46. **Wiesel SW, Tsourmas N, Feffer HL, et al.** A study of computer assisted tomography I. The incidence of positive CAT scans in an asymptomatic group of patients. Spine. 1984;9:549-51.

47. **Modic MT, Masaryk T, Boumphrey F, et al.** Lumbar herniated disc disease and canal stenosis: prospective evaluation by surface coil MR, CT, and myelography. Am J Radiol. 1986;147:757-65.

48. **Hitselberger WE, Witten RM.** Abnormal myelograms in asymptomatic patients. J Neurosurg. 1968;28:204.

49. **Modic MT, Pflanze W, Feiglin DH, et al.** Magnetic resonance imaging of musculoskeletal infections. Radiol Clin North Am. 1986;24:247-58.

50. **Traill Z, Richards MA, Moore NR.** Magnetic resonance imaging of metastatic bone disease. Clin Orthop. 1995;312:76-88.

51. **Boden SD, Davis DO, Dina TS, et al.** Abnormal magnetic-resonance scans of the lumbar spine in asymptomatic subjects. J Bone Joint Surg Am. 1990;72:403-8.

52. **Jensen MC, Brant-Zawadzki N, Obuchowski N, et al.** Magnetic resonance imaging of the lumbar spine in people without back pain. N Engl J Med. 1994;331:69-73.

53. **Bogduk N, Modic MT.** Controversy: lumbar discography. Spine. 1996;21: 402-4.

54. **Dixon JS, Bird HA, Wright V.** A comparison of serum biochemistry in ankylosing spondylitis, seronegative and seropositive rheumatoid arthritis. Ann Rheum Dis. 1981;40:404-8.

55. **Khan MA, Khan MK.** Diagnostic value of HLA B-27 testing in ankylosing spondylitis and Reiter's syndrome. Ann Intern Med. 1982;96:70-6.

56. **Malmivaara A, Hakkinen U, Aro T, et al.** The treatment of acute low back pain—bed rest, exercises, or ordinary activity? N Engl J Med. 1995;332: 351-5.

57. Agency for Health Care Policy and Research (AHCPR). Acute Low Back Problems in Adults. U.S. Department of Health and Human Services. Public Health Service. AHCPR Publication No. 95-0642. Rockville, MD; December 1994.

58. **Mazanec DJ.** Back pain: medical evaluation and therapy. Cleve Clin J Med. 1995;62:163-8.

Systemic Lupus Erythematosus

36

Daniel J. Mazanec, MD, and Seth M. Kantor, MD

KEY POINTS

Pretest Probabilities

- The prevalence of systemic lupus erythematosus (SLE) is approximately 1% in a general hospital population and about 0.14% in women aged 16 to 64 years in a hospital-based practice.

- Clinical criteria for SLE are useful in estimating the pretest probability of the disease.

Diagnostic Strategies

- The diagnosis of SLE is made by consideration of both clinical and laboratory findings.

- The antinuclear antibody (ANA) test is a highly sensitive test for lupus. A negative test makes a diagnosis of SLE very unlikely.

- Of the tests with high specificity for SLE, the anti-double-stranded DNA (anti-dsDNA) test is the most sensitive. It is the preferred test for confirmation of the diagnosis.

- In rare patients with "ANA-negative" lupus, antibodies to the Ro antigen are the most common serologic abnormality.

BACKGROUND

Systemic lupus erythematosus (SLE) is a chronic multisystem inflammatory disorder characterized by protean clinical manifestations and serologic evidence of autoimmunity. It occurs seven to nine times more commonly in women than in men, with a peak age of onset in the middle twenties (1,2). The diagnosis depends on recognition of combinations of clinical findings in association with characteristic autoantibodies. It is important to be able to recognize the discriminating ability of individual signs, symptoms, and laboratory findings when evaluating patients for the possibility of SLE.

ESTIMATING PRETEST PROBABILITY

The 1982 Revised Criteria for the Classification of Systemic Lupus Erythematosus developed by the American Rheumatism Association (American College of Rheumatology) consists of 11 criteria. When four of these criteria were noted serially or simultaneously, the criteria were found to be 96% sensitive and 96% specific when tested in SLE patients and controls (3). Although not intended for diagnostic purposes in an individual patient, the criteria are useful in predicting pretest probability of disease. Table 36-1 shows the revised criteria with their individual sensitivities, specificities, and likelihood ratios.

The prevalence of SLE in the general hospital population has been estimated at approximately 1%. This estimate is intermediate between the prevalence of SLE of 0.14% in women aged 16 to 64 years at a hospital clinic, 2% in a general community-based rheumatologist's office, and 3.6% in a large subspecialty clinic (4–6). Using an estimated disease prevalence of 1% and the sensitivity and specificity for the clinical (nonimmunologic) criteria, post-test probabilities based on increasing numbers of manifestations have been calculated (Table 36-2). The presence of four disease manifestations suggests a probability of SLE of one in three, whereas six or more manifestations suggest virtual certainty of diagnosis. For example, in the absence of other manifestations, a patient with symptoms of arthritis and leukopenia would have a probability of only 5%. These calculations assume equal weight for each criterion.

As is evident from the likelihood ratios in Table 36-1, certain clinical features, particularly malar or discoid rash or cellular casts, have higher predictive value for the diagnosis of SLE. Some authors have investigated methods to weigh individual clinical features and thereby provide more accurate estimates of pretest probability (6,7).

The diagnostic value of additional immunologic testing is greatest when the diagnosis is in doubt—that is, when two to five clinical manifestations are noted. In general, clinicians err by overemphasizing the importance of serologic abnormalities.

DIAGNOSTIC TESTS

Fluorescent Antinuclear Antibody

Of the available immunologic tests for the diagnosis of SLE, the fluorescent antinuclear antibody (ANA) test has the highest sensitivity. As noted in Table 36-3, almost all patients who meet the criteria for the

Table 36-1. The 1982 Revised Criteria for the Classification of Systemic Lupus Erythematosus and Their Operating Characteristics*

Criterion	Definition of Positive Finding	Sensitivity	Specificity	Likelihood Ratio Finding Present	Likelihood Ratio Finding Absent
		←——— % ———→			
Malar rash	Fixed erythema, flat or raised over the malar eminences, tending to spare the nasolabial folds	57	96	14	0.45
Discoid rash	Erythematous raised patches with adherent keratotic scaling and follicular plugging; atrophic scarring may occur in older lesions	18	99	18	0.83
Photo-sensitivity	Skin rash as an unusual reaction to sunlight (by patient history or physician observation)	43	96	11	0.59
Oral ulcers	Oral or nasopharyngeal ulceration, usually painless, observed by a physician	27	96	6.8	0.76
Arthritis	Nonerosive arthritis involving two or more peripheral joints, characterized by tenderness, swelling, or effusion	86	37	1.4	0.38
Serositis	Pleuritis: convincing history of pleuritic pain or rub heard by a physician or evidence of of pleural effusion; or pericarditis, documented by electrocardiographs or rub or evidence of pericardial effusion	56	86	4.0	0.51
Renal disorder	Persistent proteinuria greater than 0.5 g/d or greater than 3+ if quantification not done; or cellular casts (may be erythrocyte, hemoglobin, granular, tubular, or mixed)	51	94	8.5	0.52
Neurologic disorder	Seizures: in the absence of offending drug or known metabolic derangements (for example, uremia, ketoacidosis, or electrolyte imbalance); or psychosis in the absence of offending drug or known metabolic derangements (for example, uremia, ketoacidosis, or electrolyte imbalance)	20	98	10	0.82
Hematologic disorder	Hemolytic anemia with reticulocytosis; or leukopenia: <4000/mm^3 total on two or more occasions: or lymphopenia; <1500/mm^3 on two or more occasions; or thrombocytopenia: <100,000/mm^3 in the absence of offending drugs	59	89	5.4	0.46

*Not presented are two additional criteria among the 11 revised criteria: a positive antinuclear antibody test result and a positive finding on either of two immunologic tests.

Table 36-2. Operating Characteristics and Probability of Systemic Lupus Erythematosus Based on Increasing Number of Manifestations*

Number of Manifestations	Sensitivity	Specificity	Probability of SLE
	←——————————— % ———————————→		
0	100	0	0
1	100	52	2
2	99	81	5
3	90	94	13
4	80	98	29
5	63	99	39
6	45	100	100

SLE = systemic lupus erythematosus.
*Based on American Rheumatism Association preliminary criteria excluding lupus erythematosus cell preparation and assuming prevalence of lupus of 1% in a teaching hospital setting. These figures are not significantly different from those derived from the data used to determine the revised criteria, except that the latter data included immunologic diagnostic tests, whereas these figures do not.

diagnosis of SLE have a positive ANA. Because of its high sensitivity, the ANA has displaced the older lupus-erythematosus cell preparation (LE prep) in the initial evaluation of patients suspected of having SLE.

The ANA test is not specific for lupus. In the population on which the 1982 revised criteria are based, the specificity was only 49% (3). Because almost all of the patients in this study had an immunologic disorder of some type, this figure is falsely low when applied to the general population. As many as 20% of patients in whom SLE might be considered will have a "false-positive" ANA result.

Some have attached considerable significance to the pattern of nuclear immunofluorescence seen in the test. For example, a peripheral or rim pattern is most commonly associated with the presence of anti-double-stranded DNA (anti-dsDNA) antibodies and, therefore, was considered essentially diagnostic of SLE (3,8). However, the pattern of immunofluorescence depends on several technical factors. Furthermore, testing is available for anti-dsDNA antibodies. Therefore, the pattern of ANA immunofluorescence should not routinely be considered in the evaluation of patients for SLE.

Lupus Erythematosus Cell Preparation
Blood smears from patients with SLE, after incubation of a defibrinated sample, will often show evidence of nucleophagocytosis by neutrophils. Whereas this phenomenon is observed in more than 70% of

Table 36-3. Operating Characteristics of Laboratory Tests in the Diagnosis of Systemic Lupus Erythematosus

Diagnostic Test	Definition of Positive Result	Sensitivity	Specificity	Likelihood Ratio	
				Positive Result	Negative Result
		← % →			
Antinuclear antibody by fluorescence	Positive undiluted	99	80	5.0	0.013
Lupus erythematosus cell preparation	Two cells	73	97	25	0.25
Anti-double-stranded DNA antibody by Farr test (radio immunoassay)	≥40% binding	73 (50–91)	98 (96–100)	37	0.28
Anti-double-stranded DNA antibody by *Crithidia luciliae* assay (immuno-fluorescence)	Positive at 1:10 dilution	52 (42–69)	98 (98–100)	26	0.49

patients with SLE early in the course of their illness (3), this test has generally been replaced by ANA testing.

Anti-Double-Stranded DNA Antibody Test

The finding of serum antibody against dsDNA is highly specific (approximately 98%) for the diagnosis of SLE (3,6,8,9,10). Patients seen during disease exacerbations are more likely to have positive tests (11). Because of this high degree of specificity, some consider a positive anti-native DNA antibody test virtually diagnostic of SLE. This interpretation, however, assumes that the test is reliably done and that the substrate is not contaminated with single-stranded DNA.

Two assays for anti-dsDNA have been found to be superior: the Farr test (radioimmunoassay) and the *Crithidia luciliae* assay (immunofluorescence). The *Crithidia* assay is cheaper and more practical to perform in most hospital laboratories. The two tests have comparable specificity but the sensitivity of the *Crithidia* assay appears to be lower (12–14). Reports suggest that antibodies directed against other antigens can bind to the kinetoplast (*Crithidia* assay) resulting in a false-positive rate of as high as 10% (15). Therefore, proper test interpretation requires knowing which assay is being used.

Anti-Ro (SSA) Antibody

Antibodies to a soluble ribonuclear protein cytoplasmic antigen known as Ro or SSA have been identified in 30% to 40% of patients with SLE and 70% to 80% of patients with Sjogren's syndrome (16). As many as 62% of patients with "ANA negative" lupus have antibodies to Ro (17). Patients with ANA-negative lupus tend to have severe photosensitive dermatitis, but have a low frequency of renal or central nervous system disease. Although not specific, the detection of anti-Ro antibodies in a patient who is ANA negative and presents with these manifestations is of diagnostic importance. Anti-Ro antibodies have also been associated with congenital heart block in the offspring of women with lupus.

Lupus Band Test

Immunoglobulins and complement proteins may be found in the dermal-epidermal junction of lesional and nonlesional skin in 50% to 90% of SLE patients (18–20). Recently, this test was compared in small series of patients with and without SLE who had suspicious cutaneous disorders. The test was found to have a sensitivity of 93%, a specificity of 87%, and positive and negative likelihood ratios of 7.2 and 0.08, respectively (20). A positive test result can occur in several other rheumatic disorders (rheumatoid arthritis, Sjogren's syndrome, scleroderma) and nonrheumatic disorders (rosacea, leprosy, porphyria). In addition, the test result may be positive during active disease and negative during periods of remission (21).

Serum Complement

Total serum hemolytic complement (CH50) and individual complement components (i.e., C3 and C4) may be low in patients with active SLE owing to the presence of immune complexes. Complement testing is used primarily to monitor treatment response or to detect relapse in advance of overt symptoms or signs. These tests have low sensitivity (40%), but relatively high specificity (90%) (4). However, for diagnostic purposes, the ANA and anti-dsDNA are more useful.

Other Tests

Antibodies to an extractable nuclear antigen, Sm, have a high degree of specificity (95%–100%) for SLE but are fairly insensitive (18%–31%) (3,6,22). Antibodies to negatively charged phospholipids (false-positive serologic test result for syphilis, lupus anticoagulant, and anticardiolipin) are identified in 5% to 50% of patients with SLE (23–25). The lack of sensitivity limits the diagnostic usefulness of these tests for SLE. Serum antiribosomal P antibodies are identified in about 15% of patients suspected of having SLE who have neuropsychiatric symptoms such as organic brain syndrome, seizures, depression, or psychosis (26).

DIAGNOSTIC STRATEGIES

The first step in the diagnostic approach to SLE is to estimate the pretest probability based on the number of clinical criteria present. At the extremes (no criteria or greater than six criteria), further diagnostic testing is of little practical value. Whether the physician should pursue the question of SLE when only one or two criteria are present should be based on the nature and severity of those criteria. Certain criteria such as malar erythema, cellular casts, and discoid lupus, have relatively greater weight for the diagnosis of SLE (6,7).

The next step in the evaluation of a patient suspected of having SLE is to order an ANA. A positive result increases the odds of SLE by about five times (Table 36-3); the post-test probability will depend on the number of clinical criteria present (Table 36-4). A negative result for this sensitive test is extremely powerful in reducing the disease probability.

Given a positive ANA, a test of high specificity is generally required to confirm the diagnosis. The anti-dsDNA test has the highest sensitivity of the specific tests currently available and is the logical choice. The revised probability of SLE, based on this test result, clinical criteria, and positive ANA are also presented in Table 36-4. A positive anti-dsDNA test result in a patient with a positive ANA and two or more clinical criteria makes SLE highly likely. However, even when the anti-dsDNA is negative, the probability of SLE will still be significant if the patient has three or more clinical criteria along with the positive ANA. In such

Table 36-4. Sequential Evaluation of the Probability of Systemic Lupus Erythematosus Based on Clinical and Laboratory Data

Number of Clinical Criteria Met	Step 1 Pretest Probability of SLE	Step 2 Post-test Probability		Step 3 Post-test Probability	
		Positive ANA Result	Negative ANA Result	Positive ANA and Positive Anti-dsDNA Results	Positive ANA and Negative Anti-dsDNA Results
←			%		→
1	2	10	<1	80	3
2	5	20	<1	90	6
3	13	42	<1	96	17
4	29	67	1	98	45
5	39	76	2	99	47

ANA = antinuclear antibody; anti-dsDNA = anti-double-stranded DNA; SLE = systemic lupus erythematosus.

cases, additional tests such as measurement of anti-Sm or complement components may be helpful.

In patients for whom the probability of SLE is high, based on clinical criteria, but who are ANA negative, a determination for anti-Ro or anti-phospholipid antibodies may be helpful. A lupus band test might also be considered in this situation.

CLINICAL PROBLEMS

Clinical Problem 1
A patient has recurrent arthralgia and one or two additional findings, suggesting a possible diagnosis of SLE.

Testing Strategy and Rationale
A complete blood count (CBC), urinalysis, and ANA test should be performed. The prevalence of SLE is low in this clinical situation. Arthralgia without clinical evidence of arthritis is not one of the criteria for the diagnosis of SLE. In this case, a CBC and urinalysis should be done to look for cytopenia, proteinuria, or casts, which would increase the probability of SLE.

Because the probability of SLE is low, a highly sensitive test such as the ANA would effectively rule out the disease when the result is negative. An unexpectedly positive ANA result would require further testing with the anti-dsDNA antibody test.

Clinical Example
A 43-year-old woman reports recurrent arthralgia. Her past medical history includes an episode of acute pruritus. She has no family history of collagen vascular disease. Her physical examination is unremarkable.

The probability of SLE is estimated to be no greater than 5%. The CBC and urinalysis are normal, findings that leave the probability of SLE low. The ANA test is ordered and, if the results are negative, would reduce the post-test probability of SLE to less than 1%. An unexpectedly positive result would require further study because the revised probability of SLE would be no greater than 20%.

Clinical Problem 2
A patient has several clinical findings supporting a diagnosis of SLE.

Testing Strategy and Rationale
An ANA test should be done and then followed up with an anti-dsDNA test if the ANA result is positive.

The ANA test, because of its high sensitivity, is a powerful tool in ruling out the diagnosis. Because it lacks specificity, however, a positive test result does not confirm the diagnosis. The anti-dsDNA test has the specificity that the ANA test lacks. Because the anti-dsDNA test does not have high sensitivity, a negative result would not rule out the diagnosis of SLE. Therefore, a logical test sequence is an ANA test followed, if the results are positive, by an anti-dsDNA test.

Clinical Example

A 25-year-old woman has had two episodes of migratory polyarthritis in the preceding 12 months. She now has a skin rash that has a malar distribution. Complete blood count and differential count are normal. Platelet count is $70,000/mm^3$.

Based on these clinical findings, the probability of SLE is estimated to be approximately 20%. This estimate is higher than the probability indicated in Table 36-4 when three criteria are present (13%) and is based on the weight assigned to the malar rash—a relatively specific finding.

A positive ANA result in this case would increase the probability of SLE from approximately 20% to 55%, a significant increment, but not sufficient to confirm the diagnosis. The anti-dsDNA test, if results are positive, would provide this confirmation (i.e., post-test probability 98%).

REFERENCES

1. **Pisetsky DS.** Systemic lupus erythematosus. Med Clin North Am. 1986; 70:337-53.
2. **Alarcon-Segovia D.** Systemic lupus erythematosus. In Schumacher HR Jr, ed. Primer on Rheumatic Disease. Atlanta: Arthritis Foundation; 1988.
3. **Tan EM, et al.** The 1982 Revised Criteria of the Classification of Systemic Lupus Erythematosus. Arthritis Rheum. 1982;25:1271-7.
4. **Weinstein A, Bardwell B, Stone B, et al.** Antibodies to native DNA and serum complement (C3) levels. Am J Med. 1983;74:206-16.
5. **Richardson B, Epstein SV.** Utility of the fluorescent antinuclear antibody test in a single patient. Ann Intern Med. 1981;95:333-8.
6. **Clough JD, Elrazak M, Calabrese LH, et al.** Weighted criteria for the diagnosis of systemic lupus erythematosus. Arch Intern Med. 1984;144:281-5.
7. **Edworthy SM, Zatarain E, McShane, et al.** Analysis of the 1982 ARA Lupus Criteria Data set by recursive partitioning methodology: New insights into the relative merit of individual criteria. J Rheum. 1988;15: 1493-8.
8. **Luciano A, Rothfield NF.** Patterns of nuclear fluorescence and DNA-binding activity. Ann Rheum Dis. 1973;32:337-41.

9. **Kalmin ND, Bartholomew WR, Wicher K.** Relative values of laboratory assays in systemic lupus erythematosus. Am J Clin Pathol. 1981;75:846-51.

10. **Hughes GRV, Cohen SA, Christian CL.** Anti-DNA activity in systemic lupus erythematosus. 1971;30:259-64.

11. **Swaak AJG, Aarden LA, Statius LW, et al.** Anti-dsDNA and complement profiles as prognostic guides in systemic lupus erythematosus. Arthritis Rheum 1979;22:226-35.

12. **Permin H, Halberg P, Christiansen E.** Antibodies against double-stranded DNA in patients with connective tissue disease. Acta Med Scand. 1978;203:61-5.

13. **Sontheimer RD, Gilliam JN.** An immunofluorescence assay for double-stranded DNA antibodies using the *Crithidia luciliae* kinetoplast as a double-stranded DNA substrate. J Lab Clin Med. 1978;91:550-8.

14. **Tietz NW.** Clinical Guide to Laboratory Tests. 3rd ed. Philadelphia: WB Saunders; 1995:60-1.

15. **Fritzler MJ.** Antinuclear antibodies in the investigation of rheumatic diseases. Bull Rheum Dis. 1985;35:1-10.

16. **Tsokos GC, Pillemer SR, Klippel JH.** Rheumatic disease syndromes associated with antibodies to the Ro (SS-A) ribonuclear protein. Semin Arthritis Rheum. 1987;16:237-44.

17. **Maddison PJ, Provost TT, Reichlin M.** Serological findings in patients with "ANA-negative" systemic lupus erythematosus. Medicine. 1981;60:87-94.

18. **Monroe EW.** Lupus band test. Arch Dermatol. 1977;113:830-4.

19. **Grossman J, Callerame ML, Condemi JJ.** Skin immunofluorescence studies on lupus erythematosus and other antinuclear-antibody-positive diseases. Ann Intern Med. 1974;80:496-500.

20. **George R, Kurian S, Mnams M, Thomas K.** Diagnostic evaluation of the lupus band test in discoid and systemic lupus erythematosis. Int J Dermatol. 1995;34:170-3.

21. **Rothfield N, Marino C.** Studies of repeat skin biopsies of nonlesional skin in patients with systemic lupus erythematosus. Arthritis Rheum. 1982;25:624-30.

22. **Barada FA, Andrews BS, Davis JS IV, et al.** Antibodies to sm in patients with systemic lupus erythematosus. Arthritis Rheum. 1981;24:1236-44.

23. **Fort JG, Cowchock FS, Abruzzo JL, et al.** Anticardiolipin antibodies in patients with rheumatic diseases. Arthritis Rheum. 1987;30:752-60.

24. **Ramsey-Goldman R.** Pregnancy in systemic lupus erythematosus. Rheum Dis Clin North Am. 1988;14:169-185.

25. **Kalunian KC, Peter JB, Middlekauff HR, et al.** Clinical significance of a single test for anti-cardiolipin antibodies in patients with systemic lupus erythematosus. Am J Med.1988;85:602-8.

26. **West SG, Emlen W, Wener MH, Kotzin BL.** Neuropsychiatric lupus erythematosis: a 10-year prospective study on the value of diagnostic tests. Am J Med. 1995;99:153-63.

Temporal Arteritis

37

Seth M. Kantor, MD

KEY POINTS

Pretest Probabilities

- Temporal arteritis usually occurs in persons older than 50 years old and has an estimated prevalence of approximately 0.15% in this population.

- Jaw claudication is the most specific single symptom and increases the likelihood of disease ninefold.

- The findings of a new headache pattern, jaw claudication, and abnormal arteries are highly specific (approximately 99%) for temporal arteritis.

Diagnostic Strategies

- Measurement of the erythrocyte sedimentation rate (ESR) and temporal artery biopsy are the two best tests for establishing a diagnosis of temporal arteritis.

- Measurement of the ESR is highly sensitive but lacks specificity. In most cases, it is an efficient initial test for excluding disease. When the results of the ESR are negative, a diagnosis of temporal arteritis should be pursued with a temporal artery biopsy only when the pretest probability is very high.

- The temporal artery biopsy is highly specific, but in most centers its sensitivity is only about 80%. When the results of the biopsy are positive, the post-test probability of temporal arteritis is high.

- Owing to the potential side effects of corticosteroid therapy, the temporal artery biopsy can provide useful information even when the pretest probability of disease is high.

BACKGROUND

Temporal, or giant cell, arteritis is a vasculitis of unknown cause that occurs mostly in older patients and affects cranial or larger arteries. The catastrophic outcome of untreated temporal arteritis (TA) is blindness, which can be prevented by timely treatment with corticosteroids. It is therefore imperative that prompt diagnosis be established so that treatment can occur early in the course of the disease (1–5). In addition to preventing blindness, corticosteroid treatment quickly alleviates other symptoms. However, because of the hazards of protracted treatment with corticosteroids, particularly in elderly persons, the diagnosis should be as secure as possible before treatment is started.

Clinicians differ as to whether TA and polymyalgia rheumatica (PMR) are distinct entities or differing manifestations of one single disease (1,3,6–9). Features common to both entities include an elevated erythrocyte sedimentation rate (ESR) and the age distribution of affected people. Between 20% and 50% of patients with TA ultimately manifest symptoms of PMR. In addition, between 5% and 15% of patients with "pure" PMR without symptoms suggestive of TA have positive temporal artery biopsies.

For diagnostic and treatment purposes, however, the best clinical strategy is to consider the two syndromes as separate. Temporal artery biopsy in patients with clinical features of PMR alone is generally unnecessary. Polymyagia rheumatica is a syndrome diagnosed essentially on clinical grounds and treated with much lower dosages of corticosteroids than is TA.

ESTIMATING PRETEST PROBABILITY

Temporal arteritis occurs mostly in persons older than 50 years of age, and the incidence continues to increase with each subsequent decade. It is seen approximately two times more frequently in women. In Olmsted County, Minnesota, the prevalence of TA was 133 per 100,000 in persons 50 years of age and older (10). The incidence varies from a low of 1.4 cases in the group consisting of persons 50 to 59 years old, to almost 30 cases per 100,000 per year in the group consisting of persons 70 to 79 years old (2,10).

In elderly patients who present with headache, visual disturbance, jaw claudication, symptoms of PMR, fever, and a tender or swollen temporal artery, the diagnosis of TA is extremely likely. However, most often patients present with less classic presentations (Table 37-1).

As many as 40% of patients present with only nonspecific systemic symptoms, such as fever, anorexia, or weight loss without headache or polymyalgic symptoms (1–5,10–14). In such cases, a malignancy may be suspected or these symptoms may be elicited after evaluation for a fever of undetermined origin (15,16). Headache, although a classic symptom suggestive of TA, is nonspecific; the recent onset of a new headache pattern has more diagnostic importance.

Unless several specific findings are present, pretest probability based on the history and examination is typically less than 50%. Jaw

Table 37-1. **Sensitivity of Clinical Manifestations in the Diagnosis of Temporal Arteritis**

Symptom or Sign	Occurrence (%)
Headache	65–80
Fever	45–67
Abnormal artery	37–57
Visual symptoms	22–41
Weight loss/anorexia/fatigue	20–79
Polymyalgia rheumatica	20–52
Scalp tenderness	20–40
Depression/mental deterioration	12–25
Jaw claudication	11–38

claudication correlates strongly with a positive biopsy and is reported to increase the likelihood of TA ninefold (17). The presence of clusters of symptoms may also be helpful in establishing a diagnosis; for example, the finding of a new headache, jaw claudication, and abnormal arteries in combination has a sensitivity of 34%, specificity of more than 99%, and a positive likelihood ratio of 47 (18). The finding of abnormal arteries and cotton wool spots in combination is also highly specific, but its sensitivity is less than 40% (13,14,19).

DIAGNOSTIC TESTS

Erythrocyte Sedimentation Rate
Because virtually all studies of TA have used the Westergren ESR (11,20), this method is the preferred technique. It is also preferred for its greater range, because many patients with TA present with an ESR of more than 100 mm/h. Although the normal range is most often quoted as 0–20 mm/h, an ESR greater than 30 mm/h generally may be considered abnormal. In most patients with TA, the ESR is at least 40 mm/h.

For the diagnosis of TA, the ESR has a strikingly high sensitivity approaching 99% (11,17,20). Rare biopsy-proven cases of TA with visual loss have been noted with a normal ESR (21). However, the ESR is not very specific because it can be elevated by many infectious, inflammatory or rheumatic disorders that can mimic TA. In addition, the ESR tends to increase with age. For patients in whom TA is clinically suspected, the specificity of the ESR is estimated to be 50% to 70% (Table 37-2) (13,20).

Temporal Artery Biopsy
Because in most clinical series of patients with TA the diagnosis is based on a positive temporal artery biopsy, the sensitivity and speci-

Table 37-2. Operating Characteristics of Erythrocyte Sedimentation Rate and Biopsy in the Diagnosis of Temporal Arteritis

Diagnostic Test	Definition of Positive Result	Sensitivity	Specificity	Likelihood Ratio	
				Positive Result	Negative Result
		←—— % ——→			
Westergren ESR	>30 mm/h	99	50–70	2.5	0.02
Temporal artery biopsy	Mononuclear cell infiltrate and disruption of internal elastic lamina	80	95	16	0.21

ficity of this test may be overestimated. However, the finding of a mononuclear inflammatory cell infiltrate in the wall of the temporal artery with fragmentation of the internal elastic membrane is highly characteristic of TA. Multinucleated, so-called giant cells are less frequently observed. When all three findings are present, the specificity of the biopsy approaches 99%, although in actual practice it is uncommon to see all the typical features.

The value of the temporal artery biopsy is limited by its imperfect sensitivity, with estimates ranging from 50% to 91% (1,2,11,13, 22–25). In part, the differences cited depend on whether patients who have only PMR symptoms were included in the study. In addition, pathologic findings of arteritis may not be continuous, and "skip lesions" of normal artery in tissue specimens may be seen (26). Thus, biopsy length and the number of sections examined may influence the result; characteristic pathologic lesions are detected only by examining multiple transverse or longitudinal sections in some 30% of patients. Approximately 5% of patients with TA are believed to have unilateral arteritis. Allowing for such disparities in technique and interpretation, the estimated sensitivity of the biopsy is 80% in most centers. Adherence to careful clinical protocols and performing biopsy of the contralateral temporal artery when the results of temporal artery biopsy of one artery are negative may increase the sensitivity to 90% (27,28).

Color Duplex Ultrasonography

Recently, the technique of color duplex ultrasonography has been applied to the diagnosis of TA. In a recent study, the technique was found to be 93% sensitive using identification of an area of stenosis, occlusion, or halo as the criterion; the finding of a dark halo, which may be caused by edema of the artery wall, was the most specific finding (29). If confirmed by other studies, this technique may be quite useful to guide decisions about whether to perform biopsy (30). It may also change the approach to therapy in situations in which biopsy is not possible.

DIAGNOSTIC STRATEGIES

Because TA is associated with potential severe morbidity (i.e., blindness) and because this morbidity is completely preventable with proper treatment, TA requires a strategy sensitive for the diagnosis of early disease. However, the diagnostic strategy must also have high specificity (few false-positive results) because treatment with moderately high doses of steroids (e.g., 40–60 mg of prednisone daily) may cause problems (the incidence of significant side effects approaches 30%) (31,32). Elderly persons are particularly prone to the metabolic side effects of corticosteroids, especially osteoporosis, vertebral collapse, and cataracts.

Temporal arteritis is often difficult to diagnose on the basis of the clinical presentation alone. Unless several specific findings are present, pretest probability after the history and physical examination is generally less than 50%. Because of the need for therapy and the nonspecificity of symptoms and signs, the clinician must use the laboratory to develop an effective clinical approach to this disorder.

Because measurement of the ESR is a simple and highly sensitive test, it is useful in the diagnosis of TA (see Tables 37-2 and 37-3). At all but very high pretest probabilities, a normal ESR generally excludes the diagnosis of TA. However, because the ESR is so nonspecific, a temporal artery biopsy is often performed to confirm the diagnosis when the ESR is elevated. The biopsy is used in this setting as confirmation so that both the physician and patient may be comfortable in initiating and continuing therapy that has the potential for significant side effects (32). When the pretest probability of disease is very high and the ESR is positive for TA, biopsy may not be necessary. However, positive results from a biopsy may be useful if complications develop during treatment; steroids might be confidently continued only with a highly certain diagnosis.

Biopsy should be done if the diagnosis of TA is suspected in patients older than 50 years of age in whom the ESR is greater than 30 mm/h with signs or symptoms suggestive of TA. Even if the ESR is normal, a biopsy should also be done when the clinical presentation suggests a high likelihood of disease.

If the results of a unilateral biopsy are negative, then the diagnosis becomes less likely. However, even though the results of a unilateral biopsy may be negative, in 5% to 10% of patients with TA the results of a biopsy of the contralateral artery would be positive [27].) When the

Table 37-3. Post-test Probabilities for Erythrocyte Sedimentation Rate and Biopsy in the Diagnosis of Temporal Arteritis

Diagnostic Test	Pretest Probabilities					
	20%		50%		80%	
	Positive Result	Negative Result	Positive Result	Negative Result	Positive Result	Negative Result
	←——————————————— % ———————————————→					
ESR alone	38	<1	71	2	91	6
Biopsy alone	80	5	94	17	98	46
Biopsy (ESR positive)	91	11	98	34	99	68
Biopsy (ESR negative)	6	<1	21	<1	51	1

ESR—erythrocyte sedimentation rate.

initial pretest probability of TA is high (e.g., 80%) and the results of the ESR are positive, many clinicians would empirically treat for TA if the results of the unilateral biopsy are negative, because the post-test probability of disease is still high (~68%) (see Table 37-3). Depending on the clinical presentation and the potential risk associated with corticosteroid therapy, others would perform contralateral temporal artery biopsy or follow the patient clinically to watch for the subsequent development of symptoms, at which point a repeat biopsy may be more likely to yield positive results.

In a patient with vague constitutional symptoms for whom the diagnosis of TA is being considered but is believed to be unlikely, the ESR is a useful initial test. If the results are normal, no further diagnostic testing for TA is necessary. If the ESR is elevated and no other causes for an elevated ESR are found, a biopsy may provide diagnostic information. If the results of the biopsy are positive, treatment is warranted and an unexpected cause for the patient's symptoms has been found. If the results of the biopsy are negative, other diagnoses should be considered (see Table 37-3).

CLINICAL PROBLEMS

Clinical Problem 1
An elderly patient has jaw claudication.

Testing Strategy and Rationale
A Westergren ESR should be performed. If the ESR is elevated, a biopsy may still be useful, although in the future, ultrasonography may be the next step. If the ESR is even minimally elevated, the

post-test probability of TA is more than 95% and the diagnosis of TA is almost certain. Treatment may be given to such patients even if the results of the biopsy are negative. If the ESR is unexpectedly normal, a positive or negative result on biopsy would still be useful diagnostically. In such a case when the ESR is unexpectedly normal, post-test probability is approximately 13%. A negative biopsy result reduces the probability of TA to approximately 3%, whereas a positive biopsy result should establish the diagnosis. True jaw claudication is the clinical symptom that most closely predicts the presence of TA on biopsy (17,18), giving a pretest probability of as high as 90%.

Clinical Example

A 70-year-old man is experiencing fatigue and low-grade fever. He gives a history of jaw pain that occurs when he chews his food and of intermittent double vision. Based on this clinical information, the likelihood of TA is high (~90%). A Westergren ESR is done, and the ESR is 80 mm/h. The post-test probability is now ~96%. Because clinical suspicion is high, a temporal artery biopsy does not need to be done, although a positive biopsy result may still be helpful if treatment complications ensue.

Clinical Problem 2

An elderly patient reports symptoms of proximal myalgia and stiffness.

Testing Strategy and Rationale

A Westergren ESR should be performed. If the ESR is elevated, a temporal artery biopsy should be considered, depending on any additional, associated symptoms.

Polymyalgia rheumatica should be suspected in elderly patients with proximal myalgia and stiffness. An elevated ESR supports that diagnosis, but it could also indicate TA. If other symptoms suggestive of TA are present, the pretest probability of this disorder warrants a biopsy. On the basis of an elevated ESR alone (without associated symptoms of TA), the probability of TA is no greater than 20%. Treatment with low-dose corticosteroids for PMR and close clinical observation would be a safe approach. Subsequent visual loss in such patients is very rare.

Clinical Example

A 72-year-old woman reports experiencing proximal myalgia and stiffness for the last 8 weeks. She has trouble getting out of a chair and climbing stairs. She also reports scalp tenderness. On physical examination, her temporal artery is somewhat nodular. The ESR is

Continued

75 mm/h. A diagnosis of PMR can be made on the basis of the typical symptoms and elevated ESR. Because of the presence of a nodular artery and an elevated ESR, the probability of TA is sufficiently high (75%) to warrant a biopsy.

REFERENCES

1. **Goodwin J.** Progress in gerontology: polymyalgia rheumatica and temporal arteritis. J Am Geriatr Soc. 1992;40:515-25.
2. **Nordberg E, Nordberg C, Malmvall BE, et al.** Giant cell arteritis. Rheum Dis Clin North Am. 1995;21:1013-26.
3. **Michet CJ, Evans JM, Fleming KC, et al.** Common rheumatologic diseases in elderly patients. Mayo Clin Proc. 1995;70:1205-14.
4. **Font C, Cid MC, Coll VB, et al.** Clinical features in patients with permanent visual loss due to biopsy-proven giant cell arteritis. Br J Rheumatol. 1997;36:251-4.
5. **Liu GT, Glaser JS, Schatz NJ, Smith JL.** Visual morbidity in giant cell arteritis clinical characteristics and prognosis for vision. Ophthalmology. 1994;101:1779-85.
6. **Brooks RC, McGee SR.** Diagnostic dilemmas in polymyalgia rheumatica. Arch Intern Med. 1997;157:162-8.
7. **Myklebust G, Gran JT.** A prospective study of 287 patients with polymyalgia rheumatica and temporal arteritis: clinical and laboratory manifestations at onset of disease and at the time of diagnosis. Br J Rheumatol. 1996;35:1161-8.
8. **Cohen MD, Ginsburg WW.** Polymyalgia rheumatica. Rheum Dis Clin North Am. 1990;16:325-39.
9. **Chuang TY, Hunder GC, Ilstrup DM, Jurland LT.** Polymyalgia rheumatica: a 10-year epidemiologic and clinical study. Ann Intern Med. 1982;97:672-80.
10. **Huston K, Hunder G, Lie JT, et al.** Temporal arteritis: a 25-year epidemiologic, clinical and pathologic study. Ann Intern Med. 1978;88:162-7.
11. **Kachroo A, Tello C, Bais R, Panush RS.** Giant cell arteritis: diagnosis and management. Bull Rheum Dis.1996;45:2-5.
12. **Gur H, Rapman E, Ehrenfeld M, Sidi Y.** Clinical manifestations of temporal arteritis: a report from Israel. J Rheumatol. 1996;23:1927-31.
13. **Hunder GG, Bloch DA, Michel BA, et al.** The American College of Rheumatology 1990 criteria for the classification of giant cell arteritis. Arthritis Rheum. 1990;33:1122-8.
14. **Desmet GD, Knockaert DC, Bobbaers HJ.** Temporal arteritis: the silent presentation and delay in diagnosis. J Intern Med. 1990;227:237-40.
15. **Fernandez-Herlihy L.** Temporal arteritis: clinical aids to diagnosis. J Rheumatol. 1988;15:1797-1801.
16. **Healey L, Wilske K.** Presentation of occult giant cell arteritis. Arthritis Rheumatol. 1980;23:641-3.

17. **Hayreh SS, Podhajsky PA, Raman R, Zimmerman B.** Giant cell arteritis: validity and reliability of various diagnostic criteria. Am J Ophthalmol. 1997;123:285-96.

18. **Rodriquez-Valverde V, Sarabia JM, Gonzalez-Gay MA, et al.** Risk factors and predictive models of giant cell arteritis in polymyalgia rheumatica. Am J Med. 1997;102:331-6.

19. **Melberg NS, Grand MG, Dieckert JP, et al.** Cotton-wool spots and the early diagnosis of giant cell arteritis. Ophthalmology. 1995;102:1611-4.

20. **Kyle V.** Laboratoy investigations including liver in polymyalgia rheumatica/giant cell arteritis. Baillieres Clin Rheumatol. 1991;5:475-84.

21. **Neish PR, Sergent JS.** Giant cell arteritis: a case with unusual neurologic manifestations and a normal sedimentation rate. Arch Intern Med. 1991; 151:378-80.

22. **Ashton-Key M, Gallagher PJ.** Surgical pathology of cranial arteritis and polymyalgia rheumatica. Ballieres Clin Rheum. 1991;5:387-404.

23. **Hall S, Lie JT, Kurland LT, et al.** The therapeutic impact of temporal artery biopsy. Lancet. 1983; 2:1217-20.

24. **Allsop C, Gallagher P.** Temporal artery biopsy in giant-cell arteritis. Am J Surg Pathol. 1981;5:317-23.

25. Temporal artery biopsy [Editorial]. Lancet 1983;1:396-7.

26. **Klein R, Campbell RT, Hunder GG, Carney JA.** Skip lesions in temporal arteritis. Mayo Clin Proc. 1979; 51:504-10.

27. **Ponge T, Barrier JH, et al.** The efficacy of selective unilateral temporal artery biopsy versus bilateral biopsies for diagnosis of giant cell arteritis. J Rheumatol. 1988;15:997-1000.

28. **Hall S, Hunder G.** Is temporal artery biopsy prudent? Mayo Clin Proc. 1984;59:793-6.

29. **Schmidt WA, Kraft HE, Vorpahl K, et al.** Color duplex ultrasonography in the diagnosis of temporal arteritis. N Engl J Med. 1997;337:1336-42.

30. **Hunder GG, Weyand CM.** Sonography in giant cell arteritis. N Engl J Med. 1997;337:1385-6.

31. **Kyle V, Hazleman BL.** Treatment of polymyalgia rheumatica and giant cell arteritis. II. Relation between steroid dose and steroid associated side effects. Ann Rheumatol Dis. 1989;48:662-6.

32. **Buchbinder R, Detsky AS.** Management of suspected giant cell arteritis:a decision analysis. J Rheumatol. 1992;19:1220-8.

Osteoporosis

38

Erica Friedman Asch, MD, and Lawrence G. Smith, MD

KEY POINTS

Pretest Probabilities

- Important risk factors to assess the likelihood of osteoporosis and subsequent fractures include patient age, gender, ethnicity, hormonal status, history of previous fractures, weight, use of medications, medical history, and family history of osteoporosis.

Diagnostic Strategies

- Postmenopausal women without risk factors who are already receiving estrogen replacement and men without risk factors require no further diagnostic testing for osteoporosis.

- For postmenopausal women who are undecided about hormone replacement therapy, bone density measurement may help decide on the value of hormonal or other treatments.

- Patients at unclear or intermediate risk for osteoporosis should undergo bone density measurement to facilitate a treatment decision.

- Because patients with established osteoporosis or those at very high risk for osteoporosis should receive antiresorptive therapy, bone density measurement may not be absolutely necessary. However, measurement may be useful to verify the diagnosis, to assess fracture risk, and to establish a baseline to allow subsequent assessment of treatment efficacy.

- Dual energy x-ray absorptiometry (DXA) of the hip and spine is the current method of choice for measuring bone density.

- Biochemical markers of bone turnover may be useful in monitoring the response to treatment and also may be helpful in the diagnostic evaluation of some patients.

BACKGROUND

Osteoporosis is defined as a skeletal disease characterized by low bone mass and microarchitectural deterioration of bone tissue with increased bone fragility and predisposition to fracture. It is a consequence of aging. Peak bone mass, which is largely genetically determined, occurs by the third decade; by the fifth decade, osteoclastic bone resorption exceeds osteoblastic bone formation, and gradual bone loss occurs. With menopause and estrogen deficiency, bone loss is accelerated. In patients with a low peak bone mass or with genetic or environmental factors that hasten bone loss, osteoporosis develops earlier. Nutritional or hormonal deficiency (estrogen or testosterone), immobilization, use of bone-toxic medications, chronic liver or renal disease, and endocrine diseases can result in a low peak bone mass or hasten bone resorption. Table 38-1 lists factors responsible for a low peak bone mass or increased bone resorption or both.

Osteoporosis is manifest clinically when the patient presents with a fracture with minimal or no trauma or reports chronic back pain secondary to kyphosis from vertebral wedge fractures. Once fractures have occurred and significant bony architectural abnormalities exist, further bone loss can be prevented, but the biomechanical competence of the skeleton cannot be repaired. The key to management is either prevention or early diagnosis and treatment.

The economic and financial burden of osteoporosis is significant: It is estimated that 20 million Americans have osteoporosis. Osteoporosis seems to meet Frame and Carlson's criteria (1) for a disease that should be screened for in a population; it is common, it is an important cause of morbidity and mortality, and tests are available that are safe and

Table 38-1. Risk Factors for Osteoporosis

Factors that decrease peak bone mass *and* increase bone resorption		Factors that decrease only peak bone mass
Female gender	Family history of osteoporosis	Caucasian or Asian descent
Hypogonadism		Short, thin body habitus
Immobilization	Ogligomenorrhea	Late onset menarche
Excess caffeine intake	Amenorrhea	
Cigarette use or alcohol abuse	Calcium or vitamin D deficiency	**Factors that increase only bone resorption**
Renal hypercalciuria	High-protein diet	Early onset menopause
Hyperthyroidism	Renal insufficiency	Achlorhydria
Cushing syndrome or exogenous steroid use	Malabsorption	Cirrhosis (especially primary biliary cirrhosis)
Chemotherapy	Hyperparathyroidism	Multiple myeloma
Anticoagulants	Inflammatory arthritis (rheumatoid arthritis or systemic lupus erythematosus	
	Anticonvulsants	

accurate in detecting low bone mass. In addition, therapy is available to prevent further bone loss and decrease the fractures that are the clinical consequences of osteoporosis.

Because the sensitivity of history and physical examination is only 60% to 75% in detecting severe osteoporosis and presumably even lower in milder disease, other methods must be used to identify those patients with established osteoporosis. Measurement of bone mineral content by one of several radiographic modalities is the primary method for diagnosis. Because the bone mass of age- and gender-matched patients with fractures overlaps with the bone mass of those without, bone mass measurement is not a diagnostic test for fracture. However, it measures the most important risk factor for future fractures and should be used for risk stratification, analogous to measurement of blood pressure or cholesterol to assess the risk of stroke or coronary disease. Osteoporosis-related fractures are uncommon until bone mass is significantly below the peak levels seen in young adults. Several different criteria for defining osteoporosis have been proposed. The most accepted is that of the World Health Organization, which defines osteoporosis as a bone density that is at least 2.5 standard deviations (SD) below the mean peak bone mass of gender-matched young normals (2,3). Osteoporosis is defined in this way because more than 99% of osteoporotic fractures occur at or below this bone density. However, because other factors also affect fracture incidence, some patients with osteoporosis defined in this way do not have fractures. Osteopenia is defined as a bone density between 1 and 2.5 SD below the mean peak bone mass of gender-matched young normals. Decisions about therapy for osteopenia should incorporate information about the patient's risk factors for subsequent bone loss (see Table 38-1) and about the presence or absence of other risk factors for fracture (4,5) (Table 38-2).

ESTIMATING PRETEST PROBABILITY

Several studies have shown that individual items from a patient's history or physical examination may not be accurate predictors of bone mass or fracture risk. Factors that independently predict risk of osteoporosis or low bone density include age, weight, height, onset of menarche or menopause, smoking history, family history of osteoporosis (especially having an affected first-degree relative), activity level, and dietary calcium intake. Individually these factors are not precise enough to stratify patients and only account for 25% to 40% of the variability in a patient's bone mineral density, depending on the set of risk factors used, and the site of bone mass measurement. Female gender, Asian or Caucasian descent, small body frame, and hormonal deficiency increase the likelihood of osteoporosis as well.

Table 38-2. Risk Factors for Fracture

Risk Factor	Relative Risk
For vertebral fracture*	
Lowest tertile of bone density (any site)	3.8–5.8
Increasing age (each 10-year increase)	2.0–2.3
One previous vertebral fracture	4.1–5.3
Two or more previous vertebral fractures	11.8
For hip fracture†	
Low bone density (each 1 SD decrease)	1.6
Maternal history of hip fracture	1.6–2.7
Muscle weakness (quadriceps)	2.1
Any fracture in patients older than 50 years	1.5–1.9
Weight loss >25% (since age 25 years)	2.0
Resting heart rate >80 bpm	1.7
Sedentary (<4 h/d standing)	1.7
Poor depth perception	1.5
Tall (at age 25 years)	1.2
Low calcium intake	1.5
Increasing age (each 10-year increase)	2.0
Long hip axis length (each 1 SD increase)	1.8
Cigarette smoking or excess caffeine intake	1.3

*Data from Ross PD, Davis JW, Epstein RS, Wasnich RD. Preexisting fractures and bone mass predict vertebral fracture incidence in women. Ann Intern Med. 1991;114:919-23.

†Adapted from data from Cumming SR, Nevitt MC, Browner WS, et al. Risk factors for hip fracture in white women. Study of Osteoporotic Fractures Research Group. N Engl J Med. 1995; 332:767-73.

An osteoporosis SCORE questionnaire (Simple Calculated Osteoporosis Risk Estimation) has been developed (Table 38-3) and validated for postmenopausal women who are at least 50 years old to help stratify patients with low or high bone mineral density (6). The SCORE divides women into two groups, those likely to have a femoral neck bone density 2 or more standard deviations below the mean of young normals and those whose bone density is likely to be normal or mildly osteopenic. Using these six questions, SCORE was 89% sensitive and 50% specific. No other formula using risk factors to predict likelihood of osteoporosis has been standardized for any other populations. Several other studies attempted to evaluate the predictive value of historical and anthropometric risk factors. In general, risk factor analysis alone has poor predictive value in identifying women with a low bone mass. In one study of perimenopausal women, all risk factors accounted for only 35% of the total variance in vertebral bone mass, and their model correctly classified just 73% of the women with a low bone mass (7).

Table 38-3. Osteoporosis Evaluation SCORE Sheet*

Question	How to Grade It	Enter Number
1. What is your current age (in years)?	Take the number in the tens column and multiply by 3	
2. What is your race or ethnic group?		
African-American	Enter 0	
Caucasian, Hispanic, Asian	Enter 5	
Native American, Other	Enter 5	
3. Have you been treated for or been told you have rheumatoid arthritis?		
Yes or No	If yes, enter 4	
4. Since the age of 45 years, have you experienced a fracture at any of the following sites?		
Hip Yes or No	If yes, enter 4	
Rib Yes or No	If yes, enter 4	
Wrist Yes or No	If yes, enter 4	
5. Do you currently take or have you ever taken estrogen?		
Yes or No	If no, enter 1	
Add score from questions 1–5		Subtotal _____
6. What is your current weight (lb)?	Take the numbers in the tens and hundreds column and subtract from the subtotal	
		Final Score _____

*Final scores of 6 or greater are associated with increased likelihood of osteoporosis (see text).
SCORE = Simple Calculated Osteoporosis Risk Estimation.
Republished with permission from Lydick E, Cook K, Turpin J, et al. Development and validation of a simple questionnaire (SCORE) to facilitate identification of women likely to have low
bone density. Am J Managed Care. 1998;4:37-48.

In another study, risk factor analyses also performed poorly when used
to predict vertebral fractures, with a sensitivity of 63% and a specificity
of 39% (8). Most risk factor assessment would permit some "risk" stratification for those with suspected osteoporosis and could help to guide
decisions about testing.

In some clinical situations, a diagnosis of osteoporosis can be made
with relative certainty. For example, findings of a vertebral compression fracture or a fracture with minimal trauma, height loss, thoracic

kyphosis, and radiographic osteopenia strongly suggest that osteoporosis is present.

DIAGNOSTIC TESTS

Ideally, diagnostic tests for osteoporosis would accurately predict the likelihood of fracture. However, because fractures depend not only on bone fragility, but also on the type and amount of force exerted on the bone, such testing is not practical. The currently available diagnostic tests for osteoporosis include measurements of bone mineral content, which provide a static measure of lifetime bone metabolism, and urine or blood assays, which are dynamic measures of bone formation or resorption or both.

The best predictor of fracture risk at any given site is a bone mineral content measurement at that site. Because of differences in bone loss in different types of bone, measurement of both trabecular (spine) and cortical (hip or wrist) bone are more sensitive for diagnosing osteoporosis than measurement of one site alone. In one study, about one third of perimenopausal women had osteoporosis at only one site (hip or spine) and a normal bone density at the other site, so the sensitivity of bone density measurement would be lower if measurements were done at only one site (9). Thus, although it is more expensive, measurement of both spine and hip bone mineral content is desirable. In perimenopausal or early postmenopausal women or in patients with corticosteroid excess, trabecular bone is predominately lost, so that measurement of the spine should be most useful. Because most measurement techniques can produce a false elevation in spine bone density related to osteophytes, scoliosis, vertebral fractures, or aortic calcification, the presence of these confounding factors makes hip or wrist measurement more accurate. In patients with hyperparathyroidism or calcium or vitamin D disorders, measurement of cortical bone (hip or wrist) is more sensitive for detecting bone loss. For each "standard deviation" decrease in bone density, the fracture risk increases by 1.5 to 2.2, depending on the region (spine compared with hip) and risk model used (see Table 38-2).

Table 38-4 lists the various modalities for measuring bone density. Sensitivity and specificity data are not presented because results using these tests have not been routinely compared with a "gold standard." Instead, this table presents information on the precision and accuracy of the available tests. Precision is defined as the coefficient of variation—that is, the standard deviation divided by the mean, for repeated measurements done over a short period in young, healthy adults. Accuracy is the coefficient of variation for measurements of bone mineral content also measured by in vitro measurement of ash bone weight.

Table 38-4. Techniques for Bone Mass Measurement

Technique	Site	Precision (%)	Accuracy (%)	Radiation (mrem)	Time (min)	Cost ($)
Dual energy x-ray absorptiometry	Spine, hip, forearm, total body	0.5–2	3–5	1–3	3-7	$100–$300
Radiographic absorptiometry	Hand, calmcaneus	1–2	6	<5	<5	$100–$200
Single-photon absorptiometry	Proximal and distal radius, calcaneus	1–3	5	10–20	15	$75
Dual energy photon absorptiometry	Spine, hip, total body	2–4	4–10	5	20–40	$100–$150
Quantitative computed tomography	Spine	2–5	5–20	100–1000 (single vs. dual)	10–15	$100–$200
Quantitative ultrasonography	Calcaneus, patella, tibia, and phalanges	3–6	*	0	5–10	~$40

*Quantitative ultrasonography measures the velocity and attenuation of sound, which correlate with bone density. Quantitative ultrasonography does not measure bone mineral content, so it cannot be compared with the ash weight of bone to allow determination of accuracy.

Data assessing the ability of bone mass measurements to distinguish patients at risk for fracture from those not at risk show that this technique has a 60% to 80% specificity for predicting fracture, depending on the criteria used for defining osteoporosis, the site of the fracture, and the site used for measuring bone mineral content (10,11). Each of the various methods used to measure bone mass is discussed briefly below.

Plain Radiography

As a measurement of bone mineral content (BMC), plain radiography is relatively insensitive (sensitivity, 50%–70%), because bone density must decrease between 25% to 40% before osteopenia can be seen.

Dual Energy X-ray Absorptiometry

Dual energy x-ray absorptiometry (DXA or DEXA) is the current method of choice for measuring bone mineral content at both trabecular and cortical sites because of its high precision and accuracy. It also has the fastest scan times and least radiation. Although "peripheral" DXA is available, there are concerns about its correlation with hip and spine measurements (12).

Radiographic Absorptiometry
Radiographic absorpitometry is readily available because it uses a standard radiography equipment, but it is limited to measurement of the fingers.

Single Photon Absorptiometry
Single photon absorptiometry is also limited because it only measures peripheral sites (forearm).

Dual Photon Absorptiometry
Dual photon absorptiometry can measure axial and appendicular sites; however, it is less precise than other methods because of problems related to radioisotope decay.

Quantitative Computed Tomography
Quantitative computed tomography of the lumbar spine is less accurate and less precise than other methods and involves ten times more radiation than other modalities, so it is rarely the method of choice. However, in patients with osteophytes or anatomic abnormalities, it can more accurately assess the bone density of the spine than can other modalities.

Quantitative Ultrasonography
Quantitative ultrasonography (QUS) is a new method for measuring bone mineral content of peripheral sites (calcaneus, patella, and tibia). It is fast and inexpensive, and it does not involve radiation exposure. Reports suggest that findings of ultrasonography may be influenced by microarchitectural characteristics as well as by bone density (13). Prospective studies have shown that the diagnostic sensitivity of QUS for the prediction of hip fractures is similar to that of hip density measurements obtained by DXA (14).

Biochemical Markers
Biochemical markers of bone turnover provide a dynamic measurement of bone growth or bone loss or both. These blood and urine markers represent products secreted by osteoblasts or osteoclasts or are products released from the bone matrix during bone resorption. Because most cases of osteoporosis result from increased bone resorption, markers of osteoclast activity or matrix breakdown are most useful.

Of the currently available assays, the urine amino-terminal telopeptide of type I collagen (NTX) appears to be the most sensitive and specific measure of bone matrix breakdown; however, both biologic and assay variability are relatively great (15). This variability limits the usefulness of this assay in the diagnosis of osteoporosis. However, in patients with borderline bone density measurements, an elevated NTX level is predictive of "more" bone loss and a better response to treatment (16). Because levels of these markers change more quickly than measurements of bone density, they may be useful in monitoring response to treatment (12).

DIAGNOSTIC STRATEGIES

The purpose of screening for osteoporosis is to identify the disorder and classify patients into fracture-risk categories to determine treatment strategies. Because the predictive value of information obtained from the history and physical examination is limited, if accurate measurement of bone density is needed for a treatment decision, it should generally be measured directly rather than estimated indirectly using risk factors.

For postmenopausal women without risk factors for osteoporosis and without a history of fracture who are taking estrogen replacement and for men without risk factors for osteoporosis, no additional evaluation or treatment is necessary. If these women are undecided about whether to receive hormone replacement, a bone density measurement may help decide on the value of hormonal or other treatment. If patients are unwilling to take medications, no other workup is needed. These patients should have adequate intake of calcium and vitamin D and a regular weight-bearing exercise regimen, regardless of their risk for osteoporosis.

For patients with osteoporosis or with significant risk factors for osteoporosis or fracture, antiresorptive therapy is indicated to treat or prevent osteoporosis. If possible, measurement of bone mineral density is useful to verify the diagnosis, assess the fracture risk or establish a baseline measurement or both to allow subsequent verification of treatment efficacy. (Of note, the accuracy of bone mass measurements in predicting subsequent fractures is better than measurement of cholesterol level to predict the risk of heart disease.)

For patients in whom the risk for osteoporosis is uncertain, a bone density measurement is indicated to facilitate a treatment decision. Whenever bone density measurement is necessary, DXA of the hip and spine is the current test of choice. Although QUS is rapidly evolving, at this time it is uncertain if it will replace DXA, be used in a complementary manner to DXA, or serve as a "pre-DXA" diagnostic test (13).

Biochemical markers of bone turnover, particularly NTX, can be useful in certain clinical situations. At present, because of the marked variability, these tests seem most useful in monitoring the response to treatment. They may have a limited role in helping to guide decisions about treatment in selected cases—for example, for those with border-line results on bone mineral density testing.

CLINICAL PROBLEMS

Clinical Problem 1
A woman with risk factors for osteoporosis asks for advice regarding preventive therapy.

Testing Strategy and Rationale
In general, women with risk factors for osteoporosis should receive hormone replacement therapy to prevent bone loss and the future development of osteoporosis and fractures. If the patient is uncertain about starting hormone replacement therapy or if the risk of osteoporosis is not clear, determining a baseline bone density may facilitate the decision.

Clinical Example
A 52-year-old white woman requests advice on prevention of osteoporosis. She is still menstruating, but her periods are becoming less regular. She enjoys excellent health. She has always been thin, has always exercised regularly, has never smoked, and has never taken any medications except a multi-vitamin. Her 75-year-old mother recently was hospitalized for a hip fracture.

This patient has risk factors for osteoporosis and fracture and should receive hormone replacement therapy provided that she agrees to the treatment and has no strong contraindications. She should also be advised to continue her exercise program and maintain an adequate intake of calcium and vitamin D. If she is uncertain about hormone replacement therapy or wishes to assess her risk of fractures better, bone density measurement should be assessed by DXA to facilitate the decision.

Clinical Problem 2
A man with significant risk factors for osteoporosis requests your help in assessing his risk of fractures.

Testing Strategy and Rationale
In a man with significant risk factors for previous, present, and/or future bone loss, a measurement of bone mineral content is necessary to predict the presence of osteoporosis and risk of subsequent fracture. If bone density testing shows osteoporosis or osteopenia in a patient with continued risk factors for bone loss, therapy with antiresorptive agents such as alendronate or calcitonin is indicated

Continued

to prevent fracture. Follow-up with a repeat bone density measurement is indicated to confirm the response to treatment.

Clinical Example

A 32-year-old man with a 10-year history of active Crohn disease is concerned about the possible side effects of the prednisone he has taken to control his gastrointestinal symptoms. He is chronically underweight with active symptoms on most days. He has taken prednisone on a daily basis for the past 4 years and intermittently for 7 years before that. He has no other active medical problems.

A DXA scan is ordered, and if bone mineral density is reduced, antiresorptive therapy should be initiated.

REFERENCES

1. **Frame PS, Carlson SJ.** A critical review of periodic health screening using specific screening criteria. Part 2: selected endocrine, metabolic, and gastrointestinal diseases. J Fam Pract. 1975;2:123-9.
2. The WHO Study Group (1994). Assessment of fracture risk and its application to screening for postmenopausal osteoporosis: synopsis of a WHO report. Osteoporos Int. 1994;4:368-81.
3. **Kanis JA, Melton LJ III, Christiansen C, et al.** The diagnosis of osteoporosis. J Bone Miner Res. 1994;9:1137-41.
4. **Ross PD, Davis JW, Epstein RS, Wasnich RD.** Preexisting fractures and bone mass predict vertebral fracture incidence in women. Ann Intern Med. 1991;114:919-23.
5. **Cummings SR, Nevitt MC, Browner WS, et al.** Risk factors for hip fracture in white women. Study of Osteoporotic Fractures Research Group. N Engl J Med. 1995;332:767-73.
6. **Lydick E, Cook K, Turpin J, et al.** Development and validation of a simple questionnaire (SCORE) to facilitate identification of women likely to have low bone density. Am J Managed Care. 1998;4:37-48.
7. **Hansen MA, Overgaard K, Riis BJ, Christiansen C.** Potential risk factors for development of postmenopausal osteoporosis examined over a 12-year period. Osteoporosos Int. 1991;1:95-102.
8. **Kleerekoper M, Peterson E, Nelson D, et al.** Identification of women at risk for developing postmenopausal osteoporosis with vertebral fractures: role of history and single photon absorptiometry. Bone Mineral. 1989;7:289-99.
9. **Pouilles JM, Tremollieres R, Ribot C.** Spine and femur densitometry at the menopause: are both sites necessary in the assessment of the risk of osteoporosis? Calcif Tissue Int. 1993;52:344-7.
10. **Duboeuf F, Braillon P, Chaput MC, et al.** Bone mineral density of the hip measured with dual-energy x-ray absorptiometry in normal elderly women and in patients with hip fracture. Osteoporosos Int. 1991;1:242-9.

11. **Prince RL, Price RI, Henzell S, et al.** Distal limb bone density measure by DEXA: reproducibility and clinical utility. In: Christiansen C, Overgaard K, Osteopress AS. Osteoporosis. Copenhagen; 1990:750-1.

12. **Scheiber LB, Torregrosa L.** Evaluation and treatment of postmenopausal osteoporosis. Semin Arthritis Rheum. 1998;27:245-61.

13. **Kroger H, Reeve J.** Diagnosis of osteoporosis in clinical practice. Ann Med. 1998;30:278-87.

14. **Bauer DC, Gluer CC, Cauley JA, et al.** BUA predicts fractures strongly and independently of densitometry in older females: a propspective study. Arch Intern Med. 1997;157:629-34.

15. **Gertz BJ, Shao P, Hanson DA, et al.** Monitoring bone resorption in early postmenopausal women by an immunoassay for cross-linked collagen peptides in urine. J Bone Miner Res.1994;9:135-42.

16. **Chestnut CH, Bell NH, Clark GS, et al.** Hormone replacement therapy in postmenopausal women: urinary N-telopeptide of Type I collagen monitors therapeutic effect and predicts response of bone mineral density. Am J Med. 1997;102:29-37.

Endocrinologic Problems

Hypercalcemia

James P. Corsetti, MD, PhD, and Dean A. Arvan, MD

39

KEY POINTS

Pretest Probabilities

- Primary hyperparathyroidism and malignancies account for most cases of sustained hypercalcemia.

- More than half of all patients with primary hyperparathyroidism are asymptomatic when hypercalcemia is first discovered.

- With the exception of a history of renal calculi, signs and symptoms of hypercalcemia lack sufficient sensitivity or specificity to be useful in the differential diagnosis.

Diagnostic Strategies

- Routine tests such as serum albumin, chloride, alkaline phosphatase, and blood hemoglobin assessments, alone or in combination, are of some value in differentiating hypercalcemia owing to malignancy from that caused by primary hyperparathyroidism.

- The newer assays for intact parathyroid hormone (PTH) greatly improve the ability to distinguish between the two common causes of hypercalcemia.

BACKGROUND

The increasing use of automated laboratory testing has led to more frequent identification of patients with hypercalcemia in both ambulatory and hospital settings. Data indicate that the prevalence of hypercalcemia in ambulatory patients varies from 0.1% to 2.2% (1–6), whereas in hospitalized patients it has ranged from 0.3% to 7.8% (2, 7–11). Determining the cause of hypercalcemia in the asymptomatic patient may be difficult. The lack of gold standards to determine the cause of hypercalcemia, other than surgery to establish the diagnosis of hyperparathyroidism, has led to the development of several tests, the utility and reliability of which have not often been subjected to critical evaluation.

The most frequent causes of hypercalcemia include primary hyperparathyroidism, malignancy, use of thiazide diuretics, sarcoidosis, renal disease, the milk-alkali syndrome, immobilization, and thyroid disease. Primary hyperparathyroidism and malignancy account for about 80% to 90% of all cases in adults (5–7,11–13). Primary hyperparathyroidism may result from parathyroid adenoma, hyperplasia, or rarely, carcinoma. Cancer of the breast accounts for about half of the cases of hypercalcemia associated with malignancy. Cancer of the lung, kidney, and urogenital tract, as well as hematologic malignancies, such as multiple myeloma and lymphoma, account for most remaining cases.

This chapter emphasizes diagnostic procedures useful in distinguishing between the two major causes of hypercalcemia: primary hyperparathyroidism and malignancy. However, this separation may not always be absolute, because of their coexistence in some patients (14).

ESTIMATING PRETEST PROBABILITY

Among ambulatory patients, hypercalcemia caused by primary hyperparathyroidism occurs approximately twice as frequently as hypercalcemia caused by malignancy, accounting for 30% to 60% of all cases. The reverse is generally true among hospitalized patients, in whom 30% to 70% of cases are associated with malignancy (1,3,4,7–9, 12,13,15,16). Primary hyperparathyroidism is more frequent in women and increases significantly after the age of 40 years, generally peaking between the ages of 60 and 70 years. The clinical presentation of primary hyperparathyroidism more often includes an array of mild constitutional manifestations rather than the classic complications such as osteitis fibrosa cystica. Additionally, the number of asymptomatic cases has increased (1,5,6,13,16–18).

A variety of symptoms (e.g., polyuria, mental status changes, gastrointestinal distress, weakness, bone pain, constipation, weight loss, anorexia, and fatigue) and conditions (e.g., renal calculi, peptic ulcer disease, and hypertension) have been attributed to primary hyperparathyroidism. Up to two thirds of patients with primary hyperparathyroidism have been reported to have more than one of these findings (18–20). However, the sensitivity of each individual finding is low, and its absence does not help rule out the diagnosis. Furthermore, given their common occurrence in patients with malignancy, they are of little help in distinguishing between the two common causes of hypercalcemia. Only the presence of renal calculi, which occurs in 29% of patients with hypercalcemia caused by primary hyperparathyroidism and in only 4% of patients with hypercalcemia caused by malignancy, has a sufficiently powerful positive likelihood ratio (7.3) to be of any use.

DIAGNOSTIC TESTS

Serum Calcium

Total serum calcium is a routine measurement in clinical laboratory practice. It consists of three fractions: free or ionized (47%), protein-bound (40%, about 80% bound to albumin), and complexed (13%). Ionized calcium is the key physiologic mediator of parathyroid hormone (PTH) secretion. Some studies have concluded that measurement of the ionized fraction may be a better indicator of primary hyperparathyroidism than total calcium in patients with intermittent or borderline elevations in total calcium (21–23). However, because total calcium determinations appear to be adequate for most patients, and ionized calcium determinations are not readily available in many laboratories, utilization of total calcium in this setting will likely continue (24).

Several factors must be considered before a diagnosis of hypercalcemia is made. Some adjustment for changes in albumin concentration is necessary. Several "correction" formulas have been proposed. One practical formula adopted by some is the addition or subtraction of 0.9 mg/dL to the measured value of total calcium for each 1 g/dL change in albumin above or below the normal mean albumin concentration (generally 4.2 g/dL) (25). Prolonged (several minutes) tourniquet application during phlebotomy produces venous stasis and capillary fluid shifts, which can elevate the total serum calcium by as much as 1 mg/dL. Ingestion of a high-calcium meal before sampling can have a similar effect. Use of certain drugs, such as thiazides, commonly leads to mild hypercalcemia. Spurious results due to interfering serum substances are less common. The effect of these variables has been shown by the finding that as many as 53% of patients initially thought to be hypercalcemic were found to be normocalcemic on correctly obtained repeat samples (1,12).

In most laboratories, a calcium level greater than 10.4 mg/dL is accepted as being above "normal." However, because hypercalcemia is generally defined as a total serum calcium level greater than two standard deviations above the mean of a healthy normal population of specified age-range and sex, a small proportion of patients with primary hyperparathyroidism will be classified as normal, and some nondiseased patients will be labeled as hypercalcemic.

Recent studies have shown that the distribution of serum calcium in hypercalcemic patients with primary hyperparathyroidism appears to be similar to that of patients with malignancy (11,26). Therefore, except for the rare patient with carcinoma who shows extreme hypercalcemia, the level of total serum calcium is of no help in the differential diagnosis of hypercalcemia.

Serum Parathyroid Hormone

Several factors must be considered when interpreting serum PTH levels. Parathyroid hormone circulates in several molecular forms. Rapid cleavage of the intact hormone in the liver and kidney produces an N-terminal peptide that is biologically active, but has a half-life of less than 10 minutes; and a C-terminal peptide that is biologically inactive, has an average half-life of about 1 hour, and accumulates significantly at creatinine clearances of less than 40 mL/min (11,27,28).

Parathyroid hormone has been measured by various radioimmunoassay methods. Different antibodies yield varying specificities for these heterogeneous PTH peptides. This problem and the lack of a highly purified human PTH reference standard have made it difficult in the past to compare test results accurately among laboratories or within the same laboratory over time. However, recent technical improvements in the measurement of the biologically active intact human PTH have substantially increased the utility of PTH assays in the differential diagnosis of hypercalcemia (28). A two-site, double antibody immunoradiometric assay, which includes a system for separating biologically active from inactive PTH molecules before analysis, has been found superior to any other assay in distinguishing hypercalcemic patients with primary hyperparathyroidism from those with malignancy (29). Patients with proven or presumed primary hyperparathyroidism have values nearly always (69 of 70, or 99%) above the upper limit of normal, whereas those with hypercalcemia of malignancy nearly always have values below the lower limit of normal (37 of 40, or 93%). It must be emphasized, however, that these estimates are not applicable to patients with renal insufficiency. They may, therefore, have elevated C-terminal mid-region or intact PTH values, regardless of their parathyroid status. Average values for the sensitivity of various serum PTH assays from hospitalized patients with documented primary hyperparathyroidism are given in Table 39-1.

Serum Chloride

Increased serum chloride levels are seen in some patients with primary hyperparathyroidism. This is believed to result from impairment in renal tubular bicarbonate reabsorption (PTH effect) leading to a mild hyperchloremic metabolic acidosis. The serum chloride level may be particularly helpful in distinguishing patients with primary hyperparathyoidism from those with malignancy in whom a tendency toward hypochloremic alkalosis is seen (2,17,18,20,30,31).

Serum Phosphate

Classic primary hyperparathyroidism is associated with a decreased serum phosphate level caused by the PTH-mediated reduction in renal tubular reabsorption of phosphate. However, many factors, such as

Table 39-1. Frequency of Various Laboratory Test Findings in the Diagnosis of Primary Hyperparathyroidism Compared with Malignancy in Patients with Hypercalcemia

Diagnostic Test	Result Indicating Primary HPT	Frequency		Likelihood Ratio	
		In Primary HPT	In Malignancy	Positive Result*	Negative Result*
		←———— % ————→			
Parathyroid hormone (PTH) assay					
C-terminal	>normal range	86	9	9.6	0.15
N-terminal	>normal range	40	0	∞	0.60
C&N terminal	>normal range	67	5	13	0.35
Intact PTH	>6.3 pmol/L	99	7	14	0.07
Albumin	>4.0 g/dL	81	16	5.1	0.23
Chloride	>102 mmol/L	71	28	2.5	0.40
Alkaline phosphatase	<96 units/L	66	33	2.0	0.51
Hemoglobin					
Men	>14.1 g/dL	79	25	3.2	0.28
Women	>13.0 g/dL	71	30	2.4	0.41

HPT = hyperparathyroidism.
*These ratios indicate the relative likelihood of the findings in hypercalcemia caused by primary hyperparathyroidism (primary HPT) compared with malignancy.

renal failure, dietary intake of phosphates, use of antacids, and vomiting, may influence the serum phosphate level, leading to either false-positive or false-normal results. When the lower limit of normal is used as the cutoff point, average sensitivity and specificity values for primary hyperparathyroidism are too low to be helpful in distinguishing these patients from those with malignancy (35% and 49%, respectively) (18,23,30,32–35).

Chloride/Phosphate Ratio

The chloride/phosphate ratio has been proposed for use in the differential diagnosis of hypercalcemia. Initial studies tended to suggest that when a ratio of 33 is used as a cutoff, excellent differentiation of primary hyperparathyroidism from all other causes of hypercalcemia was obtained (sensitivity, 94%–96%; specificity, 97%–100%) (34,35). Although subsequent studies have yielded sensitivities ranging from 73% to 95%, the findings from others have been less impressive (2,17,30). Some investigators have suggested that the chloride/phosphate ratio may be less useful than chloride levels alone (26).

Alkaline Phosphatase

The alkaline phosphatase may be elevated in patients with primary hyperparathyroidism as well as in those with malignancy (18,26,33). For the most part, serum levels of this enzyme are greater in patients with malignancy than in those with primary hyperparathyroidism. The alkaline phosphatase level is also of little value in differentiating patients with primary hyperparathyroidism or malignancy from those with other causes of hypercalcemia.

Other Laboratory Tests

Several other tests, including serum albumin and hemoglobin determinations, have been used in the differential diagnosis of hypercalcemia (Table 39-1). Several investigators have developed multivariate discriminant functions using as many as 18 clinical variables in an attempt to improve the identification of hypercalcemic subgroups (20,26,31,34–37). In one study (26), it was found that by using albumin, PTH, and chloride measurements in a logistic discriminant function, a 95% classification accuracy could be achieved in distinguishing patients with primary hyperparathyroidism from those with malignancy. We caution against relying too heavily on such approaches for two reasons. First, data and formulas generated in one setting are not necessarily transferable to another (see Chapter 4). Second, the presence of renal failure significantly distorts the relationships among various tests.

Confirmatory testing for malignancy-associated hypercalcemia has been assisted in recent years by the discovery of parathyroid hormone-related protein (PTHrP). This is a protein with sufficient amino terminal sequence homology with PTH to mimic its actions via PTH receptors. It is now known to be the major mediator of hypercalcemia in humoral hypercalcemia of malignancy (38,39), and it has been found to be elevated in 55% to 78% of such patients (6). Its determination is most useful in and should be restricted to a setting in which the previously described test results tend to rule out hyperparathyroidism, and there is no obvious malignancy to account for hypercalcemia. An elevated PTHrP level would be strongly suggestive of occult malignancy. However, it should be noted that in rare cases, malignant neoplasms have been reported to secrete PTH alone or together with PTHrP, which further complicates the diagnostic evaluation (5,39).

DIAGNOSTIC STRATEGIES

Clinical findings from the history and physical examination together with routine biochemical tests are usually sufficient to establish the cause of hypercalcemia when it is caused by an established malignancy, hyperthyroidism, the milk-alkali syndrome, renal insufficiency, or sarcoidosis. The major issue of differential diagnosis rests in distinguishing between primary hyperparathyroidism and malignancy in patients who are either asymptomatic or have vague constitutional symptoms. If the serum calcium level is borderline, it should be repeated for confirmation (11), and/or an ionized Ca should be ordered (21, 22). In many cases, the repeat value will fall within the limits of normal and remain within those limits.

Of the various tests commonly done, the albumin, chloride, alkaline phosphatase, and hemoglobin determinations may be helpful. Malignancy-related hypercalcemia is frequently associated with low albumin and hemoglobin levels, a low-normal or low chloride level, and a significantly elevated alkaline phosphatase level. On the other hand, hypercalcemia in association with normal levels of albumin and hemoglobin, a high-normal chloride level, and slightly elevated alkaline phosphatase level suggest primary hyperparathyroidism.

Confirmatory testing for hyperparathyroidism is provided by simultaneous determination of serum PTH and calcium levels. An elevated PTH value, using an improved double-antibody assay, significantly increases the likelihood of primary hyperparathyroidism. Confirmatory testing for humoral hypercalcemia of malignancy is provided by determination of serum PTHrP level.

CLINICAL PROBLEM

An asymptomatic patient has an elevated serum calcium level.

Testing Strategy and Rationale

A blood count and assessments of serum creatinine or blood urea nitrogen, albumin, chloride, and alkaline phosphatase should be obtained. The results of these tests would suggest which of the confirmatory tests should be ordered.

Clinical Example

A 48-year-old woman has a serum calcium of 10.9 mg/dL on a routine biochemical screen. She reports having occasional leg cramps but no other symptoms. An older sister died from metastatic breast carcinoma at the age of 45 years. The patient has no abnormal physical findings. In particular, the breast examination is normal. A repeat serum calcium is 11.2 mg/dL, and renal function is normal.

Continued

Given this information, one could estimate the likelihood of primary hyperparathyoidism to be about one in three. Albumin and alkaline phosphatase determinations should be obtained. If the results are 4.2 g/dL and 95 U/L, respectively, then, on the basis of the data given in Table 39-1, the revised likelihood of primary hyperparathyroidism would be about 80%. A PTH measurement using a two-site immunoradiometric assay should then be obtained. A positive result would increase the post-test probability of primary PTH to about 99%.

REFERENCES

1. **Harrop JS, Bailey JE, Woodhead JS.** Incidence of hypercalcaemia and primary hyperparathyroidism in relation to the biochemical profile. J Clin Pathol. 1982;35:395-400.
2. **Wong ET, Freier EF.** The differential diagnosis of hypercalcemia: an algorithm for more effective use of laboratory tests. JAMA. 1982;247(1):75-80.
3. **Boonstra CE, Jackson CE.** Hyperparathyroidism detected by routine serum calcium analysis. Ann Intern Med. 1965;63:468.
4. **Boonstra CE, Jackson CE.** Serum calcium survey for hyperparathyroidism: results in 50,000 clinic patients. Am J Clin Pathol. 1971;55:523.
5. **Heath H III.** Primary hyperparathyroidism: recent advances in pathogenesis, diagnosis, and management. Adv Intern Med. 1992;37:275-93.
6. **Kaye TB.** Hypercalcemia: how to pinpoint the cause and customize treatment. Postgrad Med. 1995;97:153-5, 159-60.
7. **Fiskin RA, Heath DA, Bold AM.** Hypercalcemia: a hospital survey. Q J Med. 1980;196:405-18.
8. **McLellan G, Baird CW, Melick R.** Hypercalcaemia in an Australian hospital adult population. Med J Aust. 1968;2:354-6.
9. **Finnis WA, Cohanim M, Yendt ER.** Unsuspected hypercalcemia among adults in hospital. Can Med Assoc J. 1981;125:561-4.
10. **Burt M, Brennan MF.** Incidence of hypercalcemia and malignant neoplasm. Arch Surg. 1980;115:704-7.
11. **Klee GG, Kao PC, Heath H III.** Hypercalcemia. Endocrinol Metab Clin North Am. 1988;17:573.
12. **Christenssom T, Hellstrom K, Wengle B, et al.** Prevalence of hypercalcaemia in a health screening in Stockholm. Acta Med Scand. 1976;200:131-37.
13. **Heath H, Hodgson SF, Kennedy MA.** Primary hyperparathyroidism: incidence morbidity, and potential impact in a community. N Engl J Med. 1980;302:189-93.
14. **Kaplan L, Katz AD, Ben-Isaac, et al.** Malignant neoplasms and parathyroid adenoma. Cancer. 1971;28:401-7.
15. **Lee DB, Zawada ET, Kleeman CR.** The pathophysiology and clinical aspects of hypercalcemic disorders. West J Med. 1978;129(4):278-320.
16. **Mundy GR, Cove DH, Fisken R, et al.** Primary hyperparathyroidism: changes in the pattern of clinical presentation. Lancet. 1980;1:1317-20.

17. **Lafferty FW.** Primary hyperparathyroidism. Arch Intern Med. 1981;141: 1761-6.

18. **Mallette LE, Bilezikian JP, Heath DA, Aurbach GD.** Primary hyperparathyroidism: clinical and biochemical features. Medicine. 1974;53(2):127-46.

19. **Roberts JW.** Symptomatic hyperparathyroidism. Surg Clin North Am. 1982;62(2):225.

20. **Fisken RA, Heath DA, Somers S, Bold AM.** Hypercalcemia in hospital patients. Lancet. 1981;I:202-7.

21. **Benson L, Ljunghall S, Groth T, et al.** Optimal discrimination of mild hyperparathyroidism with total serum calcium, ionized calcium and parathyroid hormone measurements. Upsala J Med Sci. 1987;92:147-76.

22. **Forster J, Monchik JM, Martin HF.** A comparative study of serum ultrafiltrable, ionized, and total calcium in the diagnosis of primary hyperparathyroidism in patients with intermittent or no elevation in total calcium. Surgery. 1988;104:1137-42.

23. **Schmidt-Gayk H, Haerdt H.** Differential diagnosis of hypercalcemia: laboratory assessment. Rec Res Cancer Res. 1994;137:122-37.

24. **Ladenson JII, Lewis JW, McDonald JM, et al.** Relationship of free and total calcium in hypercalcemic conditions. J Clin Endocrinol Metab. 1979;48(3):393.

25. **Berry EM, Gupta MM, Turner SJ, Burns RR.** Variation in plasma calcium with induced changes in plasma specific gravity, total protein, and albumin. Br Med J. 1973;II:640-3.

26. **Boyd JC, Ladenson JH.** Value of laboratory tests in the differential diagnosis of hypercalcemia. Am J Med. 1984;77:863-72.

27. **Slatopolsky E, Martin K, Morrissey J, Hruska K.** Current concept of the metabolism and radioimmunoassay of parathyroid hormone. J Lab Clin Med. 1982;99(3):309-16.

28. **Kao PC, van Heerden JA, Grant CS, et al.** Clinical performance of parathyroid hormone immunometric assays. Mayo Clin Proc. 1992;67:637-45.

29. **Blind E, Schmidt-Gayk H, Scharla S, et al.** Two-site assay of intact parathyroid hormone in the investigation of primary hyperparathyroidism and other disorders of calcium metabolism compared with a midregion assay. J Clin Endocrinol Metab. 1988;67:353-60.

30. **Kvetny J, Orthman-Brask H, Frederiksen PK, et al.** Hypercalcemia due to primary hyperparathyroidism or malignant disease. Acta Med Scand. 1982;212:163.

31. **Lind L, Ljunghall S.** Serum chloride in the differential diagnosis of hypercalcemia. Exp Clin Endocrinol. 1991;98:179-84.

32. **Kao PC, Jiang NS, Klee GG, Purnell DC.** Development and validation of a new radioimmunoassay for parathyrin (PTH). Clin Chem. 1982; 28(1):69-74.

33. **Omenn GS, Roth SI, Baker WH.** Hyperparathyroidism associated with malignant tumors of nonparathyroid origin. Cancer. 1969;24(5):1004-11.

34. **Reeves CD, Palmer F, Bacchus H, Longerbeam JK.** Differential diagnosis of hypercalcemia by the chloride/phosphate ratio. Am J Surg. 1975;130:166-71.

35. **Palmer FJ, Nelson JC, Bacchus H.** The chloride-phosphate ratio in hypercalcemia. Ann Intern Med. 1974;80:200.

36. **Johnson KR, Howarth AT, Hamilton M, Mascall GC.** Laboratory differentiation of hypercalcemic patients. Clin Chem. 1982;28(2):333-8.

37. **Frolich A, Friis Nielsen B, Conradsen K, McNair P.** Filtering clinically significant hypercalcemia from non-significant hypercalcemia at the laboratory level. Scand J Clin Lab Invest. 1993;53:215-23.

38. **Law F, Ferrari S, Rizzoli R, Bonjour JP.** Parathyroid hormone-related protein: physiology and pathophysiology. Adv Nephrol Necker Hosp. 1994;23:281-94.

39. **Moseley JM, Gillespie MT.** Parathyroid hormone-related protein. Crit Rev Clin Lab Sci. 1995;32:299-343.

Hypercortisolism: Cushing Syndrome

40

Edgar R. Black, MD

KEY POINTS

Pretest Probabilities

- Clinical signs and symptoms are helpful in estimating the probability of hypercortisolism.

- The presence of proximal weakness, spontaneous ecchymoses, hypokalemia, or osteoporosis substantially increases the likelihood of hypercortisolism.

Diagnostic Strategies

- The single-dose overnight dexamethasone suppression test is an excellent screening test in the diagnosis of Cushing syndrome when the probability of disease is low. A normal result virtually establishes the absence of disease.

- An elevated 24-hour urinary free cortisol excretion or midnight plasma cortisol level confirms the diagnosis of Cushing syndrome when the pretest probability of disease is high.

- Radiographic examination of the sella turcica or adrenal glands is not a useful test in the initial evaluation of hypercortisolism.

BACKGROUND

Hypercortisolism occurs only rarely but is often considered a possible diagnosis in patients who have the common findings of obesity, hypertension, or diabetes mellitus. Physicians may feel compelled to perform laboratory tests to rule out Cushing syndrome as a treatable cause for these common clinical conditions.

Cushing syndrome (i.e., sustained hypercortisolism) may result from several processes, including adrenocorticotropic hormone (ACTH)–producing pituitary tumors; autonomous benign or malignant adrenal tumors; or extrapituitary tumors producing ectopic ACTH or corticotropin releasing hormone (CRH). The pituitary syndrome, Cushing disease, is the most common of the three types—accounting for approximately 70% of cases in several series (1–3)—and generally affects women of childbearing age. The other two forms occur with nearly equal frequency, but adrenal tumors are more common in children, and the syndromes from ectopic hormones generally occur in older persons. Cushing syndrome may also result from the use of exogenous corticosteroids.

This chapter emphasizes establishing the diagnosis of Cushing syndrome rather than the differentiation of the various causes of hypercortisolism.

ESTIMATING PRETEST PROBABILITY

Patients with Cushing syndrome usually present with features attributable to sustained hypercortisolism. In patients who present with a classic picture of Cushing syndrome—for example, moon facies, central obesity, plethora, red striae, ecchymoses, proximal muscle weakness, and osteoporosis—a rather certain clinical diagnosis can be made. However, such classical presentations are uncommon. The diagnosis of the syndrome can be complicated further by the atypical presentation sometimes seen in patients with ectopic ACTH production, who are more likely to present with hypokalemic metabolic alkalosis and edema than with obesity, striae, and hypertension. This difference probably is owing to higher levels of cortisol and to the shorter duration of the illness in this latter subgroup.

Reliable information concerning the incidence and prevalence of Cushing syndrome is not available. Certainly, the disease is rare and the prevalence in the general population is less than 1 case per 1000 persons (4). The usefulness of clinical information in assessing the probability of Cushing syndrome was studied by Nugent (5), and the sensitivity and specificity for the most helpful signs and symptoms are shown in Table 40-1. By expressing this information as likelihood ratios and assuming a disease prevalence of 0.1%, in patients presenting with central obesity, weakness, plethora, acne, striae, hirsutism, ecchymoses, osteoporosis, and edema, but without the other findings, the calculated probability of the disease is approximately 95%. Similarly, in patients presenting with the four specific findings of hypokalemia, weakness, ecchymoses, and osteoporosis, the probability of the disease is approximately 80% using only these four findings and assuming that these occur independently. On the other hand, in patients presenting with three or four of the less specific findings, such as hypertension, edema, and hirsutism, the likelihood of the disease is still relatively low (<3%).

Table 40-1. Operating Characteristics of Clinical Signs and Symptoms in the Diagnosis of Hypercortisolism

Diagnostic Finding	Sensitivity	Specificity	Likelihood Ratio	
			Finding Present	Finding Absent
	←———— % ————→			
Central obesity	90	71	3.1	0.14
Weakness	65	93	9.3	0.38
Plethora	82	69	2.6	0.26
WBC >11,000	58	70	1.9	0.60
Acne	52	76	2.1	0.63
Pigmented striae	46	78	2.1	0.69
Diastolic BP >105 mm Hg	39	83	2.3	0.73
Pitting edema	38	83	2.2	0.75
Hirsutism	50	71	1.7	0.70
Ecchymoses	53	94	8.8	0.50
Potassium <3.7	25	96	6.2	0.78
Oligomenorrhea	72	49	1.4	0.57
Abnormal GTT	88	23	1.1	0.52
Generalized obesity	3	38	0.05	2.5
Osteoporosis (early diagnosis)	26	94	4.8	0.79
Osteoporosis (late diagnosis)	64	97	21	0.37

BP = blood pressure; WBC = white blood cell; GTT = glucose tolerance test.
Adapted from Nugent CA, Warner HR, Dunn JT, Tyler FH. Probability theory in the diagnosis of Cushing syndrome. J Clin Endocrin Metab. 1964;24:621.

The accurate identification of some patients with "pseudo-Cushing syndrome" can be particularly problematic. Many persons with major depression have abnormal cortisol regulation, although cortisol hypersecretion, if present, is usually minimal. Nevertheless, it can be difficult to distinguish patients with major depression and obesity, hypertension, and diabetes mellitus from those with true Cushing syndrome (4).

DIAGNOSTIC TESTS

Two general types of diagnostic tests are used in the evaluation of possible Cushing syndrome: those that measure baseline cortisol levels or production rate, and those that test the suppressibility of the pituitary-adrenal axis. Although radiographic examinations of the sella turcica and adrenal glands may be used as part of the evaluation of those with proven Cushing syndrome, they should not be a part of the initial evaluation.

Plasma Cortisol

In normal persons, plasma cortisol levels show frequent fluctuations in magnitude and a diurnal variation, with higher levels occurring during morning hours. This variability makes the diagnosis of hypercortisolism using plasma values difficult (6). Because the diurnal variation in cortisol secretion results in lower afternoon levels and because patients with Cushing syndrome often have a decreased diurnal variation, most studies of the utility of plasma cortisol levels examine afternoon or evening specimens. Results published in one review (6) and listed in Table 40-2 show sensitivities of 83% for afternoon (4 PM to 9 PM) cortisol levels and 96% for midnight cortisol levels, respectively. Using persons in whom disease is suspected instead of "normals" as the appropriate controls, the 4 PM cortisol level has a specificity of 67% (7) and the midnight cortisol level has a specificity of 96% (8). A recent study reported a sensitivity of 100% for

Table 40-2. Operating Characteristics of Diagnostic Tests for Hypercortisolism

Diagnostic Test	Definition of Positive Result*	Sensitivity	Specificity	Likelihood Ratio	
				Positive Result	Negative Result
		←———— % ————→			
Measurement of plasma cortisol levels (4 PM–9 PM)	>13–20 µg/dL	83 (48–100)	67[†]	2.5	0.16
Measurement of plasma cortisol levels (midnight)	>6–15 µg/dL	96 (68–100)	96[†]	24	0.04
Measurement of 24-hour urinary free cortisol	>20–181 µg/dL	94 (78–100)	91[†] (75–100)	10	0.07
Measurement of 24-hour urinary 17-hydroxysteroids	>6–14 mg/dL	89 (65–100)	73[†] (46–100)	3.3	0.15
MRI of sella turcica	Abnormal pituitary	40	90	4	0.67
CT of sella turcica	Abnormal pituitary	20	75	0.8	1.1
Abdominal CT scan	Abnormal adrenal	40	~95	8	0.63

MRI = magnetic resonance imaging; CT = computed tomography.

*Steroid assays are performed by various techniques (e.g., colorimetric, fluorimetric, competitive protein binding) that produce different definitions of positive results but have similar sensitivity and specificity. In interpreting tests, it is important to be aware of the assay used and the normal range for the assay.

[†]Controls are persons in whom the disease is suspected.

midnight cortisol levels when measurements were done in hospitalized patients who had been sleeping until the minutes before phlebotomy (9). This report again demonstrated the limited utility of cortisol levels measured at other times of the day.

Urinary Free Cortisol

In contrast with standard plasma cortisol levels, measurement of 24-hour urinary free cortisol excretion has the potential diagnostic benefit of assessing cortisol production over time. Urinary free cortisol levels are often elevated in patients with hypercortisolism both because of excess steroid production and because saturation of cortisol-binding globulins permits rapid glomerular filtration of plasma cortisol. Crapo (6) demonstrated that 24-hour urinary free cortisol enables the clinician to differentiate almost completely between patients with Cushing syndrome and controls in whom the disease is suspected. As listed in Table 40-2, the test has a sensitivity of 94% and a specificity of 91% in control groups consisting of persons in whom Cushing syndrome is suspected. The specificity is more than 99% in "normal" controls and is 95% in obese patients.

The specificity of this test can decrease dramatically in patients experiencing "stress" and during pregnancy. Elevated urinary free cortisol levels have been found in 30% to 40% of patients with acute illness, awaiting surgery (10), or with depression (11). Elevated levels also are common during pregnancy (10). Thus, positive test results obtained under these circumstances tend to be less helpful in the diagnosis. Measuring the amount of creatinine in the specimen may help determine the adequacy of the collection.

Urinary Cortisol Metabolites

Determination of 24-hour urinary excretion of cortisol metabolites is another method of assessing cortisol production. Measurement of 17-hydroxysteroids (17-OHCS) has been studied in the diagnosis of Cushing syndrome. This assay is relatively sensitive but fairly nonspecific, especially in obese persons (see Table 40-2) (6). Some authors (12) have suggested that specificity can be improved to more than 95% by normalizing the milligrams per day of urinary 17-OH steroids excreted adjusted per gram of urine creatinine.

Single-Dose Dexamethasone Suppression Test

The single-dose overnight dexamethasone suppression test (DST) is a simple method of determining pituitary suppressibility by corticosteroids. The test is performed by administering 1 mg of dexamethasone orally at about midnight and measuring the plasma cortisol at 8:00 AM the following morning. At times, a hypnotic is prescribed to ensure restful sleep. The test result is considered positive if the morning cortisol level is more than a predetermined value, usually between 3.5 to 10 mg/dL, depending on assay type and institution. (As noted in the foot-notes for Tables 40-2 and 40-3, the definition of an abnormal test result can vary considerably based on the steroid assay used. Thus, in inter-preting test results, it is necessary to be familiar with the assay that is used. The ranges for abnormal test results in Tables 40-2 and 40-3 reflect studies reviewed for this chapter.)

The single-dose DST has been found to be extremely sensitive (>98%) and moderately specific (approximately 85%–90%) (see Table 40-3) (6,13,14). False-negative results probably are caused by episodic low rates of cortisol secretion that occur in cases unrelated to dexamethasone administration. False-positive results may occur in obese patients, patients who consume excessive ethanol, those receiving treatment with phenytoin or potent estrogens, and those with severe depression. Patients taking spironolactone can also have false-positive results with the fluorescent assays for cortisol (15).

Low-Dose Dexamethasone Suppression Test

The low-dose DST is considered the definitive test for confirming the diag-nosis of Cushing syndrome (16). The test is performed by administering

Table 40-3. Operating Characteristics of Suppression Tests in the Diagnosis of Hypercortisolism

Diagnostic Test	Definition of Positive Result*	Sensitivity	Specificity	Likelihood Ratio Positive Result	Negative Result
		← % →			
Single-dose DST	>3.5–10 μg/dL	98 (84–100)	85 (63–92)	6.5	0.02
Low-dose DST					
Using measurement of urinary 17-hydroxysteroids	>4.0 mg/dL	94 (67–100)	~98[†]	47	0.06
Using measurement of urinary free cortisol levels	>0.019–0.025 mg/dL	95	97 (95–100)	32	0.05
Using measurement of plasma cortisol levels	>1.5–2 μg/dL	90–98	100	∞	0.06
DST with CRH stimulation	>1.4 μg/dL	100	100[†]	∞	0

DST = dexamethasone suppression test; CRH = corticotropin releasing hormone.

*Steroid assays are performed by various techniques (e.g., colorimetric, fluorimetric, competi-tive protein binding) that produce different definitions of positive test results but similar sen-sitivity and specificity results. In interpreting tests, it is important to be aware of the assay used and the normal range for the assay.

[†]Controls are patients in whom the disease is suspected.

dexamethasone, 0.5 mg every 6 hours for eight doses, and measuring the 24-hour urine excretion of 17-OH corticosteroids during the final 24 hours of dexamethasone administration. Patients with Cushing syndrome fail to suppress cortisol production and excrete more than 4 mg/dL of 17-OH steroids during this period. This test is highly sensitive (approximately 95%) and extremely specific (approximately 98%) (see Table 40-3), even in persons in whom the disease is suspected (16). Rarely, in patients with hypercortisolism, the test result is false-negative owing to delayed metabolism of dexamethasone (17), which results in a marked increase in plasma dexamethasone levels over those usually obtained. The elevated dexamethasone levels may then cause adrenal suppression in some patients with hypercortisolism, particularly in those with Cushing syndrome. False-positive results for this test may occur in patients with severe depression (18) or in those taking phenytoin. Measurement of urinary free cortisol levels during this suppression test is also sensitive and specific (see Table 40-3).

Kaye and Crapo (19) discuss encouraging initial findings from techniques that have been used to simplify the low-dose test. Recent studies report a sensitivity of 90% to 98% and a specificity of approximately 100% using the plasma cortisol value that is measured after completing the dexamethasone administration (9,18).

Dexamethasone Suppression and Corticotropin Releasing Hormone Stimulation

This recently described test uses the low-dose DST followed by administration of CRH. It is based on the limited suppressibility of cortisol production by dexamethasone and the enhanced responsiveness to CRH that results from Cushing syndrome. It appears to be most useful in difficult patients with mild abnormalities of glucocorticoid metabolism, such as those with "pseudo-Cushing" syndrome. In the initial report, using a cutoff cortisol level of 38 nmol/L (1.4 mg/dL) after CRH administration, the test was 100% sensitive and 100% specific in identifying the 39 patients with Cushing syndrome and the 19 with "pseudo-Cushing" syndrome (18).

Radiographic Studies

Evaluation of the Sella Turcica

The sella turcica and pituitary gland can be examined using magnetic resonance imaging (MRI) and computed tomography (CT). The sensitivity of these methods is inversely related to the size of the tumor, with sensitivity being lowest for microadenomas. Magnetic resonance imaging appears to be the better imaging technique. Initial results with MRI were very encouraging (20,21). In a more recent report using gadolinium-enhanced scans (22), although MRI correctly identified the five patients with macroadenomas, it identified abnormalities in only 51%

of the 45 patients with microadenomas and in 6 patients the lesion noted on MRI did not correspond to the adenoma found at surgery. In addition, 10% of "normal" controls had pituitary lesions compatible with adenomas. Given these results, and the knowledge that approximately 70% of patients with hypercortisolism have pituitary lesions, the overall sensitivity of MRI in the initial evaluation of suspected hypercortisolism is only about 35% to 40%.

In their review, Kaye and Crapo (19) summarized the results of several series describing the use of CT scans in patients with hypercortisolism resulting from pituitary causes and report a test sensitivity of 47% and specificity of 74%. More recent reports suggest that sensitivity may be only approximately 20% (22). The low sensitivity reflects the difficulty in detecting microadenomas, and the false-positive scans result from finding nonsecreting cysts as well as from scanning artifacts. Again, the overall sensitivity for CT in the initial evaluation would be less than 20%, because not all patients with suspected hypercortisolism have a pituitary cause for their disease.

Abdominal Imaging

Computed tomography and MRI of the adrenal glands are useful in detecting adrenal tumors in patients with hypercortisolism. Significant bilateral adrenal enlargement can be detected by CT in 50% of cases of ectopic-ACTH production and in about 10% of patients with Cushing disease (23). Therefore, in the initial evaluation of a typical group of patients in whom Cushing syndrome is suspected, abdominal CT has a sensitivity of 40%. The specificity of these radiographic procedures should approach 95%—in some patients the results of scanning will be false-positive owing to the detection of nonpathologic adrenal adenomas (24,25). Computed tomography is reported to be helpful in identifying cysts and myelolipomas, and MRI is useful in differentiating adrenal adenomas from carcinomas (24).

Other Tests

Because the focus of this chapter is on the diagnosis of hypercortisolism and not on establishing its specific cause, tests such as measurement of ACTH levels, CRH stimulation, metapyrone testing, inferior petrosal sinus sampling, or imaging studies for "occult" tumors are beyond the scope of this discussion. For information on these tests, readers may consult a recent review (2).

DIAGNOSTIC STRATEGIES

Studies are often performed to rule out the diagnosis of Cushing syndrome in persons with hirsutism, hypertension, and obesity, when in fact the disease is uncommon and the pretest probability of disease is generally low. However, in patients with several of the specific clinical signs or symptoms, such as hypokalemia, proximal weakness, ecchymoses, or osteoporosis, the pretest probability of disease is much higher (i.e., >50%).

When the pretest probability of hypercortisolism is low (e.g., <50%), the overnight single-dose DST is an excellent method for ruling out the disease, because the test is highly sensitive (>98%) and normal study results virtually preclude the diagnosis (Table 40-4). However, because false-positive results may occur, an abnormal DST result obtained under these circumstances necessitates additional testing with a more specific test such as the 24-hour urinary free cortisol. These false-positive DST results may occur more frequently in patients with depression or obesity.

When the pretest probability of disease is high (e.g., >50%, the diagnosis may be confirmed using a test with high specificity, such as the 24-hour urinary free cortisol or measurement of the midnight plasma cortisol level. If the results are positive, additional testing is needed to determine the cause of the hypercortisolism.

Table 40-4. Post-test Probabilities for Diagnostic Tests in the Diagnosis of Hypercortisolism

Diagnostic Test	Pretest Probability					
	20%		50%		80%	
	Positive Result	Negative Result	Positive Result	Negative Result	Positive Result	Negative Result
	←			%		→
Single-dose DST	62	1	87	2	96	9
Measurement of plasma cortisol levels (4 PM–9 PM)	39	6	72	20	91	50
Measurement of plasma cortisol levels (midnight)	86	1	96	4	99	14
Measurement of 24-hour urinary free cortisol	72	2	91	6	98	21
Measurement of 24-hour urinary 17-hydroxysteroids	45	4	77	13	93	37
Low-dose DST	92	2	98	6	99	20
MRI of sella turcica	50	14	80	40	94	73
Abdominal CT scan	66	14	89	39	97	72

DST = dexamethasone suppression test; MRI = magnetic resonance imaging; CT = computed tomography.

In cases in which the metabolic abnormalities are mild and tests give conflicting results, the low-dose DST combined with CRH stimulation may provide useful information. Radiographic studies such as MRI scanning of the pituitary gland or imaging of the adrenal glands are not helpful initial diagnostic examinations because of their low sensitivities.

CLINICAL PROBLEMS

Clinical Problem 1

A patient with obesity, hypertension, and diabetes mellitus who does not have the specific clinical findings of weakness, hypokalemia, ecchymoses, or osteoporosis is evaluated for possible Cushing syndrome.

Testing Strategy and Rationale

An overnight single-dose DST should be obtained, followed by a 24-hour urinary free cortisol measurement if the initial test result is positive.

The pretest probability of disease is low (<20%) in these patients, and a normal DST result virtually rules out the diagnosis. With a positive test result, the post-test probability of disease would be in an intermediate range and the patient should be further evaluated with a more specific test such as the 24-hour urinary free cortisol measurement. If this test result is negative, the probability of disease is again low, whereas a positive result would yield a high post-test probability of disease.

Clinical Example

A 35-year-old woman with central obesity, acne, hirsutism, plethora, and oligomenorrhea is evaluated at a general medical practice. She has not noted spontaneous ecchymoses but does have pigmented striae. She is hypertensive and has dependent edema. Based on disease prevalence and her findings, the disease probability can be estimated to be approximately 20% and further testing is recommended. An overnight single-dose DST is ordered. If the results of this test are normal, no further testing is indicated.

Clinical Problem 2

A patient presents with moon facies, central obesity, and several specific clinical findings such as weakness, ecchymoses, and osteoporosis.

Testing Strategy and Rationale

One of the specific tests, such as measurement of 24-hour urinary free cortisol or midnight cortisol level, should be done.

In patients with these findings, the probability of disease is relatively high (as much as 80%), and the diagnosis should be made using the measurement of 24-hour urinary free cortisol or midnight plasma cortisol level. Other tests for the disease produce lower post-test probabilities of disease. If the results of these two tests are negative, the probability of disease is reduced to less than 20%.

Clinical Example
An obese young woman presents with weakness, ecchymoses, hypokalemia, and osteoporosis. Based on the presence of the specific clinical findings, the probability of Cushing syndrome is estimated to be more than 80%. A 24-hour urinary free cortisol determination is performed, and if the results are positive, the diagnosis is confirmed.

REFERENCES

1. **Gold EM.** The Cushing syndromes: changing views of diagnosis and treatment. Ann Intern Med. 1979;90:829-44.
2. **Orth DN.** Cushing's syndrome. N Engl J Med. 1995;332:791-803.
3. **Biemond P, deJong FH, Lamberts SWJ.** Continuous dexamethasone infusion for seven hours in patients with the Cushing Syndrome. Ann Intern Med. 1990;112:738-42.
4. **Labhart A.** Clinical Endocrinology. New York: Springer-Verlag; 1974:340.
5. **Nugent CA, Warner HR, Dunn JT, Tyler FH.** Probability theory in the diagnosis of Cushing syndrome. J Clin Endocrin Metab. 1964;24:621-7.
6. **Crapo L.** Cushing syndrome: a review of diagnostic tests. Metabolism. 1979;28:955-77.
7. **Eddy RL, Jones AL, Gilliland PF, et al.** Cushing syndrome: a prospective study of diagnostic methods. Am J Med. 1973;55:621-63.
8. **Ernest I.** Steroid excretion and plasma cortisol in 41 cases of Cushing Syndrome. Acta Endocrinol. 1966;51:511-25.
9. **Newell-Price J, Trainer P, Perry L, et al.** A single sleeping midnight cortisol has 100% sensitivity for the diagnosis of Cushing's syndrome. Clin Endocrinol. 1995;43:545-50.
10. **Espiner EA.** Urinary excretion in stress situations and in patients with Cushing Syndrome. J Endocrinol. 1966;35:29-44.
11. **Carroll BJ, Curtis GC, Davies BM, et al.** Urinary free cortisol excretion in depression. Psychol Med. 1976;6:43.
12. **Streeten DHP, Stevenson CT, Dalakos TG, et al.** The diagnosis of hypercortisolism: biochemical criteria differentiating patients from lean and obese normal subjects and from females on oral contraceptives. J Clin Endocrinol Metab. 1969;29:1191-211.
13. **Montwill J, Igoe D, McKenna TJ.** The overnight dexamethasone test is the procedure of choice in screening for Cushing's syndrome. Steroids. 1994;59:296-8.

14. **Fok ACK, Tan KT, Jacob E, Sum CF.** Overnight (1 mg) dexamethasone suppression testing reliably distinguishes non-cushingoid obesity from Cushing's syndrome. Steroids. 1991;56:549-51.

15. **Aron DC, Tyrrell JB, Fitzgerald PA, et al.** Cushing syndrome: problems in diagnosis. Medicine. 1981;60:25-35.

16. **Liddle GW.** Tests of pituitary-adrenal suppressibility in the diagnosis of Cushing syndrome. J Clin Endocrinol Metab. 1960;20:1539-60.

17. **Caro JF, Meikle AW, Check JH, Cohen SN.** Normal suppression to dexamethasone in Cushing disease: an expression of decreased metabolic clearance for dexamethasone. J Clin Endocrinol Metab. 1978;47:667-70.

18. **Yanovski JA, Cutler CG, Chrousos GP, Nieman LK.** Corticotropin-releasing hormone stimulation following low-dose dexamethasone administration: a new test to distinguish Cushing's syndrome from pseudo-Cushing's states. JAMA. 1993;269:2232-8.

19. **Kaye TB, Crapo L.** The Cushing syndrome: an update on diagnostic tests. Ann Intern Med. 1990;112:434-44.

20. **Mampalam TJ, Tyrrell JB, Wilson EB.** Transphenoidal microsurgery for Cushing disease: a report of 216 cases. Ann Intern Med. 1988;109:487-93.

21. **Peck WW, Dillon WP, Norman D, et al.** High-resolution MR imaging of pituitary microadenomas at 1.5 T: experience with Cushing disease. AJR Am J Roentgenol. 1989;152:145-51.

22. **Hall WA, Luciano MG, Doppman JL, et al.** Pituitary magnetic resonance imaging in normal human volunteers: occult adenomas in the general population. Ann Intern Med. 1994;120:817-20.

23. **White FE, White MC, Drury PL, et al.** Value of computed tomography of the abdomen and chest in investigation of Cushing syndrome. Br Med J. 1982;284:771-4.

24. **Osella G, Terzolo M, Borretta G, et al.** Endocrine evaluation of incidentally discovered adrenal masses (incidentalomas). J Clin Endocrinol Metab. 1994;79:1532-9.

25. **Carpenter PC.** Cushing syndrome: update of diagnosis and management. Mayo Clin Proc. 1986;61:49-58.

Hyperthyroidism and Hypothyroidism   **41**

James G. Dolan, MD, and Steven D. Wittlin, MD

KEY POINTS

Pretest Probabilities

- Sensitive clinical indices exist for the diagnosis of both hyperthyroidism and hypothyroidism in ambulatory patients. Little information exists on the diagnostic value of these indices in patients with serious nonthyroidal illnesses.

Diagnostic Strategies

- The ultrasensitive, third-generation thyroid-stimulating hormone (TSH) immunoradiometric assay is the best test to establish or exclude thyroid dysfunction both in ambulatory patients and in patients with severe nonthyroidal illnesses.

- To diagnose hyperthyroidism when the ultrasensitive TSH assay is not available, the free triiodothyronine (T3) assay, free thyroxine (T4) assay, or free T4 index should be used in ambulatory patients. The free T4 assay or T4 index is best in patients with severe nonthyroidal illnesses.

- To diagnose hypothyroidism when the ultrasensitive TSH assay is not available, the TSH by radioimmunoassay (RIA) is the best test in both ambulatory populations and in patients with severe nonthyroidal illnesses.

- Serum T4 assays are less expensive but less accurate in the diagnosis of either hyperthyroidism or hypothyroidism. Free T4 and free T3 indices calculated from total serum hormone and T3 resin uptake results are acceptable alternatives to direct free-hormone measurements.

BACKGROUND

The measurement of circulating thyroid hormone levels is an integral part of the workup of patients with suspected thyroid disease. In addition, because abnormalities of thyroid hormone secretion can result in

473

widespread clinical manifestations, the question of thyroid dysfunction must be addressed in the workup of a variety of patient symptoms. Because a patient's general state of health has a major bearing on the use and interpretation of thyroid function studies, this chapter discusses test use in two settings: for the general ambulatory population and for patients with severe nonthyroidal illnesses.

ESTIMATING PRETEST PROBABILITY

Weighted clinical indices have been developed for the diagnosis of both hyperthyroidism and hypothyroidism. This type of index maximizes the diagnostic usefulness of clinical information because the evidence provided by both abnormal and normal findings is appropriately considered. These clinical indices were derived in ambulatory populations. The value of clinical signs and symptoms for the diagnosis of thyroid dysfunction in patients with severe underlying disease is unknown.

Hyperthyroidism

The best available estimates of the prevalence and annual incidence of hyperthyroidism in the general population are 0.3% and 0.05%, respectively (1). Crooks and colleagues developed a clinical index for the diagnosis of hyperthyroidism in patients suspected of having the disease (Table 41-1). In their original population, the index achieved a sensitivity of 100% and a specificity of 88% using a cutoff score of 10. Gurney and colleagues (3) studied the index in a population that included only women. The original Crooks index had a sensitivity of 95% and a specificity of 68%, whereas the modified index had values of 95% and 89%, respectively.

Because hyperthyroidism can present subtly in older patients with fewer of the "typical" symptoms, clinical findings are less sensitive in the elderly. In a recent study, tachycardia, fatigue, and weight loss were the most common symptoms in older patients with hyperthyroidism (4). Hyperthyroidism in this age group may also present with atrial fibrillation. In a retrospective study of hyperthyroidism in patients over the age of 60 (5), the Crooks index achieved a maximum sensitivity of 62%. Data were not available to calculate specificity. When some minor adjustments were made, the sensitivity increased to 75%.

Hypothyroidism

The best available estimate of the prevalence of hypothyroidism in the general population is 0.35% (1). Billewicz and colleagues (6) developed a weighted clinical index for use in patients with suspected hypothyroidism (Table 41-2). In the original population, this index achieved a sensitivity of close to 100%, but with a specificity of just 50% (6). A

Table 41-1. Crooks Index*

Symptom or Sign	Present	Absent
Dyspnea on effort	+1	0
Palpitations	+2	0
Tiredness	+2	0
Preference for heat	−5	0
Preference for cold	+5	0
Indifferent to temperature	0	0
Excessive sweating	+3	0
Nervousness	+2	0
Appetite increased	+3	0
Appetite decreased	−3	0
Weight increased	−3	0
Weight decreased	+3	0
Palpable thyroid	+3	−3
Thyroid bruit	+2	−2
Exophthalmos	+2	0
Lid retraction	+2	0
Lid lag	+1	0
Hyperkinetic movements	+4	−2
Fine finger tremor	+1	0
Hands hot	+2	−2
Hands moist	+1	−1
Atrial fibrillation	+4	0
Heart rate		
<80 bpm	−3	0
80–90 bpm	0	0
>90 bpm	+3	0

*Euthyroid if 10 or less; hyperthyroid if more than 10.
Republished with permission from Crooks J, Murray IPC, Wayne EJ. Statistical methods applied to the clinical diagnosis of thyrotoxicosis. Q J Med. 1959;28:211-34.

more recent study from India found that similar sensitivity and specificity could be achieved with the index, but using a lower cutoff than in Billewicz's study. This finding could reflect population differences, inclusion of a different spectrum of cases, or use of different criteria to define disease (7). The usefulness of this index in the elderly ambulatory population is not known.

DIAGNOSTIC TESTS

The operating characteristics of thyroid function tests, using average values or best estimates obtained from the available literature (8–20), are summarized in Table 41-3 (p 477). Values are given separately for

Table 41-2. Billewicz Index*

Symptom or Sign	Present	Absent
Diminished sweating	+6	−2
Dry skin	+3	−6
Cold intolerance	+4	−5
Weight increase	+1	−1
Constipation	+2	−1
Hoarseness	+5	−6
Paresthesias	+5	−4
Deafness	+2	0
Slow movements	+11	−3
Coarse skin	+7	−7
Cold skin	+3	−2
Periorbital puffiness	+4	−6
Pulse rate <75 bpm	+4	−4
Delayed relaxation, ankle jerk	+15	−6

*Euthyroid if 30 or less; hyperthyroid if more than 30.

Republished with permission from Billewicz WZ, Chapman RS, Crooks J, et al. Statistical methods applied to the diagnosis of hypothyroidism. Q J Med. 1969;38:255-66.

test performance in diagnosis of hyperthyroidism or hypothyroidism, as well as for patients who are ambulatory or hospitalized with severe nonthyroidal illnesses.

Thyroid Hormone Assays

Tests frequently used to assess thyroid function are measurements of thyroid hormone concentrations in the blood. The thyroid gland releases two active hormones—T4 and T3. Following release, T4 is converted in peripheral tissues to T3 and several metabolically inactive compounds. In healthy persons, peripheral conversion of T4 accounts for most circulating T3. Both T4 and T3 are largely bound to serum proteins, primarily thyroid-binding globulin (TBG). The small amount of unbound hormone is the metabolically active form. A variety of conditions, including pregnancy, liver disease, oral contraceptive use, narcotic use, and heredity, may increase the serum TBG levels. This can result in increased total serum hormone concentrations with normal free, physiologically active levels (21).

Tests are readily available to measure total (bound and unbound) T3 and T4. To adjust for variations in the total hormone concentration attributable to altered amounts of serum-binding proteins, direct and indirect measurements of free T4 and free T3 can be used. The most widely employed indirect method is the free T4 index (FT4I), which is proportional to the serum free T4 concentration. To calculate this

Table 41-3. Operating Characteristics of Diagnostic Tests in the Diagnosis for Hyperthyroidism and Hypothyroidism

Disease, Population, and Test	Sensitivity	Specificity	Likelihood Ratio	
			Positive Result	Negative Result
	←————%————→			
Hyperthyroidism				
Ambulatory patients				
Total T4	90	91	10	0.11
Free T4, Free T4 index	95	95	19	0.05
Third generation TSH	>99	>99	>99	<0.01
Total T3	87	90	8.7	0.14
Free T3	97	97	32	0.03
Severe nonthyroidal illness				
Total T4	90	80	4.5	0.12
Free T4, Free T4 index	95	97	32	0.05
Third generation TSH	99	95	20	0.01
Hypothyroidism				
Ambulatory patients				
Total T4	90	80	4.5	0.12
Free T4, Free T4 index	90	90	9	0.11
TSH	99	99	99	0.01
Severe nonthyroidal illness				
Total T4	60	70	2.0	0.57
Free T4, Free T4 index	60	80	3.0	0.50
TSH	99	95	20	0.01

T4 = thyroxine; TSH = thyroid-stimulating hormone; T3 = triiodothyronine.

index, the total T4 concentration is multiplied by the T3 resin uptake (T3RU), which is a measure of the number of unoccupied binding sites on thyroid-binding serum proteins. Free T4 levels are becoming increasingly available and are commonly measured by enzymatic immunoassays (MEIA). A free T3 index (FT3I) can also be determined by substituting the total T3 concentration for the total T4 concentration in the calculation.

Thyroid Stimulating Hormone

Thyroid hormone release is regulated by TSH, which is produced in the pituitary and subject to modulation by T3 and T4. Thyroid-stimulating hormone secretion is stimulated by a hypothalamic hormone, thyrotropin-releasing hormone (TRH). The serum TSH level is the most widely available test with high sensitivity and specificity for hypothyroidism, in either ambulatory or ill populations (Table 41-3).

The recent development of ultrasensitive, third-generation TSH assays capable of detecting 0.01 to 0.03 mU/mL of circulating TSH has made it possible to use a low serum TSH level in the diagnosis of hyperthyroidism.

Thyrotropin Releasing Hormone Stimulation Test

The TRH stimulation test measures the change in serum TSH concentration in response to the administration of synthetic TRH. In hyperthyroidism, the TRH stimulation test is considered to be 100% sensitive; that is, a normal response completely excludes the diagnosis. Unfortunately, the specificity is less than 100%. Hence, the diagnosis cannot be unequivocally made on the basis of a positive test. The TRH stimulation test is also useful in the evaluation of suspected secondary hypothyroidism.

Other Tests

Thyroid gland function can also be assessed by measuring the uptake of radioactive iodine, the RAIU test. Although the RAIU test is necessary for the diagnosis of certain forms of thyroiditis, serum hormone measurements are now preferred in the assessment of thyroid function because of lower cost, convenience, and the avoidance of radiation to the patient.

Confounding Factors

Nonthyroidal illnesses have been found to have a variety of effects on thyroid physiology and, consequently, on the use and interpretation of thyroid function tests (19, 22–28). The most common finding is reduced peripheral conversion of T4 to T3. However, elevated T4 levels, decreased T4 levels, decreased TSH levels, and depressed TSH responsiveness to TRH have all been reported during nonthyroidal illnesses. Thyroid-stimulting hormone levels can increase transiently during the recovery phase of acute illnesses.

Several pharmacologic agents also interfere with the interpretation of thyroid function tests. These include iodine-containing compounds such as radiographic contrast agents, phenytoin, oral contraceptives, corticosteroids, dopamine, methadone, and lithium (29).

Age does not appear to have a significant effect on peripheral thyroid hormone levels with the possible exception of a slight decrease in T3 levels in older men. Reports of decreased thyroid hormone levels in elderly populations most likely represent the effect of concurrent nonthyroidal illnesses in the patients examined (30). An increased prevalence of elevated TSH levels has been reported in women beginning at age 45 years (31); some of these cases may represent subclinical hypothyroidism (32).

DIAGNOSTIC STRATEGIES

If available, the best test of thyroid function in any patient suspected of thyroid disease is a third-generation TSH assay (Table 41-4). This test is equivalent to a TRH stimulation test in the diagnosis of hyperthyroidism and to the older TSH radioimmunoassay (RIA) in the diagnosis of hypothyroidism.

If a third-generation TSH assay is not available, the free T3, free T4, or the free T4 indices are all acceptable substitutes in the workup of suspected hyperthyroidism in ambulatory populations. In patients with severe nonthyroidal illnesses, the free T4 or the free T4 index should be used.

Table 41-4. Post-test Probabilities for Selected Diagnostic Tests in the Diagnosis of Hyperthyroidism and Hypothyroidism

Disease, Population, and Test	Pretest Probabilities					
	20%		50%		80%	
	Positive Result	Negative Result	Positive Result	Negative Result	Positive Result	Negative Result
	←————————————————— % —————————————————→					
Hyperthyroidism						
Ambulatory patients						
Total T4	71	3	91	10	98	31
Free T4, Free T4 index	83	1	95	5	99	17
Third-generation TSH	96	<1	99	1	>99	4
Free T3	89	<1	97	3	>99	11
Severe nonthyroidal illness						
Total T4	53	3	82	11	95	33
Free T4, Free T4 index	89	1	97	5	>99	17
Third-generation TSH	83	<1	95	1	99	4
Hypothyroidism						
Ambulatory patients						
Total T4	53	3	82	11	95	33
TSH	96	<1	99	1	>99	4
Severe nonthyroidal illness						
Total T4	33	13	67	36	89	70
TSH	83	<1	95	1	99	4

T4 = thyroxine; TSH = thyroid-stimulating hormone; T3 = triiodothyronine.

For the diagnosis of hypothyroidism, both methods of measuring TSH perform equally well, and the serum TSH is the best test for hypothyroidism in all patient populations. The serum T4 assay, using a cutoff lower than the usual laboratory defined level, has fair sensitivity but low specificity (8).

CLINICAL PROBLEMS

Clinical Problem 1
A patient presents with two or three symptoms suggesting hyperthyroidism.

Testing Strategy and Rationale
A pretest probability estimate using the Crooks Index should be developed, and a sensitive TSH test should be obtained. The clinical diagnosis of hyperthyroidism can be difficult, and the physician's estimate of pretest likelihood should be assisted by the Crooks Index, which may lower the probability enough to make further workup unnecessary. If further workup is required, a sensitive TSH assay is the best available test.

Clinical Example
A 34-year-old married woman presents with symptoms of anxiety, weight loss, palpitations, and fatigue for the past four months. There is no clear history of heat intolerance. On examination, she has a slightly enlarged thyroid but no thyroid bruit, eye changes, or abnormal movements except for a fine tremor of her outstretched hands. Her hands are cool and moist. Her pulse rate is 88 beats/min and regular.

This patient has perhaps a 10% probability of hyperthyroidism. Her score on the Crooks index is five and falls in the euthyroid range, which reduces the probability of hyperthyroidism. Although the likelihood of hyperthyroidism is relatively low, the patient and her physician may decide that further testing to exclude the diagnosis is indicated. The best test in this situation is an ultrasensitive, third-generation TSH assay. A normal value in this situation would definitively exclude the diagnosis of hyperthyroidism. Free T4 or free T3 levels would be acceptable alternatives if an ultrasensitive assay were not available.

Clinical Problem 2
A patient presents with clinical findings suggestive of hypothyroidism.

Testing Strategy and Rationale

The pretest probability should be calculated using the Billewicz index, and a TSH level should be ordered. A serum TSH level, regardless of the assay used, is the best test to exclude or confirm hypothyroidism at any pretest probability.

Clinical Example

A 67-year-old man is admitted to the hospital because of worsening chronic congestive heart failure. Over the past 3 to 4 months, he has had a marked increase in his symptoms of dyspnea and fatigue. He has also gained 10 lb and reports feeling constantly cold. His family reports that his walking seems slower. His examination reveals a pulse rate of 66 beats/min, bibasilar rales, a soft S3, and 2+ pretibial edema. His thyroid gland appears normal.

Based on these findings, the diagnosis of hypothyroidism is considered with a probability of 50%. At an intermediate probability of hypothyroidism in a patient with a severe nonthyroidal illness, the best laboratory test is a TSH assay, sensitivity 99%, specificity 95% (Table 41-3). If the TSH is elevated, the probability of hypothyroidism is about 95%. If the TSH is normal, the probability is approximately 1%.

REFERENCES

1. **dos Remedios LV, Weber PM, Feldman R, et al.** Detecting unsuspected thyroid dysfunction by the free thyroxine index. Arch Intern Med. 1980; 140:1045-9.

2. **Crooks J, Murray IPC, Wayne EJ.** Statistical methods applied to the clinical diagnosis of thyrotoxicosis. Q J Med. 1959;28:211-34.

3. **Gurney C, Hall R, Harper M, et al.** Newcastle thyrotoxicosis index. Lancet. 1970;2:1275-8.

4. **Trivalle C, Doucet J, Chessagne P, et al.** Differences in the signs and symptoms of hyperthyroidism in older and younger patients. J Am Geriatr Soc. 1996;44:50-3.

5. **Davis PJ, David FB.** Hyperthyroidism in patients over the age of 60 years. Medicine. 1974;53:161-81.

6. **Billewicz WZ, Chapman RS, Crooks J, et al.** Statistical methods applied to the diagnosis of hypothyroidism. Q J Med. 1969;38:255-66.

7. **Seshadri MS, Samuel BU, Kanagasabapathy AS, et al.** Clinical scoring system for hypothyroidism—is it useful? J Gen Intern Med. 1989; 4:490-2.

8. **Goldstein BJ, Mushlin AI.** Use of a single thyroxine test to evaluate ambulatory medical patients for suspected hypothyroidism. J Gen Intern Med. 1987;2:20-4.

9. **Marsden P, McKenon CG.** Serum triiodothyronine concentration in the diagnosis of hyperthyroidism. Clin Endocrinol. 1975;4:183-9.

10. **Sawin CT, Chopra D, Albano J, Azizi F.** The free triiodothyronine (T3) index. Ann Intern Med. 1978;88:474-7.

11. **Wiersanga WM, Touber JL.** Thyroid function tests. II. Studies in patients with thyroid disease. Neth J Med. 1980;23:200-9.

12. **Howorth PJN, MacLagan NF.** Clinical application of serum total thyroxine estimation, resin uptake, and free thyroxine index. Lancet. 1969;1:224-8.

13. **de Los Santos ET, Starich GH, Mazzaferri EL.** Sensitivity, specificity, and costeffectivensss of the sensitive thyrotropin assay in the diagnosis of thyroid disease in ambulatory patients. Arch Intern Med. 1989;149:526-32.

14. **Seth J, Beckett G.** Diagnosis of hyperthyroidism—the newer biochemical tests. Clin Endocrinol Metab. 1985;14:373-96.

15. **Seth J, Kellet HA, Caldwell G, et al.** A sensitive immunoradiometric assay for serum thyroid stimulating hormone. A replacement for the thyrotropin releasing hormone test? Br Med J. 1984;289:1334-6.

16. **Caldwell G, Kellett HA, Gow SM, et al.** A new strategy for thyroid function testing. Lancet. 1985;1:1117-9.

17. **Spencer CA, Lai-Rosenfeld AO, Guttler RB, et al.** Thyrotropin secretion in thyrotoxic and thyroxine treated patients: assessment by a sensitive immunoenzymometric assay. J Clin Endocrinol Metab. 1986;63:349-55.

18. **Klee GG, Hay ID.** Assessment of sensitive thyrotropin assays for an expanded role in thyroid function testing. Proposed criteria for analytic performance and clinical utility. J Clin Endocrinol Metab. 1987;64:461-71.

19. **White GH.** Recent advances in routine thyroid function testing. Crit Rev Clin Lab Sci. 1987;24:315-62.

20. **Surks MI, Ocampo E.** Subclinical thyroid disease. Am J Med. 1996;100: 217-23.

21. **Borst GC, Eil C, Burman KD.** Euthyroid hyperthyroxinemia. Ann Intern Med. 1983;98:366-78.

22. **Gooch BR, Isley WL, Utiger RD.** Abnormalities in thyroid function tests in patients admitted to a medical service. Arch Intern Med. 1982;142:1801-5.

23. **Kaplan MM, Larsen PR, Crantz FR, et al.** Prevalence of abnormal thyroid function test results in patients with acute medical illnesses. Am J Med. 1982;72:9-16.

24. **Wong ET, Bradley SG, Schultz AL.** Elevation of thyroid-stimulating hormone during acute nonthyroidal illness. Arch Intern Med. 1981;141:873-5.

25. **Chopra IJ, Soloman DH, Hepner GW, et al.** Misleadingly low free thyroxine index and usefulness of reverse triiodothyronine measurement in nonthyroidal illnesses. Ann Intern Med. 1979;90:905-12.

26. **Gavin LA, Rosenthal M, Cavalieu RR.** The diagnostic dilemma of isolated hyperthyroxinemia in acute illness. JAMA. 1979;242:251-3.

27. **Chopra IJ, VanHerle AJ, Chua Teco GN, Nguyen AH.** Serum free thyroxine in thyroidal and nonthyroidal illness: a comparison of measurements by radioimmunoassay, equilibrium dialysis, and free thyroxine index. J Clin Endocrinol Metab. 1980;51:135-43.

28. **Spencer C, Eigen A, Shen D, et al.** Specificity of sensitive assays of thyrotropin (TSH) used to screen for thyroid disease in hospitalized patients. Clin Chem. 1987;33:1391-6.

29. **Wenzel KW.** Pharmacologic interference with in vitro tests of thyroid function. Metabolism. 1981;30:717-32.

30. **Evered DC, Tunbridge WMG, Hall R, et al.** Thyroid hormone concentrations in a large scale community survey. Effect of age, sex, illness, and medication. Clin Chem Acta. 1978;83:223-9.

31. **Tunbridge WMG, Evered DC, Hall R, et al.** The spectrum of thyroid disease in a community: the Whickham Survey. Clin Endocrinol. 1977;7:481-93.

32. **Woeber KA.** Subclinical thyroid dysfunction. Arch Intern Med. 1997;157:1065-8.

Thyroid Nodules

42

James G. Dolan, MD, and Steven D. Wittlin, MD

KEY POINTS

Pretest Probabilities

- Solitary palpable thyroid nodules are a common clinical finding, with an age-dependent prevalence ranging from 1% to 5%. The proportion of all single thyroid nodules that are malignant is estimated to be 5% to 10%.

- Patient age and sex are significant historical risk factors for all types of thyroid malignancy. Family history is important in cases of medullary carcinoma. A history of low-dose irradiation to the thyroid region may be associated with an increased risk of subsequent thyroid cancer.

Diagnostic Strategies

- Fine-needle aspiration is the best test for evaluating a solitary thyroid nodule when the probability of malignancy is low to intermediate.

- When the probability of malignancy for a solitary nodule is high, surgical exploration is the best course to follow.

BACKGROUND

Palpable thyroid nodules are common, and their prevalence increases with age from approximately 1% in persons aged 10 to 20 years old to approximately 5% in persons aged 70 to 80 years old (1–3). Nodules are four times more common in women than men (4).

Most thyroid nodules are benign lesions, predominantly follicular adenomas. Other causes of benign thyroid nodules include cysts, multinodular goiters, and focal thyroiditis. Sometimes, however, a thyroid nodule is caused by thyroid cancer. The most common form of thyroid cancer is papillary carcinoma, which accounts for 60% to 70% of reported cancers. Follicular carcinomas occur in approximately 20% of patients with thyroid cancer, undifferentiated tumors in 15%, and medullary carcinoma in 5%.

The baseline prevalence of cancer in all patients with solitary thyroid nodules has been estimated to be approximately 5% to 10% (5).

The goal in evaluating a patient with a solitary thyroid nodule detected on physical examination is to differentiate benign from malignant nodules. Because surgery is the recommended approach to suspected cancerous nodules, the diagnostic process must also minimize the number of surgical procedures that result from false-positive diagnoses. This chapter summarizes the approach to the diagnosis of thyroid nodules based on the operating characteristics of available tests.

ESTIMATING PRETEST PROBABILITY

Patient age, sex, family history, and history of irradiation to the head or neck are historical factors that modify the likelihood of thyroid cancer in a patient with a solitary thyroid nodule.

Although the prevalence of thyroid nodules increases with age, several studies have recorded a disproportionate number of cases of thyroid cancer in younger patients, ranging from 33% to 48% of all tumors discovered during surgery (6–8). The validity of these findings has been questioned, and the true relation between age and thyroid cancer is unknown (9). Data from the Framingham study indicate that the chance that a thyroid nodule is malignant is about twice as high for men as it is for women (10). Family history is important in the diagnosis of medullary carcinoma of the thyroid.

An increased risk of thyroid malignancy has been reported in people who received low doses of thyroid irradiation, usually several decades earlier during infancy or childhood for some benign condition such as thymic enlargement, acne, or enlarged tonsils. The prevalence of thyroid malignancy in these patients has ranged from 4% to 7% (11–13). Maxon and colleagues (1) have calculated a dose-related, absolute-risk estimate that can be used if the dosage of irradiation that was used is known. Although generally accepted as a risk factor (2,9), the association between previous low-dose thyroid irradiation and subsequent thyroid cancer has been challenged by Royce and colleagues (14), who showed in a controlled fashion that the prevalence of thyroid malignancy was not increased in a group of patients who received irradiation compared with an age-matched and sex-matched control group. Large amounts of thyroid irradiation—for example, doses used in ^{131}I ablative therapy or in cancer radiation therapy—have not been associated with an increased incidence of thyroid cancer, probably because most of the gland is destroyed.

Some clinical signs are helpful in estimating the likelihood of malignancy in a patient with a solitary thyroid nodule. Because thyroid malignancies rarely secrete clinically significant amounts of thyroid hormone, evidence of hyperthyroidism considerably reduces the probability of cancer. Similarly, thyroid cancer is less likely if there are multiple nodules rather than a single palpable nodule. A palpably hard nodule has a sensitivity of 42% and a specificity of 89% for cancer, whereas fixation to surrounding tissues has a sensitivity of 31% and a specificity of 94% (15). Most other individual clinical findings are of no diagnostic value because they are as common in patients with cancer as in those without cancer. Constellations of clinical findings may be more useful. In a recent study, a clinical categorization based on the presence of one or more "high risk" signs and symptoms including rapid tumor growth, a very firm nodule, fixation to adjacent structures, vocal cord paralysis, enlarged regional lymph nodes, or distant metastases achieved a sensitivity of 55% and a specificity of 94% (16).

DIAGNOSTIC TESTS

Radioisotope Scanning

The use of radioactive scanning techniques is based on the observation that cancerous thyroid tissue picks up smaller amounts of the iodine or technetium radioisotopes commonly used in the scanning than does normal tissue. Therefore, thyroid cancers have been characterized as being "cold" on scans (i.e., showing little or no radioactive uptake), and cold nodules are considered to be possibly malignant. The operating characteristics of thyroid scintiscans are summarized in Table 42-1. The sensitivity of radioiodine scanning is approximately 83% (14,17–23), and that of technetium scanning is approximately 93% (21–26). False-negative results are caused by the occasional occurrence of a "hot" nodule that is malignant and interference from surrounding tissues obscuring the lack of uptake in a malignant nodule.

The specificities of thyroid scintiscans for malignancies are very low: 25% for radioiodine scans and 15% for technetium scans. The major reason for this poor specificity is that, in addition to malignant nodules, many other thyroid lesions also show reduced uptake of the radioisotopes. The diagnostic usefulness of radionuclide scanning is severely compromised by this lack of specificity. Because more than 80% of solitary thyroid nodules are "cold," a large proportion of positive scans are falsely positive (27). Although a negative test result is helpful in reducing the likelihood of carcinoma, a positive radionuclide scan does not substantially change the likelihood of thyroid cancer.

Ultrasonography

Ultrasonography can be used for several purposes. This test can define the size and exact location of a nodule and allows changes in size over time to be accurately assessed with little discomfort or risk to the patient. Because thyroid cysts are rarely malignant, finding a simple

Table 42-1. Operating Characteristics of Diagnostic Tests for Thyroid Cancer

Diagnostic Test	Definition of Positive Result	Sensitivity	Specificity	Likelihood Ratio	
				Positive Result	Negative Result
		←——— % ———→			
Scintiscan	Cold, solitary nodule				
Iodine 131		83	25	1.1	0.68
Technetium 99m		93	15	1.1	0.47
Ultrasonography	Solid or mixed lesion	95	18	1.2	0.28
Thyroid hormone suppression	Decrease in size or disappearance of the nodule	85	25	1.1	0.6
Fine-needle aspiration	Aspirate suspicious or positive for malignancy	82	88		
	Malignant			61	
	Suspicious			3.5	
	Benign			0.19	

cyst is thought to be good evidence against malignancy; for this reason, ultrasonography is useful as a primary test for the diagnosis of a malignant thyroid nodule.

The sensitivity of ultrasonography for detecting malignancy is 95%. However, its specificity is only 18%, reflecting that although most thyroid malignancies are noncystic, most noncystic thyroid nodules are caused by benign lesions (20,22,28–31). Furthermore, approximately 80% of thyroid nodules are noncystic. Thus, the diagnostic utility of ultrasonography is similar to that of radionuclide scanning.

Thyroid Hormone Suppression

Thyroid hormone suppression is used as a test for the diagnosis of thyroid cancer based on the assumption that thyroid malignancies are not responsive to thyroid-stimulating hormone (TSH), whereas benign nodules are. Therefore, if a patient is given exogenous thyroid in doses sufficient to completely suppress TSH secretion, a benign, TSH-dependent nodule should shrink or disappear over time. In contrast, an autonomous malignant thyroid nodule should be unaffected and remain stable or continue to grow during this period.

If no change or growth of the nodule is considered to be positive criterion for malignancy, the thyroid suppression test has a sensitivity of approximately 85% and a specificity of approximately 25% (25,32–35).

Again, as with the other tests discussed so far, the low specificity of the thyroid suppression test limits its diagnostic utility.

Fine-Needle Aspiration

The fourth and final diagnostic test is fine-needle aspiration of the nodule. This procedure involves inserting a 22- to 25-gauge needle, usually without anesthesia, into the nodule and aspirating. The aspirate is then fixed on a slide and examined cytologically. Complications are rare. Fine-needle aspiration has replaced thyroid biopsy with larger needles because it is just as effective but is less expensive and less dangerous (25).

Fine-needle aspiration cytology has been shown to discriminate well if the aspirate is interpreted as definitely benign or definitely malignant. However, in between 20% and 40% of patients, malignancy cannot be ruled out based on the aspirate and is read as suspicious for malignancy. Because follow-up studies have shown that approximately 25% of patients whose aspirate is interpreted as suspicious have thyroid cancer, it is generally recommended that this finding be considered a positive test result and that operative resection be performed. If both malignant and suspicious cytologic findings are considered positive results, the reported sensitivity of fine-needle aspiration ranges between 70% and 100%, with a mean of 82% (95% CI, 79% to 97%), and the reported specificity ranges from 28% to 100%, with a mean of 88% (CI, 78% to 97%) (16,24,25,36–44). It should be emphasized that interpretation of the fine-needle aspirate is critically dependent on the skill of the cytopathologist.

The problem with judging the diagnostic usefulness of the fine-needle aspirate on the basis of its sensitivity and specificity alone is that the uncertainty in interpreting a suspicious result masks the impact of an aspirate read as benign or malignant. This problem can be avoided by calculating individual likelihood ratios (see Chapter 3) for each test result (45). Using this approach, the likelihood ratios for malignant, suspicious, and benign aspirates are approximately 61* (CI, 38 to 84), 3.5 (CI, 1.2 to 5.7), and 0.19 (CI, 0.08 to 0.31), respectively.

In approximately 10% to 20% of patients, a fine-needle aspirate may be inadequate for cytologic interpretation. In this situation, the best approach is a repeat aspiration followed by an ultrasonography-guided procedure, if necessary.

---

*Several studies have reported no false-positive results for malignant aspirates. This makes it mathematically impossible to calculate a likelihood ratio because the calculation would require dividing by zero. In these cases, a likelihood ratio of 99 was used.

DIAGNOSTIC STRATEGIES

Table 42-2 lists the post-test probabilities of thyroid cancer in a solitary thyroid nodule based on the results of radioactive iodine and technetium scintiscans, ultrasonography, response to thyroid suppression, and fine-needle aspiration in euthyroid patients. Thyrotoxic patients and patients with clinically apparent multinodular glands are generally considered to be free of malignancy and have not been included in series investigating solitary thyroid nodules. When the probability of malignancy is low or intermediate, the fine-needle aspiration is the best diagnostic test. An aspirate interpreted as definitely benign markedly reduces the probability of malignancy, whereas an aspirate interpreted as definitely malignant indicates that surgical removal of the nodule is warranted. An aspirate suspicious for malignancy does not substantially change the likelihood of disease. In this setting, the best approach may be to repeat the aspiration. If the repeat aspirate is malignant or suspicious for malignancy, surgical removal is generally recommended. If the repeat aspirate is benign, the best management strategy is close clinical observation.

At a high pretest probability (e.g., 80%), none of the tests reviewed is sufficiently powerful to substantially reduce the probability of malignancy, and surgical removal of the nodule is indicated.

Table 42-2. Post-test Probabilities of Malignancy for Diagnostic Tests in the Diagnosis of Thyroid Cancer

Diagnostic Test	Pretest Probabilities					
	20%		50%		80%	
	Positive Result	Negative Result	Positive Result	Negative Result	Positive Result	Negative Result
	←			%		→
Scintiscan						
Iodine-131	22	15	53	40	82	73
Technetium-99m	21	10	52	32	81	65
Ultrasonography	22	6	54	22	82	53
Thyroid hormone suppression	22	13	53	38	82	71
Fine-needle aspirate						
Malignant cells identified	94		98		>99	
Suspicious for malignancy	47		78		93	
Benign	5		17		44	

CLINICAL PROBLEM

A patient is noted to have an isolated solitary thyroid nodule.

Testing Strategy and Rationale

A fine-needle aspiration of the nodule should be performed. In patients with a solitary nodule who are not "high risk" based on signs or symptoms, the probability of malignancy is low and most of their thyroid nodules are benign. The best test in such patients is fine-needle aspiration.

Clinical Example

On routine physical examination, an otherwise healthy 67-year-old woman is found to have a 2-cm thyroid nodule. The nodule is firm and freely moveable. No cervical adenopathy or evidence of thyroid dysfunction is found. The likelihood that the nodule represents a thyroid cancer is at most approximately 5%. A negative fine-needle aspirate would reduce the probability of malignancy to 1%. At this level, further clinical observation is the best strategy, with no further diagnostic tests. An aspirate showing definitely malignant cells would raise the probability of thyroid cancer to approximately 75%, confirming the need for surgical removal. An aspirate read as suspicious for malignancy would increase the probability of cancer to about 15%, indicating the need for further evaluation.

REFERENCES

1. **Maxon HR, Thomas SR, Saenger EL, et al.** Ionizing irradiation and the induction of clinically significant disease in the human thyroid gland. Am J Med. 1977;63:967-78.
2. **Rojeski MT, Gharib H.** Nodular thyroid disease. N Engl J Med. 1985;313:427-36.
3. **Mazzaferri EL.** Management of a solitary thyroid nodule. N Engl J Med. 1993;328:553-9.
4. **Vander JB, Gaston EA, Dawber TR.** Significance of solitary nontoxic thyroid nodules. N Engl J Med. 1954;251:970-3.
5. **Mazzaferri EL.** Thyroid cancer in thyroid nodules: finding a needle in the haystack. Am J Med. 1992;93:359-62.
6. **Woolner LB, Beahrs OH, Black BM, et al.** Classification and prognosis of thyroid carcinoma. Am J Surg. 1961;102:354–87.
7. **Cady B, Sedgwick CE, Meissner WA, et al.** Changing clinical, pathologic, therapeutic, and survival patterns in differentiated thyroid carcinoma. Ann Surg. 1976;184:541-53.
8. **Hoffman GL, Thompson NW, Heffron C.** The solitary thyroid nodule. Arch Surg. 1972;105:379-85.

9. **Mazzaferri EL, de Los Santos ET, Rofagha-Keyhani S.** Solitary thyroid nodule: diagnosis and management. Med Clin North Am. 1988;72:1177-212.

10. **Klonoff DC, Greenspan FS.** The thyroid nodule. Adv Intern Med. 1982;27: 101-26.

11. **Reketoff S, Harrison J, Karanfilski BT, et al.** Continuing occurrence of thyroid carcinoma after irradiation to the neck in infancy and childhood. N Engl J Med. 1975;292:171-5.

12. **Pincus RA, Reichlin S, Hempelmann LH.** Thyroid abnormalities after radiation exposure in infancy. Ann Intern Med. 1967;66:1154-64.

13. **Schneider AB, Favus MJ, Stachura ME, et al.** Incidence, prevalence, and characteristics of radiation-induced thyroid tumors. Am J Med. 1978;64: 243-52.

14. **Royce PC, MacKay BR, DiSabella PM.** Value of post-irradiation screening for thyroid nodules. JAMA. 1979;242:2675-8.

15. **Haff RC, Schecter BC, Armstrong RG, Evans WE.** Factors increasing the probability of malignancy in thyroid nodules. Am J Surg. 1976;131:707-9.

16. **Hamming J, Goslings B, van Steenis GJ, et al.** The value of fine-needle aspiration biopsy in patients with nodular thyroid disease divided into groups of suspicion of malignant neoplasms on clinical grounds. Arch Intern Med. 1990;150:113-6.

17. **Kendall LW, Condon RE.** Prediction of malignancy in solitary thyroid nodules. Lancet. 1969;1:1071.

18. **Messaris G, Kyriakou K, Vasilopoulos P, Tountas C.** The single thyroid nodule and carcinoma. Br J Surg. 1974;61:943-4.

19. **Reichelt HG, Brase A, Hundeshagen H, Stender HS.** Xeroradiographic studies in 150 patients with solitary scintigraphically nonfunctioning nodules of the thyroid gland. Radiology. 1977;125:689-92.

20. **Brown L, Kantounis S.** The thyroid nodule: view from the community hospital. Am J Surg. 1975;129:532-6.

21. **Clark OH, Demling R.** Management of thyroid nodules in the elderly. Am J Surg. 1976;132:615-9.

22. **Katz AD, Zager WJ.** The malignant "cold" nodule of the thyroid. Am J Surg. 1976;132:459-62.

23. **Liechty RD, Stoffel PT, Zimmerman DE, Silverberg SG.** Solitary thyroid nodules. Arch Surg. 1977;112:59-61.

24. **Thijs LG.** Diagnostic ultrasound in clinical thyroid investigation. J Clin Endocrinol Metab. 1971;32:709-16.

25. **Ryo UY, Arnold J, Colman M, et al.** Thyroid scintigram: sensitivity with sodium pertechnetate Tc99m and gamma camera with pinhole collimator. JAMA. 1976;235:1235-8.

26. **Gershengorn MC, McClung MR, Chu EW, et al.** Fine-needle aspiration cytology in the preoperative diagnosis of thyroid nodules. Ann Intern Med. 1977;87:265-9.

27. **Ashcraft MW, Van Herle AJ.** Management of thyroid nodules: II. Scanning techniques, thyroid suppressive therapy, and fine needle aspiration. Head Neck Surg. 1981;3:297-322.

28. **Ashcraft MW, Van Herle AJ.** Management of thyroid nodules: I. History and physical examination, blood tests, x-ray tests, and ultrasonography. Head Neck Surg. 1981;3:216-30.

29. **Rosen IB, Walfish PG, Miskin M.** The application of ultrasound to the study of thyroid enlargement. Arch Surg. 1975;110:940-4.

30. **Blum M, Weiss B, Hernberg J.** Evaluation of thyroid nodules by A-mode echography. Radiology. 1971;101:651-6.

31. **Blum M, Goldman AB, Herskovic A, et al.** Clinical applications of thyroid echography. N Engl J Med. 1972;287:381-4.

32. **Thomas CG Jr, Buckwalter JA, Staab EV, et al.** Evaluation of dominant thyroid masses. Ann Surg. 1976;183:463-9.

33. **Molitch ME, Beck JR, Dreisman M, et al.** The cold thyroid nodule: an analysis of diagnostic and therapeutic options. Endocr Rev. 1984;5:185-99.

34. **Glassford GH, Fowler EF, Cole WH.** The treatment of nontoxic nodular goiter with desiccated thyroid: results and evaluation. Surgery. 1965;58: 621-6.

35. **Hill LD, Beebe HG, Hipp R, et al.** Thyroid suppression. Arch Surg. 1974; 108:403-5.

36. **Al-Sayer HM, Krukowski ZH, Williams VM, Matheson NA, et al.** Fine needle aspiration cytology in isolated thyroid swellings: a prospective two year evaluation. BMJ. 1985;290:1490-2.

37. **Cusick E, MacIntosh CA, Krukowski ZH, et al.** Management of isolated thyroid swellings: a prospective six-year study of fine needle aspiration cytology in diagnosis. BMJ. 1990;301:318-21.

38. **de los Santos ET, Keyhani-Rofagha S, Cunningham JJ, Mazzaferri EL.** Cystic thyroid nodules. The dilemma of malignant lesions. Arch Intern Med. 1990;150:1422-7.

39. **Dwarakanathan A A, Staren ED, D'Amore MJ, et al.** Importance of repeat fine-needle biopsy in the management of thyroid nodules. Am J Surg. 1993;166:350-2.

40. **Grant C, Hay I, et al.** Long-term follow up of patients with benign thyroid fine-needle aspiration cytologic diagnoses. Surgery. 1989;106:980-5.

41. **Hawkins F, Bellido D, et al.** Fine needle aspiration biopsy in the diagnosis of thyroid cancer and thyroid disease. Cancer. 1987;59:1206-9.

42. **Norton LW, Wangensteen SL, et al.** Utility of thyroid aspiration biopsy. Surgery. 1982;92:700-5.

43. **Piromalli D, Martelli G, et al.** The role of fine needle aspiration in the diagnosis of thyroid nodules: analysis of 795 consecutive cases. J Surg Oncol. 1992;50:247-50.

44. **Ramacciotti C E, Pretorius HT, et al.** Diagnostic accuracy and use of aspiration biopsy in the management of thyroid nodules. Arch Intern Med. 1984;144:1169-73.

45. **Sackett DL, Haynes RB, Tugwell P.** Clinical Epidemiology. A Basic Science for Clinical Medicine. Boston: Little, Brown and Company; 1985;108-26.

Breast Cancer

43

Ruth W. Kouides, MD, MPH, and Alvin I. Mushlin, MD, ScM

KEY POINTS

Pretest Probabilities

- The probability of breast cancer Increases with age and is greater in women with a personal or a strong family history of breast cancer and those who have not previously had a negative mammogram. The probability of cancer in a young woman without any risk factors is about 0.1%, whereas it exceeds 10% for an older patient with risk factors.

- For a woman with a breast mass that is clinically evident on physical examination, the chance of malignancy is approximately 20%.

- Findings on physical examination are useful in further estimating the probability of cancer in a palpable mass. When the mass has benign characteristics, the chance of malignancy is 5% to 10%.

DIAGNOSTIC STRATEGIES

- Screening mammography has proved to be beneficial in decreasing breast cancer mortality in women aged 50 to 74 years. Physical examination alone is not sensitive enough to exclude the presence of cancer.

- In the evaluation of breast masses, a triple-stage assessment consisting of physical examination, imaging with mammography, and fine-needle aspiration can be used in deciding whether to proceed to surgical removal. A benign result on all three components of this triple test may obviate the need for surgery in many individuals.

- When the clinical suspicion of breast cancer is high based on presenting signs or physical examination findings, a biopsy should be done. Imaging tests may guide the surgical approach, but negative tests do not lower the probability of disease enough to eliminate the need for biopsy.

BACKGROUND

Breast cancer is the most common cancer and the second most common cause of cancer death in American women. Overall, the risk that a woman will have breast cancer during her lifetime is approximately 12.5%, or 1 in 8 (1). An estimated 178,700 new cases of breast cancer occurred, and 43,500 breast-cancer deaths occurred among U.S. women in 1998 (1). As presented in this chapter, evidence exists that early detection of breast cancer reduces mortality and improves survival in women aged 50 to 74 years; evidence of benefit in other age groups is not established.

ESTIMATING PRETEST PROBABILITY

The elements of the clinical history that are most helpful in estimating the likelihood of cancer in an asymptomatic population or in a patient presenting with a breast mass are 1) age of the patient; 2) a previous history of breast cancer; and 3) a positive family history (2). The chance of cancer is higher for older women but lower for women who have had a previous negative screen (Table 43-1). A previous history of breast cancer elevates the chances of developing cancer in the other

Table 43-1. Risk of Breast Cancer Based on Age and Mammographic Interpretation

Age (y)	Type of Screening	Pretest Probability of Breast Cancer	Post-test Probability of Breast Cancer Based on Age and Mammographic Interpretation			
			Additional Evaluation Needed	Suspicious for Malignancy	Malignant	Normal
			←————————————————— % —————————————————→			
30–39	Initial	0.10	1.0	9.0	57	0.02
	Subsequent	0.04	1.0	11	100	0.01
40–49	Initial	0.30	2.0	30	87	0.04
	Subsequent	0.16	4.0	34	100	0.04
50–59	Initial	0.60	5.0	39	92	0.04
	Subsequent	0.24	6.0	43	100	0.06
60–69	Initial	1.30	7.0	54	90	0.08
	Subsequent	0.34	8.0	52	100	0.10
≥70	Initial	1.40	7.0	63	97	0.10
	Subsequent	0.34	8.0	52	100	0.10

Republished with permission from Kerlikowske K, Grady D, Barclay J, et al. Likelihood ratios for modern screening mammography: risk of breast cancer based on age and mammographic interpretation. JAMA. 1996;276:39-43.

breast tenfold. A woman with a first-degree relative who had breast cancer is two to three times more likely to develop breast cancer. A woman with both a sister and mother with breast cancer is about 14 times more likely to develop breast cancer (3). A woman with the BRCA-1 gene has a 16% chance of developing breast cancer by age 40 and an 86% chance by age 80 (4). Therefore, a 40-year-old woman with neither a previous history of breast cancer nor a positive family history has a probability of cancer of about 0.1%, the prevalence usually reported in general screening studies. In contrast, a 60-year-old woman with a positive family history and previous mastectomy has a probability exceeding 10%.

These estimates include both cases that have accumulated undetected over time (prevalent cases) and those newly occurring (incident cases). Once a woman has been screened and found to be free of cancer, the chances that a malignancy will be present the next year are much lower. For example, a 40-year-old woman with a previous negative mammogram has a 0.04% chance of breast cancer in the next year.

Physical examination of the breast mass for moveability, border characteristics, and consistency helps estimate the probability of the presence of cancer. A lump detected either by the patient or by a physician carries a 20% risk of cancer overall unless there are indications that the finding is benign (5). However, the usual characteristics of benign lesions are not completely reliable because cancers may present with similar findings: Three of five cancers are freely moveable, two of five have regular borders on palpation, and an equal proportion feel soft or cystic (Table 43-2) (6).

Using the operating characteristics from Table 43-2, the probability of cancer in a nonmoveable breast mass would be about 50%, whereas the likelihood of malignancy would be reduced from 20% to about 14% if the mass were moveable. When a breast mass has irregular borders

Table 43-2. Operating Characteristics of Physical Examination Findings in Evaluating Breast Masses for Cancer

Physical Finding	Sensitivity	Specificity*	Likelihood Ratio	
			Positive Result	Negative Result
	← % →			
Not soft or cystic	62	~90	6.2	0.42
Irregular borders	60	~90	6.0	0.44
Not freely moveable	40	~90	4.0	0.67

*Based on the assumption that almost all benign disease of the breast have "benign" physical findings.

or is not soft or cystic, the probability of cancer approaches 60%. Conversely, the probability of cancer would be reduced to approximately 10% if the borders were regular or the mass were soft or cystic. When the initial presentation is late in the disease course and a breast mass is accompanied by enlarged axillary lymph nodes, the probability of malignancy exceeds 50%.

The accuracy of breast physical examination is highly dependent on the size of the tumor and the age of the woman screened. The accuracy of self-examination is dependent, in addition, on the compliance of the person and her facility and training in this technique.

When no mass is present, certain other breast conditions may suggest malignancy. For example, in one study slightly fewer than 10% of patients with a nipple discharge had carcinoma (7).

DIAGNOSTIC TESTS

Two clinical situations require consideration in the use of available diagnostic studies in relationship to breast cancer: 1) screening for breast cancer in asymptomatic women, and 2) evaluation of palpable breast masses.

SCREENING FOR BREAST CANCER

Breast Self-Examination
The sensitivity of breast self-examination (BSE) is approximately 26%. The efficacy of BSE in reducing breast cancer mortality is unproven (8,9). The 5-year results of the USSR/WHO randomized study has found higher physician visit and biopsy rates in women in the BSE group without a difference in the average tumor size or nodal status (9). Therefore, the value of BSE in reducing breast cancer mortality is yet to be determined.

Clinical Breast Examination
The sensitivity of clinical breast examination (CBE) varies with the size of the tumor. The sensitivity of CBE is about 88% for lesions larger than 1 cm, but only 34% to 55% for lesions smaller than 1 cm. Specificity ranges from 89% to 96% (Table 43-3). The addition of CBE to mammography does not reduce breast cancer mortality beyond that achieved by mammography alone (10).

Mammography
Screening mammography is the only approach proven to decrease breast cancer mortality. For women aged 50 to 74 years, mortality is reduced by 25% to 30% (11–12); the benefit for women 40 to 49 years is still controversial (11–14). Possible explanations for the failure to show a benefit for

Table 43-3. Operating Characteristics of Screening Tests and Procedures in the Diagnosis of Breast Cancer

Diagnostic Test	Sensitivity	Specificity	Likelihood Ratio	
			Positive Result	Negative Result
	←	%	→	
Breast self-examination	26	—	—	—
Clinical breast examination	34–88	89–96	3.1–22	0.12–0.74
Mammography	71–95	90–99	(see Table 43-1)	

mammography for younger women in the clinical trials to date are an insufficient sample size, utilization of older technology, the predominant use of 2-year screening intervals, and the bias of intention to treat analysis related to noncompliance and contamination. It is also possible that the lack of benefit is because more aggressive tumors in younger women may decrease the window of opportunity to detect the tumor before it has spread. Trials are currently underway in Europe to determine the value of mammography screening for women in their forties.

Techniques for mammography have improved since its introduction in the 1960s, with the most marked changes occurring around 1985. These improvements include use of a dedicated unit and techniques to ensure low radiation doses. Film-screen mammography requires less radiation and gives more precise tissue definition than xerography. In addition to technical concerns, there is considerable variability in the interpretation of mammograms by radiologists. The sensitivity between readers may vary within a 40% range (15). Physicians are encouraged to use the high-volume centers that meet accreditation standards (16). The sensitivity of mammography in the breast cancer mortality trials ranged from 83% to 95%, and the specificity varied from 93.5% to 99.1% (17). Although these trials were begun between 1963 and 1982, and therefore reflect older technology, more recent mammography series reported similar results with sensitivities of 71% to 92% and specificities of 90% to 98% (17). The accuracy of mammography is lower for younger women. In one study, the sensitivity was 93.2% in women 50 years old or older compared with 83.5% in women between 40 and 49 years of age (18). Having dense breasts worsened the sensitivity of mammography in older women (98.4% versus 83.7%), but not for younger women (18). Double reading of mammograms may improve the sensitivity up to 10% (19). Similarly, there is a trend toward improved mortality in clinical trials that required two-view instead of one-view mammography (11).

The mammogram interpretation is affected by hormone replacement therapy (HRT). Hormone replacement therapy increases the density of postmenopausal breast tissue. The increased density may be asymmetric and therefore lead to worry and possible biopsy (20–23). A small study showed a trend toward lower sensitivity and specificity for users of HRT compared to nonusers and former users (24).

Mammograms are not typically interpreted as positive or negative; therefore, using likelihood ratios (Chapter 3) rather than sensitivities and specificities is helpful. For example, a first mammogram that is read as "additional evaluation needed" has a likelihood ratio of 7.1 (95% CI, 5.9 to 8.3) for malignancy compared to likelihood ratios of 124 (CI, 86 to 172) and 2209 (CI, 643 to 12,715) for mammograms read as "suspicious for malignancy" and "malignant," respectively (25). Table 43-1 summarizes the post-test probability of breast cancer according to age and mammographic interpretation in a screening situation. The relatively low post-test probabilities for cancer among the various abnormal readings implies that many women without disease need further evaluation.

EVALUATION OF ABNORMAL MAMMOGRAMS AND PALPABLE MASSES

Diagnostic and Digital Mammography

To evaluate further an abnormality on a screening mammogram or on physical examination, additional mammographic views are used. These views may include the entire breast from another orientation or a compression-spot view of the suspicious area.

Digital mammography is currently being evaluated for its ability to distinguish malignant from benign lesions. This technique uses a computerized mammographic image that can be manipulated (e.g., removing background density in efforts to identify underlying lesions). Also, computerized protocols can "read" the mammograms and may improve the uniformity of interpretation (26–29). The final contribution of digital mammograms is yet to be determined, but there is particular hope that it will improve the evaluation of patients with dense breasts.

Ultrasonography

When a mass has already been located via palpation, ultrasonic B-scanning machines can differentiate cystic from solid lesions. In separating cystic from solid lesions, the overall accuracy approaches 100%, making fine-needle aspiration of cystic lesions an alternative to surgical procedures in many patients.

There is increased interest in use of ultrasonography to distinguish benign from malignant lesions and thereby reduce biopsy rates. Preliminary reports using microbubble techniques to demonstrate vessels and shunts within lesions and quantitative ultrasonography to measure flow velocities are promising (30,31). Ultrasonography on solid breast nodules showed a sensitivity of 98.4% and a specificity of 67.8% for cancer (32). Because the criteria for a positive study were not clearly determined a priori in these studies, these findings need to be replicated. Furthermore, ultrasonography is operator dependent, and these results may not apply in all settings.

Ultrasonographic examination for the detection of axillary node involvement to potentially obviate the need for a nodal dissection has been explored. However, its low sensitivity, approximately 70%, limits this application at this time (33,34).

Tissue Diagnosis

Currently, three approaches are used to obtain tissue diagnosis in the evaluation of suspicious lesions: fine-needle aspiration, core biopsy, and open, excisional biopsy.

Fine-Needle Aspiration

Without local anesthesia, a fine needle can be passed into a localized mass, and material can be aspirated through a syringe for cytologic examination. Ultrasonography or stereotactic techniques can be used to evaluate nonpalpable mammographically detected lesions. Several passes through a lesion while maintaining "negative" pressure on the syringe improves sampling. Material adequate for cytologic examination has been obtainable in almost all samples when ultrasonography or stereotactic guidance was used (35–38). In most series, the sensitivity has been between 88% and 95%, with specificity between 92% and 99% (Table 43-4) (35–38). An aspirate that shows atypical cells or an inadequate specimen requires further investigation, usually with excisional biopsy. Between 24% and 71% of samples read as atypical were found to be malignant on further workup (35–38).

In some cases, cytologic examination of nipple discharge may be the only technique that leads to the diagnosis. In one small series of women with nipple discharge, cytologic examination of the fluid had a low sensitivity (55%) but a high specificity (100%) (39).

Core Needle Biopsy

With a core biopsy, local anesthetic is used and a small cut is made in the skin, followed by insertion of a large-bore needle that cuts a sample of tissue. The main advantage of the core biopsy over fine-needle aspiration (FNA) is that it provides a tissue sample, rather than a cellular aspirate. In some cases, prognostic indicators such as estrogen receptor status can also be determined. The core biopsy technique is more traumatic, and there has been concern that fewer samples might be obtained compared with FNA. However, more than 92% of lesions have been adequately sampled using core biopsy techniques (23,40). Stereotactic or ultrasonographic guidance for the biopsy, radiologic

Table 43-4. Operating Characteristics of Tests and Procedures in the Diagnosis of Breast Cancer Among Patients with Palpable Masses and Mammographic Abnormalities

Diagnostic Test	Sensitivity	Specificity	Likelihood Ratio Positive Result	Likelihood Ratio Negative Result
	←————— % —————→			
Mammography	80 (79–88)	90 (85–93)	8.0	0.22
Ultrasonography	98	68	3.1	0.02
Fine-needle aspiration*	95 (88–96)	98 (92–99)	48	0.05
Core biopsy*	93 (88–98)	98 (97–100)	47	0.07
Magnetic resonance imaging	95 (92–100)	65 (37–73)	2.7	0.08
Nuclear imaging				
Palpable lesion	93 (88–96)	90 (62–95)	9.3	0.07
Nonpalpable lesion	64 (60–77)	96 (75–100)	16	0.38

*When adequate material is obtained.

imaging of the specimen to verify that calcifications were sampled, and pathologic examination of frozen sections may all enhance sample rates. The sensitivity of core biopsy is 88% to 98%, and its specificity is 97% to 100% (23,40).

Excisional Biopsy
Excisional biopsy remains the gold standard. When inadequate specimens are obtained with less invasive techniques, a surgical biopsy is required. For nonpalpable lesions, needle localization is necessary. Again, in cases of biopsy for nonpalpable lesions (e.g., suspicious calcifications on mammography), specimen radiography ensures that the questionable area was indeed sampled.

Magnetic Resonance Imaging
Magnetic resonance imaging (MRI) of the breast is currently characterized by excellent sensitivity (92%–100%), but low specificity (37%–73%) for cancer (41–45). There is no agreement on the optimal techniques (breast coils, contrast enhancement), interpretation, and role in the workup of breast abnormalities for MRI (46). Limitations include false-positives caused by fibrocystic disease, mastitis, and other inflammatory processes and false-negatives with ductal carcinoma in situ (DCIS) because calcifications do not appear on MRI images. Potential roles include evaluation of dense breasts or tissue surround-

ing breast implants and preoperative staging to look for multifocal disease.

Nuclear Imaging

Thallium-201 and technetium-99m-sestamibi scans have been used to evaluate palpable breast masses and mammograms that show abnormalities. Thallium has a sensitivity of 91% to 96% with a specificity of 95% for palpable masses (47,48), compared with a sensitivity of 77% when further evaluating cases with only mammographic abnormalities (49). Technetium similarly has sensitivities of 88% to 94% for palpable lesions (50–56), compared with 60% to 64% for nonpalpable lesions (53,54). Both have inadequate sensitivities (27%–64%) to evaluate axillary nodal status (48,57). Image resolution is inadequate for independent biopsy localization.

Positron Emission Tomography

Positron emission tomography (PET) scanning with radiolabeled 2-[^{18}F] fluoro-2-deoxy-D-glucose has been evaluated to detect axillary lymph-node involvement. However, PET scanning has a sensitivity of only 33% in those with the smallest tumors, who are the most likely candidates for avoiding a nodal dissection (58). Because PET scanning relates to physiologic activity, it holds promise in providing insight about tumor aggressiveness and responsiveness to therapy (59).

Computed Tomography

The higher radiation dose associated with computed tomography compared with mammography limits its applicability. However, it may have a role in the diagnosis of local recurrence after conservative therapy. In this situation, test sensitivity is reported at 91% and specificity at 85% (60).

DIAGNOSTIC STRATEGIES

Mammography is the screening test of choice. Many practitioners supplement mammography with physician examination and patient self-examination, although the utility of these strategies is unproven. Most current recommendations suggest annual mammography for women aged 50 to 74 years. The role of screening mammography in those aged 40 to 49 years is controversial.

If the results of mammography are positive on an initial screen in a 50-year-old woman, the probability that she has cancer is about 9%. As seen in Table 43-1, her pretest probability is 0.6%, and a positive mammogram means that her risk of cancer varies from 5% to 92%, depending on the mammographic interpretation. A tissue diagnosis with or without radiologic localization is needed. A negative mammography study in a screening situation provides reassurance that the patient is free of detectable breast cancer, reducing the likelihood of cancer to less than 0.1%.

In evaluating a patient with a palpable mass, in cases in which the pretest probability of cancer is higher, positive mammography results give a correspondingly higher post-test probability than when used for screening. Positive studies make tissue diagnosis imperative. On the other hand, a mammogram revealing no signs of malignancy is only somewhat reassuring because the probability of cancer is still approximately 5%, with further studies often indicated. However, if the physical examination suggests a cystic structure that is confirmed by ultrasonography and aspiration reveals no malignant cells, then a benign diagnosis can be made with substantial certainty. In such instances, nothing more need be done if follow-up can be ensured.

When the clinical suspicion of malignancy is especially high, based on physical examination findings, a negative result on any of the studies is not sufficiently accurate to advise against biopsy. Diagnostic procedures are useful only for localization or planning surgical technique. Any planned imaging should be done before biopsy because of the potential confusion in interpreting mammograms when postoperative hematomas are present.

CLINICAL PROBLEMS

Clinical Problem 1
A middle-aged woman with a positive family history of breast cancer has a breast examination during her routine health maintenance evaluation, the results of which are normal.

Testing Strategy and Rationale
A screening mammogram should be obtained. Several studies have demonstrated the life-saving effect of mammography screening in women older than 50 years of age, and mammography remains the best test to determine that an occult breast cancer is not present. On the basis of her family history, the prior probability of an occult tumor would be about 3%. Because breast physical examination is about 50% sensitive, the probability of cancer may still be approximately 2% after a normal examination. However, if the results of mammography are normal, the chance of an occult malignancy would be reduced to less than 1%.

Clinical Example
A 55-year-old woman visits her primary care physician for her annual health evaluation. She has a family history of breast cancer.

Her self-examinations at home and the results of the physician's examination are normal. Mammography should be ordered.

Clinical Problem 2
A patient has a breast mass that feels cystic.

Testing Strategy and Rationale
Further testing is indicated. One approach would be to proceed directly to an excisional biopsy, but a less invasive alternative strategy is possible. This would begin by obtaining a mammogram. A mammogram positive for malignancy would be followed by biopsy. If the mammogram is normal, a fine-needle aspiration would complete the "triple test" of physical examination, mammogram, and cytologic examination. (The sensitivity and specificity of a triple test are approximately 97% and 94%, respectively.) (61)

Clinical Example
A 45-year-old woman with no known risk factors for breast cancer presents with the history of having detected a painless lump in the right breast. Physical examination reveals a moveable, regular mass that feels cystic.

Multiple benign characteristics on physical examination lower the probability of cancer to less than 5%, but further testing is indicated. Mammography is performed and the results are normal, reducing the probability of breast cancer to approximately 1%. If a subsequent aspiration of the mass is performed and is negative, the probability of malignancy becomes very low, approximately 0.2%. Another mammogram within a short interval is usually recommended after such an evaluation, although the yield of this approach is controversial (62).

REFERENCES

1. **Landis SH, Murray T, Bolden S, Wingo PA.** Cancer statistics. CA Cancer J Clin. 1998;48:6-29.
2. **Marchant DJ.** Epidemiology of breast cancer. Clin Obstet Gyn. 1982;25:387-92.
3. **Sattin RW, Rubin GL, Webster LA, et al.** Family history and the risk of breast cancer. JAMA. 1985;253:1908
4. **King M, Rowell S, Love SM.** Inherited breast and ovarian cancer. JAMA. 1993;269:(15)1975
5. **Baker LH.** Breast cancer detection demonstration project: five year summary. CA Cancer J Clin.1982;32:194-225.
6. **Venet L, Strax P, Venet W, Shapiro S.** Adequacies and inadequacies of breast examinations by physicians in mass screening. CA Cancer J Clin. 1971;28:1546

7. **Atkins H, Wolff B.** Discharges from the nipple. Br J Surg. 1964;51:602-6.

8. **Ellman R, Moss SM, Coleman D, Chamberlain J.** Breast self-examination programmes in the trial of early detection of breast cancer: ten year findings. Br J Cancer. 1993;68:(1)208-12.

9. **Semiglazov VF, Moiseyenko VM, Bavli JL, et al.** The role of breast self-examination in early breast cancer detection (results of the 5-years USSR/WHO randomized study in Leningrad). Eur J Epidemiol 1992;8:(4)498-502.

10. **Baines CJ, Miller AB, Bassett AA.** Physical examination: its role as a single screening modality in the Canadian National Breast Screening Study. Cancer 1989;63:1816-22.

11. **Kerlikowske K, Grady D, Rubin SM, et al.** Efficacy of screening mammography. A meta-analysis. JAMA. 1995;273:149-54.

12. **Elwood JM, Cox B, Richardson AK.** The effectiveness of breast cancer screening by mammography in younger women (published errata appear in Online J Curr Clin Trials 1993 Mar 5;Doc No 34 and 1994 Mar 31;Doc No 121). Online J Curr Clin Trials 1993;Doc No 32.

13. **Shapiro S, Venet W, Strax P, Venet L.** Chapters 1-5. In Abeloff MD, Boyer SH, Green GM, et al. Periodic Screening for Breast Cancer. Baltimore: The Johns Hopkins University Press; 1995:1-57.

14. **Smart CR, Hendrick RE, Rutledge JH, Smith RA.** Benefit of mammography screening in women ages 40 to 49 years. Cancer. 1995;75:1619-26.

15. **Beam CA, Layde PM, Sullivan DC.** Variability in the interpretation of screening mammograms by US radiologists. Findings from a national sample. Arch Intern Med 1996;156:209-13.

16. **Paquelet JR.** Medicare, mammography, and the Mammography Quality Standards Act of 1992. Radiology. 1994;190:47-9A.

17. **Mushlin AI, Kouides RK, Shapiro DE.** Estimating the accuracy of screening mammography. Am J Prev Med. 1998; 14:143-53.

18. **Kerlikowske K, Grady D, Barclay J, et al.** Effect of age, breast density, and family history on the sensitivity of first screening mammography. JAMA. 1996;276:33-8.

19. **Anderson ED, Muir BB, Walsh JS, Kirkpatrick AE.** The efficacy of double reading mammograms in breast screening. Clin Radiol 1994;49:248-51.

20. **Kaufman Z, Garstin WI, Hayes R, et al.** The mammographic parenchymal patterns of women on hormonal replacement therapy. Clin Radiol. 1991;43:389-92.

21. **Cyriak D, Wong CH.** Mammographic changes in postmenopausal women undergoing hormonal replacement therapy. AJR Am J Roentgenol. 1993; 161:1177-83.

22. **Laya MB, Gallagher JC, Schreiman JS, et al.** Effect of postmenopausal hormonal replacement therapy on mammographic density and parenchymal pattern. Radiology 1995;196:433-7.

23. **Frayne J, Sterrett GF, Harvey J, et al.** Stereotactic 14 gauge core-biopsy of the breast: results from 101 patients. Aust N Z J Surg. 1996;66:585-91.

24. **Laya MB, Larson EB, Taplin SH, White E.** Effect of estrogen replacement therapy on the specificity and sensitivity of screening mammography. J Natl Cancer Inst 1996;88:643-9.

25. **Kerlikowske K, Grady D, Barclay J, et al.** Likelihood ratios for modern screening mammography. Risk of breast cancer based on age and mammographic interpretation. JAMA. 1996;276:39-43.

26. **Ema T, Doi K, Nishikawa RM, et al.** Image feature analysis and computer-aided diagnosis in mammography: reduction of false-positive clustered microcalcifications using local edge-gradient analysis. Med Phys. 1995;22: 161-9.

27. **Huo Z, Giger ML, Vyborny CJ, et al.** Analysis of speculation in the computerized classification of mammographic masses. Med Phys. 1995;22: 1569-79.

28. **Wei D, Chan HP, Helvie MA, et al.** Classification of mass and normal breast tissue on digital mammograms: multiresolution texture analysis. Med Phys. 1995;22:1501-13.

29. **Chang YH, Zheng B, Gur D.** Computerized identification of suspicious regions for masses in digitized mammograms. Invest Radiol. 1996;31: 146-53.

30. **Kedar RP, Cosgrove D, McCready VR, et al.** Microbubble contrast agent for color Doppler US: effect on breast masses (Work in progress). Radiology. 1996;98:679-86.

31. **Richter K, Heywang-Kobrunner SH.** Sonographic differentiation of benign from malignant breast lesions: value of indirect measurement of ultrasound velocity. AJR Am J Roentgenol. 1994;825-31.

32. **Stavros AT, Thickman D, Rapp CL, et al.** Solid breast nodules: use of sonography to distinguish between benign and malignant lesions. Radiology. 1995;196:123-34.

33. **Vaidya JS, Vyas JJ, Thakur MH, et al.** Role of ultrasonography to detect axillary node involvement in operable breast cancer. Eur J Surg Oncol. 1996;22:140-3.

34. **Walsh JS, Dixon JM, Chetty U, Paterson D.** Colour Doppler studies of axillary node metastases in breast carcinoma. Clin Radiol. 1994;49:189-91.

35. **Gordon PB, Goldenberg SL, Chan NH.** Solid breast lesions: diagnosis with US-guided fine-needle aspiration biopsy. Radiology. 1993;189:573-80.

36. **Mitnick JS, Vazquez MF, Pressman PI, et al.** Stereotactic fine-needle aspiration biopsy for the evaluation of nonpalpable breast lesions: report of an experience based on 2, 988 cases. Ann Surg Oncol. 1996;3:185-91.

37. **Vazquez MF, Mitnick JS, Pressman P, et al.** Stereotactic aspiration biopsy of nonpalpable nodules of the breast. J Am Coll Surg. 1994;178:17-23.

38. **Saarela AO, Kiviniemi HO, Rissanen TJ, Paloneva TK.** Nonpalpable breast lesions: pathologic correlation of ultrasonographically guided fine-needle aspiration biopsy. J Ultrasound Med. 1996;15:549-53.

39. **Dunn JM, Lucarotti ME, Wood SJ, et al.** Exfoliative cytology in the diagnosis of breast disease. Br J Surg. 1995;82:789-91.

40. **Nguyen M, McCombs MM, Ghandehari S, et al.** An update on core needle biopsy for radiologically detected breast lesions. [Review] [17 refs]. Cancer. 1996;78:2340-5.

41. **Stomper PC, Herman S, Klippenstein DL, et al.** Suspect breast lesions: findings at dynamic gadolinium-enhanced MR imaging correlated with mammographic and pathologic features. Radiology. 1995;197:387-95.

42. **Gilles R, Meunier M, Lucidarme O, et al.** Clustered breast microcalcifications: evaluation by dynamic contrast-enhanced subtraction MRI. J Comput Assist Tomogr. 1996;20:9-14.

43. **Heiberg EV, Perman WH, Herrmann VM, Janney CG.** Dynamic sequential 3D gadolinium-enhanced MRI of the whole breast. Magn Reson Imaging. 1996;14:337-48.

44. **Bone B, Aspelin P, Bronge L, et al.** Sensitivity and specificity of MR mammography with histopathological correlation in 250 breasts. Acta Radiol. 1996;37:208-13.

45. **Cross MJ, Harms SE, Cheek JH, et al.** New horizons in the diagnosis and treatment of breast cancer using magnetic resonance imaging. Am J Surg. 1993;166:749-53.

46. **Heywang-Kobrunner SH.** Contrast-enhanced magnetic resonance imaging of the breast. Invest Radiol. 1994;29:94-104.

47. **Waxman AD, Ramanna L, Memsic LD, et al.** Thallium scintigraphy in the evaluation of mass abnormalities of the breast. J Nucl Med. 1993;34:18-23.

48. **Cimitan M, Volpe R, Candiani E, et al.** The use of thallium-201 in the preoperative detection of breast cancer: an adjunct to mammography and ultrasonography. Eur J Nucl Med. 1995;22:1110-7.

49. **Lee VW, Sax EJ, McAneny DB, et al.** A complementary role for thallium-201 scintigraphy with mammography in the diagnosis of breast cancer. J Nucl Med. 1993;34:2095-100.

50. **Khalkhali I, Cutrone J, Mena I, et al.** Technetium-99m-sestamibi scintimammography of breast lesions: clinical and pathological follow-up. J Nucl Med. 1995;36:1784-9.

51. **Khalkhali I, Cutrone JA, Mena IG, et al.** Scintimammography: the complementary role of Tc-99m sestamibi prone breast imaging for the diagnosis of breast carcinoma. Radiology. 1995;196:421-6.

52. **Taillefer R, Robidoux A, Lambert R, et al.** Technetium-99m-sestamibi prone scintimammography to detect primary breast cancer and axillary lymph node involvement. J Nucl Med. 1995;36:1758-65.

53. **Villanueva-Meyer J, Leonard MH, Jr., Briscoe E, et al.** Mammoscintigraphy with technetium-99m-sestamibi in suspected breast cancer. J Nucl Med. 1996;37:926-30.

54. **Palmedo H, Grunwald F, Bender H, et al.** Scintimammography with technetium-99m methoxyisobutylisonitrile: comparison with mammography and magnetic resonance imaging. Eur J Nucl Med. 1996;23:940-6.

55. **Lind P, Gallowitsch HJ, Kogler D, et al.** Tc-99m-tetrofosmin scintimammography: a prospective study in primary breast lesions. Nuklearmedizin. 1996;35:225-9.

56. **Palmedo H, Schomburg A, Grunwald F, et al.** Technetium-99m-MIBI scintimammography for suspicious breast lesions. J Nucl Med. 1996;37:626-30.

57. **Lam WW, Yang WT, Chan YL, et al.** Detection of axillary lymph node metastases in breast carcinoma by technetium-99m sestamibi breast scintigraphy, ultrasound and conventional mammography. Eur J Nucl Med. 1996;23:498-503.

58. **Avril N, Dose J, Janicke F, et al.** Assessment of axillary lymph node involvement in breast cancer patients with positron emission tomography

using radiolabeled 2-(fluorine-18)-fluoro-2-deoxy-D-glucose. J Natl Cancer Inst. 1996;88:1204-9.

59. **Feig SA.** Strategies for improving sensitivity of screening mammography for women aged 40 to 49 years [Editorial comment]. JAMA. 1996;276:73-4.

60. **Hagay C, Cherel PJ, de Maulmont CE, et al.** Contrast-enhanced CT: value for diagnosing local breast cancer recurrence after conservative treatment. Radiology. 1996;200:631-8.

61. **Yiangou C, Davis J, Livni N, et al.** Diagnostic role of cytology in screen-detected breast cancer. Br J Surg. 1996;83:816-9.

62. **Gwin JL, Jr., King B, Hudson KB, Bell JL.** Interval mammography after needle localization biopsy of breast abnormalities that are pathologically benign. Am J Surg. 1995;170:323-6.

Genitourinary Problems

Secondary Amenorrhea **44**

Joseph A. Aloi, MD, Julia E. Connelly, MD, and John T. Philbrick, MD

KEY POINTS

Pretest Probabilities

- The history and physical examination, including clinical assessment of the patient's estrogen status, usually directs attention to the most likely cause of secondary amenorrhea.

- Hypothalamic-pituitary dysfunction associated with weight loss, emotional stress, or strenuous exercise is the most common cause of pathologic secondary amenorrhea.

- Pituitary tumors are not common in a primary care setting; however, they are more likely when amenorrhea is accompanied by galactorrhea, headache, or changes in vision.

Diagnostic Strategies

- Pregnancy and hypothyroidism must be ruled out before further evaluation is undertaken.

- When the pretest probability is not high for a specific condition, the initial diagnostic strategy should be to determine estrogen status.

- If the pretest probability is high for a specific condition, the diagnostic strategy often can be tailored to confirm the diagnosis.

- Prolactin testing should be reserved for patients who are hypoestrogenic or who have galactorrhea, headache, or changes in vision.

BACKGROUND

Secondary amenorrhea is defined as the cessation of menstruation for at least 3 months in a nonpregnant woman who previously has had normal menstrual cycles. Although recommendations for evaluation vary, a rational strategy should focus on patient characteristics and define the site of the functional abnormality. Diagnosis is important because therapy should ameliorate the underlying abnormality, dimin-

509

ish the sequelae related to the hypoestrogenemia (e.g., osteoporosis), or to unopposed estrogen (e.g., endometrial hyperplasia), and treat infertility if present.

A complete review of the requirements necessary for normal menstruation is beyond the scope of this chapter. However, the essential features include the following: 1) hypothalamic gonadotropin-releasing hormone (GnRH) stimulates secretion of follicle-stimulating hormone (FSH) and luteinizing hormone (LH) from the pituitary; 2) FSH stimulates the ovary and results in increasing levels of 17 beta-estradiol; 3) estradiol exerts a positive feedback effect at the pituitary and contributes to the midcycle increase in FSH and LH; 4) ovulation follows the LH surge and the corpus luteum is formed from the collapsing follicle; 5) estradiol and progesterone secretion increase in the corpus luteum; 6) estradiol causes endometrial proliferation; 7) the combined effect of estradiol and progesterone converts a proliferative endometrium to secretory; and 8) menstruation follows progesterone withdrawal from an estrogenized endometrium (1,2).

ESTIMATING PRETEST PROBABILITY

A population-based survey in Sweden demonstrated that the yearly incidence of secondary amenorrhea of more than 3 months' duration was 3.3% (3). The incidence and the cause of secondary amenorrhea vary among clinical settings. Table 44-1 provides summary information about the causes of secondary amenorrhea in patients seen in two gynecology referral clinics (4,5). Such information is not available from primary care settings, where the frequency of hypothalamic-pituitary dysfunction, ovarian failure, and hypothyroidism is probably higher, whereas the frequency of hyperprolactinemia and tumors is lower (6).

The most common cause of secondary amenorrhea in women during their reproductive years is pregnancy. The postpartum period may also cause secondary amenorrhea; however, the menses will return to normal within 3 months after delivery in 90% of patients who are not breast-feeding (7). Oral contraceptives may also affect menstrual patterns. When these contraceptives are discontinued, menses usually return to normal within 6 months. Studies suggest that oral contraceptives do not cause amenorrhea but may temporarily mask its development in women who previously had oligomenorrhea (8).

Hypothalamic-pituitary dysfunction is probably the most common cause of secondary amenorrhea seen in primary care settings. Emotional stress (9), strenuous exercise (especially running) (10,11), and weight loss (12) are frequently associated with such dysfunction. These patients have either normal or low estrogen levels. Estrogen levels vary directly with the degree of weight loss and psychological distress. In studies,

Table 44-1. Frequency of Causes of Secondary Amenorrhea from Two Gynecology Referral Clinics

Cause	Study	
	Hull et al.*	Reindollar et al.†
	←———————— % ————————→	
Euestrogenic (eugonadism)		
Hypothalamic-pituitary dysfunction	20	8
Polycystic ovary disease	5	28
Asherman syndrome	—	7
Other	—	4
Hypoestrogenic (hypogonadism)		
Hypothalamic-hypopituitary	38	26
Ovarian failure	12	12
Hyperandrogenic states		
Ovarian tumor	—	1
Congenital adrenal hyperplasia	—	<1
Hyperprolactinemia		
Pituitary tumor	12	8
Drug use (chlorpromazine, thioridazone, haloperidol, metoclopramide)	—	2
Other	12	1
Hypothyroidism	1	2

*Data from Hull MGR, Knuth UA, Murray MAF, Jacobs HS. The practical value of the progestogens challenge test, serum oestradiol estimation or clinical examination in assessment of the oestrogen state and response to clomiphene in amenorrhea. Br J Obstet Gynecol. 1979;86:799-805.
†Data from Reindollar RH, Novak M, Tho SPT, McDonough PG. Adult-onset amenorrhea: a study of 262 patients. Am J Obstet Gynecol. 1986;155:531-43.

2.6% of college women (13) and 19% of female Olympic marathon runners developed secondary amenorrhea (11). The amenorrheic runners were younger, lighter, and leaner than eumenorrheic runners (11). Weight loss associated with body fat less than 22% of body weight may result in amenorrhea, as occurs in women with anorexia nervosa.

Ovarian failure occurs as a normal physiologic process in 95% of women between 45 and 55 years of age. The mean age of menopause is 51 years. Women younger than 40 years of age may develop premature ovarian failure from afollicular ovaries, resistant ovaries, and autoimmune diseases (1,14).

Secondary amenorrhea associated with polycystic ovary syndrome is more likely when obesity, hirsutism, and infertility are also present.

Hyperprolactinemia causes amenorrhea by inhibiting GnRH stimulation of LH and FSH and thereby production of estrogen. Pituitary tumors, drugs (chlorpromazine, thioridazine, haloperidol, and metoclopramide), and other factors such as hypothyroidism, uremia, nipple stimulation, and emotional stress result in elevated prolactin levels. Approximately 80% of women with elevated prolactin levels have galactorrhea, whereas only 50% of women with galactorrhea have hyperprolactinemia. Patients with prolactin levels greater than 200 ng/mL usually have macroadenomas (>10 mm) (15). The presence of headaches and visual abnormalities associated with secondary amenorrhea increases the pretest probability of a pituitary tumor.

Asherman syndrome occurs when abortions, pelvic inflammatory disease, or aggressive dilatation and curettage result in intrauterine or cervical obstruction.

Estrogen deficiency is most likely to be the cause of amenorrhea in patients whose cervix and vagina are bright pink and contain only small amounts of serous fluid. Hull (4) reports that if visual examination suggests estrogen deficiency, progesterone withdrawal tests (discussed later in this chapter) yield negative results in 94% of patients. However, of patients for whom the visual examination suggests normal estrogen levels, 61% menstruate on withdrawal from progesterone. Clinical estrogen status cannot always be determined, and it was uncertain in 26% of these patients.

DIAGNOSTIC TESTS

Accurate estimates of the sensitivity and specificity of diagnostic tests used in the evaluation of secondary amenorrhea are unavailable owing to the frequent lack of an independent gold standard, the biologic variability of many of the hormonal levels, and the rapidly evolving technology in imaging tests.

Pregnancy Tests

Current tests for pregnancy are designed to recognize the beta subunit of human chorionic gonadotropin (HCG). Median levels of HCG range from 0.13 IU/mL during the fourth week of pregnancy to 10 IU/mL during the tenth week of pregnancy. Urine tests can detect from 0.2 to 4.0 IU/mL, and serum tests can detect as little as 0.025 IU/mL. Urine tests are 90% sensitive from 14 to 21 days after the first missed menses, whereas serum radioimmunoassay tests are 90% sensitive 1 day after the first missed period. False-negative test results may occur in patients with ectopic pregnancy and threatened abortion. False-positive tests may occur with choriocarcinoma, hydatidiform mole, and other tumors that produce ectopic HCG (16).

Progesterone Challenge Test

To determine the functional state of the endometrium (e.g., whether it has become proliferative in the presence of estrogen), medroxyprogesterone (Provera) is administered orally, 10 mg/d for 5 to 10 days, and withdrawal bleeding is awaited. Hull (4) reported a significant relation between the level of 17 beta-estradiol and presence of withdrawal bleeding. Ninety-five percent of patients with 17 beta-estradiol levels greater than 100 pmol/L had withdrawal bleeding, whereas 95% with 17 beta-estradiol levels less than 100 pmol/L had no withdrawal bleeding. The absence of withdrawal bleeding in patients with clinical evidence of estrogen (approximately 39%) is explained by estrogen levels that are insufficient to stimulate proliferation of the endometrium and in a few patients by anatomic outflow obstruction. In these patients, treatment with conjugated estrogens (Premarin, 0.625 mg) for 2 weeks, followed by repeat progesterone administration can distinguish outflow obstruction from hypoestrogenemia.

Follicle-Stimulating Hormone, Luteinizing Hormone, and Prolactin

Radioimmunoassay and immunoradiometric measurements are commonly used for quantifying FSH, LH, and prolactin levels. Because standard preparations may vary among laboratories, it is important to know the normal range for each laboratory and to be cautious about comparing results from different sites. Because of the episodic nature of gonadotropin release, repeat testing may be necessary. Serum levels of FSH greater than 40 IU/L generally indicate ovarian failure; low serum gonadotropin in a woman with amenorrhea suggests hypothalamic or pituitary dysfunction. An elevated LH level with a normal FSH level (ratio LH/FSH ≥2.0) suggests polycystic ovarian syndrome (1,2). Patients with amenorrhea and elevated prolactin levels (>15–20 ng/mL) are typically deficient in estrogen (16,17).

Imaging Tests

Radiologic tests are used to diagnose prolactin-secreting pituitary adenomas and, more rarely, masses in the area of the hypothalamus (e.g., craniopharyngiomas, meningiomas, other pituitary disease). High-detail computed tomography (CT) is highly sensitive for the diagnosis of macroadenomas (>10 mm), but relatively insensitive for microadenomas as small as 3 to 4 mm in diameter. By CT alone, a functioning microadenoma (<10 mm) cannot be ruled out (18) and smaller tumors can easily be missed. Low-density areas (cysts or infarcts) present on CT may mimic microadenomas in 7% to 20% of patients without pituitary disease. Magnetic resonance imaging (MRI) is far superior to CT for imaging this part of the brain (19,20).

DIAGNOSTIC STRATEGIES

As discussed in the section on estimating pretest probability, the patient's history and physical examination provide important clues to the most likely causes of secondary amenorrhea. Conditions such as pregnancy, hypothyroidism (see Chapter 41), and hypercortisolism (see Chapter 40) need to be considered when the initial evaluation suggests that they are possible.

If the pretest probability is high for a specific condition, the diagnostic strategy should be tailored to confirm the suspected abnormality. For example, if the patient is experiencing severe emotional stress, hypothalamic-pituitary abnormalities are the probable cause. Further workup could be delayed while attempts to alleviate the patient's stress are made. Similarly, if a patient has galactorrhea associated with amenorrhea, the

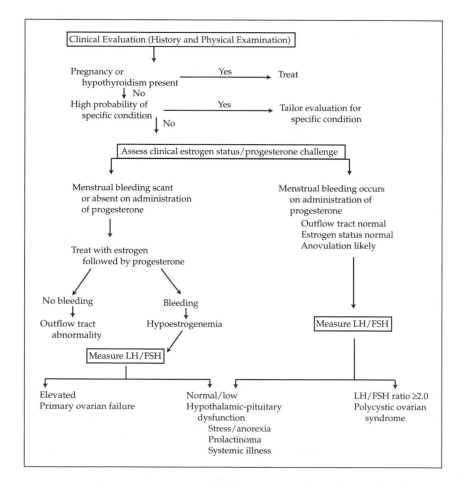

Figure 44-1. Diagnostic strategy for evaluation of secondary amenorrhea.

pretest probability of a pituitary tumor is high and the diagnosis needs to be pursued directly. The initial test should be a serum prolactin level, followed by radiologic imaging if the prolactin level is elevated.

However, if the pretest probability is not high for a specific condition, the initial diagnostic strategy requires defining the patient's estrogen status (euestrogenic or hypoestrogenic). Several methods are useful: clinical observation of the vaginal mucosa, microscopic examination of the cervical mucous, and progesterone withdrawal (which also provides information about the functional status of the endometrium). The occurrence of menstrual bleeding after treatment with progesterone provides evidence that estradiol and FSH are present. When withdrawal bleeding is scanty or does not occur, the amount of estrogen may not be adequate to cause endometrial proliferation or an obstruction to uterine outflow may be present. In such cases, the presence of uterine obstruction can be proved by the absence of withdrawal bleeding after both estrogen and progesterone are administered. Figure 44-1 shows a flow chart outlining the various diagnostic strategies.

CLINICAL PROBLEMS

Clinical Problem 1
A young patient presents with persistent amenorrhea and factors pointing to hypothalamic-pituitary dysfunction.

Testing Strategy and Rationale
Estrogen status should be determined, pregnancy excluded, progesterone challenge performed, and gonadotropin levels measured.

History and physical examination should focus on probable causes of secondary amenorrhea. Pregnancy and hypothyroidism should be considered. If signs of estrogen are present on examination, the functional state of the endometrium can be determined by the progesterone challenge test. Withdrawal bleeding demonstrates that estrogen and FSH are present. A normal or low LH level reflects hypothalamic-pituitary dysfunction.

Clinical Example
A 21-year-old female college student who runs marathons developed amenorrhea 12 months ago after having had normal menses since menarche. Her menstrual cycles had previously been regular. She takes no medications and her body weight is normal. She is not sexually active. Physical examination suggests evidence of normal estrogen levels. The results of a pregnancy test are negative. Withdrawal bleeding occurs after administration of progesterone.

Continued

Prolactin level is normal, and the LH level is low. A diagnosis of hypothalamic-pituitary dysfunction is made.

Clinical Problem 2

A sexually active woman of reproductive age reports that she has not menstruated for 4 months.

Testing Strategy and Rationale

A history should be obtained and a physical examination should be performed. A pregnancy test should be done. Estrogen status needs to be determined, and a progesterone challenge should be performed if the results of the pregnancy test are negative.

The history should elicit information on sexual history, previous gynecologic problems, and use of oral contraceptives. If the results of the pregnancy test are negative, the physical examination should assess estrogen status. If the estrogen level appears to be normal, a progesterone challenge test is indicated. Absence of withdrawal bleeding on administration of progesterone suggests that either levels of estrogen are inadequate or obstruction to outflow is present, and a combined estrogen-progesterone challenge test should be ordered.

Clinical Example

A 33-year-old woman who has a history of pelvic inflammatory disease and a recent abortion describes a 4-month history of amenorrhea. Her menstrual cycles had previously been regular. She does not exercise, has had no change in her body weight, and describes no obvious sources of stress in her life. Although sexually active without using contraceptives, the results of a pregnancy test are negative. Clinical examination suggests a normal estrogen level. No withdrawal bleeding occurs with progesterone challenge or with a combined estrogen-progesterone challenge test indicating outflow obstruction.

REFERENCES

1. **Carr BR.** Disorders of the ovary and female reproductive tract. In: Williams Textbook of Endocrinology. 8th ed. Philadelphia: WB Saunders; 1992: 733-98.

2. **Warren MP.** Evaluation of secondary amenorrhea [Clinical Review 77]. J Clin Endocrinol Metab. 1996;85:437-42.

3. **Pettersson F, Fries H, Nillius SJ.** Epidemiology of secondary amenorrhea. Am J Obstet Gynecol. 1973;117:80-6.

4. **Hull MGR, Knuth UA, Murray MAF, Jacobs HS.** The practical value of the progestogen challenge test, serum oestradiol estimation or clinical exami-

nation in assessment of the oestrogen state and response to clomiphene in amenorrhoea. Br J Obstet Gynaecol. 1979;86:799-805.

5. **Reindollar RH, Novak M, Tho SPT, McDonough PG.** Adult-onset amenorrhea: a study of 262 patients. Am J Obstet Gynecol. 1986;155:531-43.

6. **Munster K, Helm P, Schmidt L.** Secondary amenorrhea: prevalence and medical contact: a cross sectional study from a Danish county. Br J Obstet Gynaecol. 1992;99:430-3.

7. **Jaffe RB.** The menopause and perimenopausal period. In: Reproductive Endocrinology. 3rd ed. Philadelphia: WB Saunders; 1991:389-408.

8. **Archer DF, Thomas RL.** The fallacy of the postpill amenorrhea syndrome. Clin Obstet Gynecol. 1981;24:943-50.

9. **Yaginuma T.** Progress and therapy of stress amenorrhea. Fertil Steril. 1979; 32:36-9.

10. **Warren, MP.** Amenorrhea in endurance runners [Clinical Review 40]. J Clin Endocrinol Metab. 1992;75:1393-7.

11. **Glass AR, Duester PA, Kyle SB, et al.** Amenorrhea in Olympic marathon runners. Fertil Steril. 1987;48:740-5.

12. **Shangold MM.** Causes, evaluation, and management of athletic oligo-/amenorrhea. Med Clin North Am. 1985;69:83-95.

13. **Bachmann GA, Kemmann E.** Prevalence of oligomenorrhea and amenorrhea in a college population. Am J Obstet Gynecol. 1982;144:98-102.

14. **Aiman J, Smentek C.** Premature ovarian failure. Obstet Gynecol. 1985;66: 9-14.

15. **Koppelman MCS, Jaffe MJ, Rieth KG, et al.** Hyperprolactinemia, amenorrhea and galactorrhea. Ann Intern Med. 1984;100:115-21.

16. **Rippey JH.** Pregnancy tests: evaluation and current status. CRC Crit Rev Clin Lab Sci. 1984;19:353-9.

17 **Jacobs HS.** Prolactin and amenorrhea. N Engl J Med. 1976;295:954-6.

18. **Jacobs HS, Franks S, Murray MA, et al.** Clinical and endocrine features of hyperprolactinaemic amenorrhea. Clin Endocrinol. 1976;5:439-54.

19. **Wolpert SM.** The radiology of pituitary adenomas. Endocrinol Metab Clin North Am. 1987;16:553-84.

20. **Kent DL, Larson EB.** Magnetic resonance imaging of the brain and spine. Ann Intern Med. 1988;108:402-24.

Microscopic Hematuria

45

Julia E. Connelly, MD

KEY POINTS

Pretest Probabilities

- Asymptomatic microscopic hematuria is commonly found in general medical patients. Its prevalence is 5% to 13% of the general clinical population.

- Serious causes of microhematuria are reported in approximately 16.5% of referral patients but in only about 2.3% of general medical patients.

- Urologic neoplasms account for approximately 13% of the cases of microscopic hematuria among elderly patients referred to a urologist and for about 1.0% of the cases in general medical patients, but they rarely occur in patients younger than 50 years old.

Diagnostic Strategies

- In asymptomatic patients younger than 50 years old with no risk factors and in whom the results of basic laboratory studies are normal, the likelihood of lesions that present a risk to patients' health and that are treatable is so low that follow-up observation is the preferred approach.

- In patients older than 50 years old with unexplained hematuria or in patients with known risk factors, the prevalence of underlying lesions may be sufficiently high to warrant further evaluation with imaging studies such as intravenous pyelography, with cystoscopy, and in some instances, with cytologic examination of urine. The decision for or against such an approach must be made on an individual basis.

BACKGROUND

Erythrocytes are commonly found in the urine of asymptomatic patients. Deciding which patients to evaluate and determining a rational strategy for evaluation pose a problem. There are several reasons for this dilemma: 1) Erythrocytes occur in the urine of healthy persons; 2) the number of erythrocytes that defines an abnormality is controversial; 3) the degree of hematuria does not necessarily correlate with the severity of the underlying cause; and 4) a lesion identified during diagnostic testing may not be responsible for the bleeding. The purpose of this chapter is to present information that helps in deciding whether to evaluate asymptomatic patients with microscopic hematuria and to suggest diagnostic strategies.

The number of erythrocytes per high-power field that are considered abnormal is controversial. Different investigators defined an "abnormal" number of erythrocytes as being as few as two to as many as 30 erythrocytes per high-power field; these same investigators report that 4% to 7% of "normal" controls had microscopic hematuria (1–4). These data assume that urologic diseases are absent, yet the assumption may be invalid because comprehensive urologic testing was not completed in all patients. Mohr and colleagues (5) defined abnormal as one or more erythrocytes per high-power field and found that 13% of general medical patients had asymptomatic hematuria; however, only 2.3% of these patients were found to have a serious abnormality.

The number of erythrocytes per high power field also depends on the preparation technique. For office evaluation, 12 mL of urine should be centrifuged for 5 minutes, the supernatant then poured off by holding the tube down for approximately 4 seconds, leaving approximately 0.25 mL in the tube, the sediment resuspended, and one drop placed on the slide with a cover slip.

Chemical tests for erythrocytes that measure hemoglobin are more convenient than microscopic evaluation. Although older tests were insensitive (6), newer chemical strips can detect 10 erythrocytes per microliter, or approximately three to five erythrocytes per high-power field (7). Among patients with microscopic hematuria, test results are negative in about 16% of patients, are trace positive in approximately 39%, and are positive in about 45%. In patients who do not have microscopic hematuria, test results are negative in 85%, are trace positive in 14%, and are positive in 1%. The test also detects myoglobin. False-negative results increase in the presence of reducing agents, such as vitamin C (8).

For asymptomatic patients, and in taking a cautious approach, we suggest that the finding of three (3) or more RBCs per high-power field or a positive result with a newer chemical strip should be considered an abnormal finding.

ESTIMATING PRETEST PROBABILITY

Age is the most important factor to consider in deciding whether to pursue further evaluation of the patient with microscopic hematuria. The prevalence of serious urologic lesions is considerably greater in patients older than 50 years than in younger patients. In a urology referral setting, Greene (7) noted that significant lesions were found only in patients older than 50 years. (Significant lesions are abnormalities leading to morbidity or mortality or whose natural history can be influenced through early detection.) Carson and colleagues (9) reported that 16% of a group of referred patients had significant lesions—-most of whom were older than 50 years. Bladder tumors and ureteral stones accounted for most of the lesions. Golin and Howard (10) noted a mean age of 60 years among the 34 of 224 patients referred for unexplained microscopic hematuria who had significant lesions. In a population-based study, Mohr (5) reported that 2.3% had "serious" lesions: uroepithelial neoplasms occurred in patients aged 75 years and older and prostate cancers in men aged 55 years and older. One renal cell cancer was found in a 44-year-old man. Again, bladder cancers and calculi accounted for most of the serious lesions (Table 45-1).

The annual incidence of bladder cancer in patients younger than 50 years is estimated to be 1.4 per 100,000, and the incidence of renal cancer in these patients 7 per 100,000 (11). The risk of bladder cancer increases with exposure to aromatic amines, as noted in dye and chemical workers, for whom the relative risk is 2.2, and in cigarette smokers, for whom the relative risk is 2.0 (12). Tumors related to such exposure usually occur after long latency periods.

Exercise is a well-established cause of hematuria; as many as one in five marathon runners have hematuria. Such hematuria usually

Table 45-1. Distribution of Urologic Findings in Patients with Asymptomatic Microscopic Hematuria

Categories of Urologic Disease	% (range)
Serious	2.3 (0–5.3)
Uroepithelial neoplasia	0.1 (0–1.2)
Ureteral calculus	0.9 (0–2.2)
Prostate cancer	0.5 (0–4.1)
Renal neoplasia	0.4 (0–1.1)
Other	0.3 (0–1.8)
Moderately serious	18.2
Renal calculi	3.3
Urinary tract infection	0.5
Nephritis or renal insufficiency	14.4
Minor	70.5

Adapted from Mohr DN, Offord KP, Owen RA, Melton J. Asymptomatic microhematuria and urologic disease: a population-based study. J Am Med Assn. 1986;256:224.

resolves within 48 hours (13). Trauma and sports-related injury are also potential causes. Nonsteroidal medications (14) and the use of anticoagulants (15) increase the occurrence of microscopic hematuria. Glomerulonephritis is another cause of asymptomatic hematuria, as is asymptomatic urinary tract infection. The possibility of "contamination" of urine during menses must be considered when microhematuria is noted in women. Information from a complete urinalysis can also be helpful. This examination may reveal numerous leukocytes and bacteria, suggesting urinary infection. An "active" urinary sediment with casts in a patient with microhematuria suggests glomerular disease. Because asymptomatic microscopic hematuria may be intermittent, its evaluation should be based on the initial discovery.

The likelihood of finding significant urologic lesions in asymptomatic patients with microhematuria who are younger than 50 years old, have no known risk factors (e.g., chemical exposure), and for whom the results of physical examination and basic laboratory studies are normal is probably less than 1%.

DIAGNOSTIC TESTS

The operating characteristics of specific tests in the evaluation of asymptomatic microscopic hematuria have not been precisely determined. First, the data are primarily limited to patients referred to urologists for evaluation. Thus, the sensitivity of various procedures for the detection of significant lesions may be falsely high, because patients referred to specialists often have more severe disease than does the general population. Only one study is population-based, and it is a retrospective assessment (5). A second problem with these studies relates to workup bias—that is, because patients without microscopic hematuria do not undergo diagnostic procedures, it is not possible to determine to what extent microscopic hematuria and the finding of significant urologic lesions are actually related.

Intravenous Pyelography/Renal Imaging

It is the standard practice in the field of urology to perform intravenous pyelography (IVP) in patients referred for unexplained microscopic hematuria. This practice is based on the finding of silent stones (renal or ureteral) in 3% to 16% (average, 6%) of patients and the finding of renal tumors in approximately 1% (8–10). Also, advanced tumors of the urinary bladder that produce filling defects will be identified. Of patients referred for urinary tract signs or symptoms who were shown to have tumors of the urinary bladder, only one third to half were identified by IVP (16–18). Thus, if cystoscopy and IVP are both used in the evaluation of a patient with asymptomatic hematuria, the IVP must be justified on the basis of finding a significant upper tract lesion sufficiently often to warrant routine use in these patients. Thus far, no studies have been done using a decision-analysis approach to estimate the utility of performing this procedure in patients with unexplained microhematuria. Some have suggested the use of abdominal ultrasonography in the evaluation of asymptomatic microhematuria, but evidence is not sufficient to make this recommendation at the present time (19). Computed tomography may also be considered when there is concern about a renal lesion, because the sensitivity and specificity of this test are at least comparable to that of IVP in detecting a renal mass.

Cystoscopy

Cystoscopy, an invasive procedure that permits visualization of the urethra, urinary bladder, and the ureteral orifices, represents the gold standard for clinically detectable lesions of the lower urinary tract. The distribution of lesions identified among patients evaluated for microscopic hematuria is shown in Table 45-2. Between 95% and 100% of patients with significant lesions identified by cystoscopy (e.g., bladder cancer) were older than 50 years.

Cytologic Examination of Urine

Cytologic examination of the urine requires the collection of a spontaneously voided specimen, fixation in 50% alcohol, and preparation of the slide for cytologic examination by appropriate staining methods. Freshly voided morning urine specimens are generally recommended.

Of patients with established urologic malignancy of transitional cell origin, cytologic findings are positive or suspicious in as many as 80% (20,21).

Table 45-2. Nature and Frequency of Lower Urinary Tract Lesions Identified by Cystoscopy in Asymptomatic Patients with Microscopic Hematuria Referred for Urologic Evaluation

Lesion	Percent of Patients
Urethral lesions	13–25
Benign prostatic hyperplasia	8–24
Bladder cancer	2–11
Cystitis	2–4
Bladder calculus	1–2
Bladder papilloma	0–1
Prostate cancer	0–1
Miscellaneous bladder lesions	3–4

Data from Greene et al (7), Carson et al (9), and Golin and Howard (10).

Among patients in whom a urologic malignancy is suspected, the specificity of the examination does not exceed 90% (20,21). False-positive findings are observed, particularly among patients with urinary calculi and chronic infection and inflammation, and those who have received irradiation or chemotherapy. Transitional cell neoplasms of the upper urinary tract are much less likely to show positive cytologic patterns than those of the urinary bladder. These data cannot be directly applied in assessing the role of cytologic examination of urine in the patient with unexplained microscopic hematuria.

Abdominal Radiography

A plain radiograph of the abdomen or "KUB" (kidney, ureter, and bladder) may be useful in evaluating younger patients when the most common explanation for asymptomatic microscopic hematuria is a renal calculus. The sensitivity is approximately 85%; about 15% of renal calculi are not radio-opaque. However, its specificity may be limited by phleboliths, which cause false-positive results.

Other Diagnostic Procedures

Among patients with the finding of microscopic hematuria, other diagnostic procedures may be indicated depending on the physical examination, routine laboratory tests, other findings on urinalysis, and the results of urologic studies. Recent studies suggest that special microscopic evaluation of erythrocytes can distinguish glomerular from nonglomerular sources. In younger patients, this procedure may aid in the evaluation of possible glomerulonephritis (22). Other procedures include biopsy of the kidney or prostate or additional imaging studies of the kidneys or the retroperitoneal structures. The various indications for these procedures are beyond the scope of this chapter.

Combination Testing

Appleton and colleagues (23) reported 5-year follow-up on 84 patients with microscopic hematuria, average age of 59 years, who had previously had normal findings on complete urologic evaluation, including IVP, cystoscopy, and cytologic examination of urine. Thirteen patients died of nonurologic disorders, yet urologic neoplasms developed in no patients on re-evaluation after 5 years, suggesting that the full evaluation is sensitive for such neoplasms.

DIAGNOSTIC STRATEGIES

As noted previously in this chapter, several factors limit our ability to recommend strategies for evaluating microscopic hematuria. First, experts do not agree on what amount of hematuria is abnormal; second, lesions identified during the evaluation may not be responsible for the hematuria; third, the literature lacks good data on the sensitivity and specificity of the various diagnostic procedures; fourth, the benefits of early detection and treatment of lesions identified in asymptomatic patients are unknown; and last, because important lesions may occasionally be present in both the upper and lower urinary tract, no single test is sufficient when a workup is necessary.

With these limitations in mind, we suggest the following approach for the evaluation of microscopic hematuria:

1. Abnormal microscopic hematuria may be defined as three or more erythrocytes per high-power field or a positive chemical test result for hemoglobin.
2. In the absence of risk factors for urinary tract stones or cancer, the asymptomatic patient younger than 50 years old requires only a plain radiograph of the abdomen (KUB) and measurement of serum creatinine to assess renal function. If the results of the KUB are positive, IVP is needed, but if the results of the KUB are normal, clinical follow-up is advised.
3. If the patient has risk factors for cancer or is older than 50 years, evaluation using imaging techniques such as IVP, cystoscopy, and possibly urine cytologic examination are justified because cancer risk is reasonably high in such patients.

CLINICAL PROBLEMS

Clinical Problem 1
A young healthy patient has asymptomatic microscopic hematuria.

Testing Strategy and Rationale
A plain radiograph of the abdomen (KUB) should be obtained. If abnormalities are found on the radiograph, IVP should be performed. A complete urinalysis should also be done, and serum creatinine should be measured.

In young patients without risk factors, the prevalence of significant disease when asymptomatic microscopic hematuria is found is less than 1%. The most common explanation is renal calculus. The plain abdominal radiograph can exclude this possibility fairly well, given its sensitivity of approximately 85% and the already low pretest probability of disease. A positive result may best be followed by IVP to confirm the diagnosis. Because glomerulonephritis may occur in asymptomatic patients, performing a complete urinalysis and serum creatinine measurement is advised.

Clinical Example

A 30-year-old man is found to have asymptomatic microscopic hematuria. Urinalysis is otherwise normal. He is not a long-distance runner, has no history of nephrolithiasis, does not smoke cigarettes, and takes no medications. A plain radiograph of the abdomen is obtained, and serum creatinine is measured. If the results of both are negative, further testing would not be performed owing to the low prevalence of significant disease in patients in this age group.

Clinical Problem 2

A patient older than 50 years has unexplained microscopic hematuria.

Testing Strategy and Rationale

Intravenous pyelography should be done, the lower urinary tract should be evaluated with cystoscopy or cytologic examination of urine or both.

In patients older than 50 years, serious illnesses including malignancy are sufficiently common to justify a thorough evaluation. Intravenous pyelography can be used to evaluate the upper tract but must be supplemented by cystoscopy or cytologic examination of urine or both, given the possibility of bladder cancer.

Clinical Example

A 65-year-old man is found to have asymptomatic microscopic hematuria. He has had no exposure to chemicals or tobacco. The results of IVP are normal, reducing substantially the likelihood of a renal calculus or carcinoma. Cystoscopy is then scheduled to evaluate for bladder cancer.

REFERENCES

1. **Addis T.** The number of formed elements in the urinary sediment of normal individuals. J Clin Invest. 1926;2:409-15.
2. **Sanders C.** Clinical urine examination and the incidence of microscopic haematuria in apparently normal males. Practioner. 1963;192-7.
3. **Wright WT.** Cell counts in urine. Arch Intern Med. 1959;103:76-8.
4. **Fromm P, Gross M, Fromm J, et al.** Factors associated with microhematuria in asymptomatic young men. Clin Chem. 1986;32:2013-5.
5. **Mohr DN, Offord KP, Owen RA, Melton J.** Asymptomatic microhematuria and urologic disease: a population-based study. J Am Med Assn 1986;256:224-9.
6. **Freni SC, Heederik GJ, Hol C.** Centrifugation techniques and reagent strips in the assessment of microhematuria. J Clin Pathol. 1977;30:336-40.

7. **Greene LF, O'Shaughnessy EJ, Hendricks ED.** Study of five hundred patients with asymptomatic microscopic hematuria. J Am Med Assn. 1956;161:610-3.

8. **Arm JP, Peile EB, Rainford DJ, et al.** Significance of dipstick haematuria. 1. Correlation with microscopy of the urine. Br J Urol. 1986;58:211-7.

9. **Carson CC, Segura JW, Greene LF.** Clinical importance of microhematuria. J Am Med Assn. 1979;241:149-50.

10. **Golin AL, Howard RS.** Asymptomatic microscopic hematuria. J Urol. 1980;124:389-91.

11. **Resseguie LJ, Nobrega FT, Farrow GM, et al.** Epidemiology of renal and ureteral cancer in Rochester, Minnesota, 1950-1974 with special reference to clinical and pathologic features. Mayo Clin Proc. 1978;53:503-10.

12. **Cole AL, Hoover R, Friedell GH.** Occupation and cancer of the lower urinary tract. Cancer. 1972;29:1250-60.

13. **Reid AI, Hosking DH, Ramsey EW.** Haematuria following a marathon run: source and significance. Br J Urol. 1987;59:133-6.

14. **Kraus SE, Siroky MB, Babayan RK, Krane RJ.** Hematuria and the use of nonsteroidal anti-inflammatory drugs. J Urol. 1984;132:288-90.

15. **Schuster GA, Lewis GA.** Clinical significance of hematuria in patients on anticoagulant therapy. J Urol. 1987;137:923-5.

16. **Kreel L, Elton A, Habershon R, et al.** Use of intravenous urography. Br Med J 1974;4:31-33.

17. **Jonsson K, Owman T.** Roentgenographic aspects of haematuria. Scand J Urol Nephrol. 1976;10:229-34.

18. **Lang EK.** The roentgenographic assessment of bladder tumors: a comparison of the diagnostic accuracy of roentogenographic techniques. Cancer. 1969;23:717-24.

19. **Aslaksen A, Gadeholt G, Gothlin JH.** Ultrasonography versus intraenous urography in the evaluation of patients with microscopic haematuria. Br J Urol. 1990;66:144-7.

20. **Foot NC, Papanicolaou GN, Holmquist ND, et al.** Exfoliative cytology of urinary sediments: a review of 2,829 cases. Cancer. 1958;127-37.

21. **Colon VF, Schumann GB.** Fine-needle aspiration cytology. Am Fam Phys. 1980;21:89-93.

22. **Hyodo T, Miyagawa I, Iino A, et al.** Diagnostic revolution of microhematuria by real time confocal scanning laser microscope: HIM method, third report. Nephron. 1995;70:171-9.

23. **Appleton GVN, Lutchman GD, Charlton CAC.** A 5-year follow-up of undiagnosed hematuria. B J Urol. 1986;58:526-7.

Urinary Incontinence　　　　　**46**

Steven A. Rich, MD, and Fitzhugh C. Pannill III, MD

KEY POINTS

Pretest Probabilities

- In ambulatory, community-living older women with established incontinence, the prevalence of stress incontinence approaches 60%, and that of detrusor abnormalities is less than 25%.
- These figures are reversed in long-term care facilities, where women have a greater frequency of chronic illness, disability, and neurologic diagnoses associated with detrusor hyperreflexia and instability.
- In both community and institutional settings, overflow incontinence accounts for between 8% and 14% of incontinence in women.
- Symptoms traditionally associated with stress incontinence (i.e., leakage on coughing or exercise) or detrusor instability (i.e., urinary frequency, urgency, or nocturia) change the probability of either diagnosis very little. Upper motor neuron signs indicate a higher likelihood of detrusor instability or detrusor hyperreflexia.
- Symptoms of straining, decreased stream, or bladder fullness increase the probability of overflow incontinence. Finding a palpable bladder is highly specific for overflow incontinence.

Diagnostic Strategies

- Community-living women without upper motor neuron signs and with a positive full-bladder stress test are likely to have stress incontinence.
- In women with neurological findings and multiple chronic illnesses who live in long-term care facilities, a bedside cystometric study showing uninhibited contractions generally indicates detrusor instability or detrusor hyperreflexia.
- Bedside cystometric techniques change the disease probability sufficiently to direct behavioral and pharmacologic therapies for urinary incontinence. Evaluation for possible surgical therapy for stress incontinence may require the higher sensitivity of multichannel cystometrics to exclude the presence of detrusor instability.

Continued

- Difficult catheterization, a postvoid residual (PVR) of more than 100 mL, or a high (>500 mL) bladder capacity on bedside cystometrics indicates a probable diagnosis of overflow incontinence.

BACKGROUND

Urinary incontinence is a major geriatric problem with social, economic, and medical morbidity (1,2). It increases social isolation, precipitates institutionalization, and is a predisposing factor for urinary infections, decubitus ulcers, and other health problems (1). Incontinence-related health care costs have been estimated to exceed $10 billion annually (3).

The International Continence Society defines urinary incontinence as "involuntary urine loss that is a social or hygienic problem, and that is objectively demonstrable"(4). An effective diagnostic strategy must objectively demonstrate incontinence and classify the cause into therapeutically relevant types.

Urinary incontinence resulting from several bladder and bladder-outlet processes is referred to as *established incontinence* (1,5). Incontinence in elderly patients can also be caused by several reversible medical conditions referred to as *transient incontinence*. These processes include urinary tract infections, vaginitis, drugs, fecal impactions, and spinal cord compression (1,3). Elderly patients may also have incontinence in response to psychological factors such as depression (6). Environmental barriers to toileting, combined with functional impairments, frequently cause what is called *functional incontinence*. Transient and functional causes may coexist with established or urologic causes. Therefore, a complete evaluation of incontinence requires that all transient and functional causes are identified by a comprehensive history and physical examination before bladder or outlet causes are postulated (1,6).

One frequent cause of established incontinence is detrusor instability. The diagnosis implies that the patient has uncontrollable contractions of the detrusor or bladder muscle, usually at low bladder volumes. To cause incontinence, these contractions must be strong enough to overcome urethral resistance. These contractions result either from a decrease in the normal central nervous system inhibition of the detrusor muscle (seen in large cerebrovascular accidents, Alzheimer disease, normal pressure hydrocephalus, and other upper motor neuron diseases) or from increases in bladder sensory stimulation caused by local inflammatory conditions (prostatic hypertrophy, urinary tract infection, or vaginitis) (1,5). When uncontrolled detrusor contractions occur in the setting of established neurologic disease, such as a stroke, the accepted term is detrusor hyperreflexia (4). With increasing age, uninhibited detrusor contractions may be documented in as many as 10% of continent women and 30% of continent men (7,8).

A second cause of established incontinence is overflow incontinence. In this case, the detrusor contractions are inadequate to overcome urethral pressures, except at extremely high bladder volumes. Either abnormally weak detrusor contractions caused by lower motor neuron disease (the "acontractile bladder" of diabetes) or abnormally high urethral pressures (an obstruction caused by urethral stricture, prostatic hypertrophy, or carcinoma) may be responsible (1,5). A high postvoid residual (PVR) is common in these patients. There is no generally accepted maximum volume that is normal for a PVR. A volume of greater than 100 mL is frequently considered to be abnormal; however, PVR volumes of 100 mL may be found in 7% to 40% of continent men and in 12% to 40% of continent women (6,9).

Stress incontinence, or sphincter weakness, is the third cause of established incontinence. In this condition, lower than normal urethral pressures are inadequate to prevent urine leakage during periods of increased intra-abdominal pressure or small detrusor contractions. This can result from postsurgical damage to the sphincter muscle itself or, more commonly, from changes in the pelvic geometry, muscle tone, and urethral mucosal thickness in menopausal women (1,5,10).

Combinations of established incontinence are present in as many as 40% of women in some studies (11,12). Most common is detrusor instability and stress incontinence (1,3). Resnick (13) described a form of overflow incontinence with a hyperactive bladder, "detrusor hyperactivity with impaired contractility," in as many as 38% of institutionalized, debilitated women.

Patients with functional incontinence or transient causes of incontinence are not analyzed specifically in the following discussion. It should be noted that patients with normal objective tests of bladder function are frequent in all studies of geriatric patients with incontinence (11,12,14). These cases most likely represent transient or functional conditions not detected before testing. The remainder of the discussion focuses on diagnostic strategies to identify the three causes of established incontinence. Because few incontinent men have been described in the literature and most incontinent patients in the community are women (1), our analysis focuses on women.

ESTIMATING PRETEST PROBABILITY

Detrusor instability is present in 7% to 65% of women, stress incontinence in 25% to 60%, and overflow incontinence in 6% to 14% (11,12,15). Detrusor instability and hyperreflexia are more common in long-term care populations (16), whereas stress incontinence predominates among community-living women (14). In some studies of outpatients, as many as 78% of incontinent women have some evidence of stress-induced leakage (14). Several studies also document mixed detrusor instability and stress incontinence in l0% to 4l% of patients (11,12,14). At least l3% of women in several studies (11,12,14) have normal urologic evaluations; as noted above, these patients may have transient or functional incontinence.

Using information from several sources (11,12,14), we computed the sensitivity, specificity, and likelihood ratios of clinical symptoms and signs in determining diagnoses of established incontinence in elderly women (Table 46-1). Certain symptoms, such as urge incontinence with detrusor instability and loss with coughing for stress incontinence, are classically attributed to specific diagnoses of established incontinence (1,2). The available literature shows that most symptoms are fairly common in all incontinent patients, regardless of ultimate diagnosis (11,12,14,17). A meta-analysis of symptom-based diagnosis of urinary incontinence in more than 6000 patients showed an extremely wide range of reported sensitivities and specificities for stress incontinence, detrusor instability, and mixed incontinence (18). Urinary symptoms are also common in many older continent persons (19), making the picture even more confusing. The history is valuable in case finding and in assessing the degree of disability the patient is experiencing.

Table 46-1. Operating Characteristics of Clinical Signs and Symptoms in the Diagnosis of Urinary Incontinence in Elderly Women

Disease	Signs and symptoms	Sensitivity	Specificity*	Likelihood Ratio Positive Result	Likelihood Ratio Negative Result
		← % →			
Detrusor instability	Frequency	69	34	1.0	0.91
	Urge incontinence	77	36	1.2	0.64
	Nocturia	56	54	1.2	0.81
	Upper motor neuron signs	31	91	3.4	0.76
Stress incontinence	Loss of urine with coughing or exercise	57	58	1.4	0.74
Overflow incontinence	Straining	43	95	8.6	0.60
	Decreased stream	71	77	3.1	0.38
	Bladder fullness	36	79	1.7	0.81
	Any of the above three	89	58	2.1	0.19
	Palpable bladder	62	99	62	0.38

*Specificities were calculated using symptoms of incontinent patients without these diagnoses.

However, the presence or absence of most individual symptoms does little to change the probability of any specific diagnosis.

A notable exception is a woman who has straining or decreased stream on urination. In this situation the probability of overflow incontinence rises dramatically (12). The absence of any of the three major symptoms of overflow (i.e., straining, decreased stream, or bladder fullness) makes this diagnosis quite unlikely. In fact, when none of these symptoms is present in women, it may be possible to exclude the diagnosis of overflow incontinence.

Physical findings are generally nonspecific, with the exception of upper motor neuron signs that increase the likelihood of detrusor instability or hyperreflexia. A palpable bladder virtually confirms overflow incontinence, although its absence does not exclude the diagnosis (12).

DIAGNOSTIC TESTS

Cystometrics

Multichannel cystometrics, often called urodynamic testing, is the "gold standard" of incontinence testing. However, standard multichannel testing is costly, relatively invasive, and carries some risk of infection. It generally requires referral to a specialist with access to appropriate technology. Older patients, in particular, have more difficulties with these tests.

The multichannel cystometrogram is essentially a record of the intravesicular pressure at increasing bladder volumes. A catheter is inserted into the bladder, and sterile water or carbon dioxide (CO_2) is instilled at a constant rate. Additional catheters, or transducers, monitor changes in intra-abdominal pressure. Intra-abdominal pressure increases are subtracted electronically from simultaneous intravesicular pressure changes to provide a measurement of pressure generated by the detrusor muscle alone. If the normal slow-rising curve of recorded pressure with increasing volume is interrupted by sharp, large (>15 cm of H_2O) pressure waves that the patient cannot inhibit, detrusor instability or hyperreflexia is present (1,2). These waves represent uninhibited bladder contractions. Some patients have detrusor instability only with provocative maneuvers, giving cystometrics a sensitivity of about 98%. The presence of uninhibited bladder contractions have been documented in 15% to 30% of continent elderly (7,8), and we estimate the test's specificity to be about 85%.

An abnormally high bladder capacity (>500 mL) with low bladder pressures suggests overflow incontinence, as do high PVR volumes (>100 mL). Differentiation between an atonic bladder and obstruction depends on the detrusor pressure, sphincter pressures, and cystoscopic and/or radiological evaluation of bladder outlet and urethra. The sensitivity and specificity of the cystometrogram for overflow incontinence has not been firmly established, but it appears unlikely that all patients with overflow will be detected. Men, in particular, can have obstruction that may be missed on cystometrics if bladder pressures and volumes are normal. Additionally, 6% to 12% of continent men and women have PVRs more than 100 mL (7,8). Consequently, we estimate that the cystometrogram is about 90% sensitive and 95% specific for overflow incontinence.

Office Procedures

Work by Ouslander (20) has established that a combination of bedside cystometrics and full-bladder stress test can be an effective substitute for cystometrics in an office setting. This simplified, single-catheter examination allows both detrusor instability and stress incontinence to be identified easily (21).

In bedside cystometrics with full-bladder stress testing, the patient voids fully, the bladder is catheterized with sterile technique, and any residual urine is drained. A PVR volume and urine for urinalysis with or without culture can be obtained. Using a catheter-tipped syringe as a funnel, the bladder is filled by gravity with sterile saline in 50-mL aliquots until the patient feels bladder fullness, a contraction or leakage occurs, or a total volume of 600 mL is reached. A normally compliant bladder can easily be filled with the syringe held less than 15 cm above the bladder. If a contraction occurs, the fluid level in the syringe rises. More than a 15-cm increase above baseline indicates detrusor instability in the absence of abdominal muscle contractions or a patient-induced Valsalva maneuver. The bladder capacity at fullness, any contractions, and the ease of urethral catheterization are recorded, and the catheter is removed. With the bladder still full, the patient coughs vigorously. If no leakage occurs in the lithotomy position, the cough is repeated with the patient in the standing position while tissue paper is held over the urethral meatus to catch any leakage. Small amounts of leakage occurring during coughing are diagnostic of stress incontinence. The patient then voids, and by subtracting the voided volume from the bladder capacity, the PVR can be calculated and compared with the initial value obtained. A PVR of more than 100 mL strongly suggests overflow incontinence, as does a bladder capacity of more than 500 mL. Difficulty with catheterization implies possible obstruction.

The bedside technique does not monitor the intra-abdominal pressure. The results must be interpreted with caution in a noncooperative patient when voluntary contractions of the abdominal muscles may be interpreted as uninhibited detrusor contractions (21). Rarely, detrusor contractions initiated by coughing can be mistaken for sphincter weakness. This can be avoided if only leakage occurring immediately with coughing is considered a positive test for stress incontinence.

Some patients with detrusor instability have false-negative test results. In one study the sensitivity was increased, with comparable specificity, by performing maneuvers (coughing and listening to running water) to provoke detrusor contractions during bedside cystometrics (22). Repeating the test on different days and using any uninhibited detrusor contractions on either test as a positive result increased the sensitivity to 92.3%, at the cost of reducing the specificity to 54.2% (23).

Table 46-2 summarizes the operating characteristics and likelihood ratios of both the bedside cystometrics and the full-bladder stress test, done as a single test with no provocative maneuvers (14,17,20). The stress test has a sensitivity of 85% and a specificity of 85% when compared with urologic measurements in detecting stress incontinence (14,17). Compared with standard multichannel cystometrics, the bedside cystometrics examination has a sensitivity of 72% and a specificity of 79% for detrusor instability (20). The efficacy of the PVR or other characteristics of the bedside exam in the diagnosis of overflow incontinence has not been studied as extensively. There is no established normal maximum PVR urine volume (9). Because some patients with obstructions can maintain normal bladder emptying, the sensitivity of the PVR for obstruction or overflow incontinence may be as low as 66% (11). Because some continent women have residual urine volumes over 100 mL, we estimate the specificity at about 88%.

Table 46-2. Operating Characteristics of Diagnostic Tests for Established Incontinence in Elderly Women

	Sensitivity	Specificity	Likelihood Ratio	
			Positive Result	**Negative Ratio**
	←————— % —————→			
Stress incontinence				
Full-bladder stress test	85	85	5.7	0.18
Detrusor instability				
Formal cystometrics	98	85	6.5	0.09
Bedside cystometrics	72	79	3.4	0.35
Overflow incontinence				
Cystometrography	90	95	18	0.11
Postvoid residual volume >100 mL	66	88	5.5	0.39

Other Tests

A variety of other examinations have been suggested for urinary incontinence, including urethral pressure profiles, simultaneous bladder-urethral pressure measurements, and urethral electromyography. Each of these has its place in selected patients, specifically in planning therapy. Uroflowmetry, cystometry, supine static urethral pressure profilometry, and lateral stress cystography demonstrated poor ability to discriminate between continent and incontinent women; therefore, these are not recommended as initial assessment tests (24).

Ambulatory urodynamic monitoring is currently a research tool in academic urodynamic centers. Advances in technology may make this a more common technique in the near future. As a result of longer monitoring time, the number of uninhibited detrusor contractions detected is expected to increase with an increased sensitivity for detrusor instability. A concern is a potential decrease in specificity due to the presence of uninhibited contractions in many continent patients (25). Substantial data in healthy persons will be needed to assess the role of this technique.

Although there may be a role for routine cystoscopy in men, because of the pretest probability of prostatic hypertrophy, most incontinent women who do not have symptoms and signs of obstruction do not need this testing. Women with some types of neurologic disease, such as multiple sclerosis, commonly have sphincter-detrusor dysynergy and require nonroutine evaluations (1).

DIAGNOSTIC STRATEGIES

Women with incontinence need a comprehensive history and focused physical examination. The presence of incontinence and the degree of severity should be assessed, and the transient and functional causes of incontinence should be identified. A suggested format for this evaluation is presented in the clinical practice guideline developed through the Agency for Health Care Policy and Research (AHCPR) (26).

In patients with no risk factors for transient or functional incontinence or in those with persistence of symptoms after correction of these factors, a cause needs to be determined to direct therapy. The operating characteristics of historical information make this information unsuitable as the sole basis of therapy. The addition of bedside cystometrics allows more accurate diagnosis and appropriate treatment with behavioral and pharmacologic therapy for stress incontinence and detrusor instability.

Consideration should be given to referring patients with potentially serious conditions before evaluation with bedside cystometric and full-bladder stress testing. Such patients would be those with symptoms of overflow or obstruction, a history of recent pelvic surgery or irradiation, frequent urinary tract infections or hematuria, marked pelvic prolapse, or possible cancer. If several signs of overflow are present on bedside testing (difficulty with catheterization, PVR over 100 mL, and bladder capacity >500 mL) referral for more indepth evaluation is appropriate.

The remaining patients can be evaluated on the basis of office testing alone. The conclusions from bedside cystometrics and full-bladder stress testing depend on the pretest probability of each disorder as estimated from population characteristics.

Table 46-3 shows the post-test probability of these tests in different populations with varying prevalences of established incontinence. The full-bladder stress test is very helpful in ambulatory, well, elderly women (prevalence stress incontinence of 60%) in whom the post-test probability of stress incontinence after a positive test is about 90%. In populations with lower prevalence, stress incontinence may not be as effectively diagnosed by this test alone, as the post-test probability after a positive test is not as high. However, a negative stress test effectively excludes stress incontinence in these lower prevalence populations, with a post-test probability below 10%.

The corollary holds true for bedside cystometrics with detrusor instability. In populations of healthy elderly women, a normal test

Table 46-3. Post-test Probability for Diagnostic Tests in the Evaluation of Established Incontinence

Diagnostic Test	Pretest Probability	Post-test Probability	
		Positive Result	Negative Result
	←————————— % —————————→		
Full-bladder stress test in diagnosis of stress incontinence			
In institutionalized patients	20	59	4
In frail patients	40	79	11
In healthy patients	60	90	21
Bedside cystometrics in diagnosis of detrusor instability			
In healthy patients	20	46	8
In frail patients	40	69	19
In institutionalized patients	60	84	34
Postvoid residual >100 mL in diagnosis of overflow incontinence			
In patients with no symptoms	5	23	2
In unselected patients	12	42	5
In patients with symptoms	23	65	10

excludes the diagnosis of detrusor instability fairly effectively (post-test probability <10%), although a positive test is less helpful. In high prevalence populations (i.e., institutionalized patients), a positive test confirms the diagnosis (post-test probability 84%), but a negative test does not exclude it.

Ouslander evaluated the use of bedside cystometrics and stress test in a study of 261 community and institutionalized elderly incontinent patients (27) and demonstrated that the bedside evaluation could eliminate the need for urological evaluation in up to half of these incontinent patients. Once a diagnosis is established, the response to behavioral or pharmacologic therapy may be monitored through patient symptoms, or through the use of voiding diaries. These are available for both ambulatory and institutional use (26).

Patients with pure stress incontinence by bedside testing may ultimately need to be considered for continence surgery. The AHCPR Guideline suggests reserving surgical options for patients who fail pharmacologic and behavioral treatment. In such situations, the higher sensitivity of multichannel cystometrics for detecting detrusor instability may be justified. Failure to detect detrusor instability preoperatively has been associated with 71% of failed surgeries for stress incontinence (29).

Table 46-3 also examines the difficult issue of overflow incontinence. Women, especially ambulatory patients, with no symptoms of overflow, as mentioned earlier, have a prior probability of overflow incontinence of less than 5%. Twelve percent illustrates the estimated prevalence in unselected patients. Women with symptoms of overflow have a prior probability as high as 23%. As Table 46-3 indicates, an abnormal PVR does not increase the post-test probability sufficiently to confirm the diagnosis of overflow, even in the high prevalence group. However, if the PVR is normal, the post-test probability is low enough to exclude the diagnosis, except in the high prevalence group. Therefore, patients with several obstructive symptoms or a PVR over 100 mL probably require further urologic evaluation. Asymptomatic patients with a normal PVR have a very small chance of overflow incontinence.

CLINICAL PROBLEMS

Clinical Problem 1
A frail, elderly woman has frequent urinary incontinence.

Testing Strategy and Rationale
Perform bedside cystometric evaluation. In patients in whom the probability of detrusor instability is high, bedside cystometrics are

indicated. A positive test results in a high post-test probability that detrusor instability is present.

Clinical Example

An 85-year-old woman, who lives in a nursing home, is brought to the physician's office by her granddaughter for evaluation of urinary incontinence along with urinary frequency and urgency. She has a history of cerebrovascular disease and moderately severe osteoarthritis. On examination evidence is found of previous strokes and osteoarthritis that limits her ambulation to slow walking. There are no other gynecological or rectal abnormalities. Her urinalysis is normal.

Bedside cystometrics show a bladder capacity of 150 mL, with the test terminated by a large contraction. PVR is 35 mL; stress test is normal. A diagnosis of probable detrusor hyperreflexia is made (because of associated neurologic abnormalities), and it is recognized that her arthritis may be causing some functional incontinence as well. Treatment with an anticholinergic antispasmotic agent is begun, and the nursing home staff is asked to provide a bedside commode.

Clinical Problem 2

An elderly, otherwise healthy woman has urinary incontinence during physical activity.

Testing Strategy and Rationale

After completing the history and physical examination, a bedside cystometric testing with a full-bladder stress test should be obtained. The pretest probability of stress incontinence in this community-living healthy woman is well over 60%. A positive full-bladder stress test should confirm the diagnosis with adequate accuracy. If the bedside cystometric component of the test does not show detrusor instability, the patient can be treated for stress incontinence. If surgical intervention for stress incontinence is planned, many would suggest obtaining the more sensitive multi-channel cystometrics to further reduce the probability of detrusor instability.

Clinical Example

A 65-year-old otherwise healthy woman presents with incontinence and urinary frequency. Her only medication is hormone replacement therapy. Most of her incontinence occurs during physical activity. Examination and urinalysis suggest no urological, rectal, or gynecological abnormalities. Bedside cystometrics are ordered and demonstrate a bladder capacity of 400 mL, with easy

Continued

filling. The full-bladder stress testing is positive. The patient voids 390 ml, and the calculated PVR is 10 mL. A diagnosis of stress incontinence is made, and Kegel exercises and alpha agonists are prescribed.

During 6 months of follow-up and documented compliance, she notes improvement, but not resolution, of the incontinence. She has stopped doing exercises because of the problem. She has palpitations with any increased doses of alpha agonist. She is referred for multichannel cystometrics, which confirms pure stress incontinence with no detrusor instability, and a retropubic urethropexy is scheduled.

REFERENCES

1. **Williams ME, Pannill FC.** Urinary incontinence in the elderly. Ann Intern Med. 1982;97:895-907.

2. **Ouslander J, ed.** Urinary incontinence. Clin Geriatr Med. 1986;2:639-886.

3. **Hu, TW.** Impact of urinary incontinence on health-care costs. J Am Geriatr Soc. 1990;38(3):292-5.

4. **Abrams P, Blaivas JG, Stanton SL, Anderson JT.** Standardization of terminology of lower urinary tract function. Neurourol Urodyn 1988;7:403-27

5. **Resnick NM, Yalla SV.** Management of urinary incontinence in the elderly. N Engl J Med. 1985;313:800-5.

6. **Ory MG, Wyman JE, Yu L.** Psychosocial factors in urinary incontinence. Clin Geriatr Med. 1986;2:657-72.

7. **Brochlehurst JC, Dillane JB.** Studies of the female bladder in old age. I. Cystometrogram in non-incontinent women. Gerontol Clin. 1986;8:285-305.

8. **Staskin DR.** Age-related physiologic and pathologic changes affecting lower urinary tract function. Clin Geriatr Med. 1986;2:701-10.

9. **Urinary Incontinence Guideline Panel.** Urinary incontinence in adults: clinical practice guideline. AHCPR publication no. 92-0038. Rockville, Maryland: Agency for Health Care Policy and Research, Public Health Service, United States Department of Health and Human Service; 1992:16

10. **Green TH.** Urinary stress incontinence: differential diagnosis, pathophysiology and management. Am J Obstet Gynecol. 1975;122:368-400.

11. **Pannill FC, Williams TF, Davis R.** Evaluation and treatment of urinary incontinence in long term care. J Am Geriatr Soc. 1988;36:902-10.

12. **Hilton P, Stanton SL.** Algorithmic method for assessing urinary incontinence in elderly women. Br Med J. 1981;282:940-3.

13. **Resnick NM, Yalla SV.** Detrusor hyperactivity with impaired contractile function. JAMA. 1987;257:3076-81.

14. **Diokno AC, Wells TJ, Brink CA.** Urinary incontinence in elderly women: urodynamic evaluation. J Am Geriatr Soc. 1987;35:943-6.

15. **Castleden CM, Duffin HM, Asher MS.** Clinical and urodynamic studies in 100 elderly incontinent patients. Br Med J. 1981;282:1103-5.

16. **Resnick NM, Yalla SV, Laurino E.** The pathophysiology of urinary incontinence among institutionalized elderly persons. N Engl J Med. 1989; 320:1-7.

17. **Wells TJ, Brink CA, Diokno AC.** Urinary incontinence in elderly women: clinical findings. J Am Geriatr Soc. 1987;35:933-9.

18. **Jensen JK, Neilsen FR, Ostergard DR.** The role of patient history in the diagnosis of urinary incontinence. Obstet Gynecol. 1994;83:904-10

19. **Brochlehurst J, Fry J, Griffiths L, Kalton G.** Dysuria in old age. J Am Geriatr Soc. 1971;19:582-92.

20. **Ouslander J, Leach G, Abelson S, et al.** Single versus multichannel cystometry in the evaluation of bladder function in an incontinent geriatric population. J Urol. 1988;140:1482-6.

21. **Ouslander J, Leach G, Staskin DR.** Simplified tests of lower urinary tract function in the evaluation of geriatric urinary incontinence. J Am Geriatr Soc. 1989;37:706-14.

22. **Fonda D, Brimage PJ, D'Astole M.** Simple screenig for urinary incontinence in the elderly: comparison of simple and multichannel cystometry. Urology. 1993;42:536-40

23. **Sand PK, Brubaker LT, Novak T.** Simple standing incremental cystometry as a screening method for detrusor instability. Obstet Gynecol. 1991;77: 453-7

24. **Diokno AC, Normolle DP, Brown MB, Herzog AR.** Urodynamic tests for female geriatric urinary incontinence. Urology. 1990;36;431-9

25. **van Waalwijk van Doorn ES, Meier AH, Ambergen AW, Janknegt RA.** Ambulatory urodynamics: extramural testing of the lower and upper urinary tract by Holter monitoring of cystometrogram, uroflowmetry and renal pelvic pressures. Urol Clin North Am. 1996;23:345-71

26. **Urinary Incontinence Guideline Panel.** Urinary incontinence in adults: Clinical practice guideline. AHCPR publication no. 92-0038. Rockville, Maryland: Agency for Health Care Policy and Research, Public Health Service, United States Department of Health and Human Service; 1992: 14-5

27. **Ouslander J, Leach G, Staskin D, et al.** Prospective evaluation of an assessment strategy for geriatric incontinence. J Am Geriatr Soc. 1989;37:715-24.

28. **Urinary Incontinence Guideline Panel.** Urinary incontinence in adults: clinical practice guideline. AHCPR publication no. 92-0038. Rockville, Maryland: Agency for Health Care Policy and Research, Public Health Service, United States Department of Health and Human Service; 1992: 18-9

29. **Sand PK, Bowen LW, Ostergard DR, Brubaker L. Panganiban R.** The effect of retropubic urethropexy on detrusor stability. Obstet Gynecol. 1988; 71:818-22

Nonpalpable Prostate Cancer   **47**

Michael J. Barry, MD

KEY POINTS

Pretest Probabilities

- Microscopic prostate cancer is found at autopsy in almost half of men in their seventies.

- The prevalence of prostate cancer greater than 0.5 mL in volume, which is more likely to cause morbidity and mortality, ranges from approximately 5% for men 40 to 49 years old to 15% for men older than 70 years of age.

Screening Strategies

- Prostate-specific antigen (PSA) tests can find many cancers earlier than digital rectal examination. However, PSA measurements have suboptimal sensitivity and specificity, and clinical trials have not yet proved whether PSA screening does more good than harm. Thus, in clinical practice, a shared decision-making approach to PSA testing with individual patients is reasonable.

- Transrectal ultrasonography is insufficiently sensitive and specific to be used as a primary screening test.

- Although digital rectal examination is relatively insensitive in detecting prostate cancer, this technique does detect tumors missed by PSA testing.

BACKGROUND

Prostate cancer is an important health problem among older men. In the United States, 184,500 new cases and 39,200 deaths from this malignancy were expected in 1998 (1). After a striking increase in the incidence of prostate cancer between 1989 and 1993, probably largely as a result of aggressive early detection efforts, incidence of this disease has been falling (2).

Early detection of prostate cancer, particularly with the tumor marker prostate-specific antigen (PSA), results in a "stage shift" toward a

greater proportion of nonmetastatic prostate cancers, many still localized to the prostate gland. Theoretically, these localized tumors should
be curable with aggressive treatment such as radical prostatectomy or
radiation therapy. However, a stage shift alone is insufficient evidence
to conclude that early detection of any cancer reduces mortality (3), and
some features about the epidemiology and natural history of prostate
cancer raise particular concerns about whether its early detection
results in better outcomes.

First, prostate cancers that are never destined to cause morbidity
and mortality are extraordinarily common. The high ratio of incidence
to mortality hints at the degree of overdiagnosis that exists in the "PSA
era," and detection of many cancers not destined to cause harm will
dilute the benefit of early detection. To some extent, the slow growth
of most localized prostate cancer, with average doubling times of 3 to
4 years (4), is responsible for this reservoir of harmless cancer. Ideally,
only cancer destined to cause harm would be detected and treated, but
current screening and staging technologies do not allow for such specificity. Moreover, the impact of aggressive treatment on the natural history of prostate cancer is uncertain, because no clinical trials with adequate statistical power have explored this issue. Nonexperimental
data suggest somewhat better outcomes with aggressive treatment,
but the differences are small enough to be potentially explained by
case selection (5).

In addition to estimating pretest and post-test probability with
prostate cancer screening, one must also consider to what extent early
detection of prostate cancer does more good than harm. Potential harm
may come from anxiety raised by suspicious test results and, in some
cases, from the detection of cancer itself; the small but finite risks of
prostatic biopsies performed as follow-up to suspicious screening test
results; and the morbidity and mortality of aggressive treatment. Given
the uncertain benefits of screening, many experts advise against routine early detection efforts and instead recommend a shared decision-
making approach with individual patients (6).

ESTIMATING PRETEST PROBABILITY

Estimating the pretest probability of prostate cancer depends on what
one considers the target of such screening. Autopsy studies reveal a
high, age-dependent prevalence of prostate cancer; but many of these
latent cancers are small, well differentiated, and unlikely to cause
future morbidity and mortality. However, even larger volume cancer is
common at autopsy. Although the ideal target of screening would only
be cancer destined to cause future morbidity and mortality, accurately
differentiating such tumors from less aggressive tumors is not possible
with current technology. Moreover, some cancer found by screening

may have already spread beyond the prostate capsule and may not be amenable to cure with current treatment technologies. Although these cancers may be easy to find and have considerable potential to do future harm, it is not clear that their early detection improves outcomes. Table 47-1 provides the pretest probabilities of prostate cancer of different extents according to age, based on a synthesis of data from autopsy studies (7).

Because digital rectal examinations (DREs) have relatively low sensitivity, these pretest probabilities serve as reasonable estimates even among men with normal DREs. However, suspicious results of a DRE modestly increase the odds of intracapsular tumors and considerably increase the odds of extracapsular tumors; DRE also helps detect tumors that are missed by PSA measurements (7).

SCREENING TESTS

The screening tests that can be considered for the early detection of prostate cancer among men who have already had a normal DRE are measurement of serum PSA and transrectal ultrasonography (TRUS).

Prostate-Specific Antigen

Prostate-specific antigen is a glycoprotein that can be measured in serum and can be elevated not only in the setting of prostate cancer but in benign diseases of the prostate as well, such as benign prostatic hyperplasia (BPH) and prostatitis. Prostate-specific antigen can also be elevated for weeks after an episode of acute urinary retention, prostatic biopsy, or prostatectomy. Ejaculation can increase the level of PSA in

Table 47-1.   Estimated Age-Specific Prevalence of Prostate Cancer in Eight Autopsy Studies

Patient Age	Prevalence of Prostate Cancer for Tumor Volume		
	<0.5 mL	>0.5 mL Intracapsular	>0.5 mL Extracapsular
y	←――――――― % ―――――――→		
40–49	7.2	3.5	1.3
50–59	9.0	4.4	1.6
60–69	13.2	6.4	2.4
70–79	23.4	11.4	4.2
80+	25.8	12.6	4.6

Republished with permission from Coley CM, Barry MJ, Fleming C, Mulley AG. Early detection of prostate cancer. Part I. Prior probability and effectiveness of tests. Ann Intern Med. 1997; 126:394-406.

some men for a day or two (8,9). Digital rectal examination, however, does not cause a clinically important elevation in PSA levels (10).

The sensitivity and specificity of PSA measurement are poorly defined. Few studies perform a "gold standard" test such as prostate biopsy to evaluate the diagnostic performance of PSA; usually only men with an elevated PSA level (or suspicious DRE results) have biopsy. If the small latent cancer that is so common at autopsy is included in sensitivity calculations, the sensitivity of PSA will obviously be very low. The most helpful estimates of PSA sensitivity may be those that reflect the ability of the test to detect cancers destined to present clinically at some future time. To this end, Gann and colleagues (11) measured "baseline" PSA in banked frozen plasma from men recruited into a large cohort study. They found that the PSA level was elevated at more than 4.0 ng/mL in 73% of men who presented with a clinical prostate cancer diagnosis within the next 4 years of follow-up, and in 46% within the next 10 years of follow-up (11). In the same study, the PSA level was 4.0 ng/mL or less in 91% of men who did not present with prostate cancer over the next 10 years; however, in interpreting this specificity estimate, one must bear in mind that the mean age of participants in this study was relatively young (63 years). The specificity of PSA measurement is in fact age dependent, because older men with a higher prevalence of BPH will have higher false positive rates. When older men who have lower urinary tract symptoms consistent with BPH are tested with PSA measurement, the specificity of the test decreases to 50% to 80% (12,13). These lower urinary tract symptoms do not appear to increase the pretest probability of prostate cancer (14). Table 47-2 provides estimates of the likelihood ratios associated with an elevated or normal PSA level for both intracapsular and extracapsular prostate cancer (7).

Both the pretest probability of prostate cancer and the false-positive rate of PSA increase with age, effects which tend to cancel each

Table 47-2. Estimated Likelihood Ratios for Results of Prostate-Specific Antigen Testing

PSA Level	Likelihood Ratio	
	Intracapsular Tumor	Extracapsular Tumor
≤ 4.0 ng/mL	0.8–1.0	0.1–0.5
4.1–10.0 ng/mL	1.4–2.8	3.2–5.1
>10 ng/mL	0.4–3.0	24–50

PSA = prostate-specific antigen.
Adapted from Coley CM, Barry MJ, Fleming C, Mulley AG. Early detection of prostate cancer. Part I. Prior probability and effectiveness of tests. Ann Intern Med. 1997;126:394-406.

other out in terms of the post-test probability of prostate cancer. The probability of prostate cancer for a PSA level greater than 4.0 ng/mL is estimated at 32% for those aged 50 to 59 years, 29% for those aged 60 to 69 years, and 34% for those aged 70 to 79 years, with an overall average of 31%. These values were derived from a large screening study using volunteer participants and may be overestimates because men with a higher pretest probability of cancer or suspicious DRE result joined the study (15). Among men in this study with an elevated PSA level and a normal DRE, the predictive value for cancer dropped to 21% (14).

The imperfect sensitivity and relatively high false-positive rate for PSA has prompted efforts to develop more sensitive and specific screening strategies. To increase sensitivity, some authorities recommend considering total PSA levels greater than 2.5 ng/mL to be suspicious (16), but this lower threshold decreases test specificity considerably. To increase specificity, experts sometimes recommend correcting total PSA for the volume of the prostate measured by ultrasonography ("PSA density") (17) or focusing on changes in PSA over time rather than on total PSA ("PSA velocity") (18). Oesterling and colleagues (19) have suggested using "age specific reference ranges" to interpret total PSA (Table 47-3). This approach trades specificity for sensitivity among younger men, who have longer life expectancies and presumably more to gain from early detection of a prostate cancer; and sensitivity for specificity among older men, who have shorter life expectancies and presumably less to gain from early detection of a prostate cancer. Most recently, measurements of both free and total PSA (most PSA circulates complexed to macromolecules) have been proposed as a way of enhancing specificity for men with equivocal total PSA levels (2.6–10.0 ng/mL) (16,20,21). Men with prostate cancer tend to have lower ratios of free to total PSA than men with BPH; as a result, some men with equivocal total PSA

Table 47-3. Age-Specific Reference Ranges for Total Serum Prostate-Specific Antigen

Age (y)	Reference Range
40–49	0.0–2.5 ng/mL
50–59	0.0–3.5 ng/mL
60–69	0.0–4.5 ng/mL
70–79	0.0–6.5 ng/mL

Adapted with permission from Oesterling JE, Jacobsen SJ, Chute CG, et al. Serum prostate-specific antigen in a community-based population of healthy men: establishment of age-specific reference ranges. JAMA. 1993;270:860-4.

levels may be spared a biopsy unless their ratio of free to total PSA is low (often <25%). However, this approach appears to improve specificity only slightly, at the cost of some sensitivity. In the absence of good outcome data, no one approach to using PSA can yet be considered optimal.

Transrectal Ultrasonography

Some clinicians have used TRUS as a primary screening test for prostate cancer. However, more recent appreciation of its poor sensitivity and specificity has generally led to its abandonment as a primary screening test (7). Its role now is to follow up on suspicious DRE or PSA results. Even in this situation, the poor sensitivity of TRUS makes most urologists perform prostate biopsies even if the study appears normal.

SCREENING STRATEGIES

Because of the lack of data on whether prostate cancer screening does more good than harm, experts disagree on whether it should be done routinely. The American Cancer Society recommends offering PSA screening (22), whereas the US Preventive Services Task Force recommends against it (23). Primary care physicians also split on the issue (24). Even advocates of PSA screening recommend against it in men with less than a 10-year life expectancy (e.g., older than 74 years old for men with average comorbidity) who are unlikely to benefit. Owing to this uncertainty, the American College of Physicians–American Society of Internal Medicine recommends that clinicians have a discussion with men in their fifties and sixties about prostate cancer and the availability of PSA for early detection and, on the basis of these conversations, make individual decisions about PSA testing. These discussions may be particularly important for men with lower urinary tract symptoms who may be worried about developing prostate cancer and men with risk factors for prostate cancer. Patients should be informed about the known risks of screening and aggressive treatment, as well as about the uncertain benefits. Although the early detection of prostate cancer has not been shown to reduce mortality in clinical trials, neither has it been shown that early detection does not reduce mortality.

If after deciding to screen for prostate cancer, it is found that the PSA test results are abnormal, a TRUS is often done next, and any suspicious areas that are detected on the ultrasonogram are biopsied. In addition, even if the ultrasonogram is normal, a set of six or more systematic biopsies are usually obtained from normal-appearing areas of the prostate. Some experts advocate a repeat set of biopsies even if the first set is normal (25).

CLINICAL PROBLEMS

Clinical Problem 1

An elderly man who also has significant comorbid disease notices worsening lower urinary tract symptoms and thus inquires about screening tests for prostate cancer.

Testing Strategy and Rationale

The primary care physician lets the patient know that an underlying prostate cancer is possible but that the symptoms are most likely caused by BPH and that the risk of cancer is not increased by these symptoms. Also, for an elderly patient with significant comorbid disease(s), it is unlikely that early detection of prostate cancer would reduce his risk of dying of prostate cancer and might in fact cause considerable morbidity.

Clinical Example

A 75-year-old man with stable angina presents to his primary care physician with slowly increasing lower urinary tract symptoms. He asks about PSA testing. Digital rectal examination reveals only a symmetrically enlarged prostate. His symptoms are not particularly bothersome. After a discussion of potential risks and benefits, they decide together to pursue a strategy of "watchful waiting."

Clinical Problem 2

A patient in his fifties requests PSA testing for early detection of prostate cancer.

Testing Strategy and Rationale

Owing to the uncertainties about the relative risks and benefits of screening, individual decisions about PSA testing must be made. Patients should be made aware of the risks of screening and associated treatments as well as of the potential benefits.

If a PSA measurement is done and the result is considered equivocal, some clinicians would recommend a biopsy, others would obtain serial tests to assure stability, and still others would suggest a free PSA measurement and perform a biopsy if the free to total PSA ratio is less than 25%. Again, the physician and patient need to decide together about next steps.

Clinical Example

A 58-year-old man whose father died of prostate cancer inquires about PSA testing. After discussing the pros and cons of testing with his physician, he decides that he is willing to accept the possible consequences of screening so that he might possibly reduce his risk of dying of prostate cancer.

A PSA measurement is done, and his PSA level is found to be 3.8 ng/mL. Although the result is not greater than the commonly used threshold of 4.0 ng/mL, it is above the age-specific reference range for men in their fifties. In this situation, after further discussion, the physician and patient decide together to follow the PSA level with repeat testing. Other reasonable approaches would be to perform a biopsy or to defer the biopsy pending a free PSA measurement.

REFERENCES

1. **Landis SH, Murray T, Bolden S, Wingo PA.** Cancer statistics, 1998. CA Cancer J Clin. 1998;48:6-29.
2. **Wingo PA, Landis S, Ries LAG.** An adjustment to the 1997 estimate for new prostate cancer cases. CA Cancer J Clin. 1997;47:239-42.
3. **Sackett DL, Holland WW.** Controversy in the detection of disease. Lancet. 1975;23:357-9.
4. **Schmid HP, McNeal JE, Stamey TA.** Observations on the doubling time of prostate cancer: the use of serial prostate-specific antigen in patients with untreated disease as a measure of increasing cancer volume. Cancer. 1993;71:2031-40.
5. **Lu-Yao GL, Yao S.** Population-based study of long-term survival in patients with clinically localised prostate cancer. Lancet. 1997;349:906-10.
6. American College of Physicians. Screening for prostate cancer. Ann Intern Med. 1997;126:480-4.
7. **Coley CM, Barry MJ, Fleming C, Mulley AG.** Early detection of prostate cancer. Part I. Prior probability and effectiveness of tests. Ann Intern Med. 1997;126:394-406.
8. **Tchetgen M-B, Song JT, Strawderman M, et al.** Ejaculation increases the serum prostate-specific antigen concentration. Urology. 1996;47:511-516.
9. **Herschman JD, Smith DS, Catalona WJ.** Effect of ejaculation on serum total and free prostate-specific antigen concentrations. Urology. 1997;50:239-43.
10. **Crawford ED, Schutz MJ, Clejan S, et al.** The effect of digital rectal examination on prostate-specific antigen levels. JAMA. 1992;267:2227-8.
11. **Gann PH, Hennekens CH, Meir JS.** A prospective evaluation of plasma prostate-specific antigen for detection of prostatic cancer. JAMA. 1995;273:289-94.
12. **Oesterling JE, Rice DC, Glenski WJ, Bergstralh EJ.** Effect of cystoscopy, prostate biopsy, and transurethral resection of prostate on serum prostate-specific antigen concentration. Urology. 1993;42:276-82.
13. **Sershon PD, Barry MJ, Oesterling JE.** Serum prostate-specific antigen discriminates weakly between men with benign prostatic hyperplasia and patients with organ-confined prostate cancer. Eur Urol. 1994;25:281-7.

14. **Catalona WJ, Richie JP, Ahmann FR, et al.** Comparison of digital rectal examination and serum prostate specific antigen in the early detection of prostate cancer: results of a multicenter clinical trial of 6,630 men. J Urol. 1994;151:1283-90.

15. **Richie JP, Ratliff TL, Catalona WJ, et al.** Effect of patient age on early detection of prostate cancer with serum prostate-specific antigen and digital rectal examination. Urology 1993;42:365-74.

16. **Catalona WJ, Smith DS, Ornstein DK.** Prostate cancer detection in men with serum PSA concentrations of 2.6 to 4.0 ng/mL and benign prostate examination: enhancement of specificity with free PSA measurements. JAMA. 1997;277:1452-5.

17. **Benson MC, Whang IS, Pantuck A, et al.** Prostate specific antigen density: a means of distinguishing benign prostatic hypertrophy and prostate cancer. J Urol. 1992;147:815-6.

18. **Carter HB, Pearson JD.** PSA velocity for the diagnosis of early prostate cancer. Urol Clin North Am. 1993;20:665-71.

19. **Oesterling JE, Jacobsen SJ, Chute CG, et al.** Serum prostate-specific antigen in a community-based population of healthy men: establishment of age-specific reference ranges. JAMA. 1993;270:860-4.

20. **Partin AW, Oesterling JE.** The clinical usefulness of percent free-PSA. Urology. 1996;48:1-3.

21. **Catalona WJ, Partin AW, Slawin KM, et al.** Use of the percentage of free prostate-specific antigen to enhance differentiation of prostate cancer from benign prostatic disease: a prospective multicenter clinical trial. JAMA. 1998;279:1542-7.

22. **vonEschenbach A, Ho R, Murphy GP, et al.** American Cancer Society guideline for the early detection of prostate cancer: Update 1997. CA Cancer J Clin. 1997;47:261-4.

23. U.S. Preventive Services Task Force. Screening for prostate cancer. Guide to Clinical Preventive Services. 2nd ed. Baltimore: Williams and Wilkins; 1996:119-34.

24. **Barry MJ, Roberts RG.** Indications for PSA testing. JAMA. 1997;277:955.

25. **Keetch DW, Catalona WJ, Smith DS.** Serial prostate biopsies in men with persistently elevated serum prostate specific antigen values. J Urol. 1994;151:1571-4.

Impotence

48

Edgar R. Black, MD

KEY POINTS

Pretest Probabilities

- Impotence is a relatively frequent problem in ambulatory care and has multiple causes, including psychogenic, endocrine, vascular, neurologic, and urologic causes.
- A thorough history and physical examination should provide sufficient information about the likely cause to guide the diagnostic evaluation.

Diagnostic Strategies

- Diagnostic tests are best targeted according to possible etiologic factors rather than applied to all patients.
- Patients with a high probability of psychogenic impotence are unlikely to need laboratory evaluation.
- In patients with clinical presentations suggestive of endocrinologic causes, serum testosterone measurements should be performed.
- If vascular or neurogenic causes of impotence are suspected, a nocturnal penile tumescence study should be done. Intracavernosal injections with duplex ultrasonography may also be useful for these patients.

BACKGROUND

The problem of impotence, or erectile dysfunction, is somewhat different from many of the problems presented in this text in that the diagnosis is generally made by the patient. The diagnostic strategy for the health care provider is to determine the cause of the disorder and to recommend appropriate treatment. This chapter focuses only on erectile dysfunction and does not cover other types of male sexual problems, such as premature ejaculation.

Impotence is generally defined as the inability over time to consistently achieve or maintain an erection of sufficient rigidity for sexual

549

activity. One must recognize that brief, sporadic episodes of erectile failure are common occurrences often related to psychological stress.

ESTIMATING PRETEST PROBABILITY

The physiology of erectile function involves the complex interaction of psychobiologic processes. Thus, impotence can be caused by one or more separate disorders including psychogenic, vascular, neurologic, endocrine, or urologic diseases. The prevalence of impotence varies with age; data from Kinsey (1) show a prevalence of 1.3% at age 35, 6.7% at age 50, and 55% at age 75. Another study showed a 34% prevalence in a medical outpatient population having an average age of about 60 years (2). More recent results from the Massachusetts male aging study reported that 5% of males aged 40 years and 15% of those aged 70 years had complete impotence and that 17% and 34%, respectively, had moderate impotence (3).

A more important classification is the relative proportions of the various causes of impotence. This information is difficult to assess because of obvious referral bias in many series and lack of a consistently applied gold standard. In addition, some patients may refuse diagnostic evaluation; in the series reported by Slag and colleagues (2), half of the patients with impotence chose not to be studied. The results of four large series are summarized in Table 48-1 and show that psychogenic impotence is very frequent, as is impotence caused by drug therapy, diabetes, and endocrinologic factors (2,4–6). A more recent

Table 48-1. Prevalence of Various Causes of Impotence

Causes	Study			
	Slag (2) (n = 120)	Spark (4) (n = 105)	Montague (5) (n = 154)	Maatman (6) (n = 200)
	←————————————— % —————————————→			
Psychogenic	14	14	40	28
Depression	—	—	5	—
Endocrine				1
Pituitary-testosterone	23	33	6	—
Other (e.g., thyroid)	6	2	—	—
Vascular disease	—	3	7	5
Neurologic disease	6	—	4	2
Diabetes mellitus	9	7	19	41
Drug therapy	25	7	2	1
Other illness	4	7	8	4
Local urologic problems	6	—	8	1
Uncertain	7	27	1	17

study again showed the high prevalence of psychogenic causes; 39.7% in a series of 406 consecutive patients evaluated in a urology-based male sexual dysfunction center were believed to have psychogenic impotence, 28.8% had organic causes, 25.1% had combined causes, and the cause was uncertain in 6.4% (7).

In attempting to determine the cause of impotence, information from the history and physical examination is critical. The comprehensive history should include data concerning the onset of impotence, situations when erections do occur, possible precipitating events, libido, the presence of symptoms suggestive of associated disorders (e.g., diabetes mellitus), and a list of medications that the patient is currently taking. The physical examination should emphasize inspection of the genitalia—for example, for Peyronie disease, determination of testicular size, and assessment of vascular and neurologic function. Wesson and colleagues (8), using criteria outlined by Magee (9), correctly identified the "final" cause for impotence in 25 of 29 cases (79%). The errors occurred both because of misclassification and assigning mixed causes (e.g., vascular and neurologic), when only one process appeared to be occurring. Unfortunately, because none of these patients had endocrine dysfunction, the use of primary information in making this distinction is uncertain. However, classifications may be developed based on history and physical examination that allow initial evaluation and therapy to proceed (8,9).

Psychogenic impotence is generally characterized by a sudden onset of erectile failure, often in younger (<age 60 years) healthy men, usually with an identifiable psychological problem, such as premature ejaculation or situational anxiety. These men maintain the ability to masturbate and often notice spontaneous erections when awakening or with psychic erotic stimuli.

Vascular impotence typically involves a gradual progression of decreasing firmness of erection, generally associated with peripheral vascular disease. However, it may occasionally be the sole manifestation of pelvic vascular disease. Because the pressure in the erect penis is a result of an equilibrium between the perfusion pressure from dilated cavernosal arteries and the resistance to outflow through compressed venules, vascular impotence may result from either diminished perfusion or excessive outflow (i.e., veno-occlusive disease) (10). In some series, veno-occlusive disease accounts for more than half of the cases of vasculogenic impotence. Although veno-occlusive dysfunction may be primary or secondary, degeneration of the cavernosal smooth muscle has been suggested as the most common cause (11).

Neurologic impotence shows intermittent progression of symptoms in association with neurologic diseases, such as spinal cord injury, multiple sclerosis, or peripheral neuropathy (e.g., in association with diabetes mellitus or alcohol abuse). Ellenberg (12) noted that 82% of impotent patients with diabetes had neuropathy, whereas only 14% of potent patients had similar findings.

Endocrine (pituitary-testosterone) impotence, as described by Spark (4), is frequently associated with small or soft testes, decreased libido, and loss of secondary sexual characteristics. Impotence may also be associated with hyperthyroidism or hypothyroidism. Recent articles have questioned whether the association between low testosterone levels and impotence in older men is cause-and-effect or two independent processes (13). In older patients with impotence and low testosterone levels, normalization of testosterone values does not necessarily result in return of potency (14,15).

Certain medications are frequently associated with impotence. However, the pathophysiology in these cases is not always clear; the cause may often be either psychogenic or pharmacologic.

Not all patients can be placed into one of these diagnostic categories, and some may have multiple factors. Nevertheless, the major challenge in evaluation is to determine the primary cause of the impotence, and subsequently, the appropriate treatment.

DIAGNOSTIC TESTS

The number and variety of diagnostic tests available to evaluate impotence reflects the difficulty in making a definite diagnosis and the lack of consensus about an optimal evaluation. The sensitivity and specificity data discussed in the following sections have been derived, when possible, using impotent patients as controls. For example, test characteristics for penile blood pressure measurements have been calculated using "nonvascular" patients with impotence for controls.

Plasma Testosterone and Prolactin

Plasma testosterone levels are measured using radioimmunoassay techniques. Because testosterone is secreted in a pulsatile fashion every 20 to 30 minutes, a single specimen is within 20% of the mean value two thirds of the time (16). Normal ranges may vary among laboratories, but the lower limit for normal is usually 300 to 350 ng/dL. The sensitivity of testosterone measurement in patients with pituitary-testosterone impotence is more than 95%. Spark (4) reports that 36 of 37 (97%) patients in whom the cause of impotence was endocrinologic had abnormally low testosterone levels. Maatman and Montague (17) found the test to have a similar sensitivity and a specificity of 97%, using 220 ng/dL as the lower limit of normal (Table 48-2). Because testosterone is transported in serum bound to proteins, a free testosterone assay may be indicated in some clinical situations (18).

Prolactin-secreting pituitary tumors are an unusual cause of impotence and are responsible for fewer than 5% of cases. Impotence

Table 48-2. Operating Characteristics of Diagnostic Tests for Impotence

Diagnostic Test	Definition of Positive Result	Sensitivity	Specificity	Likelihood Ratio	
				Positive Result	Negative Result
		← ——— % ——— →			
Plasma testosterone measurement	Varies	97	97	32	0.03
Penile blood pressure	Penile/ brachial ratio <0.75–0.8	~90	50–70	1.8–3.0	0.14–0.20
Duplex ultrasonography					
Arterial disease (maximum flow)	Varies	~85	~95	~17	~0.16
Venous leak (diastolic flow)	Varies	~90	~70	~3	~0.14
Nocturnal penile tumescence		Uncertain, estimated 80–95	Uncertain, estimated 80–95	~4–19	~0.05–0.25
Cystometric evalution		82	90	8.2	0.20
Biothesiometry		85	39	1.4	0.38
Bulbocavernosus reflex	>38 ms	55–70	Estimated 95	11–14	0.32–0.47

appears to be a late clinical manifestation such that when these patients present with impotence, they generally are found to have depressed serum testosterone levels along with the elevated prolactin levels. All eighteen of the patients reported by Carter and colleagues (19) and seven of eight reported by Spark and colleagues (4) had these findings. These men generally fail to respond to testosterone therapy unless the hyperprolactinemia is treated. Therefore, although determination of prolactin is important in the evaluation of low serum testosterone levels, current evidence does not support its routine determination in patients with suspected organic impotence.

Penile Pulse and Blood Pressure

The determination of penile pulse and blood pressure is an attempt to detect impotence caused by vascular disease. Calculating test characteristics is difficult because of the use of different techniques and ways of determining a positive test—for example, penile to brachial pressure ratios compared with absolute pressure difference between penile and brachial pulses. The lack of a gold standard (i.e., angiography or improvement after reconstructive surgery) is also a problem. These measurements can be confusing because the penis has three sets of paired arteries, but the two cavernous arteries seem primarily responsible for potency. Thus, studies may measure a normal dorsal artery when the cause of the impotence may in fact be an occluded cavernous vessel. These studies can also be problematic because studies of a flaccid penis may not adequately reflect the hemodynamics of an erect penis.

Canning and colleagues (20) found diminished potency in a group of 31 patients with vascular disease when the penile pulse was not detectable. Interestingly, Abelson (21) found normal penile blood pressures using Doppler techniques in two of six impotent patients with diabetes who did not have palpable penile pulses. The sensitivity for Doppler blood pressure measurements in determining vascular impotence varies from 85% to 100% (22,23), and specificity ranges between 50% and 70% depending on the control group used (see Table 48-2). Some studies (24) suggest that penile plethysmography provides a more accurate assessment of total penile blood flow; however, good data on test operating characteristics are not available.

Intracavernous Injections

The intracavernous injection of various vasoactive substances, such as papaverine or prostaglandin E_1 (alprostadil), have been used with increasing frequency in the diagnosis and treatment of impotence (25,26). These agents cause erections either by relaxing vascular smooth muscle directly or blocking adrenergically induced tone (27). Therefore, patients with impotence who do not develop full erections in response to these injections probably have either significant arterial insufficiency or severe veno-occlusive dysfunction—that is, excessive venous outflow ("leak"). Patients with other forms of impotence generally develop a firm erection after an injection; however, severe anxiety may result in a false-positive test result.

Color Duplex Ultrasonography

Color duplex ultrasonography may be combined with papaverine or prostaglandin injections to study changes in the caliber of the cavernosal arteries and the rate of blood flow (28). Arteriogenic (inflow) impotence is assessed by determining the maximum flow after an injection. Veno-occlusive dysfunction can be evaluated by measuring diastolic velocity, because a venous leak is associated with increased diastolic flow.

For arteriogenic impotence, various values have been used for defining an abnormal test; however, most studies use values less than 25 to 35 cm/s to identify arterial inflow disease. One study reported a sensitivity of 80% and a specificity of 96% when a value below 30 cm/s was used to define a positive test (29). In a study using angiography as the "gold-standard," 11 of 12 (91%) of those whose peak flow was less than 35 cm/s had arterial disease (30).

For venous leakage, diastolic velocities of more than 5 to 7 cm/s are generally used to define a positive test. Findings on duplex ultra-sonography seem to correlate well with cavernosography, which is a more invasive study used in the diagnosis of veno-occlusive disease. Using a cutoff of 7 cm/s, investigators noted this test to have a sensitivity of 94% and specificity of 69% compared with cavernosography (29) (see Table 48-2).

To increase the accuracy of these tests, it is important to ensure complete trabecular smooth muscle relaxation (31). This can be done by using multiple injections of vasoactive agents. Others have suggested using audiovisual sexual stimulation in addition to injections (32). The timing of measurements and conducting unilateral measurements compared with bilateral measurements can also impact the test's accuracy.

Nocturnal Penile Tumescence

Nocturnal penile tumescence (NPT) measures the occurrence of penile erection during sleep. In patients with intact neurohumoral-vascular systems, nocturnal erections occur four to five times nightly, usually during rapid eye movement (REM) sleep. Erections that are present upon awakening are likely related to this, rather than to a full bladder (33). Nocturnal monitoring attempts to measure the number of erections and also to determine changes in penile circumference and the firmness of the erection. There are various ways to study these changes, ranging from sophisticated strain gauges that measure axial rigidity to Rigiscan (Dacomed, Minneapolis, MN), Snap-gauges, or observing separation of postage stamp perforations applied circumferentially around the penis. Obviously, such testing is not needed when the patient reports normal, adequate erections in selective sexual settings, such as potency with some partners or with masturbation.

The role of nocturnal tumescence studies is to attempt to separate psychogenic from organic causes of impotence. Patients with psychogenic impotence have normal erections (positive test result), whereas patients with organic disease (e.g., vascular disease) should present with diminished or absent erections (negative test result). Karacan and colleagues (34) demonstrated the marked difference in NPT results obtained in impotent patients with diabetes compared with those obtained in patients with psychogenic impotence. Because nocturnal tumescence occurs primarily during REM sleep, sophisticated sleep monitoring may be required to be certain that this is occurring. In addition, the effect of severe psychological problems (e.g., depression) on these studies is unknown. Another problem with NPT studies is that it is difficult to equate a given change in penile circumference with potency (6). Fisher and colleagues (35) noted changes in penile circumference with full erection that varied from 15 to 45 mm. Many authors suggest waking the patient during the time of maximal tumescence to assess if the erection is sufficient for vaginal penetration.

Data on the specificity and sensitivity of this test are not available. However, normal tumescence (a positive study result) in a patient with impotence should result in a high post-test probability of psychogenic impotence. In some patients, conditions such as abnormal sensory afferent pathways may not interfere with NPT but may be an organic cause of impotence (10). Brief periods (i.e., 1–2 minutes), of full erections are usually not considered to define a positive test result (35). Unfortunately, 5% to 20% of patients without nocturnal erections during NPT studies (negative test result) do not have recognizable organic disease, and the true diagnosis is unknown (33). These patients may represent cases of psychogenic impotence with false-negative NPT results or may have undefined organic disease (true-negatives). This uncertainty precludes calculation of test characteristics. Similarly, inadequate data is available to calculate values for modifications of the formal NPT, such as use of the Snap-gauge.

Cystometric Examinations

To date, it has been difficult to assess neurologic causes of impotence. Various tests have been suggested, including evaluation of anal sphincter tone and demonstration of the bulbocavernosus reflex (BCR) (i.e., contraction of the anus when the glans penis is compressed). The use of bladder cystometrics in neurologic impotence is based on the recognition that the autonomic pathways for micturition and erection are identical. Ellenberg (12) studied potent and impotent patients with diabetes and found that cystometrics were abnormal in 37 of 45 impotent patients with diabetes (sensitivity, 82%) but were normal in 27 of 30 potent persons (specificity, 90%).

Penile Biothesiometry

Neurologic causes of impotence can also be evaluated by testing the vibratory perception threshold of the skin of the penile shaft using penile biothesiometry. This technique measures the somatic afferent component of erectile function and is often abnormal in patients with peripheral neuropathies. The threshold generally becomes higher with increasing age. Data to calculate test characteristics are limited. In one study, Padma-Nathan (36) reported a sensitivity of 85% and a specificity of 39% in the detection of neurologic impotence in 137 patients with organic impotence of varying causes.

Bulbocavernosus Reflex

Measuring the latency time of the BCR is another technique used in the evaluation of possible neurologic impotence. This technique assesses the somatic function of both afferent and efferent nerves and is obtained by applying a stimulation to the penis and then measuring the response over the bulbocavernous muscle. Although this technique is described frequently, little data is available to assess test characteristics adequately. Data from one small series of 17 patients showed this test to have a sensitivity of 55% and a specificity of 100% (37). A more recent report showed that 14 of 20 (70%) of patients with neurogenic impotence had an abnormal BCR (38).

DIAGNOSTIC STRATEGIES

It is difficult to design an optimal strategy for the evaluation of impotence because of the problems involved in establishing a definite diagnosis and uncertainty about test sensitivity and specificity. It seems clear that no single test should be performed in all patients, because of the low post-test probability associated with a positive result when the pretest probability of a particular cause is low. Rather, tests should be done to investigate the most likely diagnosis based on a thorough history and physical examination. The goal of the patient evaluation is to identify the most probable cause of the impotence, so that appropriate treatment can be prescribed.

Patients with presumed (i.e., high pretest probability) psychogenic impotence should receive psychosexual counseling. Additional diagnostic evaluation or therapeutic interventions may be indicated if no improvement in sexual function is achieved with therapy or if other conditions are elicited during ongoing evaluation.

In patients with characteristics of endocrine disorders (e.g., small testicles and loss of libido) and in those without a definite psychogenic or organic illness, plasma testosterone levels should be measured, because the test result substantially alters the probability of endocrine impotence.

In patients with presumed neurologic or vascular disease, the return of erectile function would require treatment. Oral sildenafil (Viagra) is a newly available option (39). Other treatments include injections with a vasoactive agent, penile prosthesis, or vascular surgery, depending on the exact cause of the impotence and on the patient's preferences. Obviously, medications that may be interfering with potency should first be eliminated. If available, NPT is probably the best initial diagnostic test, in that abnormal tumescence indicates almost certain organic disease. If no contraindications are present, a therapeutic trial of sildenafil should also be an option. Finally, a modified sleep study using devices such as the Snap-Gauge or the intracavernous injection, often with duplex ultrasonography, are other alternatives.

In situations in which the cause is likely multifactorial (e.g., a patient with diabetes and with neuropathy who has a relatively sudden onset of impotence), studies such as NPT, response to sildenafil, intracavernous injection with duplex ultrasonography, or cystometrics would likely be helpful in determining the cause and the optimal therapy of the impotence. The tests used should reflect local resources and expertise. Nocturnal penile tumescence, injection, or cystometrics is likely to be a useful test in patients with suspected neurologic disease, whereas NPT or injection with duplex ultrasonography would be preferred in patients with possible vascular impotence.

As noted above, oral sildenafil has greatly altered the approach to treatment of erectile dysfunction (39). This agent works by causing increased levels of cyclic guanosine monophosphate (GMP) in penile tissue that leads to greater blood flow into the corpus cavernosa. Although it seems to be effective in many patients, additional studies may demonstrate varying effectiveness for different types of impotence. It has been suggested that it may not be effective in those with severe arterial insufficiency, loss of trabecular smooth muscle, or incompressible cavernosal veins (40).

Although the usefulness of sildenafil in treating erectile failure of various types may mean that many of the diagnostic studies discussed in this chapter are not needed before treatment with sildenafil is started, it is still necessary to be familiar with these approaches and tests. First, it is important to conduct a systematic clinical evaluation of patients presenting with impotence to determine a likely cause; second, if the response to sildenafil is found to vary with the type of impotence, then determining the probable cause can help educate the patient about the likely success of oral sildenafil; third, some third-party payors may provide coverage for sildenafil only in cases of organic impotence, thus requiring that providers be able to differentiate organic from psychogenic causes; and fourth, because some patients have contraindications to use of sildenafil (e.g., the concurrent use of nitrates), the diagnostic and therapeutic approaches discussed in this chapter still apply.

CLINICAL PROBLEMS

Clinical Problem 1
A young healthy man presents for evaluation after the sudden onset of impotence.

Testing Strategy and Rationale
No tests are required. Counseling and therapy should be initiated. In healthy persons with sudden onset of erectile failure, psy-

chogenic impotence is the most likely diagnosis. The presence of a normal examination and history of a normal libido provides additional support for this diagnosis. The onset of impotence is often related to a stressful or traumatic event. If the patient did not improve with therapy, then further evaluation, including NPT or endocrine evaluation, or a therapeutic trial may be indicated.

Clinical Example

A 35-year-old man presents with impotence of 3 months' duration. His impotence began when he lost his job. He has normal libido, and the results of the physical examination are normal. He is able to have firm erections with masturbation but not with intercourse. The most likely diagnosis is psychogenic impotence, and sexual counseling should be initiated. Further studies would be indicated only if he did not respond to therapy.

Clinical Problem 2

A patient with peripheral vascular or neurologic disease or both reports impotence.

Testing Strategy and Rationale

An NPT study should be done unless the history suggests that the impotence has another cause. Another possible approach is a trial of sildenafil. Patients with impotence related to vascular or neurologic disease or both usually present with a gradual loss of erectile function and with physical findings related to their underlying disease (e.g., decreased peripheral pulses or neuropathy). They often have normal libido but are unable to have firm erections under any circumstances. An NPT study that does not demonstrate erections makes the diagnosis of organic impotence likely, whereas normal study results indicate that the disease is probably psychogenic in origin. Intracavernous injections with duplex ultrasonography, modified sleep studies, or urinary cystometrics could serve as alternative diagnostic tests. A positive response to sildenafil, although resulting in effective treatment, would likely not indicate the cause of the erectile dysfunction.

Clinical Example

A 60-year-old man with a history of peripheral vascular disease, stable angina (he is taking nitrates), and diabetes mellitus presents with a 6-month history of impotence. He describes a gradual decrease in the firmness of erections for more than a year. Recently, he has not detected normal erections at any time. His examination reveals absent pulses in the lower extremities and decreased sensation to the knees. Genital examination is normal. This most like-

Continued

ly is a case of organic impotence caused by vascular or neurologic disease or both. Treatment with sildenafil is contraindicated. An NPT study is indicated. If no erections are noted by this study, then follow-up testing, such as duplex ultrasonography, is indicated. However, if normal erections are seen on NPT, then the likely diagnosis is psychogenic impotence, in which case counseling is indicated.

REFERENCES

1. **Kinsey AC, Pomeroy WB, Martin CE.** Sexual Behavior in the Human Male. London: WB Saunders; 1948.
2. **Slag MF, Morley JE, Elson MK, et al.** Impotence in medical clinic outpatients. JAMA. 1983;249:1736-40.
3. **Feldman HA, Goldstein I, Hatzichristou DG, et al.** Impotence and its medical and psychosocial correlates: results of the Massachusetts male aging study. J. Urol. 1994;151:54-61.
4. **Spark RF, White RA, Connolly PB.** Impotence is not always psychogenic. JAMA. 1980;243:750-5.
5. **Montague DK, James RE Jr, DeWolfe VG, Martin LM.** Diagnostic evaluation, classification, and treatment of men with sexual dysfunction. Urology. 1979;14:545-8.
6. **Maatman TJ, Montague DK, Martin LM.** Cost-effective evaluation of impotence. Urology. 1986;27:132-5.
7. **Melman A, Tiefer L, Pedersen R.** Evaluation of first 406 patients in urology department based center for male sexual dysfunction. Urology. 1988;32:6-10.
8. **Wesson LE, Sessions PA, Fried FA.** A new approach to evaluating impotence in outpatients. NC Med J. 1982;43:562-7.
9. **Magee MC.** Psychogenic impotence: a critical review. Urology. 1980;15:435-42.
10. **Krane RJ, Goldstein I, deTejada IS.** Impotence. N Engl J Med. 1989; 321:1648-59.
11. **Carrier S, Brock G, Kour NW, Lue TF.** Pathophysiology of erectile dysfunction. Urology. 1993;42:468-80.
12. **Ellenberg M.** Impotence in diabetes: the neurologic factor. Ann Intern Med. 1971;75:213-9.
13. **Korenman SG, Morley JE, Mooradian AG, et al.** Secondary hypoganadism in older men: its relation to impotence. J Clin Endocrinol Metab. 1990;71:963-9.
14. **Guay AT, Bansal S, Heatley GJ.** Effect of raising endogenous testosterone levels in impotent men with secondary hypogonadism: double blind placebo-controlled trial with clomiphene citrate. J Clin Endocrinol Metab. 1995;80:3546-52.
15. **Mulligan T, Schmitt B.** Testosterone for erectile failure. J Gen Intern Med. 1993;8:517-21.

16. **Griffin JE, Wilson JD.** Disorders of the testis. In: Petersdorf RG et al, eds. Harrison's Principles of Internal Medicine. 10th ed. New York: McGraw Hill; 1983:689-700.

17. **Maatman TJ, Montague DK.** Routine endocrine screening in impotence. Urology. 1986;27:499-502.

18. **McClure RD.** Endocrine evaluation and therapy of erectile dysfunction. Urol Clin North Am. 1988;15:53-64.

19. **Carter JN, Tyson JE, Tolis G, et al.** Prolactin-secreting tumors and hypogonadism in 22 men. N Engl J Med. 1978;299:847-52.

20. **Canning JR, Bowers LM, Lloyd FA, Cottrell TLC.** Genital vascular insufficiency and impotence. Surg Forum. 1963;14:298.

21. **Abelson D.** Diagnostic value of the penile pulse and blood pressure: a Doppler study of impotence in diabetics. J Urol. 1975;113:636-9.

22. **Engel G, Burnham SJ, Carter MF.** Penile blood pressure in the evaluation of erectile impotence. Fertil Steril. 1978;30:687-90.

23. **Dow JA, Gluck RW, Colimbu M, et al.** Multiphasic diagnostic evaluation of arteriogenic, venogenic, and sinusoidogenic impotency. Urology. 1991; 38:402-7.

24. **Kedia KR.** Vasculogenic impotence: diagnosis and objective evaluation using quantitative segmental pulse volume recorder. Br J Urol. 1984;56:516-20.

25. **Virag R, Frydman D, Legman M, Virag H.** Intracavernous injection of papaverine as a diagnostic and therapeutic method in erectile failure. Angiology. 1984;35:79-87.

26. **Porst H.** The rationale for prostaglandin E1 in erectile failure: a survey of worldwide experience. J Urol. 1996;155:802-15.

27. **Juenemann KP, Lue TB, Fournier GR Jr, Tanagho EA.** Hemodynamics of papaverine- and phentolamine-induced penile erection. J Urol. 1986;136: 158-61.

28. **Robinson LQ, Woodcock JP, Stephenson TP.** Duplex scanning in suspected vasculogenic impotence: a worthwhile exercise? Br J Urol. 1989;63:432-6.

29. **Patel U, Amin Z, Friedman E, Vale J, et al.** Colour flow and spectral Doppler imaging after papaverine-induced penile erection in 220 impotent men: study of temporal patterns and the importance of repeated sampling, velocity asymmetry and vascular anomalies. Clin Radiol. 1993;48:18-24.

30. **Benson CB, Aruny JE, Vickers MA.** Correlation of duplex sonography with arteriography in patients with erectile dysfunction. AJR Am J Roentgenol. 1993;160:71-3.

31. **Goldstein I.** Impotence. J Urol. 1994;151:1533-4.

32. **Montorsi F, Guazzoni G, Barbieri L, et al.** The effect of intracorporeal injection plus genital and audiovisual sexual stimulation versus second injection on penile color Doppler sonography parameters. J Urol. 1996;155:536-40.

33. **Wein AJ, VanArsdalen K, Malloy TR.** Nocturnal penile tumescence. In: Krane RJ, Siroky MB, Goldstein I, eds. Male Sexual Dysfunction. Boston: Little, Brown; 1983:203-11.

34. **Karacan I, Scott FB, Salis PJ, et al.** Nocturnal erections, differential diagnosis of impotence, and diabetes. Biol Psychiatry. 1977;12:373-80.

35. **Fisher C, Schiavi RC, Edwards A, et al.** Evaluation of nocturnal penile tumescence in the differential diagnosis of sexual impotence. Arch Gen Psychiatry. 1979;36:431-7.

36. **Padma-Nathan H.** Neurologic evaluation of erectile dysfunction. Urol Clin North Am. 1988;15:77-80.

37. **Herman CW, Weinberg HJ, Brown J.** Testing for neurogenic impotence: a challenge. Urology. 1986;27:318-21.

38. **Dettmers C, vanAhlen H, Faust H, et al.** Evaluation of erectile dysfunction with the sympathetic skin response in comparison to bulbocavernosus reflex and somatosensory evoked potential of the pudendal nerve. Electromyogr Clin Neurophysiol. 1994;34:437-44.

39. **Goldstein I, Lue TF, Padma-Nathan H, et al. for the Sildenafil Study Group.** Oral sildenafil in the treatment of erectile dysfunction. N Engl J Med. 1998;338:1397-404.

40. **Utiger RD.** A pill for impotence. N Engl J Med. 1998;338:1458-9.

Ovarian Cancer

49

Carmen E. Guerra, MD

KEY POINTS

Pretest Probability

- The lifetime risk of ovarian cancer is 1 in 70 (1.4%) for a woman in the United States without a family history of the disease.
- The risk of ovarian cancer increases with age; prevalence is 16 per 100,000 women for those aged 40 to 44 years and 54 per 100,000 women for those aged 75 to 79 years.
- In women with hereditary ovarian cancer syndrome, the lifetime risk of the disease is approximately 50%.

Screening Strategies

- In women at average risk for ovarian cancer, screening for the disease has no known benefit.
- Women with multiple affected relatives should receive genetic counseling and be considered for genetic testing. In some situations, screening with regular pelvic examination, transvaginal ultrasonography, and CA-125 levels may be indicated.

BACKGROUND

Ovarian cancer remains the most lethal gynecologic malignancy in the United States and is responsible for 14,500 deaths annually (1). Despite the application of aggressive cytoreductive surgical management and chemotherapeutic protocols, the 5-year survival rate remains less than 50% (1). This low rate is largely owing to the fact that ovarian malignancies are generally clinically asymptomatic in the early stages and that, at the time of diagnosis, two thirds of the patients have advanced, high-volume disease. In contrast, 90% of the patients diagnosed with localized disease are cured (1). An effective screening technique may, therefore, have an impact on the outcome of this disease. However, because of the relatively low occurrence rate of ovarian cancer (the disease affects 1 in 70 women) and the characteristics of available tests, very few with early cancer would be identified and most abnormal test results would be false-positives. Some suggest that screening may have a role in a selected, high-risk populations in which the likelihood of disease is higher; but, at present, no evidence has been shown to demonstrate that screening such a population improves the mortality rate.

ESTIMATING PRETEST PROBABILITY

Several factors have been identified that modify the risk of ovarian cancer. Family history of ovarian cancer and older age are associated with increased risk, whereas the use of the oral contraceptive medications and pregnancy reduce the risk (Table 49-1).

The strongest risk factor for ovarian cancer is a family history of the disease. Two patterns of inheritance are known: hereditary ovarian cancer syndromes and a "family history" of ovarian cancer. These two groups compose fewer than 10% of all the patients diagnosed with ovarian cancer.

Women from families with a hereditary ovarian cancer syndrome constitute the group at highest known risk for ovarian cancer. In this group, inheritance follows an autosomal dominant mode with variable penetrance, and an affected person has a 40% to 50% chance of developing ovarian cancer. Three subtypes of hereditary ovarian cancer syndrome are recognized: 1) a breast-ovarian cancer syndrome, which is associated with an inherited mutation in the BRCA1 and BRCA2 genes (2); 2) a site-specific ovarian cancer syndrome; and 3) nonpolyposis col-

Table 49-1. Risk Factors for Ovarian Cancer

Risk Factor	Relative Risk	Lifetime Risk for Ovarian Cancer* (%)
No risk factors	1.0	1.2
Oral contraceptive use	0.65	0.8
Pregnancy	0.5	0.6
One first- or second-degree relative with ovarian cancer	3.1	3.7
Two or three relatives with ovarian cancer	4.6	≥5.5
Familial ovarian cancer syndrome	Unknown	40–50

*Risk is estimated for a 50-year-old woman.

Republished with permission from Carlson KJ, Skates SJ, Singer DE. Screening for ovarian cancer. Ann Intern Med. 1994;121:124-32.

orectal cancer, endometrial cancer, and ovarian cancer syndrome, which is also known as the "Lynch II Syndrome" (3). Women with these syndromes typically present with ovarian cancer at an earlier age and two or more generations have the respective cancers.

Women with a "family history" of ovarian cancer have one or more relatives with ovarian cancer without evidence of a hereditary pattern. Estimates of relative risk for women with a family history of ovarian cancer demonstrate an odds ratio of 3.1 (95% CI, 2.2 to 4.4) for women with one affected (first- or second-degree) relative and an odds ratio of 4.6 (CI, 1.1 to 18.4) for those with two or more affected relatives (4). Using these ratios, the lifetime probability of ovarian cancer for a 50-year-old woman has been estimated to increase from 1.2% to 3.7% with one affected relative and to 5.5% with two to three affected relatives (5). A recent study in the United Kingdom based on death-certificate data found the relative risk of ovarian cancer to be 2.3 if one first-degree relative was affected and 26.7 if two first-degree relatives had ovarian cancer (6). One possible reason for the differences in risk for those with two or more affected relatives could be differing proportions of those with a "hereditary syndrome."

Increasing age is also a risk factor for ovarian cancer; disease prevalence is 15.7 cases per 100,000 women aged 40 to 44 years and increases to 54 cases per 100,000 women aged 75 to 79 years (7). Nulliparity is also associated with an increased risk of ovarian cancer. Multigravidas have relative risk of 0.5 compared with nulliparous women, and the risk decreases proportionally with increasing numbers of pregnancies. Each additional pregnancy after the first lowers a woman's risk by approximately 10% to 15% (8). Use of oral contraceptives reduces the relative risk by 30% to 60%, depending on the duration of use; the relative risk for women who ever used oral contraceptives is 0.65 (9,10).

DIAGNOSTIC TESTS

Pelvic Examination

The pelvic examination has limited usefulness in screening for ovarian malignancies, because ovarian malignancies have usually spread by the time they are palpable. The usefulness of the pelvic examination is also highly dependent on the skill of the examiner. Some of the studies that have evaluated the sensitivity and specificity of the pelvic examination have used abdominal ultrasonography as the comparative standard; however, this may have overestimated the sensitivity of the pelvic examination, because abdominal ultrasonography is not as sensitive as transvaginal ultrasonography.

In one study of 801 women aged 40 to 70 years who underwent screening pelvic examination and abdominal ultrasonography, 106 women (13%) had abnormal findings on bimanual examination. Six of these patients were discovered to have ovarian malignancies, and one additional ovarian carcinoma was detected by ultrasonography (11). Of the 106 women who had abnormal pelvic examinations, 51 had a normal abdominal ultrasonography and were believed not to have ovarian cancer based on the ultrasonographic findings and limited clinical follow-up. In another study of 1300 asymptomatic postmenopausal women who underwent pelvic examination and abdominal ultrasonography, the pelvic examination identified 10 of the 33 (30%) ovarian lesions detected by ultrasonography, all of which were benign. The bimanual examination did not identify the two ovarian malignancies (Stage I) found by transvaginal ultrasonography (12). Finally, in a study that evaluated CA-125 levels in screening for ovarian cancer in 5550 women aged 37 to 85 years, 175 women had an elevated CA-125 level and subsequently underwent serial measurement of CA-125 levels, pelvic examinations, and abdominal ultrasonography. The two examiners were able to palpate five of six ovarian cancers discovered in the study (13).

Ultrasonography

Abdominal ultrasonography relies on detection of increases of ovarian volume and changes in echogenicity that occur in patients with ovarian malignancies. It has been shown to be relatively sensitive (reported sensitivities in the range of 62%–100% [14–22]) but not very specific; in one study, this study detected 10 to 15 benign lesions for every case of ovarian cancer diagnosed at laparotomy in asymptomatic women (23). More recently, transvaginal ultrasonography has been found to be more sensitive than abdominal ultrasonography, achieving sensitivities near 100% and with reported specificities of approximately 97% (24–28).

Color flow Doppler may prove to be an important adjunct to transvaginal ultrasonography in the screening for ovarian cancer. It detects the neovascularization that characterizes most malignant tumors. Preliminary data are encouraging; one study has demonstrated a low vascular resistance in 15 of 16 patients with cancer, whereas 35 of 36 benign lesions had a normal vascular flow pattern (29). Larger studies will determine if color flow Doppler may become a useful screening method for ovarian cancer.

Another proposed approach to improving the accuracy of transvaginal ultrasonography is a sonographic morphology index. This index, proposed by the Ovarian Cancer Screening Project, is based on three structural components: ovarian volume, wall structure, and septal structure. Scores are assigned based on the appearance of these structures. A morphology index score greater than 5 (out of a maximum of 12 points) had a sensitivity of 89% and a specificity of 73%

indicating malignancy (30). Additional studies will help to determine if the use of the sonographic morphology index as a complement to transvaginal ultrasonography, perhaps in combination with color flow Doppler, significantly improves the operating characteristics of ultra-sonographic techniques in screening for ovarian cancer.

CA-125

CA-125 is a cell surface glycoprotein antigen on malignant cells derived from coelomic epithelium, i.e., müllerian ducts and cells lining the peritoneum, pleura, and pericardium. Antigen levels are elevated in approximately 80% of patients with epithelial ovarian cancers, including approximately 50% of those with stage I disease (31). Elevated CA-125 levels may predate the clinical diagnosis of ovarian cancer by as many as 3 years (32). However, CA-125 levels can be elevated in numerous benign gynecologic conditions, including pregnancy, pelvic infections, uterine leiomyomas, endometriosis, and benign ovarian tumors and cysts, as well as in advanced endometrial cancer, pancreatic cancer, cirrhosis, and pericarditis (33). It also has been shown to fluctuate during the menstrual cycle (34). At a cutoff value of 35 U/mL, the sensitivity of the CA-125 radioimmunoassay has been reported to be 61% to 96% (35–51). In many studies, sensitivity increases with increasing tumor stage. The estimated specificity of the CA-125 is reported to be 98.6% to 99.9% (52,53). Currently, CA-125 is not considered sufficiently sensitive to be used as the sole screening test for ovarian cancer. Lowering the cutoff value could improve sensitivity, but this would worsen specificity. Other tumor markers are being explored for possible use in combination with CA-125; these include CA15-3, TAG 72, M-CSF, OVX1, LSA, and NB 70K, but preliminary data suggest that increased sensitivity is again accompanied by decreased specificity (54).

In screening for ovarian cancer, the combination of serial measurement of CA-125 levels (using a cutoff value of 30 U/mL) and transabdominal ultrasonography has been reported to have a specificity of 99.9% (55) and a sensitivity of 79% at 1-year follow-up and of 58% during 2-year follow-up. A National Cancer Institute–sponsored trial to evaluate the combination of transvaginal ultrasonography and measuring CA-125 levels in screening for ovarian cancer is currently in progress (56).

Other Imaging Modalities

The role of computed tomography (CT) and magnetic resonance imaging (MRI) in screening for ovarian cancer has not been extensively evaluated. Most studies of these tests have involved further evaluation of certain abnormalities detected by ultrasonography or evaluating patients for either metastatic or recurrent disease (57). One study, involving a small number of patients, reported CT to have a sensitivity of 89% to 96% and a specificity of 44% to 83% in distinguishing malignant from benign ovarian lesions; similar results were noted for MRI (58). In another study of 63 patients, MRI had a sensitivity of 67% and a specificity of 97% in distinguishing benign from malignant ovarian lesions (59). Magnetic resonance imaging has superior soft tissue contrast compared with CT and ultrasonography. The role of spiral CT has yet to be determined.

The cross-sectional and multiplanar imaging afforded by CT and MRI, respectively, can provide important staging information in the management of ovarian cancer. At present, CT is the established primary imaging modality for ovarian cancer staging. Preoperatively, CT and MRI can also assist in the selection of the best surgical technique, the determination of whether preoperative chemotherapy is necessary, and evaluation of possible bowel involvement.

Genetic Testing

Several genetic mutations have been identified in women at highest risk for ovarian cancer. The most common type of familial ovarian cancer is the hereditary breast–ovarian cancer syndrome, and as previously noted, it is associated with inherited mutations in the BRCA1 and BRCA2 genes (2). The site-specific ovarian cancer syndrome has been hypothesized to be either a variant of the BRCA1-associated phenotype or a separate disease process. The Lynch II syndrome (or, hereditary nonpolyposis colorectal cancer, endometrial cancer, ovarian cancer syndrome) is associated with an inherited mutation of the DNA mismatch repair genes MSH2 and MLH1 (3). Genetic testing for these inherited mutations is performed at several academic medical centers for research purposes and is also now commercially available.

Because the lifetime risk of ovarian cancer for members of families with the hereditary cancer syndrome is approximately 50%, genetic testing should be considered in those in whom such a syndrome is suspected. Because of the complex issues pertaining to genetic testing, referral to a center conducting research in genetic testing or evaluation by a multidisciplinary team is suggested. Their approach to the patient should consist of several components, including performing pedigree analysis to determine if the presence of a genetic disorder is likely followed by counseling and education to arrive at a decision about testing (60).

SCREENING STRATEGIES

Although the pelvic examination is neither highly sensitive nor highly specific in detecting ovarian malignancies, particularly during the early stages of the disease, it is often used in the detection of other gynecologic disorders (including cervical cancer), and it is recommended that the adnexa be palpated during this examination. If an adnexal mass is palpated, further evaluation with transvaginal ultrasonography is indicated. If the mass is found to be a simple cyst, no further workup is indicated. If a complex cyst is found, it can be followed with a repeat pelvic examination and transvaginal ultrasonography and color flow Doppler in 6 to 12 weeks, because many of these are hemorrhagic cysts that subsequently resolve. If a complex cyst persists or increases in size, or if the examination reveals a solid mass, appropriate referral should be made. If the findings of ultrasonography are equivocal, CT or MRI of the pelvis may also be considered.

In 1995, the National Institutes of Health published its consensus on ovarian cancer screening, treatment, and follow-up (61). The consensus panel concluded that there was no available information to support widespread screening with either transvaginal ultrasonography or measurement of CA-125 levels in women without any family history of ovarian cancer. Our review did not reveal any new information to suggest changing this approach. Furthermore, in women with a first-degree relative affected with ovarian cancer and who have a lifetime risk of the disease of 5%, no prospective data are available to support screening, although this risk may be considered sufficiently high by the individual patient and her physician that screening may still be an option.

In patients with two or more first-degree relatives with ovarian cancer, the lifetime risk of the disease increases to at least 6% to 7% and the chances of having a hereditary ovarian cancer syndrome is at least 3% (61). One important step in the evaluation of these patients is consideration of genetic counseling and genetic testing based on the family history, as noted earlier in this chapter. If testing is completed and the patient is found to have one of the inherited syndromes, the patient is at high risk for ovarian cancer. Although the benefit has not been proved and the cost-effectiveness has not yet been determined, the consensus for screening these patients is to perform annual or semiannual pelvic examination and measurement of CA-125 levels and annual ultrasonography (61). The role of prophylactic oophorectomy in these patients is currently unresolved. Although overall risk is increased in those with several affected relatives but without the inherited syndrome, there are no prospective data to support screening. Thus an individualized, shared decision-making approach must be taken in such patients.

CLINICAL PROBLEMS

Clinical Problem 1
A woman with no family history of ovarian cancer or other malignancies presents for a routine physical examination.

Continued

Testing Strategy and Rationale

Such patients are perhaps the most typical of those who present to the clinician. Without further knowledge of specific risk factors for ovarian cancer, these patients have an average lifetime risk of 1.2%. No screening technique has been proved to be of benefit in these patients.

Clinical Example

A 50-year-old postmenopausal woman without a family history of ovarian cancer asks about screening tests for ovarian cancer. She has used oral contraceptives in the past and also has two adult children that resulted from two pregnancies. Her relative risk for ovarian cancer is reduced, and her lifetime risk is probably less than 0.5%. In conjunction with obtaining a Pap smear, a pelvic examination with examination of adnexa is done. If the results of the pelvic and bimanual examination are normal, no further testing is indicated, because the benefits of screening such patients have not been shown. If, however, any adnexal mass is detected, transvaginal ultrasonography should be performed.

Clinical Problem 2

A patient who has a strong family history of ovarian cancer asks about approaches to early detection of cancer.

Testing Strategy and Rationale

This patient is at highest known risk for ovarian cancer, with her lifetime risk at least 6% to 7% with two or more affected family members. The possibility of a hereditary ovarian cancer syndrome must also be considered. Depending on the family history, genetic counseling and testing may be indicated. Based on the evaluation, screening tests such as transvaginal ultrasonography, a color flow Doppler, and/or measurement of the CA-125 level should be considered in addition to performing a pelvic examination.

Clinical Example

A 40-year-old nulliparous woman whose mother, grandmother, aunt, and cousin had ovarian cancer asks about screening tests for early detection. The patient does not have any gynecologic symptoms. Detailed family history suggests a hereditary cancer syndrome. After discussions with a genetic counselor, genetic testing is performed and a genetic abnormality is identified. Given the high lifetime risk for ovarian cancer for this patient (as high as 50%), the clinician and patient decide to begin a screening program that includes periodic pelvic examination, measurement of CA-125 levels, and ultrasonography, recognizing that the benefits of such an approach have not been demonstrated.

REFERENCES

1. **Landis SH, Murray T, Bolden S, Wingo PA.** Cancer statistics, 1998. CA Cancer J Clin. 1998;48:6-29.

2. **Hall JM, Lee MK, Morrow J, et al.** Linkage analysis of early onset familial breast cancer to chromosome 17q21. Science. 1990;250:1684-9.

3. **Bronner CE, Baker SM, Morrison PT, et al.** Mutation in the DNA mismatch repair gene homolog nMLH1 is associated with hereditary nonpolyposis colon cancer. Nature. 1994;368:258-61.

4. **Kerlikowske K, Brown JS, Grady DG.** Should women with familial ovarian cancer undergo prophylactic oophorectomy. Obstet Gynecol. 1992;80:700-7.

5. **Carlson KJ, Skates SJ, Singer DE.** Screening for ovarian cancer. Ann Intern Med. 1994;121:124-32.

6. **Easton DF, Ford D, Matthews FE, et al.** The genetic epidemiology of ovarian cancer. In: Sharp F, Mason WP, Blackett T, Berek J, eds. London: Chapman and Hall; 1995:3-12.

7. **Yancik R, Ries LG, Yates JW.** Ovarian cancer in the elderly: analysis of surveillance, epidemiology and end results of program data. Am J Obstet Gynecol. 1986;154:639.

8. **Hartage P, Schiffman MH, Hoover R, et al.** A case-control study of epithelial ovarian cancer. Am J Obstet Gynecol. 1989;161:10.

9. **Whittemore AS, Harris R, Itnyre J.** The Collaborative Ovarian Cancer Group. Characteristics relating to ovarian cancer risk: collaborative analysis of 12 case-controlled studies. Am J Epidemiol. 1992;136:1184.

10. **Hankinson SE, Colditz GA, Hunter DJ, et al.** A quantitative assessment of oral contraceptive use and risk of ovarian cancer. Obstet Gynecol. 1992;75:106-9.

11. **Andolf E, Jorgensen C, Astedt B.** Ultrasound examination for detection of ovarian carcinoma in risk groups. Obstet Gynecol. 1992;75:106-9.

12. **Van Negell JR Jr, DePriest PD, Puls LE, et al.** Ovarian cancer screening in asymptomatic postmenopausal women with transvaginal ultrasonography. Cancer. 1991;68:458-62.

13. **Einhorn N, Sjovall K, Knapp RC, et al.** Prospective evaluation of serum CA-125 levels for the early detection of ovarian cancer. Obstet Gynecol. 1992;80:14-8.

14. **Finkler NJ, Benacerraf B, Lavin PT, et al.** Comparison of CA125, clinical impression and ultrasound in the preoperative evaluation of ovarian masses. Obstet Gynecol. 1988;72:659-64.

15. **Benacerraf BR, Finler NJ, Wojaechowski C, et al.** Sonographic accuracy in diagnosis of ovarian masses. J Reprod Med. 1990;35:491-5.

16. **Requard CK, Mettler FA Jr, Wick JD.** Preoperative sonography of malignant ovarian neoplasms. Am J Roentgenol. 1981;137:79-82.

17. **Herrmann UJ Jr, Locher GW, Goldhirsch A.** Sonographic patterns of ovarian tumors: prediction of malignancy. Obstet Gynecol. 1987;69:777-81.

18. **Luxman D, Bergman A, Sagi J, et al.** The postmenopausal adnexal mass: correlation between ultrasonography and pathologic findings. Obstet Gynecol. 1991;77:726-8.

19. **Andolf E, Svalenius E, Astedt B.** Ultrasonography for early detection of ovarian carcinoma. Br J Obstet Gynaecol. 1986;93:1286-9.

20. **Andolf E, Jorgensen C, Astedt B.** Ultrasound examination of ovarian carcinoma in risk groups. Obstet Gynecol. 1990;75:106-9.

21. **Goxwamy RK, Campbell S, Whitehead MI.** Screening for ovarian cancer. Clin Obstet Gynecol. 1983;10:621-43.

22. **Campbell S, Royston P, Bhan V, et al.** Novel screening strategies for early ovarian cancer by transabdominal ultrasound. Br J Obstet Gynaecol. 1990;97:304-11.

23. **Campbell S, Bhan V, Royson P, et al.** Comparison of CA125, clinical impression and ultrasound in the preoperative evaluation of ovarian masses. Obstet Gynecol. 1988;72:659-64.

24. **Gransberg S, Norsrom A, Winkland M.** Tumors in the lower pelvis as imaged by vaginal sonography. Gynecol Oncol. 1990;37:224-9.

25. **Sassone AM, Timor-Tritsch IE, Artner A, et al.** Transvaginal sonographic characterization of ovarian disease: evaluation of a new scoring system to predict ovarian malignancy. Obstet Gynecol. 1991;78:70-6.

26. **Van Negell JR Jr, DePriest DP, Puls LE, et al.** Ovarian cancer screening in asymptomatic postmenopausal ovarian size and morphology. Am J Obstet Gynecol. 1986;93:1286-9.

27. **Rodriguez MH, Platt LD, Medearis AL, et al.** The use of transvaginal ultrasonography for evaluation of postmenopausal women by transvaginal ultrasonography. Cancer. 1991;68:458-62.

28. **Bourne TH, Campbell S, Reynolds KM, et al.** Screening for early familial ovarian cancer with transvaginal ultrasonography and colour blood flow imaging. BMJ. 1993;306:1025-9.

29. **Weiner Z, Thaler I, Beck D, et al.** Differentiating malignant tumors from benign ovarian tumors with transvaginal color flow imaging. Obstet Gynecol. 1992;79:159.

30. **DePriest PD, Varner E, Powel J, et al.** The efficacy of a sonographic morphology index in identifying ovarian cancer: a multi-institutional investigation. Gynecol Oncol. 1994;55:174-8.

31. **Bast RC, Klug TL, St John ER, et al.** A radioimmunoassay using monoclonal antibody to monitor the course of epithelial ovarian cancer. N Engl J Med. 1983;309:883.

32. **Helzlsouer KJ, Bush TL, Alberg AJ, et al.** Prospective study of serum CA125 levels as markers of ovarian cancer. JAMA. 1993;269:1123-6.

33. **Kabawat SE, Bast RC, Bhan AK, et al.** Tissue distribution of a coelomic epithelium related antigen recognized by the monoclonal antibody OC125. Int J Gynecol Pathol. 1983;2:275.

34. **Pittaway DE, Fayez JA.** Serum CA125 antigen levels increase during menses. Am J Obstet Gynecol. 1987;156:75-6.

35. **Finkler NJ, Benacerraf B, Lavin PT, et al.** Comparison of serum CA125, clinical impression and ultrasound in the preoperative evaluation of ovarian masses. Obstet Gynecol. 1988;72:659-64.

36. **Einhorn N, Bast RC Jr, Knapp RC, et al.** Preoperative evaluation of serum CA 125 levels in patients with primary ovarian cancer. Obstet Gynecol. 1986;67:414-6.

37. **O'Connell GJ, Ryan E, Murphy KJ, et al.** Predictive value of CA125 for ovarian carcinoma in patients presenting with pelvic masses. Obstet Gynecol. 1987;70:930-2.

38. **Malkasian GD Jr, Knapp RC, Lavin PT, et al.** Preoperative evaluation of serum CA125 levels in premenopausal and postmenopausal patients with pelvic masses: discrimination of benign from malignant disease. Am J Obstet Gynecol. 1988;159:341-6.

39. **Vailev SA, Schlaerth JB, Campeau J, et al.** Serum CA125 levels in preoperative evaluation of pelvic masses. Obstet Gynecol. 1988;71:751-5.

40. **Chen DX, Schwartz PE, Li XG, et al.** Evaluation of CA125 levels in differentiating malignant from benign tumors in patients with pelvic masses. Obstet Gynecol. 1988;72:23-7.

41. **Einhorn N, Knapp RC, Bast RC, et al.** CA125 assay used in conjunction with CA15-3 and TAG-72 assays for discrimination between malignant and non-malignant diseases of the ovary. Acta Oncol. 1989;28:655-7.

42. **Soper JT, Hunter VJ, Daly L, et al.** Preoperative serum tumor-associated antigen levels in women with pelvic masses. Obstet Gynecol. 1990;75:249-54.

43. **Maggino T, Sopracordevole F, Matarese M, et al.** CA125 serum levels in the diagnosis of pelvic masses: comparison with other methods. Eur J Gynecol Oncol. 1987;8:590-5.

44. **Yedema C, Massuger L, Hilgers J, et al.** Preoperative discrimination between benign and malignant ovarian tumors using a combination of CA125 and CA15-3 serum assays. Int J Cancer Suppl. 1988;3:61-7.

45. **Patsner B, Mann WJ.** The value of preoperative serum CA125 levels in patients with pelvic mass. Am J Obstet Gynecol. 1988;158:873-6.

46. **Mogensen O, Mogensen B, Jakobsen A.** CA125 in the diagnosis of pelvic masses. Eur J Cancer Clin Oncol. 1989;25:1187-90.

47. **Cruickshank DJ, Fullerton WT, Klopper A.** The clinical significance of preoperative serum CA125 in ovarian cancer. Br J Obstet Gynaecol. 1987; 94:692-5.

48. **Zurawski VR, Knapp RC, Einhorn N, et al.** An initial analysis of preoperative serum CA 125 levels in patients with early stage ovarian carcinoma. Gynecol Oncol. 1988;30:7-14.

49. **Zanaboni F, Vergadoro F, Presti M, et al.** Tumor antigen CA125 as a marker of ovarian epithelial carcinoma. Gynecol Oncol. 1987;28:61-7.

50. **Brioschi PA, Irion O, Bischof P, et al.** Serum CA125 in epithelial ovarian cancer: a longitudinal study. Br J Obstet Gynaecol. 1987;94:196-201.

51. **Schilthuis MS, Aalders JG, Bouma J, et al.** Serum CA 125 levels in epithelial ovarian cancer: relation with findings at second-look operations and their role in the detection of tumor recurrence. Br J Obstet Gynaecol. 1987;94:202-7.

52. **Zurawski VR Jr, Sjovall K, Schoenfeld DA.** Prospective evaluation of serum CA125 levels in a normal population, phase I: the specificities of single and serial determinations in testing for ovarian cancer. Gynecol Oncol. 1990;36:299-305.

53. **Einhorn N, Sjoval K, Knapp RC.** Prospective evaluation of serum CA125 levels for early detection of ovarian cancer. Obstet Gynecol. 1992;80:14-8.

54. **Boente M, Godwin AK, Hogan WM.** Screening, imaging and early diagnosis of ovarian cancer. Clin Obstet Gynecol. 1994;37:377-90.

55. **Jacobs I, Davies AP, Bridges J, et al.** Prevalence screening for ovarian cancer in postmenopausal women by CA125 measurement and ultrasonography. BMJ. 1993;306:1030-4.

56. **Kramer BS, Gohagan J, Prorok PC, et al.** A National Cancer Institute sponsored screening trial for prostate, lung, colorectal and ovarian cancers. Cancer. 1993;71:589-93.

57. **Johnson RJ.** Review radiology in the management of ovarian cancer. Clin Radiol. 1993;48:75-82.

58. **Buist MR, Golding RP, Burger CW, et al.** Comparative evaluation of diagnostic methods in ovarian carcinoma with emphasis on CT and MRI. Gynecol Oncol. 1994;52:191-8.

59. **Hata K, Hata T, Manabe A, et al.** A critical evaluation of transvaginal Doppler studies, transvaginal sonography, magnetic resonance imaging, and CA 125 in detecting ovarian cancer. Obstet Gynecol. 1992;80:922-6.

60. **Berchuck A, Cirisano F, Lancaster M, et al.** Role of BRCA1 mutation screening in the management of familial ovarian cancer. Am J Obstet Gynecol. 1996;175:738-46.

61. **NIH Consensus Development Panel on Ovarian Cancer.** Ovarian cancer: screening, treatment and follow-up. JAMA. 1995;273:491-7.

Hematologic Problems

Microcytosis

50

Paul F. Griner, MD

KEY POINTS

Pretest Probabilities

- The likelihood that iron deficiency is the cause of anemia in an otherwise healthy woman is probably 80% to 90%.

- Significant microcytosis with minimal or no anemia suggests thalassemia minor; the probability of disease is 90% or greater.

Diagnostic Strategies

- When the pretest probability of iron deficiency is intermediate to high, a low serum ferritin level confirms the diagnosis.

- When the clinical suspicion of iron deficiency is low, a normal serum ferritin level generally rules out the diagnosis.

- In elderly patients and in those with chronic disease, the sensitivity of measurement of serum ferritin is decreased. Measurement of ferritin remains the most predictive test in this situation; however, the likelihood of iron deficiency does not decrease until the test result is well within the normal range.

- An elevated A_2 hemoglobin confirms the diagnosis of β-thalassemia minor.

BACKGROUND

A complete blood count (CBC) includes the determination of the mean erythrocyte (corpuscular) volume (MCV). The term microcytic anemia is used to describe anemia that is accompanied by a reduced MCV, a finding that may be noted in any illness that results in impaired hemoglobin synthesis.

The normal range for MCV is defined arbitrarily as the central 95% of the distribution of MCV among a healthy population, 80 to 96 fL in most laboratories. A high correlation exists between the MCV and the mean corpuscular hemoglobin (MCH) (1). Either may be used as a parameter for the initial evaluation of patients with anemia. Both are more accurate than the assessment of a blood smear in detecting early changes in erythrocyte size and hemoglobin content (2).

Iron deficiency is the most common cause of microcytosis and microcytic anemia. The prevalence varies with age; it is noted in as many as 14% of adult women, 2% of men, and 25% of elderly patients (3,4). Among patients with anemia, classification of those with and those without iron deficiency is important so that its cause (e.g., blood loss) may be identified and treated, so that morbidity caused by iron deficiency per se may be reduced, and so that inappropriate treatment of those whose anemia is not caused by iron deficiency may be avoided.

The thalassemic disorders are the second most common cause of microcytosis among otherwise healthy people. Depending on the disorder, many patients with these hemoglobinopathies can have minimal or no anemia. It is important to differentiate thalassemic disorders from iron deficiency so that unnecessary diagnostic studies or inappropriate treatment with iron is avoided.

Microcytosis is observed in as many as 20% to 30% of patients with anemia who have severe chronic illness. End-stage renal disease, chronic inflammatory disorders such as rheumatoid arthritis, and malignancies account for most cases. Differentiation of microctyosis with these causes from microcytosis caused by iron deficiency is important, again to avoid inappropriate therapy, although some patients with microcytosis with these causes also have iron deficiency. Various disorders of heme synthesis are responsible for the remaining cases of microcytic anemia in adults. They include known exogenous causes such as alcohol, aluminum, isoniazid, and lead, as well as sideroblastic anemia of unknown cause.

ESTIMATING PRETEST PROBABILITY

A careful medical history helps estimate the probability of a specific diagnosis from among the various causes of microcytosis. The sex of the patient, history of blood loss, dietary history, chronic illness, family and ethnic background, and potential toxic exposure are all important.

The probability of iron deficiency anemia may be as high as 80% in women with a history of heavy menses. A craving for clay, starch, or ice may increase the pretest probability to more than 90%. On the other hand, none of these findings is sufficiently sensitive to be very helpful in ruling out the diagnosis of iron deficiency anemia, even when all are absent. For the same reason, the absence of any of the physical findings that have been described in patients with iron deficiency anemia (i.e., glossitis, stomatitis, or spooned nails) is not helpful. The degree of abnormality of erythrocyte indices is helpful. When the MCV is less than 70 fL, or the MCH less than 22 pg, either iron deficiency or thalassemia minor is virtually certain.

A family history of anemia, particularly among patients of Mediterranean or Southeast Asian extraction or among black patients, increases the probability of thalassemia minor. The strongest clue to this diagnosis is the finding of pronounced microcytosis, a normal or near normal hematocrit, and a high-normal or increased erythrocyte count. When these three findings are present, the likelihood of thalassemia minor may be 90% or greater. When they are accompanied by significant morphologic abnormalities on blood smear, such as poikilocytosis, target cells, or basophilic stippling, the diagnosis of thalassemia minor is almost certain.

Hemoglobin E is another cause of microcytosis and erythrocytosis. The trait is prevalent in Southeast Asia, but cases have been recognized in the United States since the resettlement of refugees from this area. As with thalassemia minor, anemia is mild. Even those homozygous for hemoglobin E have relatively mild disease but with marked microcytosis.

Because iron deficiency is so prevalent, one needs to bear in mind that it may coexist with other causes of microcytosis. For example, microcytic anemia in patients with a known chronic illness could be caused by the illness itself, iron deficiency, or both. In complex cases, therefore, evaluation of multiple potential causes of microcytosis may be a sequential process. A history of alcohol abuse or exposure to lead increases the pretest probability of microcytic anemia caused by an exogenous agent.

DIAGNOSTIC TESTS

Tests for Iron Deficiency

Iron deficiency can be established with reasonable certainty if a significant increase in hemoglobin occurs after treatment with iron. This diagnostic method is usually not appropriate because it fails to address promptly the underlying cause of any negative iron balance (such as occult blood loss) and the possible need for identification and treatment of that cause. In addition, some patients without iron deficiency continue to take iron despite lack of benefit, and some such patients are at risk for iron overload. The absence of stainable iron in the bone marrow is highly sensitive and specific for iron deficiency, providing a satisfactory but rarely needed gold standard for the diagnosis.

Ferritin

Ferritin is a serum protein that, with some exceptions, is an accurate indicator of body iron stores (5,6). In nonelderly patients with iron deficiency not complicated by other diseases, the serum ferritin level is almost always below 12 µg/L (5,7–9). Higher levels are noted in elderly persons, and a cutoff of 45 µg/L has been suggested for people older than 65 years (4). False-negative results are often seen when iron deficiency is complicated by liver disease, malignant neoplasms, and chronic diseases, particularly those involving chronic inflammation, such as rheumatoid arthritis (6,7,10). The predictive value of serum ferritin measurement far exceeds that of other tests that have been used to help differentiate iron deficiency from other causes of microcytosis, such as transferrin saturation, erythrocyte protoporphyrin, erythrocyte volume distribution, and mean cell volume (11). Thus, at sensitivities of 90%, ferritin measurement has a specificity of 75%, whereas that of transferrin saturation is only 25%. Conversely, at a specificity of 90%, the sensitivity of ferritin measurement is 85%, whereas that of transferrin saturation is less than 50% (11) (Fig. 50-1).

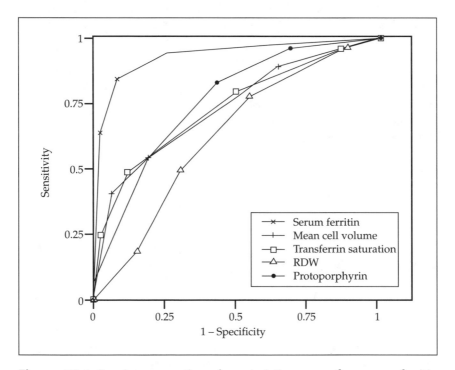

Figure 50-1 Receiver operating characteristic curves for serum ferritin radioimmunoassay, red blood cell protoporphyrin determination, transferrin saturation test, mean cell volume determintion, and red blood cell volume distribution (RDW). For each value of each test, the y-axis represents the sensitivity of the test (the proportion of patients with iron deficiency correctly identified by the test) and the x-axis (1 – specificity) of the test (the proportion of patients without iron deficiency who are falsely classified as having iron deficiency). (Republished with permission from Guyatt GH, Oxman AD, Ali M, et al. Laboratory diagnosis of iron deficiency anemia: an overview. J Gen Intern Med. 1992;7:145-53.)

Other Tests

For several decades, clinicians relied primarily on the serum iron level, total iron binding capacity, and transferrin saturation (i.e., the ratio of serum iron to total iron-binding capacity) for the assessment of body iron stores. The serum iron level is an indicator of the amount of iron available for erythropoiesis. When it is low, the explanation may be either an absolute reduction in iron stores or reduced availability of storage iron. A low transferrin saturation is thus seen not only in patients with iron deficiency but also in as many as one fourth of patients with anemia associated with chronic disease. Early studies suggested that a transferrin saturation of 16% or less detected almost cases of iron deficiency (12). Subsequent studies have shown that this is not the case. Guyatt's analysis shows that even when the cutoff is 5%, the sensitivity of this test may be no higher than 85% (11). Given concerns about both lack of sensitivity and specificity, it is logical to conclude that, compared with serum ferritin measurement, the transferrin saturation has a minimal role in the evaluation of patients with suspected iron deficiency (Table 50-1).

Other tests that have been reported to be helpful in diagnosing anemia caused by iron deficiency include free erythrocyte protoporphyrin (13), red blood cell distribution width (RDW) (14), and serum transferrin receptor (15). None are as helpful as the measurement of serum ferritin alone, particularly when its interpretation is modified for those with concomitant illness; and, even when used in combination with ferritin measurement, the addition of these tests to the predictive power of the serum ferritin level is limited (11).

Table 50-1. Operating Characteristics of Diagnostic Tests for Iron Deficiency Anemia*

Diagnostic Test	Sensitivity	Specificity	Likelihood Ratio	
			Positive Result	Negative Result
	←——— % ———→			
Ferritin (<15 µg/L)	59	99	59	0.41
Ferritin (<25 µg/L)	73	98	37	0.28
Ferritin (<100 µg/L)	94	71	3.2	0.08
Percent saturation transferrin (<10%)	49	88	4.1	0.58

*These values were derived from studies with varied populations, including those with chronic illnesses and inflammatory diseases. Including these patients in these calculations likely understates the tests' sensitivities in otherwise healthy patients with anemia.

Based on data from Guyatt GH, Oxman AD, Ali M, et al. Laboratory diagnosis of iron deficiency anemia: an overview. J Gen Intern Med. 1992;7:145-53.

Tests for Thalassemia and Similar Disorders

Red Blood Cell Count
In most cases of α- or β-thalassemia minor and hemoglobin E, a high-normal or elevated erythrocyte count is observed in conjunction with microcytosis. This finding has an estimated sensitivity of 75% and specificity of 97% and thus tends to distinguish these causes of microcytosis from iron deficiency (16,17).

Hemoglobin Electrophoresis
Globin synthesis is unbalanced in the thalassemias and is caused by either reduced α- or β-chain synthesis. Beta-thalassemia minor is by far the most common (found particularly in patients of Mediterranean descent) and is characterized by an increase in A_2 ($\alpha_2\delta_2$) hemoglobin in virtually all patients (18). Because the finding of an elevated A_2 hemoglobin level is specific, it is accepted as the gold standard for the disease. Conventional hemoglobin electrophoresis may not result in clear separation of A_2 from A_1 hemoglobin. For this reason, some laboratories use column chromatography to determine precisely the A_2 hemoglobin level.

Alpha-thalassemia minor is much less common and is not accompanied by any electrophoretic abnormality. The diagnosis depends on suspicion of thalassemia minor in patients with microcytosis who have a normal to high erythrocyte count, mild anemia, variable morphologic findings on blood smear, and family origin in an area of the world where the prevalence of the thalassemia gene is high (e.g., Southeast Asia or Africa).

Free Erythrocyte Protoporphyrin
In most cases, the tests just described can distinguish thalassemia minor from iron deficiency, lead poisoning, or anemia associated with chronic disease. The measurement of free erythrocyte protoporphyrin (FEP) is helpful in the occasional case that remains unclear because the disorders with which thalassemia minor are most often confused are accompanied by abnormalities of porphyrin metabolism. The free erythrocyte protoporphyrin level is also elevated in most patients with iron depletion (sensitivity, 80%) (11) but is only rarely elevated in patients with thalassemia minor (specificity, 97%) (13).

Red Blood Cell Distribution Width
Electronic particle counters used to calculate erythrocyte indices also generate a parameter, RDW, that reflects variation in erythrocyte size. In patients with thalassemia minor, a uniform decrease in erythrocyte size is observed (14). In patients with anemia caused by iron deficiency or chronic disease, significant variation in erythrocyte size is the rule.

DIAGNOSTIC STRATEGIES

When the pretest estimate of the likelihood of iron deficiency is intermediate to high, a low serum ferritin level is diagnostic (Table 50-2). Conversely, a normal ferritin level generally rules out iron deficiency in patients with low pretest estimates. However, in elderly patients or those with chronic illness, normal ferritin levels may be misleading when the pretest estimate is intermediate to high. As Guyatt and colleagues (4,11) have shown, in such cases the post-test probability of iron deficiency does not decrease unless ferritin values are more than 40 to 45 µg/L in elderly patients and more than 70 µg/L in patients with chronic disease (4,11). Guyatt and colleagues (11) also describe the calculation of distinct likelihood ratios for patients with and without inflammatory diseases that can further aid in the interpretation of test results. Tables 50-1 and 50-2 show the superiority of serum ferritin measurement over the percent saturation of transferrin. Ferritin measurement is superior both for confirming and for ruling out iron deficiency, regardless of the pretest estimate.

If the diagnosis remains unclear in patients with chronic disease, examination of the bone marrow for stainable iron can distinguish between iron deficiency and chronic illness as the cause of the microcytic anemia, but this is rarely necessary. A therapeutic trial of iron is a more practical approach. Patients who do not have iron deficiency will not respond, whereas those who do may or may not respond as the presence of chronic disease may prevent a response. In any case, a trial of iron benefits those who are able to respond.

In most cases, the results of the CBC are sufficient to distinguish thalassemia minor from iron deficiency or other causes of microcyto-

Table 50-2. Post-test Probabilities of Iron Deficiency Anemia Based on Serum Ferritin Measurement and Percent Saturation of Transferrin*

Diagnostic Test	Pretest Probabilities of Iron Deficiency					
	20%		50%		80%	
	Positive Result	Negative Result	Positive Result	Negative Result	Positive Result	Negative Result
	←————————————————— % —————————————————→					
Ferritin (<15 µg/L)	94	9	98	29	99	62
Ferritin (<25 µg/L)	90	6	97	22	99	52
Percent saturation transferrin (<10%)	50	13	80	37	94	69

*These results are based on studies with varied populations, including those with chronic illnesses and inflammatory diseases. Including these patients in these calculations likely understates the tests' ability to rule out disease in otherwise healthy patients with anemia.

sis. The combination of pronounced microcytosis, a high-normal or elevated erythrocyte count, and minimal or no anemia is highly predictive, giving a probability of approximately 90% for thalassemia minor. A supportive blood smear, positive family history, or ancestry from a part of the world where the disease is prevalent essentially establishes the diagnosis. The finding of increased A_2 hemoglobin confirms the diagnosis of β-thalassemia minor. Alpha-thalassemia minor and hemoglobin E can be distinguished by FEP and conventional hemoglobin electrophoresis, respectively.

Evaluation of patients for rare causes of microcytic anemia must be guided by the history. In children, possible environmental exposure to lead calls for the measurement of blood lead levels. In patients with alcoholism who have microcytic anemia without evidence of iron deficiency, a therapeutic trial of pyridoxine may be appropriate. Bone marrow examination identifies refractory sideroblastic anemia. Rare causes of microcytosis such as aluminum toxicity and zinc intoxication can be identified through identification of exposure and determination of serum levels (19,20).

CLINICAL PROBLEMS

Clinical Problem 1

A menstruating woman is found to be anemic; she has no other illness.

Testing Strategy and Rationale

A serum ferritin test should be performed. The prevalence of iron deficiency is fairly high in this population: 14% overall in adult women and possibly as high as 80% in women with heavy menses. Low erythrocyte indices would increase the possibility of iron deficiency, although they are neither highly specific nor highly sensitive for iron deficiency. In patients without complicating illness to interfere with the test results, the serum ferritin level is sensitive and specific for iron deficiency. Therefore, it can reliably confirm or exclude the diagnosis of iron deficiency.

Clinical Example

A 25-year-old woman has had two normal pregnancies and moderately heavy menses. On routine screening, the hematocrit is found to be 33% and the MCV is low-normal. Based on this information, the probability of iron deficiency is estimated to be 80%. The patient's serum ferritin level is 12 μg/L. Post-test probability is 99%. Iron supplementation is begun.

Clinical Problem 2

A patient with anemia has multiple severe chronic medical illnesses.

Testing Strategy and Rationale

A serum ferritin test should be performed. If the patient has no obvious source of iron loss, the probability that the anemia is caused by chronic disease is greater than that of iron deficiency. Such patients often have erythrocyte indices showing a mild microcytic hypochromic picture. In patients with chronic disease, the serum ferritin level may be in the normal range, and the post-test probability of iron deficiency does not decrease unless the ferritin level is in the range of 70 µg/L or more.

Clinical Example

A 56-year-old postmenopausal woman has moderately severe rheumatoid arthritis and moderate impairment of renal function. She is not receiving aspirin or other anti-inflammatory agents. A CBC reveals a hematocrit of 31%, hemoglobin of 10.5 g/dL, and MCV of 73 fL. Stool guaiacs reveal no evidence of occult bleeding. The probability of iron deficiency is estimated to be approximately 20%. Using a cutoff of 25 µg/L, the post-test probability of iron deficiency would be reduced to approximately 6% if the serum ferritin were normal but would be approximately 90% if the result was unexpectedly positive. In such patients, ferritin values in the upper range of normal (i.e., >100 µg/L) are more helpful in excluding iron deficiency than those near the lower limits of normal.

REFERENCES

1. **Croft RF, Streeter AM, O'Neill BJ.** Red cell indices in megaloblastosis and iron deficiency. Pathology. 1974;6:107-17.
2. **Beutler E.** The red cell indices in the diagnosis of iron deficiency anemia. Ann Intern Med. 1959;50:313-22.
3. **Fairbanks VF, Beutler E.** Iron deficiency. In: Williams WJ, Beutler E, Erslev AJ, Lichtman MA, eds. Hematology. New York: McGraw-Hill; 1990: 482-505.
4. **Guyatt GH, Patterson C, Ali M, et al.** Diagnosis of iron deficiency anemia in the elderly. Am J Med. 1990;88:205-9.
5. **Lipschitz DA, Cook JD, Finch CA.** A clinical evaluation of serum ferritin as an index of iron stores. N Engl J Med. 1974;290:1213-6.
6. **Jacobs A, Worwood M.** Ferritin in serum: clinical and biochemical implications. N Engl J Med 1975;292:951-6.
7. **Mazza J, Barr RM, McDonald JWD, et al.** Usefulness of the serum ferritin concentration in the detection of iron deficiency in a general hospital. Can Med Assoc J.1978;119: 884-6.

8. **Walsh JR, Fredrickson M.** Serum ferritin, free erythrocyte protoporphyrin, and urinary iron excretion in patients with iron disorders. Am J Med Sci. 1977;273:293-300.

9. **Kalmin ND, Robson EB, Bettigole RE.** Serum ferritin and marrow iron stores. N Y State J Med. 1978;78:1052-5.

10. **Cook JD.** Clinical evaluation of iron deficiency. Semin Hematol. 1982;19:6-18.

11. **Guyatt GH, Oxman AD, Ali M, et al.** Laboratory diagnosis of iron-deficiency anemia: an overview. J Gen Intern Med. 1992;7:145-53.

12. **Beutler E, Robson MJ, Buttenwieser E.** A comparison of the plasma iron, iron-binding capacity, sternal marrow iron and other methods in the clinical evaluation of iron stores. Ann Intern Med. 1958;48:60-82.

13. **Stockman JA, Weiner LS, Simon GE, et al.** The measurement of free erythrocyte porphyrin (FEP) as a simple means of distinguishing iron deficiency from beta-thalassemia trait in subjects with microcytosis. J Lab Clin Med. 1975;85:113-9.

14. **Thompson SG, Meola T, Lipken M, et al.** Red cell distribution width, mean corpuscular volume, and transferrin saturation in the diagnosis of iron deficiency. Arch Intern Med. 1988;148:2128-30.

15. **Ferguson BJ, Skikne BS, Simpson KM, et al.** Serum transferrin receptor distinguishes the anemia of chronic disease from iron deficiency anemia. J Lab Clin Med. 1992;19:118-26.

16. **Klee GG, Fairbanks VF, Pierre RV, et al.** Routine erythrocyte measurements in diagnosis of iron deficiency anemia and thalassemia minor. Am J Clin Pathol. 1976;66:870-7.

17. **Fairbanks VF, Gilchrist GS, Brimhall B, et al.** Hemoglobin E trait reexamined: a cause of microcytosis and erythrocytosis. Blood. 1979;53:109-15.

18. **Weatherall DJ, Cleff JB.** The Thalassaemia Syndromes. Oxford: Blackwell Scientific Publications; 1981.

19. **Swartz R, Dombrouski J, Burnatowska-Hledin M, Mayor G.** Microcytic anemia in dialysis patients: reversible marker of aluminum toxicity. Am J Kidney Dis. 1987;IX:217-23.

20. **Hoffman HN II, Phyliky RL, Fleming CR.** Zinc-induced copper deficiency. Gastroenterology. 1988;94:508-12.

Macrocytosis $\qquad$ **51**

Jeffrey E. Lancet, MD, and Aaron P. Rapoport, MD

KEY POINTS

Pretest Probabilities

- The probability that a patient with an elevated mean corpuscular volume (MCV) has vitamin B_{12} or folate deficiency depends on the degree of MCV elevation.

- An MCV in the range of 100 to 110 fL is most likely caused by alcoholism, infection with human immunodeficiency virus, hemopoietic stem cell disorders, liver disease, or administration of antineoplastic agents.

- As the MCV increases further, the probability of vitamin B_{12} or folate deficiency also increases, so that an MCV of greater than 130 fL is usually associated with a deficiency of one or both of these vitamins.

Diagnostic Strategies

- In patients with an MCV greater than 110 fL or in patients with a less elevated MCV who have peripheral neuropathy, unexplained cognitive dysfunction, cytopenias, hypersegmentation of neutrophils, or a condition known to mask a macrocytic response, measurement of serum B_{12} and serum or erythrocyte folate levels is indicated.

- If the B_{12} level is found to be less than 250 pg/mL, a two-step Schilling test or possibly measurement of parietal cell antibodies should be performed to determine whether pernicious anemia is present.

- A low erythrocyte folate level should prompt a search for intestinal malabsorption if there is no evidence of decreased dietary intake or increased utilization of folate.

BACKGROUND

Macrocytosis, or elevated mean corpuscular volume (MCV), is an important laboratory finding that refers to the enlargement of erythrocytes. Because hemoglobin production is not affected by the processes responsible for macrocytosis, the MCHC (mean corpuscular hemoglobin concentration) is usually normal, whereas the MCH (mean corpuscular hemoglobin) is elevated in proportion to the MCV (1).

Megaloblastic hemopoiesis is one of the major mechanisms responsible for macrocytosis. It is caused by impairment of DNA synthesis despite normal cytoplasmic growth and maturation, resulting in more time for cell growth between cell divisions and therefore in larger cells. Deficiencies of the vitamins B_{12} and folate are two common causes of megaloblastic hemopoiesis. Disorders of the hemopoietic stem cells—for example, myelodysplastic syndromes, myeloproliferative disorders, acute myelogenous leukemia, aplastic anemia, and sideroblastic anemia—are known to produce megaloblastic changes (1). In addition, drugs that interfere with metabolism or utilization of folate and cobalamin or both may induce megaloblastic changes (Table 51-1) (2).

Mild elevations of MCV are seen in hemorrhage and hemolysis owing to the early release of larger erythrocyte precursors (3). Hypothyroidism can cause an anemia that can be macrocytic in more than 50% of patients (4). High titers of cold agglutinins or high concentrations of immunoglobulins can spuriously increase the electronic MCV (5). Until recently, the most common setting in the United States in which clinicians encountered macrocytosis was ethanol abuse, with macrocytosis occurring in approximately 90% of persons with alcoholism (6), most of whom were not anemic and only one third of whom had evidence of folate deficiency. However, recent studies show that infection with human immunodeficiency virus and the use of zidovudine constitute another frequent cause of macrocytosis (7).

In contrast to other causes of macrocytosis, deficiencies of vitamin B_{12} and folate cause early elevations of the MCV that often precede significant decreases in the hemoglobin level (1).

An elevated MCV can precede clinical suspicion of pernicious anemia by as much as 6 years (8). Thus, attention to macrocytic indices allows the clinician to detect B_{12} and folate deficiencies and treat them before serious sequelae develop. The remainder of this chapter focus-

Table 51-1. Drugs That Cause Megaloblastic Anemia

Class of Drug	Specific Drug
Antifolates	Methotrexate, sulfasalazine, pyrimethamine, trimethoprim/sulfamethoxazole
Purine analogues	6-mercaptopurine, azathioprine, acyclovir
Pyrimidine analogues	5-fluorouracil, zidovudine
Ribonucleotide reductase inhibitors	Hydroxyurea, cytarabine
Anticonvulsants	Phenytoin, phenobarbital
Miscellaneous	p-Aminosalicylate, metformin, colchicine

es on the diagnosis and evaluation of these two important vitamin deficiencies.

ESTIMATING PRETEST PROBABILITY

Erythrocyte indices are so readily available that they are easily ignored. The range of the MCV in healthy persons varies slightly between different laboratories, but the MCV in patients without conditions that produce macrocytosis rarely exceeds 94 fL (9). An elevated MCV was encountered in 17% of hospitalized patients with anemia as well as in some patients without anemia (10).

The likelihood of folate or B_{12} deficiency in a patient with an elevated MCV is in proportion to the degree of the MCV elevation. When the MCV is less than 95 fL, the probability of one of these deficiencies has been estimated to be as low as 0.1% (10). The macrocytosis of alcoholism is a common cause of MCVs in the range of 95 to 110 fL (11). Beyond 110 fL, MCV elevation becomes more predictive of vitamin deficiency. Of patients with an MCV in the range of 115 to 129 fL, nearly half have B_{12} or folate deficiency, whereas nearly all patients with an MCV greater than 130 fL have a deficiency of at least one of these vitamins (12). One exception is patients who take hydroxyurea, in whom the MCV may be 130 fL or higher (13).

The MCV alone, however, is not sensitive enough for B_{12} and folate deficiency that it can be relied on as a sole screening test (14–16), and it may in fact be normal or near normal in disease states such as pernicious anemia. Coexisting iron deficiency or α- or β-thalassemic traits can mask the macrocytosis of B_{12} and folate deficiency and render the MCV normal or even low (15,17). This seems to be particularly true in elderly persons (18). Other clinical and laboratory criteria, such as peripheral neuropathy, psychosis, organic brain syndrome (see comments in Chapter 55), family history of pernicious anemia, malabsorption syndromes, hypersegmented neutrophils on the blood smear, and unexplained cytopenias may help detect patients with potential deficiencies (14,16). Hypersegmentation of neutrophils may be more sensitive than macrocytosis for detecting B_{12} and folate deficiencies. When defined as one neutrophil with six or more lobes or 5% of neutrophils with five or more lobes, hypersegmentation is 98% sensitive for megaloblastic anemia (19,20).

DIAGNOSTIC TESTS

Bone Marrow Examination

Bone marrow examination is the gold standard for the diagnosis of megaloblastic anemia and remains an essential part of the workup in selected cases of macrocytosis and anemia (9). Certain causes for macrocytosis and anemia, such as myelodysplastic and myeloproliferative disorders, may be diagnosed only through examination of the bone marrow. Some authors, however, propose that cobalamin deficiency may occur without characteristic bone marrow findings (21).

Serum B_{12} Level

Competitive binding assays for B_{12} have improved the measurement of this vitamin in serum. Microbiologic methods were laborious, and early radioimmunoassays sometimes missed B_{12} deficiency by detecting inactive cobalamin analogues (22).

With newer assays using purified intrinsic factor as the B_{12} ligand, the sensitivity of the serum B_{12} level for true B_{12} deficiency is extremely high (9), although not 100% (23). However, the serum B_{12} level is not as specific (24). Pregnant women, patients who have had partial gastrectomy, patients with folate deficiency, strict vegetarians, and a few healthy persons may have low serum B_{12} levels without any evidence of B_{12} deficiency even after long-term follow-up (9). The lower limit of the normal range for the serum B_{12} level is approximately 250 pg/mL, although it declines gradually with age (25). Use of a stricter cutoff for the serum B_{12} level (e.g., <100 pg/mL) improves specificity but reduces sensitivity from near 100% to approximately 65% (12).

Although pernicious anemia is the major cause of B_{12} deficiency, it can also result from inadequate dietary intake or defective utilization.

Methylmalonic Acid and Total Homocysteine Concentrations

The metabolites methylmalonic acid and homocysteine accumulate when mammalian cobalamin-dependent enzymatic reactions are impaired, leading to elevated serum levels of both metabolites. Elevations in serum levels of these metabolites are highly sensitive markers of true cobalamin deficiency states, in which they both tend to be elevated (26). Elevation of the serum homocysteine level alone seems to be a reliable indicator of folate deficiency (26). These tests may obviate the need for secondary tests and empiric therapeutic trials when the diagnosis is uncertain (23,26).

Methylmalonic Aciduria

The 24-hour urinary excretion of methylmalonic acid increases in B_{12} deficiency (23) because the enzyme responsible for initiating the degradation of methylmalonate to acetate requires vitamin B_{12}. As an end-product of odd-chain fatty acid oxidation and isoleucine and valine metabolism, methylmalonate accumulates when these substances are given in test quantities. Although this test is highly specific for B_{12} deficiency, its sensitivity is often low until B_{12} deficiency becomes profound (3).

Deoxyuridine Suppression Test

This sensitive test measures the impaired synthesis of thymidine, which is the biochemical defect present in both B_{12} and folate deficiency that is responsible for megaloblastosis. By selective replacement of folate or B_{12}, the assay permits determination of the missing vitamin(s). However, this test is not widely used because it requires tissue culture techniques for bone marrow aspirate and because simpler tests are available.

Schilling Test

Pernicious anemia is best diagnosed by the Schilling test. In the two-step Schilling test, the patient is administered oral crystalline radioactive B_{12} alone and then crystalline radioactive B_{12} bound to hog intrinsic factor. A large "flushing" dose of cold B_{12} is given simultaneously to block liver uptake sites and to displace radioactive B_{12} that becomes bound to tissue receptors. A 24-hour urine collection is done after each step to determine the percentage of ingested radioactive B_{12} excreted in the urine. Healthy persons excrete more than 7% to 8% of the administered radioactive B_{12} after each step. Patients with pernicious anemia (i.e., parietal cell atrophy leading to intrinsic factor deficiency) excrete less than 7% of radioactive B_{12} when it is administered alone but excrete normal amounts when given intrinsic factor as well. Patients who have low excretion patterns after both steps may have intestinal malabsorption syndromes, such as sprue, Crohn disease, or bacterial overgrowth, although many such patients have B_{12} deficiency on the basis of pernicious anemia but exhibit the transient ileal dysfunction that commonly accompanies megaloblastic anemia (22,27). Thus, many clinicians prefer to perform the Schilling test 1 week or more after parenteral B_{12} supplementation is begun.

A difficulty with the two-step Schilling test is the need to have patients complete two accurate 24-hour urine collections. A one-step, double isotope Schilling test allows patients to complete both phases of the test with one urine collection. However, this version leads to a higher frequency of indeterminate results (27). An alternative for patients who cannot perform the urine collections is the collection of a blood sample 8 to 10 hours after the start of the Schilling test and the measurement of radioactive B_{12} in the serum (9).

A potential pitfall of the Schilling test is its reduced sensitivity in the early stages of pernicious anemia. Patients may have false-negative test results because those with parietal cell atrophy tend to lose the ability to split B_{12} from the peptide bonds attaching it to food proteins before they lose the ability to absorb unbound crystalline B_{12} (28-30).

Intrinsic Factor and Parietal Cell Antibodies

Intrinsic factor "blocking-type" antibodies appear in 50% to 60% of patients with pernicious anemia (22). False-positive test results are rare but can occur after administration of radioisotopes used in nuclear imaging studies and in patients receiving exogenous B_{12} (31). Thus, the specificity of this test is highest when these antibodies are measured more than 1 week after administration of either B_{12} supplement or scintigraphic agents.

The presence of parietal cell antibodies are sensitive but nonspecific for pernicious anemia, occurring in 84% of patients with this disorder but also in approximately 50% of patients with gastritis and in 5% to 22% of healthy persons (1). This test may be useful in evaluating patients with possible pernicious anemia in that a negative test may obviate the need for performing the more cumbersome Schilling test.

Gastric Acid Secretion

When defined by a basal gastric pH greater than 6.0 and a decrease in pH of less than 1 unit after histamine challenge, achlorhydria is found in virtually all patients with pernicious anemia (1). The absence of achlorhydria thus effectively rules out pernicious anemia as a cause for B_{12} deficiency or megaloblastic anemia. Although not frequently used, this test is probably the most rapidly available screening test for pernicious anemia.

A promising new diagnostic modality for detecting pernicious anemia is the modified magnesium hydrogen breath test. This simple test has recently been reported to be highly sensitive and specific for the detection of achlorhydria in a small group of patients with known pernicious anemia (32). Larger prospective studies are needed to determine if this test is superior to other available methods for detecting achlorhydria.

Serum and Erythrocyte Folate

Serum folate levels are now measured by radioimmunoassay; earlier assays depended on cumbersome microbiologic methods. Unlike B_{12} deficiency, which can take decades to develop in adults who do not ingest B_{12} but can absorb it, folate balance is critically dependent on dietary intake. In patients who fast for several days (e.g., after surgery) a steady decline in serum folate levels may develop. For this reason, the serum folate level is not regarded as an optimal index of tissue folate status.

Erythrocyte folate is 30-fold more concentrated than serum folate, is incorporated into the cell early in erythropoiesis, and is trapped there. A low erythrocyte folate level is a strong indication of a depleted folate pool (33). The erythrocyte folate can be misleading, however, because vitamin B_{12} facilitates entry of folate into cells and promotes retention. Thus in B_{12} deficiency states one may encounter a low erythrocyte folate level, a high serum folate level, and overall normal folate stores (24). Also, because of the long lifespan of erythrocytes, the erythroctye folate level can lag behind a folate deficiency state by months. Other tests for folate deficiency such as folate clearance studies and formiminoglutamate (FIGLU) excretion are useful but not commonly used (33). When folate deficiency cannot be explained by poor dietary intake, as in patients with alcoholism who are malnourished, or by increased requirement, as in pregnant women or patients with sickle cell disease or chronic hemolytic anemia, further workup for malabsorption states should be undertaken (34).

Neutrophil Myeloperoxidase Activity

Owing to skipped cellular divisions during maturation, there appears to be an increased number of myeloperoxidase-laden granules in megaloblastic neutrophils (35). However, with evaluation of neutrophil myeloperoxidase activity, potential false-positive test results occur frequently in patients who smoke cigarettes and in those with iron deficiency (36,37). Thus, because of its limited availability and low specificity, this test is less likely to be used in the evaluation of megaloblastic changes.

DIAGNOSTIC STRATEGIES

Evaluating macrocytosis is important because this condition may be the first clue to serious yet treatable deficiencies of vitamins B_{12} and folate. Unless the MCV is greater than 110 fL, macrocytosis is not highly predictive for these conditions, yet the clinician must bear in mind that normal or near-normal erythrocyte indices are by no means sufficient to rule out these vitamin deficiencies. Mild to moderate elevations of the MCV are more specific for folate or B_{12} deficiencies when associated with peripheral neuropathy, unexplained cognitive impairment, hypersegmentation of neutrophils, or cytopenias. In any patients with one of these clinical findings or an elevation in MCV close to or more than 110 fL , serum B_{12} and serum or erythrocyte folate levels should initially be measured by radioimmunoassay. Measurement of either the serum or erythrocyte folate level should be useful in ambulatory patients, whereas measurement of the erythrocyte folate level may be preferable in acutely ill hospitalized patients.

If the serum B_{12} level is less than 250 pg/mL (184 pmol/L), a Schilling test or possibly measurement of parietal cell antibodies should be performed. Positive results for either of these tests confirms the diagnosis of B_{12} deficiency on the basis of pernicious anemia. When the clinical suspicion of pernicious anemia remains high despite normal or equivocal Schilling test results, measurement of serum methylmalonic acid and total homocysteine levels can be helpful. Bone marrow aspirate to detect megaloblastic changes may also be considered. In equivocal cases, repeating the Schilling test and measurement of serum B_{12} level months later may help clarify the diagnosis. A low serum B_{12} level (i.e., one less than 250 pg/mL) should never be ignored.

A low erythrocyte folate level may sometimes accompany primary B_{12} deficiency, but the serum folate level is usually high in such cases. If the serum folate level is low (ambulatory patients) or if the erythrocyte folate level is low while the B_{12} level is normal (ambulatory or hospitalized patients), a presumptive diagnosis of folate deficiency should be made. If the erythrocyte folate level is normal when the clinical suspicion of folate deficiency is high, measurement of a serum folate level may be useful because erythrocyte folate levels can remain normal in the early stages of folate depletion. Unless the clinical history reveals a satisfactory reason for folate deficiency, such as anticonvulsant use (inhibits folate absorption), pregnancy, or a disorder requiring increased intake (hemolytic anemia), the patient should be evaluated for malabsorption. Approximately 10% to 30% of cases of folate deficiency are accompanied by a mildly reduced B_{12} level (9,34), which usually disappears with folate administration.

Therapeutic trials to diagnose megaloblastic anemias are now generally outmoded by the aforementioned laboratory methods, which are less expensive and more reliable. These trials may be useful in parts of the world where serum vitamin assays are not readily available. In a therapeutic trial, low doses of either folate (200 µg/d) or B_{12} (1 to 2 µg/d) are given, and the reticulocyte response is compared with pretreatment values. Usually the reticulocyte count increases after 2 to 3 days of therapy and peaks after 5 to 8 days. The other vitamin is added if the reticulocyte response is not significant (1). The anemia usually resolves within 1 to 2 months, when the correct therapy has been instituted. It is important to properly diagnose B_{12} and folate deficiency because treatment of pernicious anemia with folate can result in a hematologic response but does not prevent neurologic complications.

CLINICAL PROBLEMS

Clinical Problem 1

A man with a long history of heavy alcohol intake has an elevated MCV and a low hemoglobin level.

Testing Strategy and Rationale

Both serum B_{12} level and serum or erythrocyte folate level should be measured. Many patients who abuse alcohol have macrocytosis, but usually the MCV is less than 110 fL and anemia is absent in these patients. Patients with an MCV greater than 110 fL should be evaluated for megaloblastic anemia. An examination of the blood smear should always be done. Round cell macrocytes are typically seen in the macrocytosis of alcoholism. Although folate deficiency is a much more common cause of megaloblastic anemia in patients with alcoholism than is B_{12} deficiency, levels of both should be checked. Low erythrocyte folate levels may accompany primary B_{12} deficiency.

Clinical Example
A thin, 45-year-old man with a 6-month history of heavy alcohol use comes to the emergency room. Routine studies show a hemoglobin concentration of 10 g/dL and an MCV of 116 fL. The blood film smear shows one six-lobed neutrophil and several with five lobes. The erythrocytes are large and ovoid. Measurement of serum or erythrocyte folate level and of serum B_{12} level should be done.

Clinical Problem 2
A middle-aged black patient is noted to have anemia and a mildly elevated MCV.

Testing Strategy and Rationale
The pretest probability that a patient with anemia and an MCV within or near the normal range has megaloblastic anemia is extremely low. However, black patients can have the α-thalassemic trait, which can mask the macrocytosis of megaloblastic anemia (14). An examination of the blood smear may disclose hypersegmentation of neutrophils, increasing the pretest probability of megaloblastic anemia. The serum or erythrocyte folate level and serum B_{12} level should be measured.

Clinical Example
During a routine health evaluation, a 60-year-old black man is found to have a hemoglobin of 9 g/dL and an MCV of 97 fL. The peripheral blood smear shows slightly enlarged erythrocytes and abundant five-lobed neutrophils. Basophilic stippling of the erythroctyes, which is characteristic of α- or β-thalassemia traits, is also seen. The serum B_{12} level is found to be low at 86 pg/mL, whereas the erythrocyte folate level is just slightly low at 100 ng/mL. The serum folate level is found to be high at 20 ng/mL. A Schilling test shows excretion of 0.5% of ingested labeled B_{12}, which increases to 14% when intrinsic factor is given. A diagnosis of pernicious anemia is made and parenteral B_{12} injections are begun.

REFERENCES

1. **Wintrobe MM, Lee GR, Boggs DR, et al.** Clinical Hematology. 8th ed. Philadelphia: Lea and Febiger; 1981:559-604.
2. **Beutler E, Lichtman MA, Coller BS, Kipps TJ.** Williams Hematology. 5th ed. New York: McGraw Hill; 1995:471-89.
3. **Chanarin I.** Investigation and management of megaloblastic anemia. Clin Hematol. 1976;5:747-63.
4. **Horton L, Coburn RJ, England JM, Himsworth RL.** The hematology of hypothyroidism. Q J Med. 1976;45:101-24.
5. **Hattersley PG, Gerard PW, Caggiano V, Nash DR.** Erroneous values on the Model S Coulter Counter due to high titer cold autoagglutinins. Am J Clin Pathol. 1971;55:442-6.
6. **Wu A, Chanarin I, Slavin G, Levi AJ.** Folate deficiency in the alcoholic: its relationship to clinical and haematological abnormalities, liver disease and folate stores. Br J Haematol. 1975;29:469-78.
7. **Snower DP, Weil SC.** Changing etiology of macrocytosis: zidovudine as a frequent causative factor. Am J Clin Pathol. 1993;99:57-60.
8. **Carmel R.** Macrocytosis, mild anemia, and delay in the diagnosis of pernicious anemia. Arch Intern Med. 1979;139:47-50.
9. **Chanarin I.** How to diagnose (and not misdiagnose) pernicious anemia. Blood Rev. 1987;1:280-3.
10. **Griner PF, Oranburg PR.** Predictive values of erythrocyte indices for tests of iron, folic acid, and vitamin B_{12} deficiency. Am J Clin Pathol. 1978;70: 748-52.
11. **Colman N, Herbert V.** Hematological complications of alcoholism: overview. Semin Hematol. 1980;17:164-76.
12. **McPhedran P, Barnes MG, Weinstein JS, Robertson JS.** Interpretation of electronically determined macrocytosis. Ann Intern Med. 1973;78:677-83.
13. **Charace S, Dover JG, Morre RD, et al.** Hydroxyurea: effects on hemoglobin F production in patients with sickle cell anemia. Blood. 1992;10:2555-65.
14. **Carmel R.** Pernicious anemia. Arch Intern Med. 1988; 148:1712-4.
15. **Spivak J.** Masked megaloblastic anemia. Arch Intern Med. 1982;142:2111-4.
16. **Thompson WG, Babitz L, Cassino C, et al.** Evaluation of current criteria used to measure vitamin B_{12} levels. Am J Med. 1987;82:291-4.
17. **Green R, Kuhl W, Jacobson R, et al.** Masking of macrocytosis by alpha thalassemia in blacks with pernicious anemia. N Engl J Med. 1982;307:1322-5.
18. **Pennypacker LC, Allen RH, Kelly JP, et al.** High prevalence of cebalamin deficiency in elderly outpatients. J Am Geriatr Soc. 1992;40:1197-204.
19. **Lindenbaum J, Nath B.** Megaloblastic anemia and neutrophil hypersegmentation. Br J Haematol. 1980;44:511-3.
20. **Herbert V.** Experimental nutritional folate deficiency in man. Trans Assoc Am Physicians. 1962;75:307-20.
21. **Carmel R, Sinow RM, Karnaze DS.** Atypical cobalamin deficiency. J Lab Clin Med. 1987;109:454-63.
22. **Lindenbaum J.** Status of laboratory testing in the diagnosis of megaloblastic anemia. Blood. 1983;61:624-7.

23. **Lindenbaum J, Savage DG, Stabler SP, Allen RH.** Diagnosis of cobalamin deficiency: II. Relative sensitivities of serum cobalamin, methylmalonic acid, and total homocysteine concentrations. Am J Hematol. 1990;34:99-107.

24. **Herbert V.** Biology of disease: megaloblastic anemias. Lab Invest. 1985; 52:3-19.

25. **Fairbanks VF, Elveback LR.** Tests of pernicious anemia: serum vitamin B_{12} assay. Mayo Clin Proc. 1983;58:135-7.

26. **Savage DG, Lindenbaum JL, Stabler SP, Allen RH.** Sensitivity of serum methylmalonic acid and total homocysteine determinations for diagnosing cobalamin and folate deficiencies. Am J Med. 1994;96:239-46.

27. **Fairbanks VF, Wahner HW, Phyliky RL.** Tests of pernicious anemia: the "Schilling Test." Mayo Clin Proc. 1983;58:541-4.

28. **Herbert V.** Don't ignore low serum cobalamin (vitamin B12) levels. Arch Intern Med. 1988;148:1705-7.

29. **Doscherholmen A, McMahon J.** Dual isotope Schilling test for measuring absorption of food-bound and free vitamin B_{12} [Abstract]. Clin Res. 1982; 30:772a.

30. **Doscherholmen A, McMahon J, Ripley D.** Inhibitory effect of eggs on vitamin B_{12} absorption: description of a simple ovalbumin 57 co vitamin B_{12} absorption test. Br J Haematol. 1976;33:261.

31. **Fairbanks VF, Lennon VA, Kokmen E, Howard FM.** Tests for pernicious anemia: serum intrinsic factor blocking antibody. Mayo Clin Proc. 1983;58: 203-4.

32. **Humbert P, Lopez de Soria P, Fernandez-Banares F, et al.** Magnesium hydrogen breath test using end expiratory sampling to assess achlorhydria in pernicious anemia patients. Gut. 1994;35:1205-8.

33. **Chanarin I.** Folate and cobalamin. Clin Hematol. 1985;14:629-41.

34. **Carmel R.** The laboratory diagnosis of megaloblastic anemias (medical progress). West J Med. 1978;128:294-304.

35. **Gulley ML, Bentley SA, Ross DW.** Neutrophil myeloperoxidase measurement uncovers masked megaloblastic anemia. Blood. 1990;76:1004-7.

36. **Dash S, Sen S, Behera D.** High neutrophil myeloperoxidase activity in smokers. Blood. 1991;77:1619.

37. **Reardon DM, Hewitt J.** The effect of haemoglobin on the Technicon H6000 eosinophil count. Clin Lab Haematol.1986;8:369.

Erythrocytosis

52

Barbara E. Weber, MD, MPH, and James Budd, MD

KEY POINTS

Pretest Probabilities

- In patients with erythrocytosis who smoke, there is a 98% likelihood that the disease is related to smoking owing to associated volume contraction, carboxyhemoglobinemia, or oxygen desaturation.

- Physicians frequently overestimate the likelihood of polycythemia vera and tumor-related erythrocytosis. However, as treatable causes with major morbidity, they are important to exclude, especially in nonsmokers.

- The probability that a patient with polycythemia has an increased erythrocyte mass increases as the hematocrit level increases.

Diagnostic Strategies

- The patient with a very high hematocrit level (>57% in men, >52% in women) merits a full workup, including abdominal imaging in most cases.

- In asymptomatic patients with mild erythrocytosis, normal spleen size, and normal platelet and leukocyte counts, a limited evaluation is appropriate. If a renal mass has been excluded, close clinical follow-up without further workup is probably sufficient.

BACKGROUND

Both hematocrit and hemoglobin determinations are concentration measurements: An elevated hematocrit or hemoglobin level may reflect an increased erythrocyte mass (absolute polycythemia), a reduced plasma volume (relative polycythemia), or both. This distinction has important therapeutic implications and is a central issue in the evaluation of patients with erythrocytosis.

Patients with erythrocytosis can generally be assigned to one of four pathophysiologic categories as shown in Figure 52-1. A large proportion have a relative polycythemia, caused primarily by a contracted plasma volume rather than by a true expansion of the erythrocyte mass. Typical patients in this category are men, have hypertension, are moderately obese, and often are smokers (1). The remaining patients with erythrocytosis have an increased erythrocyte mass. Many of these patients have secondary polycythemia, caused either by an appropriate erythropoietic response to tissue hypoxia or by inappropriate secretion of an erythropoietin-like substance by a neoplasm or locally ischemic renal cortex. The balance have a clonal neoplastic disorder of hematopoietic stem cells that have escaped the usual erythropoietic regulation (i.e., polycythemia vera). The term idiopathic erythrocytosis is used to describe erythrocytosis in patients who cannot be found to have either polycythemia vera or secondary polycythemia.

The physician faced with a patient with polycythemia must consider the frequency of possible causes, the characteristics of available diagnostic tests, and the utility of pursuing a specific diagnosis. The conditions for which a specific diagnosis is likely to affect treatment and prognosis significantly are polycythemia vera and erythrocytosis secondary to a neoplasm. Treatment of polycythemia vera improves sur-

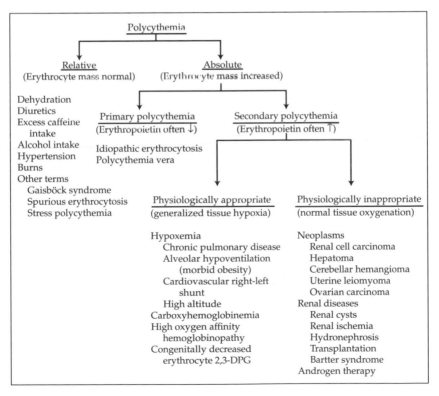

Figure 52-1. Causes of elevated hematocrit values.

vival. Renal cell carcinoma is the malignancy most commonly associated with erythrocytosis and, if present, must be detected and treated.

ESTIMATING PRETEST PROBABILITY

The history and physical examination often suggest a cause for erythrocytosis. Findings may suggest arterial oxygen desaturation caused by smoking, chronic pulmonary disease, cyanotic heart disease, or morbid obesity. Some patients have overt polycythemia vera with splenomegaly, leukocytosis, and thrombocytosis; and, rarely, patients have the classic triad of flank pain, an abdominal mass, and hematuria, suggesting renal cell carcinoma. However, even if basic laboratory data are obtained, as many as 25% of patients do not have a clear diagnosis without additional testing (2).

Several factors help estimate pretest probabilities of the various causes of polycythemia. The likelihood that a true increase in erythrocyte mass has occurred varies directly depending on the level of hematocrit elevation (Table 52-1) (3). Relative polycythemia is very unlikely in men with hematocrit levels of 60% or greater or in women with levels of 55% or more. The difference between the ranges of normal hematocrit levels in men and women is due to androgens, which both increase erythropoietin production and enhance the effect of erythropoietin on bone marrow.

Three to five percent of patients who smoke have erythrocytosis (600–1000 per 100,000 persons) (4,5), accounting for the most cases of mild to moderate elevations in hematocrit levels. Two thirds of these patients have physiologic expansion of erythrocyte mass caused by carboxyhemoglobinemia, increased oxygen affinity of remaining hemoglobin, or associated pulmonary disease. One third have a contracted plasma volume as the primary cause of the elevated hematocrit level (6). In patients with chronic obstructive pulmonary disease, the

Table 52-1. Probability of Increased Erythrocyte Mass as a Function of Hematocrit

Hematocrit		Probability
Men	Women	
← % →		
<52	<47	15
52–55	47–50	35–40
56–57	51–52	45
58–59	53–54	65
≥60	≥55	99

relation between oxygen saturation and erythrocyte mass, erythropoietin level, and hematocrit is variable (7–9).

Erythrocytosis secondary to neoplasms is rare. The annual incidence of renal cell carcinoma in the United States is less than 11 cases per 100,000 persons (10), with 1% to 5% of these having associated erythrocytosis (11). Hepatoma is even less common, with 5% to 10% of patients having associated erythrocytosis (12). Finding an abdominal mass increases the probability of such neoplasms in a patient with erythrocytosis.

Polycythemia vera has a prevalence of 10 cases per 100,000 persons. Polycythemia vera is unusual in person younger than 40 years old: 95% of patients are aged 40 years or older, and 84% are aged 50 years or older (3). Polycythemia Vera Study Group criteria for the clinical diagnosis of polycythemia vera (Table 52-2) can distinguish a homogeneous group of patients with polycythemia vera but may lead to the exclusion of atypical and early forms (13,14). Three fourths of patients with polycythemia vera have palpable splenomegaly, leukocytosis, or thrombocytosis at presentation. Splenomegaly is not a feature of causes of erythrocytosis other than polycythemia vera. Although it can be readily found by abdominal imaging, it can be missed by physical examination (15,16). Table 52-3 details test characteristics for detecting an enlarged spleen.

Thus, basic clinical information can help estimate the probability of various causes of erythrocytosis in a given patient. A polycythemic patient who smokes has roughly a 98% likelihood of smoking-related erythrocytosis. Approximately 1% of smokers with erythrocytosis have polycythemia vera, and fewer than 0.1% have tumor-related polycythemia. In nonsmokers, the prevalence of relative polycythemia is less clear, but probably still accounts for most cases of erythrocytosis. Polycythemia vera is present in approximately one third of nonsmoking patients with erythrocytosis, and physiologically appropriate sec-

Table 52-2. Polycythemia Vera Study Group Criteria for Diagnosis of Polycythemia Vera*

Category A	Category B
A1: Total erythrocyte volume Men ≥36 mL/kg Women ≥32 mL/kg	B1: Thrombocytosis, >400,000/mm^3
A2: Arterial oxygen saturation >92%	B2: Leukocytosis, >12,000/mm^3 (no fever or infection)
A3: Splenomegaly	B3: Leukocyte alkaline phosphatase score >100
	B4: Serum vitamin B_{12} >900 pg/mL

*Clinical diagnosis of polycythemia vera: A1 + A2 + A3, or A1 + A2 + any two from category B.

Table 52-3. Operating Characteristics of Diagnostic Tests Used in the Evaluation of Patients with Erythrocytosis

Test	Diagnosis	Sensitivity	Specificity	Likelihood Ratio	
				Positive Result	Negative Result
		← % →			
History					
Aquagenic pruritis	PV	40–60	high	**	**
Smoking	Smoker's polycythemia	5	98	2.5	0.97
Physical					
Abdominal examination	Splenomegaly (PV)	70	100	∞	0.30
Positive Traube space (percussion and palpation)	Splenomegaly (any cause)	46	97	15	0.56
Positive Traube space (percussion *or* palpation)	Splenomegaly (any cause)	72	68	2.3	0.41
Laboratory					
Increased erythrocyte mass	PV	90	50	1.8	0.2
Leukocyte >12,000/mm^3	PV	43	94	7.2	0.61
Platelet >400,000/mm^3	PV	63	80	3.2	0.46
Serum B$_{12}$ level >900 pg/mL	PV	36	70	1.2	0.91
Oxygen saturation >92%	PV	89	88	7.4	0.13
LAP score >100	PV	70	90	7.0	0.33
Endogenous erythroid culture	PV	89–93	65–74	2.5–3.6	0.09–0.17
Low-normal erythropoietin level	PV	64–94	96–99	16–94	0.06–0.38
High erythropoietin level	Secondary erythrocytosis	98–100	30–70	1.4–3.3	0–0.07
Imaging					
Intravenous pyelography	Renal mass	90	75–80	4.0	0.13
Abdominal CT	Renal mass	90–95	98	46	0.07
Abdominal ultrasonography	Renal mass	83–98	94	15	0.10
Radioisotope spleen scan	Splenomegaly (PV)	90	?	**	**
PVSG criteria					
"A1 + A2 + A3"*	PV	79	?	**	**

PV = polycythemia vera; LAP = leukocyte alkaline phosphate; CT = computed tomography; PVSG = Polycythemia Vera Study Group.

*See Table 52-2.

** = not available.

ondary polycythemia or nonmalignant renal disease accounts for most of the remaining cases. Tumors account for less than 1% of cases of erythrocytosis even in nonsmokers.

DIAGNOSTIC TESTS

Blood Cell Counts

For patients with polycythemia vera, the leukocyte count is greater than $12,000/mm^3$ in more than 40%, with the platelet count greater than $400,000/mm^3$ in more than 60% (3). The presence of elevations in all three cell lines and splenomegaly is highly specific for polycythemia vera. However, these elevations individually are nonspecific. Heavy cigarette smoking causes a chronic increase in the leukocyte count, with 10% of white persons who smoke having leukocyte counts greater than $11,000/mm^3$ (17). Six to twenty percent of cases of renal cell and hepatocellular carcinomas may also be associated with mild leukocytosis and thrombocytosis (11).

Blood Oxygen Saturation

Blood oxygen saturation less than 92% is sufficient to cause tissue hypoxia and erythropoietin secretion. Marrow responsiveness and erythrocyte survival determines whether erythrocytosis ensues. Oxygen saturation should be measured directly rather than extrapolated from the arterial oxygen tension and normal hemoglobin–oxygen dissociation curve, because the accuracy of extrapolated values is affected by shifts in the curve due to acid-base disturbance, abnormal hemoglobin, or 2,3-DPG deficiency. Desaturation may be positional or diurnal, and evaluation of the patient with chronic cardiopulmonary disease or morbid obesity may require supine or nocturnal measurements (18). In patients for whom the cause of secondary polycythemia is obvious (see Fig. 52-1), one should begin the evaluation with a measurement of arterial blood gas.

Other causes of erythrocytosis must be considered even in the presence of oxygen desaturation. Eleven percent of the PVSG population had oxygen saturations less than 92% (3). Thus, the diagnosis of "appropriate" secondary polycythemia should not preclude periodic re-evaluation of hematologic parameters. An increasing hematocrit level in a patient with stable cardiopulmonary disease should prompt further evaluation.

Carboxyhemoglobin

Inhaled carbon monoxide binds avidly to hemoglobin, which becomes unavailable for oxygen transport. The remaining hemoglobin molecules have increased oxygen affinity, further impairing tissue oxygen delivery. Because carboxyhemoglobin has a half-life of 4 hours, blood levels are highly variable, depending on the number of cigarettes smoked and the length of time since the last cigarette. Measurement should be done in the afternoon on a day of typical consumption. A level greater than 4% is sufficient to cause erythrocytosis.

Erythrocyte Mass and Plasma Volume

Hematocrits 60% or greater in men and 55% or more in women are virtually always associated with true polycythemia (see Table 52-1) and need not be evaluated with measurement of erythrocyte mass, especially if splenomegaly is present (19). With lesser degrees of erythrocytosis, nuclear medicine blood volume studies often demonstrate relative rather than true polycythemia. Both erythrocyte mass and plasma volume should be determined simultaneously, because one does not predict the other reliably. The "expected" mass varies with body habitus and is predicted by several nomograms (20).

Smokers commonly have both an elevated erythrocyte mass and low plasma volume. Because plasma volume changes occur quickly, such patients show a decrease in hematocrit within 4 days of abstinence (6). Such a diagnostic trial may be useful in compliant patients.

Ten percent of patients meeting PVSG criteria for polycythemia vera have normal erythrocyte masses (3). Close follow-up of hematologic parameters is therefore indicated for patients with normal erythrocyte mass who do not exhibit the features typically associated with relative polycythemia.

Hemoglobin Electrophoresis

Patient presenting with erythrocytosis infrequently have a hemoglobin variant, usually familial, with increased oxygen affinity. Oxygen delivery is impaired despite normal blood oxygen saturation, causing appropriate erythropoietin secretion. Routine hemoglobin electrophoresis is a poor screening test for such patients, because it does not differentiate most such variant molecules (21). A simple preliminary assessment can be made by measuring the partial pressure of oxygen and oxygen saturation of venous blood and plotting the point on the normal dissociation curve; a point to the left of the curve indicates increased oxygen affinity (22). Determination of the hemoglobin–oxygen dissociation curve for these cases shows a "left shift" and a P_{50} that is generally less than 20 mm Hg. (21).

Imaging Studies To Detect a Renal Mass

More than 85% of patients with renal cell carcinoma have at least one of the three findings of hematuria, flank pain, or a palpable mass. Rarely, a patient presents with erythrocytosis as the sole manifestation of disease, often at a curable stage.

Several strategies have been proposed for the detection and diagnosis of a renal mass (23–26). Table 52-3 lists the test characteristics for the various imaging modalities. Intravenous pyelography is relatively inexpensive and may detect other renal disorders that can cause erythrocytosis but may miss small central lesions and fails to distinguish cystic from solid masses. Computed tomography (CT) scanning offers higher sensitivity and specificity but at a higher cost. Ultrasonography offers intermediate sensitivity and specificity without the use of radiation or contrast. Both CT and ultrasonography can also be used to detect splenomegaly.

Erythropoietin Level

Sensitive radio-immunoassay and enzyme-immunoassay techniques for measuring erythropoietin are now readily available. Early studies suggested that the assay has excellent discriminating ability—that is, low levels of erythropoietin were found in patients with polycythemia vera, and high levels were found in those with the various secondary polycythemias. This was confirmed in a recent study showing that a low erythropoietin level had a sensitivity of 72% and specificity of 99% for distinguishing patients with polycythemia vera from those with secondary polycythemia and idiopathic erythrocytosis (27). However, a review of six other studies since 1986 showed substantial overlap in erythropoietin levels between those with polycythemia vera and those with secondary polycythemia (28). Although an elevated serum erythropoietin level effectively rules out polycythemia vera and a very low level is highly suggestive of polycythemia vera, intermediate levels are common and leave the diagnosis in doubt. These assays also may not reliably detect ectopic, erythropoietin-like substances, and therefore do not exclude a diagnosis of neoplasia.

Erythroid Tissue Culture

When erythroid cells from blood or bone marrow of polycythemia vera patients are cultured, "endogenous colonies" grow in the absence of erythropoietin, unlike cultures from patients with other types of erythrocytosis that are erythropoietin dependent. This technique may prove discriminating in the early diagnosis of polycythemia vera. In a study of 108 patients referred for evaluation of erythrocytosis, 43 of 46 patients with clear polycythemia vera formed endogenous colonies in marrow culture, whereas none of 17 patients with secondary causes of erythrocytosis did so. In half of the 45 unclassifiable patients such colonies formed, and these patients may represent cases of early polycythemia vera (13). The use of endogenous erythroid colony growth with other newer criteria for diagnosing polycythemia vera can have sensitivity as high as 94% and specificity approaching 100% (14); however, this testing is not routinely available.

Results from these techniques have been incorporated into proposed new diagnostic criteria for polycythemia vera (29). An increased erythrocyte mass (>25% above the patient's mean normal predicted value) and absence of a cause of secondary polycythemia are essential criteria. In this case, either palpable splenomegaly or the presence of a marker of clonal hematopoiesis supports the diagnosis of polycythemia vera. In the absence of both of these latter major criteria, patients must meet at least two minor criteria to secure the diagnosis. Such criteria include platelet count of more than $400,000/mm^3$, neutrophil count of more than $10,000/mm^3$, splenomegaly demonstrated by a scanning technique, characteristic BFU-E growth, and reduced serum erythropoietin value (29).

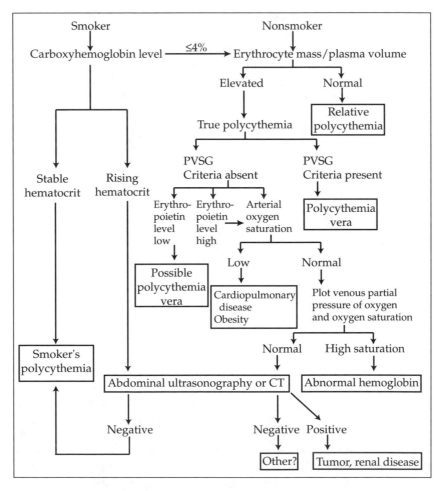

Figure 52-2. Evaluation for erythrocytosis. PVSG = polycythemia vera study group; CT = computed tomography.

DIAGNOSTIC STRATEGIES

Patients with symptoms of hyperviscosity or with a very high hematocrit level (>57% in men; >52% in women) have a high likelihood of serious disease and should receive a full evaluation as detailed in Figure 52-2. Unless initial evaluation reveals a normal erythrocyte mass or the typical syndrome of polycythemia vera, abdominal ultrasonography or CT is necessary to rule out a renal mass. If the cause of erythrocytosis remains elusive, serum erythropoietin determination or erythroid tissue culture may provide insight in some cases.

In patients with milder erythrocytosis and an elevated erythrocyte mass, absence of symptoms, normal leukocyte and platelet counts, and normal spleen size, a more limited evaluation is appropriate. Associated cardiopulmonary disease and risk factors should be addressed. A renal mass should be excluded, unless the erythrocytosis is chronic, stable, and associated with an obvious cause. However, close clinical follow-up rather than a full workup may be appropriate once a renal tumor has been excluded.

CLINICAL PROBLEMS

Clinical Problem 1

A long-term smoker, who is otherwise healthy, is found to have mild erythrocytosis.

Testing Strategy and Rationale

Carboxyhemoglobin level should be measured. Previous laboratory studies need to be reviewed to determine if the change is chronic. Abdominal ultrasonography should be done if no information on previous hematocrit levels is available or if the change is new.

In asymptomatic patients with mild erythrocytosis, only a diagnosis of polycythemia vera or tumor is likely to alter treatment or prognosis. In this smoker, the likelihood of polycythemia vera is approximately 1% and tumor-related erythrocytosis is less than 0.1%. If the results of an abdominal examination, leukocyte and platelet counts, and urinalysis are all normal, these figures are reduced even further. If the elevation in hematocrit is chronic and stable, no further evaluation is needed. If documentation of a stable hematocrit is unavailable, a renal tumor should be excluded. In the absence of positive PVSG diagnostic criteria (see Table 52-2), the possibility of early polycythemia vera can be assessed through periodic re-evaluation of hematologic parameters and abdominal examination for splenomegaly.

Continued

Clinical Example

A 42-year-old male smoker is found to have a hematocrit of 53% on routine complete blood count. He appears in excellent health and does not have dyspnea with exertion. The results of a physical examination are normal, as is the remainder of his complete blood count. A carboxyhemoglobin level of 6% supports the diagnosis of smoker's polycythemia. Abdominal imaging should be ordered only if previous complete blood count data are unavailable.

Clinical Problem 2

A nonsmoker has mild constitutional symptoms, possible splenomegaly, and moderately severe erythrocytosis and thrombocytosis.

Testing Strategy and Rationale

A full evaluation should be done (see Fig. 52-2). The patient's symptoms and degree of erythrocytosis suggest the need for prompt treatment. Polycythemia vera and tumor are important considerations. If an elevated erythrocyte mass is confirmed, the abdominal findings and thrombocytosis suggest polycythemia vera. Tumor is unlikely (<1%) but must be considered if PVSG diagnostic criteria are not met.

Clinical Example

A 55-year-old male nonsmoker presents with fatigue. He appears mildly plethoric with a normal cardiopulmonary examination. His abdomen is obese with a spleen tip palpable on deep inspiration. Hematocrit is 58%, leukocyte count is 10,800/mm³, and platelet count is 480,000/mm³. The results of urinalysis are normal.

The level of erythrocytosis indicates a 65% likelihood of true increase in erythrocyte mass, which is confirmed with formal measurement. Abdominal ultrasonography documents moderate splenomegaly and a normal left kidney. These findings are highly suggestive of polycythemia vera, and the additional finding of a normal arterial oxygen saturation would fulfill the PVSG criteria for that diagnosis.

REFERENCES

1. **Weinreb NJ, Shih CF.** Spurious polycythemia. Semin Hematol. 1975;12: 397-407.
2. **Erslev AJ, Caro J.** Pathophysiology and classification of polycythaemias. Scand J Haematol. 1983;31:287-92.
3. **Berlin NI.** Diagnosis and classification of the polycythemias. Semin Hematol. 1975;12:339-51.

4. **Isager H, Hagemp L.** Relationship between smoking and high packed cell volume and haemoglobin levels. Scand J Haematol. 1971;8:241-4.

5. **Djulbegovic B, Hadley T, Joseph G.** A new algorithm for the diagnosis of polycythemia. Am Fam Physician. 1991;44:113-20.

6. **Smith JR, Landaw SA.** Smoker's polycythemia. N Engl J Med. 1978;298: 6-10.

7. **Gallo RC, Fraimow W, Cathcart RT, Erslev AJ.** Erythropoietic response in chronic pulmonary disease. Arch Intern Med. 1964;113:559-68.

8. **Shaw DB, Simpson T.** Polycythemia in emphysema. QJM. 1961;30:135-52.

9. **Guidet B., Offenstadt G, Boffa G, et al.** Polycythemia in chronic obstructive lung disease. Chest. 1987;92:867-70.

10. **Parker Sl, Tong T, Bolden S, Wingo PA.** Cancer statistics, 1997. CA Cancer J Clin. 1997;47:5-27.

11. **Thorling EB.** Paraneoplastic erythrocytosis and inappropriate erythropoietin production: a review. Scand J Haematol. 1972;17:1-166.

12. **Moertel CG.** The liver. In: Holland JF, Frei E, eds. Cancer Medicine. Philadelphia: Lea and Febiger; 1982:1774.

13. **Lemoine F, Najman R, Baillou C, et al.** A prospective study of the value of bone marrow erythroid progenitor culture in polycythemia. Blood. 1986;68: 996-1003.

14. **Westwood N, Dudley JM, Sawyer B, et al.** Primary polycythemia: diagnosed by non-conventional positive criteria. Eur J Hematol. 1993;51:228-32.

15. **Westin J, Lanner L-O, Larsson A, Weinfell A.** Spleen size in polycythemia. Acta Med Scand. 1972;191:263-71.

16. **Barkun AN, Camus M, Green I, et al.** The bedside assessment of splenic enlargement. Am J Med. 1991;91:512-8.

17. **Friedman GD, Siegelaus AB, Seltzer CC.** Smoking habits and the leukocyte count. Arch Environ Health. 1973;26:137-43.

18. **Ward HP, Bigelow DB, Petty TL.** Postural hypoxemia and erythrocytosis. Am J Med. 1968;45:880-8.

19. **Ferrant A.** What clinical and laboratory data are indicative of polycythemia and when are blood volume studies needed? Nouv Rev Fr Hematol. 1994;36:151-4.

20. **Pearson TC, Glass UH, Wetherley-Mein G.** Interpretation of measured red cell mass in the diagnosis of polycythemia. Scand J Haematol. 1978;21: 153-62.

21. **Bunn HF, Forget BH, Ranney HM.** Human Hemoglobins. Philadelphia: WB Saunders; 1977:312-35.

22. **Lichtman MA, Murphy MS, Adamson JW.** Detection of mutant hemoglobins with altered affinity for oxygen. Ann Intern Med. 1976;84:517-21.

23. **Gatenby RA.** Diagnostic evaluation of a renal mass. Semin Oncol. 1983;10: 401-12.

24. **Pollack HM, Goldberg BB, Morales JO, Bogash M.** A systematized approach to the differential diagnosis of renal masses. Radiology 1974; 113:653-65.

25. **Stephenson TF, Iyengar S, Rashid HA.** Comparison of computed tomography and excretory urography in detection and evaluation of renal masses. J Urol. 1984;131:11-3.

26. **Pollack HM, Goldberg BB.** The kidney. In: Abdominal Gray Scale Ultrasonography. New York: John Wiley and Sons; 1977:211.

27. **Messinezy M, Westwood NB, Woodcock SP, et al.** Low serum erythropoietin—a strong diagnostic criterion of primary polycythemia even at normal hemoglobin levels. Clin Lab Haematol. 1995;17:217-20.

28. **Casadevall N.** Determination of serum erythropoietin: its value in the differential diagnosis of polycythemias. Nouv Rev Fr Hematol. 1994;36:173-6.

29. **Pearson TC, Messinezy M.** The diagnostic criteria of polycythaemia rubra vera. Leuk Lymphoma. 1996;22(Suppl 1):87-93.

Coagulation Disorders   **53**

Karai P. Balaji, MD, and Anthony L. Suchman, MD

KEY POINTS

Bleeding Disorders

Pretest Probabilities

- The risk of unsuspected disorders of plasma coagulation in asymptomatic patients is very low.
- As many as 40% of patients who present with abnormal bleeding have a coagulation disorder.

Diagnostic Strategies

- Preoperative coagulation testing with prothombin time (PT) and partial thromboplastin time (PTT) is warranted only when there appears to be an increased risk of postoperative hemorrhage based on clinical or epidemiologic grounds.
- Both the PT and PTT are accurate and complementary tests in the initial diagnostic evaluation of abnormal bleeding.
- The platelet count and bleeding time are also useful in assessing abnormal bleeding.

Hypercoagulable States

Pretest Probabilities

- Patients with recurrent thromboembolism, a positive family history, or thrombotic events at an early age should be considered for testing for inherited or acquired hypercoagulable states.

Diagnostic Strategies

- Patients who are considered for testing for hereditary or acquired hypercoagulable states should be evaluated for activated protein C resistance, proteins C and S and antithrombin III deficiency, or the lupus and anticardiolipin antibodies.

BACKGROUND

Clinicians are frequently asked to evaluate for suspected abnormalities of coagulation, both hemorrhagic diatheses as well as hypercoagulable states. This chapter examines the performance of selected laboratory tests for coagulation and discusses their use in several common clinical situations.

A vast array of tests are available for assessing blood coagulation. The two most frequently ordered tests, the activated partial thrombo-plastin time (PTT) and the prothrombin time (PT) are among the most accurate tests in laboratory medicine, but they are often ordered unnec-essarily (1,2). Other coagulation tests, such as correction studies and individual factor assays, are not discussed in this chapter. Their use, which is appropriately restricted to the detailed analysis of clinically apparent bleeding disorders, is well described in standard hematology textbooks.

ESTIMATING PRETEST PROBABILITY

Bleeding Disorders

The probability of a coagulation disorder varies greatly with the clini-cal setting. Preoperative evaluation of patients is one scenario in which coagulation studies are often performed. Major postoperative hemor-rhage is an infrequent but serious complication of surgery, the likeli-hood of which depends largely on the nature and site of the operation. Most postoperative hemorrhages result from inadequate hemostasis rather than from underlying coagulopathy. Coagulation abnormalities are rare in asymptomatic patients on evaluation before surgery. In con-trast, patients who present with abnormal bleeding have an apprecia-ble prevalence (as high as 40% [3]) of disorders related to plasma coag-ulation function. Most such patients have abnormalities of the intrinsic or combined pathways.

Clinical information can help to identify patients who may be at increased risk for coagulation disorders (4). Evaluation should include inquiry into personal and family history of abnormal or prolonged bleed-ing, either spontaneous or occurring after injuries or medical procedures; personal history of liver disease, malabsorption, or malnutrition; recent use of extended spectrum antibiotics, especially of more than 1 week's duration; and recent use of anticoagulants (4–8). Also, the skin and mucous membranes should be inspected for ecchymoses and petechiae.

Patients of Ashkenazic Jewish descent (those generally of Eastern European origin, representing approximately 80% of Jewish persons in North America) have an increased rate of asymptomatic factor XI defi-ciency, with a reported prevalence of 11% for heterozygous and 0.2% for homozygous deficiencies (5,9–11). Of those Ashkenazic patients with the deficiency, only 1% have excessive bleeding. Many of these events occur after prostate surgery (11). von Willebrand disease has a prevalence of approximately 1% in the general population (12,13). Hemophilia A and B (deficiencies of factors VIII and IX, respectively) are uncommon, with respective prevalences of 0.01% and 0.0025% among live male births.

Factor VII deficiency, which can be acquired or inherited, is associated with increased risk of bleeding. Inherited factor VII deficiency is extremely rare, with a prevalence of 2 to 3 cases per 10,000,000 persons. Acquired factor VII deficiency occurs in such conditions as hepatic insufficiency, malabsorption, malnutrition, and anticoagulation. Factor VII, which is synthesized exclusively in the liver, has a short half-life; therefore, coagulation tests can be an indicator of hepatic synthetic capacity. When postoperative hemorrhage occurs in patients with factor VII deficiency, it tends to occur after procedures that leave raw surfaces, such as dental extraction and tonsillectomy (14).

Disorders such as malabsorption that cause deficiencies of vitamin K can affect production of factors II, VII, IX, and X. Both the intrinsic and extrinsic coagulation systems can be affected.

Factor XIII deficiency is extremely rare but may cause significant bleeding if levels become very low. It may be congenital or acquired and may be associated with Henoch–Schönlein purpura, colitis, erosive gastritis, isoniazid therapy, and some leukemias (15,16). Factor XIII deficiency should be considered when patients have significant bleeding and the results of screening tests are normal.

Acquired inhibitors may also cause bleeding: In 15% to 35% of patients with hemophilia, antibodies to factor VIII develop as a result of repeated factor concentrate transfusion (17). Acquired inhibitors may also occur spontaneously or as a result of autoimmune disorders, parturition, lymphoid malignancies, certain skin disorders, and use of drugs such as penicillin (18).

Hypercoagulable States

As with bleeding disorders, hypercoagulable conditions that predispose to thromboembolic disease can be acquired or inherited. Most patients with venous thrombosis (see Chapter 9) have obvious predisposing factors such as prolonged immobilization, oral contraceptive use, postoperative states, cancer, pregnancy, or myeloproliferative disorders (19). Inherited causes were considered to account for fewer than 10% of unexplained cases (20); however, with the identification of resistance to activated protein C (APC), this frequency is now estimated to be 50% (21). Deficiencies of protein C, protein S, and antithrombin III are inherited in an autosomal-dominant pattern (22). Resistance to APC occurs in heterozygous and homozygous forms; homozygotes are at greater risk from APC resistance.

The prevalence of APC resistance (heterozygous) in the general population has been reported to be between 3% and 8% (22,23). Studies using healthy adult donors have indicated prevalences of protein C and of antithrombin deficiency that are estimated to be 3.3 and 2 per 1000 persons, respectively (24,25). Based on these studies, it may be inferred that more than 50% of affected persons never have a thrombotic episode (24,25).

In patients with venous thromboembolism, estimates of the prevalence of APC resistance range from 20% to 50% and estimates of proteins C and S and antithrombin III deficiencies range between 2% and 5% (26–28). In a European study of more than 2000 patients with venous thromboembolism, protein deficiencies were found in approximately 13%; 0.5% had antithrombin III deficiency, 3.2% had protein C deficiency, 7.3% had protein S deficiency, and 0.75% had combined deficiencies (29). In this study, approximately 20% of those with a family history of thrombosis, who were younger than 45 years, or who had recurrent thrombosis had a protein deficiency (29). The risk of thrombosis is increased when deficiencies of protein C, protein S, or antithrombin III coexist with APC resistance (30–32).

Patients with protein deficiencies may also present with certain clinical findings (33). Patients with protein C deficiency may have both recurrent superficial and deep thrombophlebitis (34). Adults with either protein C or protein S deficiency may experience skin necrosis when treated with warfarin sodium (Coumadin) (35).

Of the acquired conditions, antiphospholipid syndromes (lupus anticoagulant and anticardiolipin antibody) are probably the most common (36). Both arterial and venous thrombosis are seen with these syndromes, as is spontaneous abortion (36). In the European study mentioned above, the overall prevalence of antiphospholipid antibodies was 4.1% (29). Approximately 30% of patients with lupus have the lupus antibody. Antiphospholipid antibodies may be seen in otherwise asymptomatic persons; 7.5% of controls in one study were found to have these antibodies (37,38). Although antiphospholipid antibodies have been associated with the use of medications such as chlorpromazine, procainamide, quinidine, phenytoin, and hydralazine, drug-induced antiphospholipid antibodies are rarely associated with thrombotic events (39). Most patients with antiphospholipid antibodies do not experience significant thrombosis or have the antiphospholipid syndrome.

Other common causes of acquired hypercoagulable states are pregnancy and use of oral contraceptives. Levels of protein S decrease by 40% to 50% during pregnancy and by 20% with use of oral contraceptives (40). Activated protein C resistance was found in almost 60% of women with thromboembolic complications during pregnancy and in 30% of those who experienced thrombotic events while using oral contraceptives (41). In contrast, approximately 10% of nonpregnant controls had APC resistance. Patients with protein deficiencies are at particularly high risk for thromboembolic events during pregnancy.

DIAGNOSTIC TESTS

The activated PTT and prothrombin time PT are affected differently by deficiency of various plasma coagulation factors. Coagulation through the intrinsic system depends on factors XII, XI, IX, and VIII. Coagulation through the extrinsic (tissue-factor dependent) system requires factor VII. Both the intrinsic and extrinsic systems depend on the final common pathway that requires factors X, V, II (prothrombin), and I (fibrinogen).

Activated Partial Thromboplastin Time

The activated PTT measures the activity of the intrinsic coagulation system and the final common pathway. Table 53-1 shows the sensitivity, specificity, and likelihood ratios of the PTT in detecting clinically important deficiencies of the various components of the intrinsic clotting system (3,42–45). The sensitivity is quite high for all disorders except von Willebrand disease. Also, although factor XII deficiency prolongs the PTT, it is not associated with clinical bleeding (46). Because the normal range for the PTT is defined statistically by the normal distribution (i.e., mean value +/– 2 standard deviations), there will be, by definition, a 2.3% false-positive rate, or a specificity of 97.7%.

Artifactual prolongation of the PTT may occur when an inadequate volume of blood is obtained (47) or when blood is drawn from a catheter through which heparin is being infused. The PTT may also be prolonged if the plasma is highly turbid or icteric, the patient is polycythemic, photoelectric machines are used, or partially clotted specimens (with resulting consumption of clotting factors) are used for the test. Coumadin can also prolong PTT although proportionally less than the PT. Prolongation of the PTT can also be found in those with the lupus anticoagulant, which is associated with thromboembolic events rather than with increased bleeding. Artificial shortening of the PTT has not been reported. Minor deficiencies of one procoagulant can be masked by high levels of another, particularly factor VIII, an acute phase reactant (48).

Prothrombin Time

The PT assesses the function of the extrinsic coagulation system and common pathway (14,49). The PT is usually used to assess factor VII activity and yields evidence about the current synthetic capacity of the liver, vitamin K deficiency, and warfarin anticoagulation. The sensitivity of the PT in detecting either severe (<5%) or moderate (5%–25%) homozygous factor VII deficiency is near 100% (50,51). Factor VII levels greater than 25% are found in heterozygotes and are not associated

Table 53-1. Operating Characteristics of the Activated Partial Thromboplastin Time (PTT) in Various Clinical Situations*

Target Condition	Sensitivity	Specificity	Likelihood Ratio	
			Positive Result	Negative Result
	←——— % ———→			
Preoperative screening*				
Deficiency of				
Any intrinsic factor	98	98	49	0.02[†]
Factor VIII				
Severe (0%–5% of normal)	100	98	50	0[†]
Moderate (6%–15%)	99	98	50	0.01
Mild (16%–30%)	90	98	45	0.1
von Willebrand disease	48–100	98	24–50	0–0.53[†]
Factor IX	100	98	50	0[†]
Factor XI	100	98	50	0[†]
Factor V	100	98	50	0[†]
Factor X	100	98	50	0[†]
Evaluating clinically suspected bleeding disorder*				
Deficiency of any intrinsic factor	99	89	9	0.01[†]

*Abnormal result = PTT >2 standard deviations above the mean.
[†]Some data obtained for partial thromboplastin time, which is less sensitive than activated PTT in mild factor deficiencies (3).
From references 3, 42–45.

with increased bleeding risk (14,49). As with the PTT, the specificity of the PT is derived statistically and is slightly less than 98%. These operating characteristics vary somewhat according to the particular reagents and instruments used (52,53).

Artifactual prolongation of the PT may result from underfilling of the test tube and from extreme polycythemia (54). Artifactual shortening may occur if blood is collected in borosilicate or siliconized borosilicate tubes (54). The effect of therapeutic doses of heparin on the PT is minimal (55).

Platelet Count and Bleeding Time

The severity of bleeding is inversely related to the platelet count. Platelet counts of greater than 50,000/mm^3 generally ensure adequate hemostasis, provided that platelet function is normal. Platelet counts of less than $10,000/mm^3$ are dangerously low and can lead to spontaneous bleeding (56,57).

The bleeding time is a test of the integrity of the interaction between platelets and the vessel wall and thus helps to assess platelet function. It is highly sensitive; however, it is nonspecific in that modest abnormalities found on this test do not indicate a greatly increased risk of bleeding. In several reports, patients receiving aspirin in whom bleeding times were more than twice the normal had no increased perioperative blood loss (58–60).

Testing for Hypercoagulable States

Specific assays are available for APC resistance and deficiencies of antithrombin III, protein C, and protein S. Although the accuracy of the measurements is high, not all affected persons with low levels will have a thromboembolic event. False-positive test results may be caused by improper timing of tests. For example, in the immediate post-thrombotic state, consumption of coagulation factors may result in falsely low proteins C and S and antithrombin III levels. Therefore, it is important to check the levels of these proteins several weeks after the thrombotic episode. Because most patients with APC resistance have the same mutation, genetic testing for the factor V Leiden mutation is helpful in those identified through initial evaluation as having APC resistance.

Anticoagulants may also distort testing for hypercoagulable states. Warfarin lowers the levels of proteins C and S, although deficiencies of these factors can be detected by comparing the levels with those of other vitamin K–dependent factors. If all factors are lowered proportionately, hereditary deficiency is unlikely. Assays for antithrombin III, lupus anticoagulant, and anticardiolipin antibodies are not affected by warfarin. Proteins C and S can be measured in patients receiving heparin, but the antithrombin III assay can be distorted. Heparin may cause false-positive test results for APC resistance and the lupus anticoagulant. Functional assays are preferred because protein dysfunction can occur in the presence of apparently normal levels (19,20,22).

DIAGNOSTIC STRATEGIES

Screening for Bleeding Disorders

Despite the intuitive appeal of preoperative testing with PTT to detect unsuspected bleeding disorders that could predispose the patient to hemorrhage, in most cases such testing is not warranted for several reasons. First, coagulation disorders are rare in asymptomatic patients. Because of this low prevalence, the post-test probability after an abnormal PTT result is still too low to be clinically meaningful or useful in these patients (61,62). Second, clinical assessment is as sensitive as the PTT in detecting procoagulant deficiencies; most abnormal PTT results occur in patients with clinical evidence of bleeding risk (3,63–66). Moreover, among patients without clinical evidence of bleeding disorders, those whose preoperative PTT are prolonged are no more likely to have a postoperative hemorrhage than those whose test results are normal, indicating that the test has no predictive power in asymptomatic patients (67–69). Third, most postoperative hemorrhages result from inadequate surgical hemostasis and thus cannot be predicted by preoperative screening tests.

In patients whose clinical evaluation suggests an increased risk of a bleeding disorder, a PTT should be obtained because an abnormal result can identify patients at further increased risk for postoperative hemorrhage (68). In addition, all patients of Ashkenazic Jewish descent should be screened with the PTT because of the increased prevalence of asymptomatic factor XI deficiency in this group (5,9–11).

Like the PTT, the PT is not recommended for the routine preoperative screening of asymptomatic patients (6,70,71). The only coagulation defect that can be detected by the PT and not by the PTT is factor VII deficiency. However, inherited factor VII deficiency is extremely rare and does not carry the same degree of risk of postoperative hemorrhage as do deficiencies of factors VIII or IX (14). Acquired factor VII deficiency occurs in conditions such as hepatic insufficiency, malabsorption, and malnutrition, in which the PT offers no advantage over the history and physical examination in screening asymptomatic patients (63).

However, when clinical evaluation suggests that these conditions are present, the results of the PT may be abnormal when those of the PTT are not (3). Therefore, both tests are needed to assess patients with findings suspicious for an increased risk of bleeding and for patients in whom an adequate clinical assessment cannot be made. Tests that yield abnormal results should be repeated, and if the results are still abnormal, second-order tests should be done. The PT and PTT are also recommended for patients whose normal coagulation may be disrupted by the planned procedure—for example, insertion of a peritoneovenous shunt, prostatectomy, or procedures involving extracorporeal circulation (5).

In patients without risk factors and without a personal or family history of bleeding, the platelet count and bleeding time are not useful routine screening tests.

Abnormal Bleeding

As many as 40% of patients who report abnormal bleeding have a disorder related to plasma coagulation factors. The PTT is a powerful test for confirming and excluding disorders of the intrinsic arm and common pathway of the coagulation cascade: the post-test probability when the test result is abnormal is approximately 86% and when the test result is normal is less than 1%.

The PT is a useful test in the evaluation of abnormal bleeding, only in part because of its high sensitivity for the detection of factor VII deficiency. More important, the combined pattern of PT and PTT results usually directs attention toward specific procoagulant factors, allowing judicious use of individual factor assays and other expensive second-order tests. Therefore, both the PTT and PT are indicated in the evaluation of abnormal bleeding.

Because thrombocytopenia is a frequent cause of bleeding, measuring platelet counts is another important part of this evaluation, especially with acute bleeding. A bleeding time should be obtained in patients with abnormal bleeding whose PTT, PT, and platelet counts are normal.

Monitoring Anticoagulant Therapy

Anticoagulant therapy is monitored to maintain anticoagulation within a therapeutic range in which the risk of recurrent thrombosis is balanced against the risk of hemorrhage. Heparin treatment is monitored with the PTT. (Partial thromboplastin time monitoring is not generally required when low-molecular-weight heparin is used.) Although the limits of the therapeutic range have not been determined precisely, several observational studies have confirmed that the maintenance of the PTT within a range of 1.5 to 2.5 times the control value reduces the risks of both recurrent clotting and hemorrhagic complications of therapy (72,73). In monitoring intravenous heparin therapy, the PTT should initially be determined every 6 hours. Once the optimal dose has been determined, the PTT needs to be measured only once each day for the duration of therapy.

Oral anticoagulant therapy with warfarin is monitored with the PT. In order to achieve more precise anticoagulation, most laboratories now report results using the International Normalized Ratio (INR) method. This method allows adjustment for the potency of a laboratory's thromboplastin reagent. Use of the INR promotes obtaining appropriate anticoagulation independent of laboratory reagents and allows easier adherence to published recommendations for intensity of anticoagulation. Currently, the target for anticoagulation in patients with venous thromboembolism is to maintain an INR of 2 to 3, whereas an INR of 3 to 4 is recommended for certain patients with recurrent thromboembolic events or those with mechanical heart valves. Patients whose anticoagulation is maintained within the therapeutic ranges are less likely to experience hemorrhage and recurrent thrombosis than are those with values outside the range.

It is necessary only to simultaneously determine the PT and PTT during the transition from heparin to warfarin therapy.

Hypercoagulable States

In most patients with thromboembolic events, a complete history and physical examination identifies the precipitating factors and no further evaluation is required (19,39,74). Further testing should be considered when patients present early in life, have a positive family history, experience recurrent unexplained thromboembolism (especially if more than one site or unusual site is involved), develop warfarin-induced skin necrosis, have venous or arterial thrombosis, or have a history of recurrent fetal loss (28). Testing asymptomatic relatives of patients with hereditary hypercoagulable states is warranted given that asymptomatic patients with inherited coagulation deficiencies are at higher risk for venous thromboembolism and that short-term prophylaxis is recommended in situations in which the risk for thrombosis is increased (28,75). Some have recommended screening for APC resistance those patients with a strong family history of thromboembolic events who are considering pregnancy or the use of oral contraceptives (41).

To detect inherited and acquired deficiencies and circulatory inhibitors in these clinical settings, specific assays for APC resistance; deficiencies of antithrombin III, protein C, and protein S; or lupus and anticardiolipin antibodies are indicated. Genetic testing can identify those with inherited APC resistance, as noted previously. Tests for defects in the fibrinolytic system or dysfibrinogenemia are not generally recommended (28). Newer studies such as the thrombin antithrombin complex, prothrombin fragments 1 and 2, and modified recalcification time are being evaluated as tests for hypercoagulability (76,77), but further studies need to be completed to assess their potential value.

CLINICAL PROBLEMS

Clinical Problem 1

A patient with no history or physical findings to suggest a coagulation disorder is scheduled for surgery.

Testing Strategy and Rationale

No coagulation tests are generally indicated. The pretest probability of a coagulation disorder in patients with no risk factors is 0.01% for men and is even lower for women. For example, despite the high sensitivity and specificity of the PTT, the post-test probability after prolonged PTT is found on testing is only 0.5%, not sufficiently high to warrant additional investigation or delay of surgery.

However, if the patient's history or physical examination revealed an increased likelihood of a coagulation disorder, then studies should be performed. In patients with a history suspicious for a coagulation disorder, the pretest probability of coagulopathy is high enough that if the test results are abnormal, the post-test probability would probably be significant.

Clinical Example
A 35-year-old white man is scheduled for an elective herniorrhaphy. He has no history of prolonged or spontaneous bleeding, knows of no family members with bleeding problems, and is not of Ashkenazic Jewish descent. On physical examination, he appears healthy and has no ecchymoses, petechiae, or signs of liver disease. Neither the PTT, PT, platelet count, nor bleeding time is ordered.

Clinical Problem 2
A patient presents with recurrent, abnormal bleeding.

Testing Strategy and Rationale
Both the PTT and PT should be performed. The PTT has high sensitivity and specificity for disorders of the intrinsic coagulation system, and the PT has equivalent characteristics for clinically important deficiencies of factor VII. In addition to the excellent performance characteristics of the individual tests, the combined pattern of results may point to a specific limb of the coagulation sequence for further study.

Patients with abnormal bleeding have a pretest probability of coagulopathy of approximately 40%. Virtually all of this risk represents intrinsic or common pathway deficiencies. The pretest probability of an isolated extrinsic pathway (factor VII) deficiency is only about 0.12%.

If the results of the PTT are abnormal, the post-test probability of coagulopathy increases to about 86%. If the results of the PT are also abnormal, attention can be directed to the common pathway or to multiple factor deficiencies; however, if the results of the PT are normal, attention can be directed to the intrinsic pathway. If the results of the PTT are normal, the post-test probability of coagulopathy decreases to less than 1%.

In this case of recurrent bleeding, the suspicion for coagulation factor problems is very high and initial testing consists of the PTT and PT. If the results of both are normal, additional studies are indicated, including measurement of the platelet count and bleeding time.

Clinical Example
Because of persistent bleeding after a minor surgical procedure, a 28-year-old man is referred for evaluation. He had a similar prob-

Continued

lem 10 years earlier with a laceration that required suturing and with scratches and scrapes when he was a child. Given the chronic nature of the problem, initial evaluation is targeted to assess coagulation factors, and both a PTT and a PT are performed.

REFERENCES

1. **Mozes B, Lubin D, Modan B, et al.** Evaluation of an intervention aimed at reducing inappropriate use of preoperative blood coagulation tests. Arch Intern Med. 1989;149:1836-8.

2. **Wahlberg T, Blomback M, Hall P, Axelsson G.** Application of indicators, predictors and diagnostic indices in coagulation disorders. Methods Inf Med. 1980;19:194-200

3. **Nye SW, Graham JB, Brinkhous KM.** The partial thromboplastin time as a screening test for the detection of latent bleeders. Am J Med Sci. 1962;243:279-87.

4. **Sham RL, Francis CW.** Evaluation of mild bleeding disorder and easy bruising. Blood Rev. 1994;8:98-104.

5. **Suchman AL, Griner PF.** Diagnostic uses of the activated partial thromboplastin time and prothrombin time. In: Sox HC, ed. Common Diagnostic Tests. 2nd ed. Philadelphia: American College of Physicians; 1990:227-44.

6. **Rappaport SI.** Preoperative hemostatic evaluation: which tests, if any? Blood. 1983;61:229-31.

7. **Alperin JB.** Coagulopathy caused by vitamin K deficiency in critically ill hospitalized patients. JAMA. 1987;258:1916-9.

8. **Sattler FR, Weitekamp MR, Ballard JO.** Potential for bleeding with the new beta-lactam antibiotics. Ann Intern Med. 1986;105:924-31.

9. **Seligsohn U, Modan M.** Definition of the population at risk of bleeding due to factor XI deficiency in Ashkenazic Jews and the value of activated partial thromboplastin time in its detection. Isr J Med Sci. 1981;17:413-5.

10. **Seligsohn U.** High gene frequency of factor XI (PTA) deficiency in Ashkenazi Jews. Blood. 1978;51:1223-8.

11. **Bashevkin ML, Nawabi IU.** Factor XI deficiency in surgical patients. N Y State J Med. 1979;79:1360-2.

12. **Rodeghiero F, Castaman G, Dini E.** Epidemiological investigation of the prevalence of von Willebrand's disease. Blood. 1987;69:454-9.

13. **Werner EJ, Broxson EH, Tucker EL, et al.** Prevalence of von Willebrand disease in children: a multiethnic study. J Pediatr. 1993;123:893-8.

14. **Britten AFH, Salzman EW.** Surgery in congenital disorders of blood coagulation. Surg Gynecol Obstet. 1966;123:1333-58.

15. **Board PG, Losowsky MS, Miloszewski KJ.** Factor XIII: inherited and acquired deficiency. Blood Rev. 1993;7:229-42.

16. **Tosetto A, Castaman G, Rodeghiero F.** Acquired plasma factor XIII deficiencies [Review]. Haematologica. 1993;78(6 Suppl 2):5-10.

17. **Sohngen D, Specker C, Bach D, et al.** Acquired factor VIII inhibitors in nonhemophilic patients. Ann Hematol. 1997;74:89-93.

18. **Cohen AJ, Kessler CM.** Acquired inhibitors. Baillieres Clin Haematol 1996;9:331-54.
19. **Alving BM.** Hypercoagulable states. Hosp Pract. 1993;28:109-21.
20. **Tabernero MD, Tomas JF, Alberca I, et al.** Incidence and clinical characteristics of hereditary disorders associated with venous thrombosis. Am J Hematol. 1991;36:249-54.
21. **Svensson PJ, Dahlback B.** Resistance to activated protein C as a basis for venous thrombosis. N Engl J Med. 1994;330:517-22.
22. **Bauer KA.** Management of patients with hereditary defects predisposing to thrombosis including pregnant women. Thromb Haemost. 1995;74:94-100.
23. **Griffin JH, Evatt B, Wideman C, et al.** Anticoagulant protein C pathway defective in majority of thrombophilic patients. Blood. 1993;82:1989-93.
24. **Miletich J, Sherman L, Broze G Jr.** Absence of thrombosis in subjects with heterozygous protein C deficiency. N Engl J Med. 1987;317:991-6.
25. **Wells PS, Blajchman MA, Henderson P, et al.** Prevalence of antithrombin deficiency in healthy blood donors: a cross-sectional study. Am J Hematol. 1994;45:321-4.
26. **Doig RG, O'Malley CJ, Dauer R, McGrath KM.** An evaluation of 200 consecutive patients with spontaneous or recurrent thrombosis for primary hypercoagulable states. Am J Clin Pathol. 1994;102:797-801.
27. **Pabinger I, Kyrle PA, Heistinger M, et al.** The risk of thromboembolism in asymptomatic patients with protein C and protein S deficiency: a prospective cohort study. Thromb Haemost. 1994;71:441-5.
28. **Brigden ML.** The hypercoagulable state: who, how, and when to test and treat. Postgrad Med. 1997;101:249-52, 254-6, 259-62 passim.
29. **Mateo J, Oliver A, Borrell M, et al.** Laboratory evaluation and clinical characteristics of 2,132 consecutive unselected patients with venous thromboembolism: results of the Spanish Multicentric Study on Thrombophilia (EMET-Study). Thromb Haemost. 1997;77:444-51.
30. **Koeleman BP, Reitsma PH, Allaart CF, et al.** Activated protein C resistance as an additional risk factor for thrombosis in protein C-deficient families. Blood. 1994;84:1031-35.
31. **Garcia de Frutos P, Dahlback B.** Resistance to activated protein C as an additional risk factor in hereditary deficiency of protein S. J Clin Invest. 1994;94:923.
32. **Van Bowen HH, Reitsma PH, Rosendaal FR, et al.** Interaction of factor V Leiden with inherited AT-III deficiency. Thromb Haemost. 1995;73:1256.
33. **Engesser L, Broekmans AW, Briet E, et al.** Hereditary protein S deficiency: clinical manifestations. Ann Intern Med. 1987;106:677-82.
34. **Bovill EG, Bauer KA, Dickerman JD, et al.** The clinical spectrum of heterozygous protein C deficiency in a large New England kindred. Blood. 1989;73:712-7.
35. **DeFranzo AJ, Marasco P, Argenta LC.** Warfarin-induced necrosis of the skin. Ann Plast Surg. 1995;34:203-8.
36. **Devine DV, Brigden ML.** The antiphospholipid syndrome: when does the presence of antiphospholipid antibodies require therapy? Postgrad Med. 1996;99:105-8,113-25.

37. **Love PE, Santoro SA.** Antiphospholipid antibodies: anticardiolipin and the lupus anticoagulant in systemic lupus erythematosus (SLE) and in non-SLE disorders: prevalence and clinical significance. Ann Intern Med. 1990;112: 682-98.

38. **Kalunian KC, Peter JB, Middlekauff HR, et al.** Clinical significance of a single test for anticardiolipin antibodies in patients with systemic lupus erythematosus. Am J Med. 1988;85:602-8.

39. **Bowen KJ, Vukelja SJ.** Hypercoagulable states: their causes and management. Postgrad Med. 1992;91:117-8, 123-5.

40. **Alving BM, Comp PC.** Recent advances in understanding clotting and evaluating patients with recurrent thrombosis. Am J Obstet Gynecol. 1992; 167:1184-91.

41. **Hellgren M, Svensson PJ, Dahlback B.** Resistance to activated protein C as a basis for venous thromboembolism associated with pregnancy and oral contraceptives. Am J Obstet Gynecol. 1995;173:210-3.

42. **Hathaway WE, Assmus SL, Montgomery RR, Dubansky AS.** Activated partial thromboplastin time and minor coagulopathies. Am J Clin Pathol. 1979;71:22-5.

43. **Proctor RR, Rapaport SI.** The partial thromboplastin time with Kaolin: a simple screening test for first stage plasma clotting factor deficiencies. Am J Clin Pathol. 1961;36:212-9.

44. **Poller L.** Severe bleeding disorders in children with normal coagulation screening tests. Br Med J. 1982;285:377.

45. **Lian EC, Deykin D.** Diagnosis of von Willebrand disease: a comparative study of diagnostic tests on nine families. Am J Med. 1976;60:344-56.

46. **Capitanio AM, Sacco R, Mannucci PM.** Pseudopathologies of hemostasis and dental surgery. Oral Surg Oral Med Oral Pathol Radiol Endod. 1991;71:184-6.

47. **Peterson P, Gottfried EL.** The effects of inaccurate blood sample volume on prothrombin time and activated partial thromboplastin time. Thromb Haemost. 1982;47:101-3.

48. **Edson JR, Krivit W, White JG.** Kaolin partial thromboplastin time: high levels of procoagulants producing short clotting times or masking deficiencies of other procoagulants or low concentrations of anticoagulants. J Lab Clin Med. 1967;70:463-70.

49. **Hougie C.** One-stage prothrombin time. In: Williams WJ, Beutler E, Erslev AJ, Rundles RW, eds. Hematology. 2nd ed. New York: McGraw-Hill; 1977.

50. **Owen CA, Amundsen MA, Thompson JH, et al.** Congenital deficiency of factor VII (hypoconvertinemia). Am J Med. 1964;37:71-91.

51. **Marder VJ, Shulman NR.** Clinical aspects of congenital factor VII deficiency. Am J Med. 1964;37:182-94.

52. **Frost T, Lau KS, Jones KOA.** The Australian reference thromboplastin: I. A study in bleeding patients. Pathology. 1981;13:525-35.

53. **Charache S, Harbaugh E, Petrilik J.** Control of anticoagulant therapy by prothrombin time tests: an old problem revisited. Am Heart J. 1981;102: 804-6.

54. **Palmer RN, Kessler CM, Gralnick HR.** Warfarin anticoagulation: difficulties in interpretation of the prothrombin time. Thromb Res. 1982;25:125-30.

55. **Salzman EW, Deykin D, Shapiro M, Rosenberg R.** Management of heparin therapy: controlled prospective trial. N Engl J Med. 1975;292:1046-50.

56. **Weaver DW.** Differential diagnosis and management of unexplained bleeding. Surg Clin North Am. 1993;73:353-61.

57. Practice guidelines for blood component therapy: a report by the American Society of Anesthesiologists Task Force on Blood Component Therapy. Anesthesiology. 1996;84:732-47.

58. **Rogers RP, Levin J.** A critical reappraisal of the bleeding time. Semin Thromb Hemost. 1990;16:1-20.

59. **Diaz-Buxo JA, Donadio JV.** Complications of percutaneous renal biopsy: an analysis of 1000 consecutive biopsies. Clin Nephrol. 1975;4:223-7.

60. **Ferraris VA, Swanson E.** Aspirin usage and perioperative blood loss in patients undergoing unexpected operations. Surg Gynecol Obstet. 1983;156:439-42.

61. **Clarke JR, Eisenberg JM.** A theoretical assessment of the value of the PTT as a preoperative screening test in adults. Med Decis Making. 1981;1:40-3.

62. **Burk CD, Miller L, Handler SD, Cohen AR.** Preoperative history and coagulation screening in children undergoing tonsillectomy. Pediatrics. 1992;89:691-5.

63. **Eisenberg JM, Clarke JR, Sussman SA.** Prothrombin and partial thromboplastin times as pre-operative screening tests. Arch Surg. 1982;117:48-51.

64. **Bachmann F.** Diagnostic approach to mild bleeding disorders. Semin Hematol. 1980;17:292-305.

65 **Bevan DH.** A field guide to the bleeding disorders for the general practitioner. Practitioner. 1982;226:25-32.

66. **Robbins JA, Rose SD.** Partial thromboplastin time as a screening test. Ann Intern Med. 1979;90:796-7.

67. **Darcy MD, Kanterman RY, Kleinhoffer MA, et al.** Evaluation of coagulation tests as predictors of angiographic bleeding complications. Radiology. 1996;198:741-4.

68. **Suchman AL, Mushlin AI.** Preoperative screening with the activated partial thromboplastin time. JAMA. 1986;256:750-3.

69. **Colon-Otero G,Cockerill KJ, Bowie EJ.** How to diagnose bleeding disorders [Review]. Postgrad Med. 1991;1:90:145-50.

70. **Schwartz SO.** What routine preoperative tests for bleeding tendencies? JAMA. 1976;22:2547.

71. **Watson-Williams EJ, Chir B.** Hematologic and hemostatic considerations before surgery. Med Clin North Am. 1979;63:1165-89.

72. **Basu D, Gallus A, Hirsh J, Cade J.** A prospective study of the value of monitoring heparin treatment with the activated partial thromboplastin time. N Engl J Med. 1972;287:324-7.

73. **Hyers TH, Hull RD, Weg JG.** Antithrombotic therapy for venous thromboembolic disease. Chest. 1986;89(2)suppl:26S-35S.

74. **Macik BG, Ortel TL.** Clinical and laboratory evaluation of the hypercoagulable states. Clin Chest Med. 1995;16:375-87.

75. **Pabinger I, Brucker S, Kyrle PA, et al.** Hereditary deficiency of antithrombin III, protein C and S: prevalence in patients with a history of venous

thrombosis and criteria for rational patient screening. Blood Coagul Fibrin. 1992;5:547-53.

76. **Spillert CR, Lazaro EJ.** Modified recalcification time: a global coagulation screening test. J Natl Med Assoc. 1993;85:611-6.

77. **Boisclair MD, Lane DA, Wilde JT, et al.** A comparative evaluation of assays for markers of activated coagulation and/or fibrinolysis: thrombin-antithrombin complex, D-dimer and fibrinogen/fibrin fragment E antigen. Br J Haematol. 1990;74:471-9.

Neurologic Problems

Syncope   **54**

Susan C. Day, MD, MPH, and John M. Eisenberg, MD

KEY POINTS

Pretest Probabilities

- Pretest probabilities for causes of syncope vary with the setting, the patient's age, and underlying condition(s). A history and physical examination identify a possible cause in approximately half the patients who present with syncope.

- The most important determinant of poor prognosis is syncope of cardiac origin. Patients with this condition have increased short- and long-term morbidity and mortality, mainly owing to the underlying cardiac disease.

- When syncope is noncardiac in origin or the cause remains unknown after a focused evaluation, mortality is not increased unless a serious underlying illness is present.

Diagnostic Strategies

- The history and physical examination provide the diagnosis in most cases for which a diagnosis can be made. Except for electrocardiography, routine laboratory testing contributes little to improving diagnostic accuracy.

- Patients at risk for cardiac disease should be evaluated by echocardiography or stress testing or both. Those with low ejection fraction or ischemia should be considered for electrophysiologic testing.

- Neurologic testing should be reserved for patients with evidence of seizures or focal neurologic signs on physical examination.

- Patients without suspected cardiac disease who have recurrent syncope may be evaluated further with electrocardiographic loop recording, head-up tilt-table testing, or psychiatric examination.

- Medications may be a contributing cause of syncope, particularly in elderly persons.

- In as many as one third of patients with syncope, no diagnosis is evident after evaluation.

BACKGROUND

Syncope is a sudden, transient loss of consciousness. Diagnostic categories often overlap, making reproducible, definitive classification of the cause of syncopal episodes difficult (1–4). In as many as one third of patients presenting with syncope, a clear cause cannot be determined after diagnostic evaluation. Classifying syncope according to long-term risk to the patient and then according to the type of pathophysiologic event is most helpful (Table 54-1). Several excellent reviews summarize the pathophysiologic mechanisms that lead to syncope (1–8).

ESTIMATING PRETEST PROBABILITY

Syncope is a common problem: 20% to 30% of "normal" patients have lost consciousness at some in their lives (1). However, the clinically serious conditions that result in syncope are relatively rare in the general population. Therefore, the challenge is to identify those few patients with clinically serious conditions.

The clinician who is evaluating a patient with syncope must move from the long list of causes of syncope to an operational approach to diagnosis. Two questions should influence the diagnostic approach: 1) What are the most likely causes of syncope in a particular patient (i.e., what are the pretest probabilities)? and 2) What is the risk of a poor outcome for a particular patient, with or without further testing?

Assessing Pretest Probabilities

The pretest probability of disease is highly dependent on the setting in which the patient is seen as well as on the patient's age (3,9–13). Table 54-1 lists the causes of syncope, with the range of frequencies influenced by the study setting. Studies that drew patients from emergency room and outpatient practice settings reported a higher incidence of noncritical syncope than studies involving patients in an intensive care or an inpatient setting.

The average age of the patients in these studies ranged from 44 to 67 years old. Neurally mediated (also called neurocardiogenic, vasovagal, or vasodepressor) syncope is the most common cause of syncope in younger patients. Psychogenic causes are also common in this age group. In elderly persons, syncope is often multifactorial and exacerbated by blunted physiologic reflexes and multidrug regimens that block normal homeostatic mechanisms (5,6).

Pretest probabilities can be further refined by use of data provided by the history and physical examination. For example, tussive syncope and micturition syncope have classic clinical presentations, whereas orthostatic hypotension can be diagnosed by a characteristic decrease in blood pressure with a change in posture. Medications, especially in combination, are an important contributor to syncope in elderly per-

Table 54-1. Frequency of Causes of Syncope

Cause	Frequency (%)
Causes with critical clinical significance	19–42
Cardiopulmonary	
Bradyarrhythmias	3–9
Tachyarrhythmias	2–18
Structural heart disease	2–4
Ischemic heart disease	1–5
Pulmonary embolism	0–2
Pulmonary hypertension	0–1
Carotid sinus hypersensitivity	0–37
Central nervouse system	
Cerebrovascular disease	1–5
Seizures	0–29*
Causes with noncritical clinical significance	8–77
Central nervous system	
Migraine/other	0–2
Drug induced	0–13
Neurally mediated	
Orthostatic hypotension	3–9
Situational syncope	0–7
Vasodepressor syncope	1–59
Metabolic	0–3
Psychogenic	5–20
Unknown	5–50

*The wide range here reflects variability on whether patients with seizures are included in the population.

sons (14). Recent studies have confirmed the value of the history in differentiating syncope caused by cardiac arrhythmias or seizure from neurally mediated causes (15,16). In patients who are elderly, have a past history of heart disease, have no prodrome, have palpitations, or whose syncope is precipitated by exertion, the syncope is more likely to have a cardiac cause.

Assessing Risk in Patients with Syncope

Several cohorts of patients have been followed for 3 to 5 years to determine the long-term morbidity and mortality associated with syncope (9–13,17,18). Patients for whom the initial episode of loss of consciousness is attributed to cardiac causes are at high risk for increased overall mortality, as well as for sudden death. The risk appears to be owing to the underlying disease rather than the syncope per se (19). Patients with noncardiac or unexplained syncope do not appear to be at increased risk for sudden death.

The risk factors for sudden death have been extensively investigated in the cardiology literature and will not be reviewed here (20–23). Older patients (i.e., those older than 70 years), patients with known cardiac disease or arrhythmias, patients with recurrent syncopal events, or those who have injured themselves during the episode of loss of consciousness fall into a high-risk group of patients who should be investigated further (24–28). Martin and colleagues (29) recently developed a risk classification system for patients presenting to emergency departments with syncope. Abnormal findings on electrocardiography, history of ventricular arrhythmias, and history of congestive heart failure were independent predictors of subsequent arrhythmia or 1-year mortality (29).

DIAGNOSTIC TESTS

With the information obtained from the history and physical, a diagnosis can be made in 50% to 80% of cases for which a diagnosis ultimately can be made. Measuring the sensitivity and specificity of diagnostic tests for syncope is difficult owing to the multiple causes and the lack of a suitable gold standard. Instead, the literature measures the usefulness of tests in terms of "diagnostic yield." Table 54-2 summarizes the yield of tests frequently ordered in the evaluation of syncope. Applying this yield data to unselected patients with syncope is problematic because in several studies, diagnostic evaluations were likely targeted toward high-risk patients in whom test yield might be greater.

Electrocardiography

Electrocardiography (ECG) is relatively inexpensive, easy to perform, and safe. Its usefulness in evaluating a patient with syncope is in disclosing an arrhythmia or prolonged QT interval or in suggesting the presence of underlying cardiac disease. Approximately 2% to 11% of patients presenting with syncope have abnormal findings on ECG (9–13,30). In addition, a normal ECG lowers the probability of occult arrhythmia or ischemic disease. For these reasons, ECG is considered a useful part of the evaluation, at least for those patients older than 40 years. Stress testing should be considered when the syncopal episode was related to exercise or if ischemia is suspected (15,20).

Long-term Cardiac Monitoring

Major arrhythmias have been detected by long-term cardiac monitoring in as many as 64% of patients presenting with dizziness or syncope and in approximately 12% of healthy patients (31–36). Results of the

Table 54-2. Diagnostic Test Yield in Patients with Syncope*

Diagnostic Test	Yield (%)
Cardiac	
Electrocardiography	2–11
Cardiac monitoring	0–30
Electrophysiologic study	0–12
Neurologic	
Skull radiography	0
Electroencephalography	0–8
Brain scan / CT	
No CNS symptoms	0–2
With CNS symptoms	35
Screening laboratory tests	0–4

CT = computed tomography; CNS = central nervous system.
*Yield refers to the number of tests providing a diagnosis divided by the number of tests performed.

monitoring must be correlated with symptoms to determine the clinical significance of the arrhythmia—only about 4% of patients with syncope demonstrate this correlation (37). Most asymptomatic or transient arrhythmias do not require further evaluation, but frequent or repetitive ventricular ectopy and sinus pauses are associated with an increased risk of sudden death and should be considered clinically important, even in the absence of symptoms (18). Twenty-four-hour monitoring may not be sufficient to detect all significant cardiac events (31). The yield of cardiac monitoring can be increased by extending it to 48 hours, although the number of false-positive readings will also increase. Patient-activated event recorders with memory loops may be a more cost-effective alternative for patients believed to be at low risk for life-threatening arrhythmias and who have recurrent syncope (2,8,30). However, patient compliance and technical difficulties associated with the loop recorders limit their usefulness.

Echocardiography

The role of echocardiography in the evaluation of syncope is controversial. In a prospective series of unselected patients referred for echocardiography, the test produced few unsuspected diagnoses (38), and in a small retrospective study of patients with syncope, it failed to reveal an unsuspected cause (39). Nevertheless, echocardiography can identify patients with poor left ventricular function or wall motion abnormalities who are at increased risk for arrhythmias. Patients with normal cardiac function are unlikely to benefit from more invasive cardiac procedures such as electrophysiologic testing. In patients with syncope who have findings suggestive of valvular heart disease, echocardiography should be done to identify the nature and severity of the lesion. Echocardiography should be not be done in younger patients who have normal cardiac examinations and histories suggestive of noncardiac syncope.

Electrophysiologic Testing

In those patients for whom electrophysiologic testing (EPS) has been performed, a high test yield is reported; in as many as 68% of patients in whom EPS is performed, arrhythmias are demonstrated that might explain the episodes of loss of consciousness (13,40–42). However, the yield of EPS decreases considerably, to approximately 12%, when applied to a population of patients in whom the results of clinical evaluation, ECG, Holter monitoring, and stress tests are normal (43). Other predictors of low yield include absence of injury during the events and multiple (more than five) or prolonged episodes of syncope (44). Electrophysiologic testing is most useful in patients with known structural heart disease including coronary artery disease, congestive heart failure, or valvular disease; frequent premature ventricular contractions on ECG; or conduction system abnormalities on resting or prolonged ECG monitoring (25,41,45,46).

Electrophysiologic testing is an expensive study and has a 1% to 2% complication rate (47). It can provide important therapeutic and prognostic information in patients with unexplained syncope and should be considered in patients in whom preliminary data suggests a high risk of cardiac syncope.

Head-up Tilt-Table Testing

Head-up tilt-table testing (HUTT) is based on the observation that vasovagal syncope can be induced by keeping susceptible persons in an upright position (37). Studies of patients with unexplained syncope show an increased incidence of abnormal neurally meditated hypotension (48). There are generally two phases: a 10- to 45-minute period of passive upright tilt-table testing followed by a repeat study while the patient is receiving an isoproterenol infusion. The HUTT is still not standardized across studies; test angle, duration, and isoproterenol infusion rates vary. A summary of existing studies by Kapoor (49) showed an overall positive response rate of 66% in patients with unexplained syncope. These patients may benefit from treatment with beta-blocker therapy. However, significant limitations of HUTT must be noted, including a 20% to 30% positive rate in healthy young persons, lack of reproducibility (50), and a lack of correlation of therapeutic response with tilt-table response (51). Head-up tilt-table testing should be limited to patients without underlying heart disease who have recurrent, unexplained syncope.

Neurologic Testing

Radiography of the skull and head computed tomography (CT) have a negligible yield when performed in patients without focal neurologic symptoms (see Table 54-2). In patients with focal neurologic signs or symptoms, these imaging tests, now dominated by head CT and magnetic resonance imaging (MRI), may be useful (9,11,12).

Electroencephalography, which is frequently ordered in the evaluation of patients with syncope, demonstrates significant abnormalities in fewer than 10% of patients, and the yield decreases when patients with an initial diagnosis of seizure or central nervous system causes of syncope are excluded from consideration (9).

Psychiatric Evaluation

Psychiatric problems are common in patients with syncope. In a prospective cohort study of patients with syncope who had standard psychiatric evaluations, 20% met the criteria for at least one psychiatric disorder or alcohol or drug disorder (52). Patients with syncope who had psychiatric disorders tended to be younger, have recurrent syncope, and report prodromal symptoms. Psychiatric evaluation should be considered for patients who have recurrent, unexplained syncope.

DIAGNOSTIC STRATEGIES

The central principle in evaluating patients with syncope is that the prevalence of severe, symptomatic disease and the yield of diagnostic tests varies according to patient characteristics and setting. Most patients, particularly most younger patients, do not have syncope of critical clinical significance.

Diagnostic testing beyond the history and physical examination may be undertaken for any one of three main purposes: 1) to confirm a diagnosis made on the basis of the history and physical examination; 2) to exclude more serious causes of syncope; or 3) to establish a cause of recurrent unexplained syncope. In most cases, a diagnosis can be made based on a careful history and physical examination, together with the results of ECG.

Debate usually focuses on those tests that are costly, necessitate hospitalization, or may incur significant risk to the patient (e.g., CT or MRI, long-term ambulatory or intensive care unit cardiac monitoring, HUTT, and EPS). The decision to order these tests requires that pretest probability of disease places the patient in a high-risk category for significant complications. In the absence of a clinical suspicion of high-risk cardiac or neurologic disease, clinical follow-up is probably more appropriate than a battery of nonfocused and expensive tests.

The American College of Physicians Clinical Efficacy Assessment Project has recently published a clinical guideline for the diagnosis of syncope (53,54). Their approach, similar to that suggested here, begins with a history, physical examination, and ECG. Patients in whom a diagnosis is evident should be treated without further testing. Those in whom a specific cause is suspected should have specific diagnostic tests to confirm the diagnosis. Patients with unexplained syncope are categorized as 1) having suspected heart disease, 2) older than 60 years of age, and 3) not having suspected heart disease. For the patients in groups 1 and 2, echocardiography and stress testing should be done. In addition, carotid massage is recommended for the patients in group 2. Those with evidence of heart disease should have ambulatory or inpatient ECG monitoring, depending on clinical concern about a serious arrhythmia. Those who have nondiagnostic monitoring should be considered for EPS testing. Those who have symptoms while in normal sinus rhythm should have the arrhythmia evaluation stopped. The patients in group 3 as well as those in groups 1 and 2 with negative cardiac workups do not need further evaluation unless the syncope recurs. These patients should then be considered for HUTT, loop monitoring, and/or psychiatric evaluation.

CLINICAL PROBLEMS

Clinical Problem 1
A young patient presents after one episode of syncope in which no injury was incurred.

Testing Strategy and Rationale
A thorough history and physical examination should be performed, especially to find evidence of serious cardiac or neurologic causes of syncope, including congenital heart disease, that require further testing to confirm. If the initial clinical assessment suggests only "benign" causes of syncope (e.g., noncritical causes as shown in Table 54-1), clinical follow-up is suggested in preference to additional testing.

Clinical Example
A 30-year old man is brought to the emergency room after fainting at a funeral. The patient has no previous history of syncope nor does he have any history of known cardiac or neurologic disease. He relates a story of passing by the open casket of a close relative, becoming suddenly warm, diaphoretic, somewhat nauseated, and

then light-headed. Within seconds, he fainted. He denies palpitations, chest pain, aura, or postictal confusion, but felt fatigued for several minutes after the event. He is not taking any medication. Observers deny any seizure activity. No fecal or urinary incontinence occurred with the event. The syncopal event lasted less than 2 minutes. He is fully oriented at the time of the examination, and the results of the physical examination are negative for cardiac or neurologic findings.

On the basis of the history and normal examination, the clinician should feel confident that the patient's syncope is "low risk" and clearly vasodepressor in nature. The patient should be offered reassurance and clinical follow-up. No further testing is warranted unless the syncope recurs.

Clinical Problem 2
A middle-aged patient presents with syncope.

Testing Strategy and Rationale
Perform a rigorous history and physical examination. Any testing beyond ECG should be based on a clinical assessment indicating a high-risk problem requiring more definitive diagnosis and treatment. The older the patient, the more likely the syncope is to have a high-risk cause, but as always, clinical assessment should form the basis for a focused testing strategy.

Clinical Example
A 58-year old woman who has had no previous syncopal attacks presents for evaluation after fainting during her vacation. The patient was eating dinner in a restaurant when she began to feel hot. She began to rise from her chair to get "fresh air," when she slumped to the table, striking her chin and chipping a tooth. She was unresponsive to verbal stimuli and appeared "ashen." She awoke 1 minute after she was placed supine by friends who were unsure if a pulse was palpable. The patient denied chest pain or palpitations, postictal confusion, incontinence, or other localizing symptoms or signs. She is not taking any medications. She has smoked cigarettes for many years and had been told that her blood pressure and cholesterol are "borderline."

The history of syncope characterized by sudden onset and rapid recovery is typical of syncope that has a cardiac cause, although the setting could also be explained by neurally mediated syncope. As always, a thorough history and physical examination searching for cardiac or neurologic abnormalities should guide subsequent testing. Electrocardiography should be performed; if the tracing suggests ischemic disease, inpatient monitoring or

Continued

stress testing should be considered. Echocardiography should be considered and should definitely be performed if the physical examination reveals a cardiac abnormality. In this case, the history makes an arrhythmia a possibility and prolonged cardiac monitoring is indicated. The history does not suggest a neurologic or metabolic cause of syncope; therefore, testing to rule out these causes would not be warranted even if the results of the initial cardiac tests were negative. Electrophysiologic testing should be considered if noninvasive testing discloses cardiac abnormalities but no definitive cause for the syncope has been determined.

REFERENCES

1. **Wright KE Jr, McIntosh HD.** Syncope: a review of pathophysiological mechanisms. Prog Cardiovasc Dis. 1971;13:580-94.
2. **Manolis AS, Linzer M, Salem D, Estes III NAM.** Syncope: current diagnostic evaluation and management. Ann Intern Med. 1990;112:850-63.
3. **Wayne HH.** Syncope: physiological considerations and an analysis of the clinical characteristics in 510 patients. Am J Med. 1961;30:418-38.
4. **Benditt D, Remole S, Milstein S, Bailin S.** Syncope: causes, clinical evaluation, and current therapy. Annu Rev Med. 1992;43:283-300.
5. **Kapoor W.** Syncope in older persons. J Am Geratr Soc. 1994;42:426-36.
6. **Lipsitz LA.** Syncope in the elderly. Ann Intern Med. 1983; 99:92-105.
7. **Kapoor W.** Evaluation and management of the patient with syncope. JAMA. 1992;268:2553-60.
8. **Kapoor W.** Workup and management of patients with syncope. Med Clin. 1995;79:1153-70.
9. **Day SC, Cook EF, Funkenstein H, Goldman L.** Evaluation and outcome of emergency room patients with transient loss of consciousness. Am J Med. 1982;73:15-23.
10. **Silverstein MD, Singer DE, Mulley AG, et al.** Patients with syncope admitted to medical intensive care units. JAMA. 1982;248:1185-9.
11. **Kapoor WN, Karpf M, Wieand S, et al.** A prospective evaluation and follow-up of patients with syncope. N Engl J Med. 1983;309:197-204.
12. **Eagle KA, Black HR.** The impact of diagnostic tests in evaluating patients with syncope. Yale J Biol Med. 1983;56:1-8.
13. **Mozes B, Confino-Cohen R, Halkin H.** Cost-effectiveness of in-hospital evaluation of patients with syncope. Isr J Med Sci. 1988;24:302-6.
14. **Hanlon JT, Linzer M, MacMillan JP, et al.** Syncope and presyncope associated with probable adverse drug reactions. Arch Intern Med. 1990;150:2309-12.
15. **Calkins H, Shyr Y, Frumin H, et al.** The value of the clinical history of the differentiation of syncope due to ventricular tachycardia, atrioventricular block, and neurocardiogenic syncope. Am J Med. 1995;98:365-73.

16. **Hoefnagels WAJ, Padberg GW, Overweg J, et al.** Transient loss of consciousness: the value of the history for distinguishing seizure from syncope. J Neurol. 1991;238:39-43.

17. **Lee RT, Cook FE, Day SC, Goldman L.** Long-term survival after transient loss of consciousness. J Gen Intern Med. 1988;3: 337-43.

18. **Kapoor WN, Peterson J, Wieand HS, Karpf M.** Diagnostic and prognostic implications of recurrences in patients with syncope. Am J Med. 1987;83: 700-8.

19. **Kapoor WN, Hanusa BH.** Is syncope a risk factor for poor outcomes? Comparison of patients with and without syncope. Am J Med. 1996;100: 646-55.

20. **Ivanova LA, Mazur NA, Smirnova TM, et al.** Electrocardiographic exercise testing and ambulatory monitoring to identify patients with ischemic heart disease at high risk of sudden death. Am J Cardiol. 1980;45:1132-8.

21. **Follansbee WP, Michaelson EL, Morganroth J.** Nonsustained ventricular tachycardia in ambulatory patients: characteristics and association with sudden cardiac death. Ann Intern Med. 1980;92:741-7.

22. **Kannel WB, Sorlie P, McNamara PM.** Prognosis after initial myocardial infarction: the Framingham study. Am J Cardiol. 1979;44:53-9.

23. **Vismara LA, Vera Z, Foerster JM, et al.** Identification of sudden death risk factors in acute and chronic coronary artery disease. Am J Cardiol. 1977;39:821-8.

24. **Klein GJ, Gulamhusein SS.** Undiagnosed syncope: search for an arrhythmic etiology. Stroke. 1982;13:746-9.

25. **Kushner JA, Kou WH, Kadish AH, Moracy F.** Natural history of patients with unexplained syncope and a nondiagnostic electrophysiologic study. J Am Coll Cardiol. 1989;14:391-6.

26. **Kapoor W, Karpf M, Levey GS.** Issues in evaluating patients with syncope [Editorial]. Ann Intern Med. 1984;13:755-7.

27. **Kapoor WN, Cha R, Peterson JR, et al.** Prolonged electrocardiographic monitoring in patients with syncope. Am J Med. 1987;82:20-8.

28. **Georgeson S, Linzer M, Griffith J, et al.** Acute cardiac ischemia in patients with syncope. Gen Intern Med. 1992;7:379-86.

29. **Martin TP, Hanusa BH, Kapoor WN.** Risk stratification of patients with syncope. Ann Emerg Med. 1997;29:459-66.

30. **DiMarco JP, Philbrick JT.** Use of ambulatory electrocardiographic (Holter) monitoring. Ann Intern Med. 1990;113:53-68.

31. **Kapoor WN.** The duration of holter monitoring in patients patients with syncope: is 24 hours enough? Arch Intern Med. 1990;150:1073-8.

32. **Glasser P, Clark PI, Applebaum HJ.** Occurrence of frequent complex arrhythmias detected by ambulatory monitoring. Chest. 1979;756:565-8.

33. **Camm AJ, Martin A, Evand KE, et al.** 24-hour ambulatory monitoring: a survey of active elderly people. In: Stott FD, Rafferty EB, Sleight P, et al, eds. International Symposium on Ambulatory Monitoring. New York: Academic Press; 1977:1-7.

34. **Lipski J, Cohen L, Espinoza J, et al.** Value of Holter monitoring in assessing cardiac arrhythmias in symptomatic patients. Am J Cardiol. 1976;37: 102-7.

35. **Jonas S, Klein I, Dimant J.** Importance of Holter monitoring in patients with periodic cerebral symptoms. Ann Neurol. 1977;1:470-4.

36. **Brodsky M, Wu D, Denes P, et al.** Arrhythmias documented by 24-hour continuous electrocardiographic monitoring in 50 male medical students without apparent heart disease. Am J Cardiol. 1977;39:390-5.

37. **Kapoor WN.** Workup and management of patients with syncope. Med Clin North Am. 1995;79:1153-70.

38. **Krumholz HM, Douglas PS, Goldman L, Waksmonski C.** Clinical utility of transthoracic two-dimensional and Doppler echocardiography. J Am Coll Cardiol. 1994;24:125-31.

39. **Recchia D, Barzilai B.** Echocardiography in the evaluation of patients with syncope. J Gen Intern Med. 1995;10:649-55.

40. **Boudoulas H, Parashos G, Schaal SF, et al.** Comparison between electro-physiologic studies and ambulatory monitoring in patients with syncope. J Electrocardiol. 1983;16:91-6.

41. **Linzer M, Prystowsky EN, Divine GW, et al.** Predicting the outcomes of electrophysiologic studies of patients with unexplained syncope. J Gen Intern Med. 1991;6:113-20.

42. **Hess DS, Morady F, Scheinman MM.** Electrophysiologic testing in the evaluation of patients with syncope of undetermined origin. Am J Cardiol. 1982;50:1309-15.

43. **Gulamhusein S, Naccarelli GV, Ko PT, et al.** Value and limitations of clinical electrophysiologic studies in assessment of patients with unexplained syncope. Am J Med. 1982;73:700-5.

44. **Krol RB, Morady F, Fakes GC, et al.** Electrophysiologic testing in patients with unexplained syncope: clinical and non-invasive predictors of outcome. J Am Coll Cardiol. 1987;10:358-63.

45. **Doherty JU, Pembrook-Rogers DP, Grogan EW, et al.** Electrophysiologic evaluation and follow-up characteristics of patients with recurrent unexplained syncope and presyncope. Am J Cardiol. 1985;55:703-8.

46. **Sugrue DD, Holmes DR Jr, Gersh BJ, et al.** Impact of intracardiac electrophysiologic testing on the management of elderly patients with recurrent syncope or near syncope. J Am Geriatric Soc. 1987;35:1079-83.

47. **DiMarco JP, Garan H, Ruskin JN.** Complications in patients undergoing cardiac electrophysiologic procedure. Ann Intern Med. 1982;97:490-3.

48. **Brignole M.** Neurally mediated syncope detected by carotid sinus massage and head-up tilt test in sick sinus syndrome. Am J Carotid. 1991;68:1032-6.

49. **Kapoor WN, Smith MA, Miller NL.** Upright tilt table testing in evaluating syncope: a comprehensive literature review. Am J Med. 1994;97:78-88.

50. **deBuitleir M, Grogan EW, Picone MF, Casteen JA.** Immediate reproducibility of the tilt-table test in adults with unexplained syncope. J Cardiol. 1993;71:304-7.

51. **Lippman N, Stein KM, Lerman BB.** Differential therapeutic responses of patients with isoproterenol-dependent and isoproterenol-independent vasodepressor syncope. Heart J. 1994;128:1110-6.

52. **Kapoor WN, Fortunato M, Hanusa BH, Schulberg HC.** Psychiatric illness in patients with syncope. Am J Med. 1995;99:505-12.

53. **Linzer M, Yang EH, Estes NAM, et al.** Diagnosing syncope: part 1: value of history, physical examination and electrocardiography. Ann Intern Med. 1997;126:989-96.

54. **Linzer M, Yang EH, Estes NAM, et al.** Diagnosing syncope: part 2: unexplained syncope. Ann Intern Med. 1997;127:76-86.

Dementia

55

Wayne C. McCormick, MD, MPH, and Eric B. Larson, MD, MPH

KEY POINTS

Pretest Probabilities

- Most elderly patients with chronic dementia have dementia caused by Alzheimer disease (about approximately 65%–75%). Other types of dementia affecting this population include the dementia associated with Parkinson disease (5%), multi-infarct dementia (10%–20%), and alcohol-related dementia (5%–10%).

- In some patients who meet screening criteria for dementia, cognitive impairment is caused by or is worsened by medication side effects (5%), depression (5%), other central nervous system illness (2%), or metabolic abnormalities (2%–4%). The frequencies of these causes are greater in younger patients and in patients with dementia of short duration.

- The prevalence of multi-infarct dementia is relatively high in black persons and in patients with hypertension or diabetes or both.

- Dementia may have more than one cause or exacerbating factor; medical illnesses worsening poor cognition are common in elderly persons with dementia.

Diagnostic Strategies

- Detecting cognitive impairment is difficult unless mental status is systematically evaluated, especially in elderly patients. The bedside evaluation, combined with historical information from a reliable informant, provides most of the information needed to ascertain the cause of dementia.

- Several short mental status tests can establish or exclude a diagnosis of cognitive impairment with fairly good accuracy. For example, the Mini-Mental State Examination has a sensitivity of 87% and a specificity of 82% for detecting cognitive impairment.

- Diagnostic criteria, such as *Diagnostic and Statistical Manual of Mental Disorders (DSM-IV)*, composed of codified elements of the medical history, physical, and neurologic examination are available for the clinical diagnosis of Alzheimer disease.

- Routine evaluation of patients with dementia often includes a complete blood count and measurement of serum electrolytes, BUN, creatinine, calcium, B_{12}, and TSH levels.
- Other tests, including computed tomography or magnetic resonance imaging, should be done selectively to evaluate patients whose basic physical and neurologic examinations yield unexpected findings.
- Genetic testing and positron-emission tomography are not recommended at this time except in research investigations.

BACKGROUND

Because of the aging of the American population and the declining mortality in patients with diseases that previously caused premature death, more people are living to advanced age and are therefore susceptible to chronic diseases such as dementia. The prevalence of dementia increases exponentially with age: of persons older than 65 years, approximately 5% to 10% have dementia; of those older than 80 years, at least 20% have the disease (1); and of those older than 85 years, as many as 50% have the disease (2). Clinicians will be asked to evaluate increasing numbers of persons with cognitive impairment, most of whom will be elderly. An effective, simple, humane, and cost-effective manner for evaluating such patients should be a mainstay of practice.

Because most dementing illnesses are not curable, one might question the wisdom of evaluating patients with dementia, given the absence of curative therapies. However, treatment of symptoms and counseling of caregivers are important. Furthermore, medical illnesses that do not cause dementia and therefore go unrecognized because of it are common in persons with dementia, and treatment of these illnesses can ameliorate cognition to some extent. Cognitive derangements may occasionally be completely (in about 3% of patients) or partially (in about 10% of patients) eliminated by treatment of the underlying illness that is believed to cause dementia (3). Whether or not dementia may be reversible is almost always apparent from the history, physical examination, and routine blood tests as outlined in this chapter. The majority of reversible cases result from medication side effects, depression, and metabolic disorders. Consequently, a thorough history and physical examination followed by elimination (when possible) of drugs affecting cognition and treatment of underlying medical conditions is of pivotal importance. Although the course of Alzheimer disease (AD) and most other dementing illnesses is usually progressive, it is not necessarily inexorably downhill; even patients with "incurable" dementia may have periods of improved or stable function.

In evaluating patients with possible dementia, the clinician's task is twofold: to determine whether dementia is present and, if so, to establish the cause. Dementia is easy to miss in routine, day-to-day medical practice. In a recent study, the diagnosis was missed in 21% of patients with dementia or delirious patients on the general medical ward of a respected hospital, and conversely, 20% of patients without dementia were judged to have dementia (4). Because dementia usually is insidious in onset, it often goes unrecognized even by family members or others in daily close contact with the affected persons. Hence, routine screening for cognitive deficits, particularly in elderly patients, is a useful undertaking, especially because this screening takes only a few minutes of the clinician's time and can easily be included in the medical history.

Once screening has documented the presence of dementia, clinicians must next establish the cause. Although the possible causes of dementia are myriad, clinical reasoning in the typical case comes down to the exclusion of causes other than AD. A definitive diagnosis of AD is based on a typical clinical picture and neuropathologic findings in brain tissue samples, neuritic plaques, and neurofibrillary tangles, particularly in the hippocampus and nucleus basalis. This is the standard against which any diagnostic test for AD must be compared. Because brain tissue is almost never obtained before autopsy in those with dementia, the clinical diagnosis of AD is, by necessity, presumptive. That said, AD may well encompass a heterogeneous set of disorders, including Lewy body disease, Pick disease, and other degenerative brain conditions that are often clinically indistinguishable from AD.

ESTIMATING PRETEST PROBABILITIES

The prevalence of the causes of dementia varies in different populations. Pretest probabilities for different causes in an individual patient depend on factors such as the patient's age and race, whether the patient is hospitalized (including the type of hospital), and even the hospital specialty ward in which the patient is hospitalized (neurology, geriatrics, psychiatry). The prevalence of causes of dementia in various populations can be found in review articles (3) and are shown in Table 55-1.

Most persons with dementia who require the attention of primary care physicians are elderly outpatients. Most of these patients in whom dementia is documented by screening examinations have AD (approximately 65%–75%), and another 5% have Alzheimer-type dementia in association with Parkinson disease. Ten to twenty percent have multi-infarct dementia or alcohol-related dementia. The remainder of patients meeting criteria for dementia have cognitive impairment caused by

Table 55-1. Frequency of Causes of Dementia in Several Populations

Cause	Elderly Outpatients	Young Inpatients	Veteran Inpatients	Finnish Inpatients
	←		%	→
Alzheimer disease	64–70	42–45	49–70	23
Multi-infarct	1–4	7–11	7–22	72
Infection	—	0–4	1–3	—
Metabolic	4	0–1	2	1
Neoplasm	—	1–8	1–5	1
Normal-pressure hydrocephalus	—	4–5	2–5	1
Subdural hematoma	0–2	—	3	—
Depression	1–5	5–8	3	—
Drugs	5	2	2–4	—
Trauma anoxia	—	1–3	—	—
Huntington disease	—	2–3	1	—
Parkinson disease	5–6	—	4	2–3
Alcohol use	3–4	5–15	3–8	—
Miscellaneous	4–8	1–12	2	—
No dementia	4–13	13–15	—	—

Adapted with permission from Clarfield AM. The reversible dementias: do they reverse? Ann Intern Med. 1988;109:476-86.

medication side effects (5%–10%) or depression without true dementia (5%–10%). Other illnesses affecting the central nervous system (CNS), such as brain tumors, paraneoplastic syndrome, normal pressure hydrocephalus, subdural hematoma, transient ischemic attacks, and CNS vasculitis, are rare causes of dementia (approximately 2%) and are even less common than metabolic abnormalities (e.g., hypothyroidism, hyperparathyroidism, hyponatremia, hypoglycemia, B_{12} or folate deficiency [approximately 2%–4%]) (5,6). At least 5% to 10% of elderly patients with dementia have more than one illness capable of causing dementia and are judged to have mixed dementia, usually consisting of AD with some other cause such as multi-infarct dementia or dementia related to alcohol use.

Because the prevalence of dementia is lower in younger populations, the frequency of causes other than AD (e.g., infections, neoplasms, normal-pressure hydrocephalus, subdural hematoma, and metabolic diseases) is greater in patients younger than 65 years of age. The prevalence of AD in younger patients with dementia (mean age <65 years old) is estimated to be around 45% (7). Illnesses affecting cognition such as depression and cognitive impairment caused by medications or alcoholism are also important causes in the younger group.

Alzheimer disease is highly variable in course and presenting symptoms. However, a common presentation for AD is an elderly person with a gradual (months to years) decline in cognitive function, with recent memory being most affected and other functions being initially less affected. Clues that the condition is not AD include rapid onset (over a few months or less); mild impairment; fluctuating course; unusual or focal neurologic findings such as gait abnormalities, myoclonus, or seizures early in the course of dementia; and adverse drug reactions. These clues should be interpreted with caution in individual patients because persons with AD occasionally have rapid onset and the other features just mentioned. Multi-infarct dementia and dementias associated with vascular diseases are more common in black persons, patients with hypertension, and patients with diabetes regardless of age. This is also the case among patients on neurology wards, where neoplasms also have a higher prevalence relative to other causes. Multi-infarct dementia is more likely to have a sudden or step-wise onset, and with this type of dementia other mental functions may be affected as much as or more than memory.

DIAGNOSTIC TESTS

Mini-Mental State Examination
One of the most widely used screening examinations in the evaluation of cognitive impairment is the Mini-Mental State Exam (MMSE) (8). This examination (Table 55-2) tests a broad range of cognitive functions, including orientation, recall, attention, calculation, language manipulation, and constructional praxis. A total of 30 points is normal, and in general a score of less than 24 signifies dementia or delirium. Using this cutoff, this test has a sensitivity of 87% and a specificity of 82%. However, the test is not particularly sensitive for mild dementia, and scores are spuriously low in persons with low education level, poor motor function, or impaired vision. Age-specific norms have been established (9), and higher cutoff scores have been suggested to improve sensitivity, but this leads to lower specificity. The examination takes approximately 7 minutes to complete.

Short Portable Mental Status Questionnaire
The Short Portable Mental Status Questionnaire (SPMSQ) also takes just a few minutes to complete and thus is another quick screening tool for dementia (10). The SPMSQ has some advantages over the MMSE in that it partially adjusts for age, sex, race, education, and motor or visual impairment. Sensitivity of the SPMSQ is 82% and specificity is 92%;

Table 55-2. Mini-Mental State Examination

Patient _____

Examiner _____

Date _____

	Maximum Score	Score
Orientation	10	
What is the (year), (season), (day of month), (month), (day of week)? (1 point for each)		_____
Where are we: (state), (county), (town), (hospital), (floor)? (1 point for each)		_____
Registration	3	
Name three objects: 1 second to say each. Then ask the patient all three after you have said them. Give 1 point for each correct answer. Then repeat them until he learns all three. Count trials and record.		_____
Trials		
Attention and calculation	5	
Serials 7s. 1 point for each correct. Stop after five answers. Alternatively spell "world" backwards.		_____
Recall	3	
Ask for the 3 objects repeated above. Give 1 point for each correct.		_____
Language	9	
Name a pencil and a watch. (2 points)		_____
Repeat the following: "No ifs, ands, or buts." (1 point)		_____
Follow a three-stage command:		
Take a paper in your right hand, fold it in half, and put it on the floor. (3 points)		_____
Read and obey the following:		
Close your eyes. (1 point)		_____
Write a sentence. (1 point)		_____
Copy this design. (1 point)		_____

	Maximum Score	Score
Total score	30	_____

Interpretation: 24–30 Normal
20–23 Mild dementia
10–19 Moderate dementia
<10 Severe dementia

Republished with permission from Folstein MF, Folstein S, McHugh JR. Mini-mental state: a practical method for grading the cognitive state of patients for the clinician. J Psych Res. 1975;12:189-98.

for mild dementia, this changes to 55% and 96%, respectively. One benefit of both the MMSE and SPMSQ is that they provide immediate diagnostic information.

Diagnostic Criteria for Dementia

Once screening has documented the presence of dementia, the clinician then must take on the task of establishing the cause. Although the possible causes of dementia are myriad, clinical judgments regarding the cause of dementia usually involve the exclusion of causes other than AD. The definitive diagnosis of AD, the most common cause of dementia in developed countries, is based on a typical clinical picture and neuropathologic findings as noted earlier in this chapter. This standard is the benchmark against which any other diagnostic test for AD must be compared, even though patients with a clinical course consistent with AD have been described without these pathologic findings (11).

Systematic review of the medical history and physical, neurologic, and mental status examination remains the best method for diagnosing the cause of dementia antemortem. Historical data from a reliable informant are essential. The two most widely used diagnostic criteria are those developed by the National Institute of Neurological and Communicative Disorders and Stroke and the Alzheimer's Disease and Related Disorders Association (NINCDS-ADRDA) (12) and those found in the Diagnostic and Statistical Manual of Mental Disorders of the American Psychiatric Association (DSM-IV) (13). These diagnostic criteria, like the MMSE and SPMSQ screening examinations, represent codified elements of the history, physical, neurologic, and mental status examinations. These criteria can also be regarded as laboratory tests and can be evaluated for sensitivity and specificity in the same manner outlined previously for the MMSE and SPMSQ screening examinations.

Multi-infarct dementia, depression, and dementia associated with alcoholism are also examined for plausibility by going through the DSM-IV criteria. In a study involving experienced clinicians who assessed the reliability and validity of these criteria in diagnosing AD, the NINCDS criteria was found to have a sensitivity and specificity of 92% and 65%. Comparable figures for the DSM-IIIR criteria (the predecessor of DSM-IV) were a sensitivity of 76% and a specificity of 80% for primary degenerative dementia, the DSM-IIIR equivalent of AD (14) (Table 55-3).

Laboratory Testing and Imaging Studies

The standard laboratory tests commonly used in the evaluation of dementia are usually not diagnostic of the cause of dementia; rather they have traditionally been used to rule out causes other than AD. In fact, the main purpose served by obtaining a standard battery of labo-

Table 55-3. Operating Characteristics of Screening Tests and Clinical Criteria in the Diagnosis of Dementia

Diagnostic Test	Sensitivity	Specificity	Likelihood Ratio	
			Positive Result	Negative Result
	←——— % ———→			
For dementia				
Mini-Mental State Examination	87	82	4.8	0.16
Short Portable Mental Status Questionnaire				
Any dementia	82	92	10	0.20
Mild dementia	55	96	14	0.47
For Alzheimer disease				
NINCDS criteria	92	65	2.6	0.12
DSM-IIIR criteria	76	80	3.8	0.30

NINCDS = National Institute of Neurological and Communicative Disorder and Stroke; DSM = Diagnostic and Statistical Manual of Mental Disorders.

ratory studies should be to detect occult medical illnesses in these patients (5,6). Routine screening tests most likely to be of value include a complete blood count, measurement of serum B_{12} or cobalamin level, thyrotropin (TSH) concentration, and levels of serum electrolytes, calcium, and creatinine. One may argue that serum B_{12} should be measured only if the mean corpuscular volume (MCV) is elevated (see Chapter 51); however, there have been reports of persons with neuropsychiatric manifestations of B_{12} deficiency occurring in the absence of anemia or macrocytosis (15). These tests are justified for several reasons: They are relatively inexpensive and noninvasive, the treatments for the illnesses they diagnose can be simple and effective, and clinical diagnosis of these illnesses can be difficult in elderly persons (e.g., occult or subclinical hypothyroidism).

Computed tomography (CT) or magnetic resonance imaging (MRI) may generally be reserved for patients in whom a CNS lesion is clinically suspected. These patients include those with unexplained abnormalities on neurologic examination or a clinical history suggestive of subdural hematoma, normal-pressure (or other types of) hydrocephalus, carcinomas that commonly metastasize to brain, CNS infection, and so forth. The finding of cerebral atrophy, widened sulci, and enlarged ventricular system, although associated with AD, is also associated with aging and hence is nonspecific. Unless abnormal progression of atrophy can be documented on serial CT or MRI scans concurrent with the typical clinical course of AD, atrophy is neither sufficient nor necessary to make this diagnosis. In most cases of suspected AD, atrophy seen on neuroimaging studies has no additional diagnostic value over the history and physical examination.

Other routine blood tests such as VDRL or rapid plasma reagin, liver function tests, and erythrocyte sedimentation rate (ESR) are probably no more helpful in the workup of dementia in elderly patients than in routine general medical evaluations of elderly patients. Several other tests, used widely in the past in the evaluation of dementia, can no longer be recommended unless specific clinical indications are present; these tests include electroencephalography, lumbar puncture, radiography of the skull, and adrenocorticotropic hormone stimulation or dexamethasone suppression.

Research in the use of sophisticated radiographic techniques to diagnose the cause of dementia continues, including MRI, positron-emission tomography (PET), and single-photon emission computed tomography (SPECT). Results of early evaluations do not indicate that any of these techniques deserve widespread use in all cases. Patients with periventricular lucencies seen on CT and MRI, "leukoaraiosis," have been screened for cognitive deficits, and deficits were not consistently found among patients with this radiographic finding. Although this phenomenon is statistically associated with risk factors for vascular disease, it does not confirm any specific diagnosis (16). Positron-emission tomography has generated considerable research interest and can document unique CNS changes in persons with AD. These techniques are expensive and are not widely available outside the research setting. Thus, based on present knowledge, these new imaging techniques do not usually add to the discriminating power of the medical history, physical examination, and codified criteria outlined earlier. As the meaning of early changes seen on PET, SPECT, or MRI are understood more fully, the utility of these scans in the diagnosis of dementias can be explored in prospective trials.

The most exciting recent developments have been in genetic testing, particularly in regard to the presence of the apolipoprotein E4 allele, whether combined with imaging techniques or not (17). Carriers of this genotype are at increased risk for AD (18); however, this is by no means a definitive prognostic indicator; persons with the allele do not invariably manifest AD, nor do those without the allele avoid it. At present, knowledge of apolipoprotein E4 genotype is of unknown clinical value to both the clinician and the patient, and it cannot be recommended until further research documents the utility of genotyping (19).

DIAGNOSTIC STRATEGIES

A mental status examination, either the MMSE or SPMSQ, should be the first step in detecting dementia in high-risk patients such as the elderly. Screening of selected elderly patients in whom impaired cognition is suspected may show cognitive impairment of greater significance than was anticipated by family, friends, or clinicians.

The bedside evaluation and physical examination combined with historical information from a reliable informant provide most of the data needed to establish the cause of dementia. The likelihood of AD can be revised using diagnostic criteria such as the DSM-IV.

The use of standard laboratory diagnostic tests generally adds little to the diagnostic power of the bedside evaluation, physical examination, and history. Nevertheless, a standard battery of routine tests is warranted to detect occult medical illnesses, including a complete blood count and measurement of serum B_{12}, thyroid-stimulating hormone, electrolytes, calcium, and creatinine, with further testing to evaluate any abnormalities found. The rationale for this battery is bolstered by studies of cohorts of elderly outpatients evaluated for dementia, half of whom were found to have previously unrecognized medical illnesses; of these patients, cognitive function improved in 50% with treatment of the underlying illnesses (5,6).

Other laboratory tests such as serologic tests for syphilis, liver function tests, or measurement of sedimentation rates are probably no more helpful in the workup of dementia than in the routine evaluation of elderly patients. Electrocardiography and chest radiography should be reserved for patients in whom cardiac or pulmonary abnormalities are found on examination. Computed tomography or MRI of the brain is useful to look for suspected stroke, subdural hematoma, or brain tumor but should be reserved for patients whose neurologic examinations yielded abnormal findings or for those with atypical presentations. Several other tests, including lumbar puncture, radiography of the skull, and electroencephalography, which were widely used in the past for evaluating dementia, are no longer recommended unless there is strong clinical suspicion that they would be helpful. Genetic testing and apolipoprotein E4 typing are being studied in research settings.

CLINICAL PROBLEMS

Clinical Problem 1
An elderly patient has a gradual decline in memory over several years.

Testing Strategy and Rationale
A careful history, physical, and neurologic examination should be performed. Basic laboratory tests should be ordered. If the results of these are normal except for confirmation of the diagnosis of

Continued

dementia, no further testing is needed. Any findings on evaluation should be carefully pursued.

Clinical Example

A 76-year-old woman has been under the care of her family physician for 15 years and lives with her daughter. She is functional in daily activities and her diet is good, but the daughter has noted a gradual decline in her memory over the past 2 to 3 years. Her examination is entirely normal except for a MMSE score of 18, and the results of the complete blood count and measurement of B_{12} level, blood chemistries, and TSH are normal.

Because the general history and the findings of the physical examination are normal and because the changes in the patient's cognition have occurred over several years, the pretest likelihood of focal CNS lesions, infections, or other medical illnesses that could affect cognition is very low. No further testing is necessary. The probable diagnosis is Alzheimer disease. Observation over time will provide some confirmation of the diagnosis, but definitive confirmation requires postmortem brain examination.

Clinical Problem 2

An elderly patient presents with multiple medical or psychological problems and a relatively short history of mental deterioration.

Testing Strategy and Rationale

A careful history and physical and neurologic examination should be performed. Basic laboratory tests should be ordered. With complicating medical or psychological conditions or a short course of disease, the index of suspicion for a cause of apparent dementia other than Alzheimer disease is high. Additional testing should be based on results of the initial evaluation.

Clinical Example

A 68-year-old retired airplane mechanic is referred for dementia. He has a history of anxiety, insomnia, depression treated with tricyclic antidepressants, and hypertension currently treated with beta-blockers and diuretics. He had a myocardial infarction 10 years previously. Over the past several months he has been observed by his wife to be increasingly forgetful and inattentive.

The findings of the physical examination are normal except for rather severe high-frequency hearing loss, and the results of routine blood tests are normal. The score of the MMSE is 23. Electrocardiography shows an old inferior myocardial infarction. A review of the medical history reveals that his medication had been changed from diuretics alone to diuretics and propranolol 6 months ago. He is taking benzodiazepines for anxiety in addition to amitriptyline for depression.

The diagnostic and treatment strategies are the same in this case: Discontinue all unnecessary medications and improve sensory input with hearing aids.

REFERENCES

1. **Small GW, Liston EH, Jarvick KF.** Diagnosis and treatment of dementia in the aged. West J Med. 1981;97:469-81.

2. **Evans DA, Funkenstein HH, Albert MS, et al.** Alzheimer's disease in a community population of older persons: marked increase beyond 85 years. JAMA. 1989;262:2551-6.

3. **Clarfield AM.** The reversible dementias: do they reverse? Ann Intern Med. 1988;109:476-86.

4. **Roca RP, Klein LE, Kirby SM, et al.** Recognition of dementia among medical inpatients. Arch Intern Med. 1984;144:73-5.

5. **Larson EB, Reifler BV, Featherstone HJ, English DR.** Dementia in elderly outpatients: a prospective study. Ann Intern Med. 1984;100:417-23.

6. **Larson EB, Reifler BV, Sumi SM, et al.** Diagnostic tests in the evaluation of dementia: a prospective study of 200 elderly outpatients. Arch Intern Med. 1986;146:1917-22.

7. **Marsden CD, Harrison MJ.** Outcome of investigation of patients with presenile dementia. Br Med J. 1972;2:249-52.

8. **Folstein MF, Folstein S, McHugh JR.** Mini-mental state: a practical method for grading the cognitive state of patients for the clinician. J Psychiatr Res. 1975;12:189-98.

9. **Bleecker ML, Bolla-Wilson K, Kawas C, Agnew J.** Age-specific norms for the Mini-Mental State Exam. Neurology. 1988;38:1565-8.

10. **Pfeiffer E.** A short portable mental status questionnaire for the assessment of organic brain deficits in elderly patients. J Am Geriatr Soc. 1975;22:433-9.

11. **Perry RH, Irving D, Blessed G, et al.** Clinically and neuropathologically distinct form of dementia in the elderly. Lancet. 1989;1:166.

12. **McKhann G, Drachman D, Folstein M, et al.** Clinical diagnosis of Alzheimer's disease: report of the NINCDS-ADRDA work group. Neurology. 1984;34:939-44.

13. American Psychiatric Association. Task Force on DSM-IV. Diagnostic and Statistical Manual of Mental Disorders. 4th ed. Washington, DC: American Psychiatric Association; 1994.

14. **Larson EB, Kukull WA, Reifler BV, et al.** The validity of 3 clinical diagnostic criteria for Alzheimer's disease. Neurology. 1990;40:1364-9.

15. **Lindenbaum J, Heathton EB, Savage DG, et al.** Neuropsychiatric disorders caused by cobalamin deficiency in the absence of anemia or macrocytosis. N Engl J Med. 1988;318:1720-8.

16. **Rao SM, Mittenberg W, Bernardin L, et al.** Neuropsychological test findings in subjects with leukoaraiosis. Arch Neurol. 1989;46:40-4.

17. **Reiman EM, Caselli RJ, Yun LS, et al.** Preclinical evidence of Alzheimer's disease in persons homozygous for the E4 allele for apolipoprotein E. N Engl J Med. 1996;334:752-8.

18. **Roses AD.** Apolipoprotein E genotyping in the differential diagnosis, not prediction, of Alzheimer's disease. Ann Neurol. 1995;38:6-14.

19. **Gledmacher DS, Whitehouse PJ.** Evaluation of dementia. N Engl J Med. 1996;335:330-336.

Index

Note: "f" following page number indicates figure; "t" indicates table.